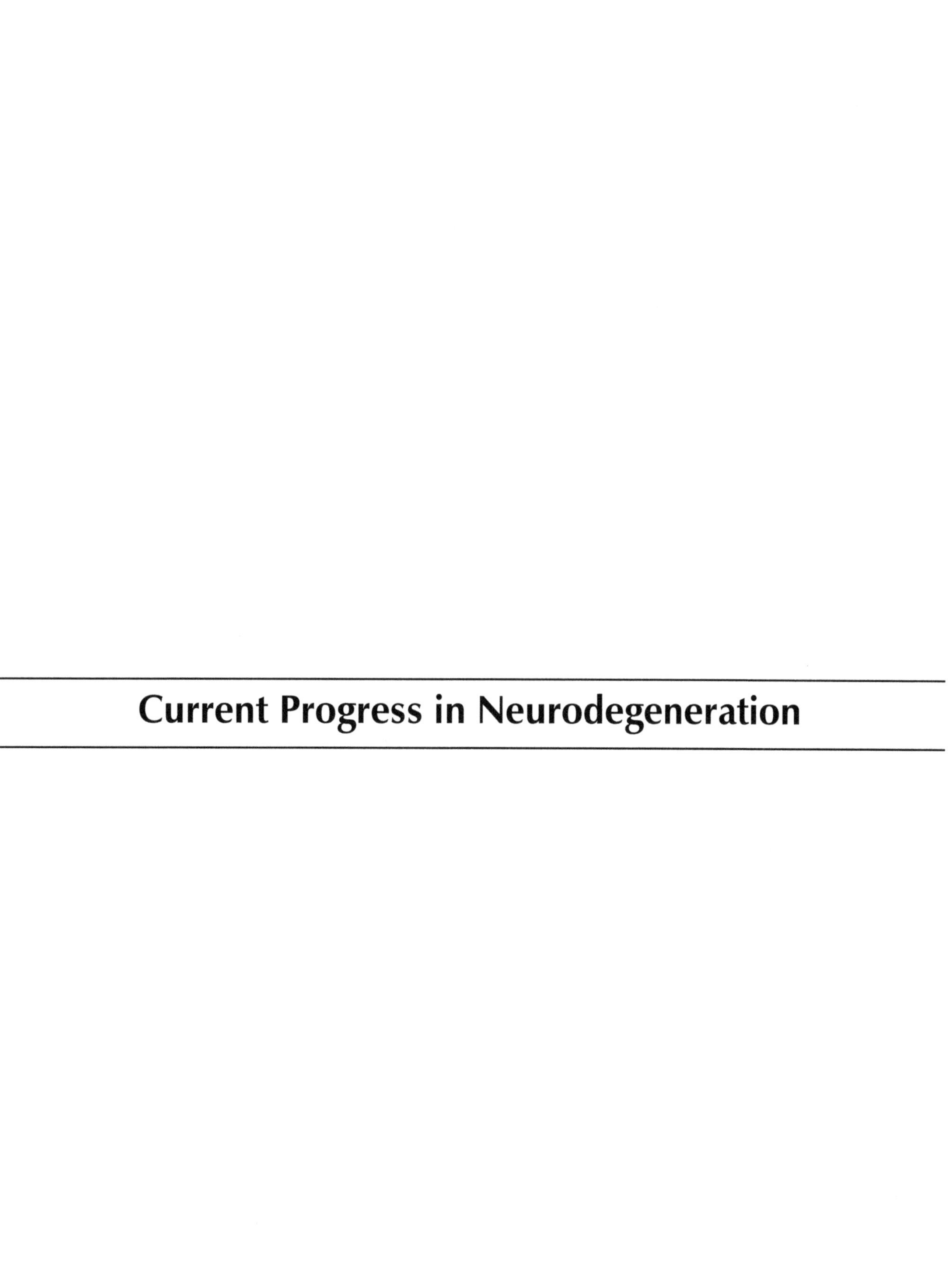

Current Progress in Neurodegeneration

Current Progress in Neurodegeneration

Editor: Elena Poole

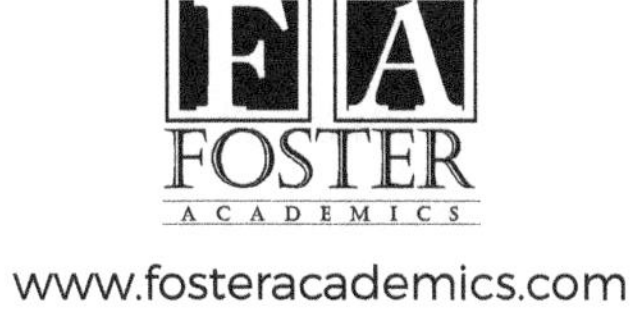

www.fosteracademics.com

www.fosteracademics.com

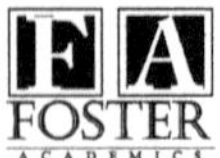

Cataloging-in-Publication Data

Current progress in neurodegeneration / edited by Elena Poole.
p. cm.
Includes bibliographical references and index.
ISBN 978-1-63242-723-6
1. Nervous system--Degeneration. 2. Degeneration (Pathology). 3. Nervous system--Diseases.
4. Nervous system--Degeneration--Treatment. I. Poole, Elena.
RC394.D35 C87 2019
616.804 7--dc23

Foster Academics,
118-35 Queens Blvd., Suite 400,
Forest Hills, NY 11375, USA

ISBN 978-1-63242-723-6 (Hardback)

Contents

Preface

The main aim of this book is to educate learners and enhance their research focus by presenting diverse topics covering this vast field. This is an advanced book which compiles significant studies by distinguished experts in the area of analysis. This book addresses successive solutions to the challenges arising in the area of application, along with it; the book provides scope for future developments.

A progressive loss of neural function and structure, which includes neuron death, occurs through a process known as neurodegeneration. It leads to several diseases, such as Huntington's disease, Parkinson's disease, amyotrophic lateral sclerosis and Alzheimer's disease. These diseases are not reversible and curable, resulting in progressive degeneration and death of neuron cells. The primary risk factor of neurodegeneration is aging. Protein misfolding, genetics, programmed cell death, intracellular mechanisms, etc. are some of the mechanisms by which neurodegeneration occurs. This book is compiled in such a manner, that it will provide in-depth knowledge about the mechanism of neurodegeneration. There has been rapid progress in the understanding of neurodegeneration and neurodegenerative diseases. Scientists and students actively engaged in neuroscience, will find this book full of crucial and unexplored concepts.

It was a great honour to edit this book, though there were challenges, as it involved a lot of communication and networking between me and the editorial team. However, the end result was this all-inclusive book covering diverse themes in the field.

Finally, it is important to acknowledge the efforts of the contributors for their excellent chapters, through which a wide variety of issues have been addressed. I would also like to thank my colleagues for their valuable feedback during the making of this book.

Editor

1

No apparent transmission of transgenic α–synuclein into nigrostriatal dopaminergic neurons in multiple mouse models

Namratha Sastry[1,3], Wang Zheng[1], Guoxiang Liu[1], Helen Wang[1,4], Xi Chen[1], Michael Cai[2,5], Parth Contractor[1,6], Carmelo Sgobio[1], Lixin Sun[1], Chengsong Xie[1] and Huaibin Cai[1*]

Abstract

Background: α–synuclein (α–syn) is the main component of intracytoplasmic inclusions deposited in the brains of patients with Parkinson's disease (PD) and certain other neurodegenerative disorders. Recent studies have explored the ability of α–syn to propagate between or across neighboring neurons and supposedly "infect" them with a prion–like mechanism. However, much of this research has used stereotaxic injections of heterologous α–syn fibrils to induce the spreading of inclusions in the rodent brains. Whether α–syn is able to transmit from the host cells to their neighboring cells in vivo is unclear.

Methods: Using immunestaining, we examined the potential propagation of α–syn into nigrostriatal dopaminergic (DA) neurons in three lines of transgenic mice that overexpress human wild–type α–syn (hα–syn) in different neuron populations.

Results: After testing for three different routes by which hα–syn propagation might occur, we were unable to find any evidence that hα–syn behaved like a prion and could be transmitted overtime into the DA neurons initially lack of hα–syn expression.

Conclusions: In transgenic mice hα–syn does not have the ability to propagate at pathologically significant levels between or across neurons. It must be noted that these observations do not disprove the studies that show its prion–like qualities, but rather that propagation is not detectable in transgenic models that do not use any injections of heterologous proteins or viral vectors to induce a spreading state.

Keywords: Parkinson's disease, α-synuclein, Propagation, Dopaminergic neurons, Transgenic mice

Background

Parkinson's disease (PD) is the second most common neurodegenerative disease, causing debilitating motor and non–motor symptoms [1, 2]. PD is pathologically characterized by the death of nigrostriatal dopaminergic neurons in the ventral *substantia nigra pars compacta* (SNc) of the midbrain, as well as the presence of intracytoplasmic inclusions known as Lewy bodies (LBs) and Lewy neurites (LNs). The main component of these inclusions is α–synuclein (α–syn) [3]. α–syn is a small 140 amino acid protein that is thought to play a role in synaptic vesicle release [4]. Both missense and multiplication mutations of α–syn are linked to early onset familial forms of PD [5]. How mutant α–syn leads to SNc DA neuron loss and LB/LN formation has been under intense investigation ever since.

PD patient brains seem to show a stereotypical appearance of LB/LN pathology that can be mapped into various stages of disease evolution: lesions first appear in the glossopharyngeal and vagal nerves, continue to the SNc DA neurons, and eventually cover the primary sensory and motor cortices [6]. Subsequent studies have hypothesized that α–syn intercellular propagation may be responsible for this stereotypical pathology and have provided evidence both in vitro and in vivo [7–10]. The

* Correspondence: caih@mail.nih.gov
[1]Transgenics Section, Laboratory of Neurogenetics, National Institute on Aging, National Institutes of Health, Building 35, Room 1A112, MSC 3707, 35 Convent Drive, Bethesda, MD 20892-3707, USA
Full list of author information is available at the end of the article

in vivo studies have primarily focused on using intracerebral inoculations of diseased brain homogenate or preformed α–syn fibrils to study development and progression of PD pathology [9, 10]. In wild–type control mice, injections of preformed fibrils of α–syn are sufficient to initiate LB/LN pathology in regions anatomically connected to the site of injection [9]. Such intracerebral injections can also accelerate the formation of LBs and LNs in otherwise asymptotic mice [10] and can be seen over serial passages of inoculations [11]. This has been further confirmed by a study where inoculation with homogenate from either A53T human α–syn transgenic mouse brains or multiple system atrophy patient brains resulted in disease pathology in mice that do not otherwise develop any spontaneous illness [12]. Moreover, this phenomenon has been studied in primates, and propagation is evident in macaque monkeys in addition to rodents [13]. Increasing evidence thus suggests that α–syn potentially behaves in a prion–like manner, where mutated α–syn can be transmitted from cell to cell and spread the pathology [14].

While these studies provide very compelling results to show the prion–like qualities of α–syn, much of the methodology involves artificial injections and inoculations. This triggered us to determine if α–syn propagation could be observed in mice that overexpress human wild–type α–syn (hα–syn), without the need for any injections. Therefore, we generated multiple lines of transgenic mice that overexpress hα–syn in different neuron populations inside and outside of the SNc. We then examined three different routes by which α–syn may propagate into the SNc DA neurons, including long–range propagation from anatomically separated regions, short–distance transmission from presynaptic spiny projection neurons (SPNs), and neighboring DA neurons. Unlike previous inoculation experiments, we found no evidence that α–syn could propagate and possess prion–like qualities in any of our three modes of study, thus questioning α–syn propagation as the method of disease progression in PD.

Methods

Ethics statement

This study was carried out in strict accordance with the recommendations in the Guide for the Care and Use of Laboratory Animals of the National Institutes of Health. The protocol was approved by the Institutional Animal Care and Use Committees of the National Institute of Child Health and Human Development, NIH (Permit Number: 13–040). All surgery was performed under ketamine anesthesia, and all efforts were made to minimize suffering.

Animals

To generate *tetO–SNCA* transgenic mice, human wild–type α-syn (*SNCA*) cDNA coding region was inserted into the mouse prion protein (pPrP)–tetO gene expression vector (a gift from Dr. David Borchelt, University of Florida, Gainesville, FL), which is controlled by the tetracycline-responsive promoter (tetP) [15]. The tetO-SNCA expression construct was then purified and microinjected into fertilized oocytes derived from C57BL/6 J mice. The founder mice were crossed with wild-type C57BL/6 J mice to produce the F1 generation. *Pitx3–tTA* knock–in mice were created as described previously [16]. *Drd1a–rtTA* mice were obtained from Jackson Laboratories (Bar Harbor, ME). All mice were housed in a 12 h light/dark cycle and fed regular diet *ad libitum*. All mouse work follows the guidelines approved by the Institutional Animal Care and Use Committees of the National Institute of Child Health and Human Development, NIH.

Genotyping

Genomic DNA was prepared from tail biopsy using DirectPCR Lysis Reagent (Viagen Biotech, Inc., Los Angeles, CA) and subjected to PCR amplification using specific sets of PCR primers for each genotype, including *Pitx3–tTA* transgenic mice (*Pitx3*–F: GACTGGCTTG CCCTCGTCCCA and *Pitx3*–R: GTGCACCGAGGCCC-CAGATCA), *tetO–SNCA* transgenic mice (PrpEx2–F: TACTGCTCCATTTTGCGTGA and SNCA–R: TCCAG AATTCCTTCCTGTGG), *Drd1a–rtTA* transgenic mice (14915–F: ACCGGAAGTGCTTTCCTTCT and 14916–R: CGACTTGATGCTCTTGATCTTCC).

Immunohistochemistry and light microscopy

Mice were sacrificed and then perfused via cardiac infusion with 4 % paraformaldehyde in cold PBS, followed by post–fixation in the same solution overnight. To obtain sections, brain tissues were removed and submerged in 30 % sucrose for 24 h and sectioned at 30 μm thickness using a cryostat (Leica CM1950, Buffalo Grove, IL). Antibodies specific to TH (rabbit polyclonal, 1:1000, Pel–Freez, Rogers, AR), human α–synuclein (mouse monoclonal, syn211, 1:500, Santa Cruz Biotech, Santa Cruz, CA) were used as suggested by manufacturers. Alexa 488 and Alexa 546–conjugated secondary antibodies (1:500, Life Technologies, Grand Island, NY) were used to visualize the staining. Fluorescence images were captured using a laser scanning confocal microscope (LSM 510; Zeiss, Thornwood, NJ). The images were presented as either a single optic layer after acquisition in z–series stack scans at 2–3 μm intervals from individual fields or displayed as maximum intensity projections to represent confocal stacks.

Image analysis

For the quantitative co–localization assessments, images from serial sections were taken and exported to ImageJ (NIH, Bethesda, MD) for imaging analyses. Each image was split into individual channels for SNCA (488 nm) and TH (546 nm). Cell bodies positive for TH were first selected using the polygon selection tool and then subjected to measurement by mean optical intensities. The mean intensities were then compared to the identical regions in SNCA channel. SNCA intensities below a set threshold were counted as being negative. The overall percentages of positive SNCA cells were then compared between the ages of 1 m and 16–18 m.

Stereology

According to the mouse brain in stereotaxic coordinates (3rd edition, Keith B.J. Franklin and George Paxinos), a series of coronal sections across the midbrain (30 μm per section, every fourth section from Bregma -2.54 mm to -4.24 mm) were chosen and processed for TH staining as described above and visualized using a widefield microscope (Axio Imager A1; Zeiss). We examined 16 sections per brain at 40x magnification. The number of TH positive neurons was assessed using the Optical Fractionator Workflow in Stereo Investigator 11 (MicroBrightField Inc, Williston, VT). The sampling scheme was designed to have coefficient of error (CE) less than 10 % in order to get reliable results. A pilot counting of samples was performed to achieve a total marking of >200 cells, which generally yields CE <10 %. Once the pilot cells counting had completed, the CE was calculated. The counting parameters would be adjusted based on the CE value. To achieve CE <10 %, normally 12 series sections with total 100 counting frames and on average 2 cells per frame would be counted. The final parameters for these studies were: grid size 150x120μm and frame size 50x50μm. Three or more mice were used per genotype at each time point.

Tissue fractionation and Western blot

Striatum tissues were homogenized with 10 volumes of sucrose buffer (0.32 M sucrose, 1 mM NaHCO3, 1 mM MgCl2, and 0.5 mM CaCl2, plus protease and phosphatase inhibitor cocktails) and centrifuged at 10,000 g for 10 min. Protein concentrations in supernatant were measured by BCA (Thermo Fisher Scientific). Proteins were size–fractioned by 4–12 % NuPage BisTris–polyacrylamide gel electrophoresis (Life Technologies) using MES running buffer (Life Technologies). After transfer to nitrocellulose membranes, the membranes were immunoblotted with the appropriate dilutions of the primary antibody: human α–syn (syn211, 1:1000; Santa Cruz Biotechnology, Santa Cruz, CA) and α–tubulin (DM1A, 1:2000; Santa Cruz Biotechnology, Santa Cruz, CA. Signals were visualized with fluorescent secondary antibodies and quantified with ImageJ.

Statistical analysis

Statistical analysis was performed using Graphpad Prism 5 (Graphpad Software Inc. La Jolla, CA). Data were presented as mean ± SEM. Statistical significances were determined by comparing means of different groups and conditions using unpaired Student t–test or one–way ANOVA with post hoc Tukey test.

Results

Transgenic hα–syn is unable to undergo long–range propagation

We generated a new line of human wild–type α–syn (*SNCA*) transgenic mice under the control of tetracycline operator (*tetO*): *tetO–SNCA*. The expression of transgenic *SNCA* assumes to be regulated by the *tetracycline transactivator* (*tTA*) in a "tet–off" gene expression system [17]. However, immunostaining revealed substantial expression of hα–syn in multiple brain regions, including the hippocampus, cerebellum, and cortex, independent of *tTA* (Fig. 1a). Our first test for propagation utilized the "leaky" expression of hα–syn present in *tetO–SNCA* transgenic mice. We wanted to see whether the tyrosine hydroxylase (TH)–positive SNc DA neurons that were initially devoid of hα–syn (Fig. 1a) would show any hα–syn accumulation with age. Potentially, these other tissues or residual hα–syn from the cerebrospinal fluid can aid in "infecting" the SNc DA neurons. If propagation can occur in this long–range fashion, hα–syn might accumulate in SNc DA neurons at advanced ages. We checked for this expression at 1 and 18 months of age (Fig. 1b). At 1–month–old, we found a few hα–syn–positive puncta distributed in the SNc region; some were spotted inside of SNc DA neurons (Fig. 1b, inset). Any additional hα–syn present at later ages would have been evidence for propagation. However, at 18 months of age, we were unable to see any apparent propagation (Fig. 1b). The lack of any substantial accumulation of hα–syn in the SNc DA neurons indicates that no long–range propagation is evident for *tetO–SNCA* mice.

Since the transcription factor paired–like homeodomain 3 (*Pitx3*) is only expressed by subpopulations of midbrain DA neurons [18], previously we inserted tetracycline transactivator (*tTA*) coding sequence into the 3'–untranslated region of mouse *Pitx3* gene to generate *Pitx3–tTA* knock–in mice, allowing *tTA* selectively expressed in midbrain DA neurons [16]. In this so–called "tet–off" system, tTA can turn on the expression of any transgene under the control of tetracycline operator (*tetO*) [16]. In the absence of such a transgene, this line of mice has no transgenic expression in the midbrain (Fig. 1a, b).

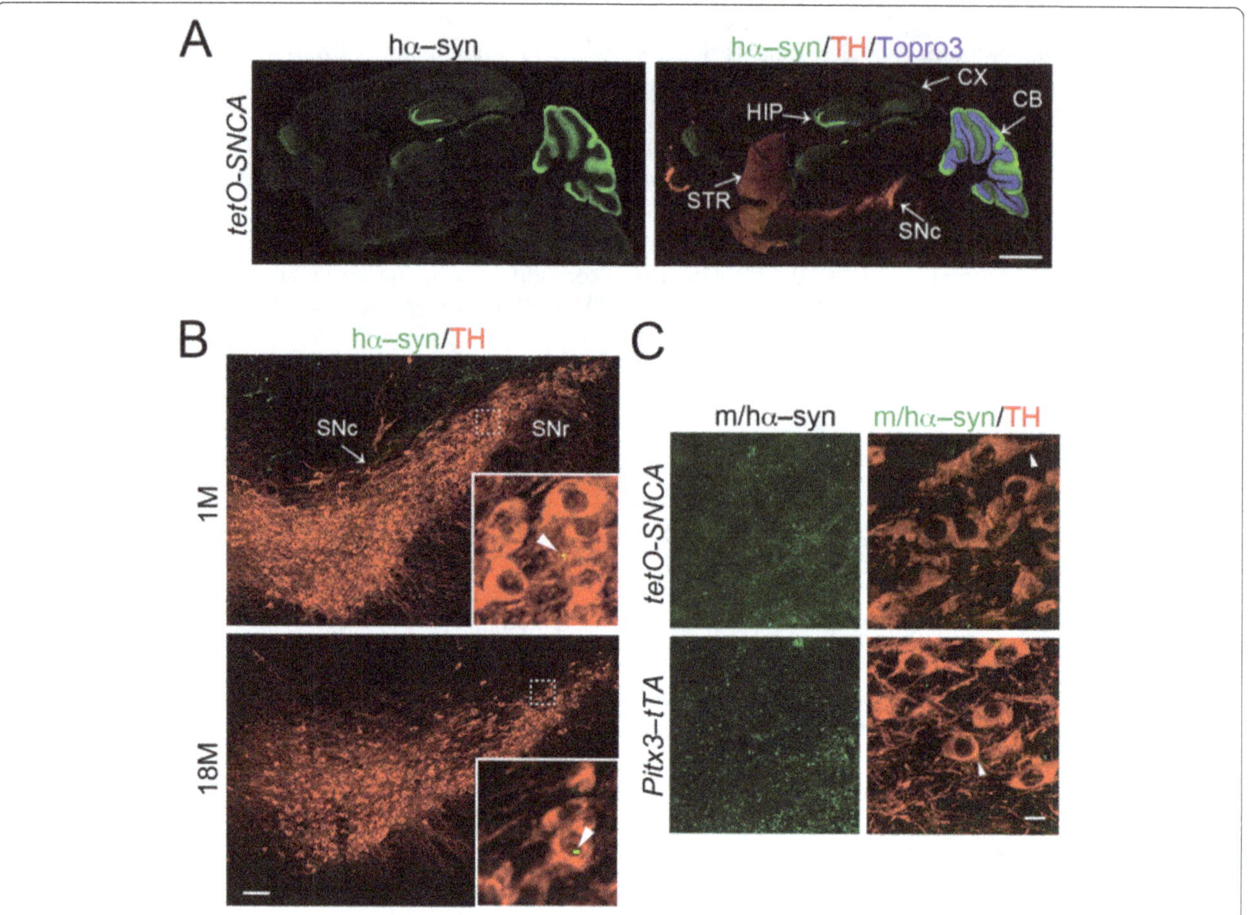

Fig. 1 No propagation of α-syn into the nigrostriatal DA neurons of tetO-*SNCA* single transgenic mice. **a** Sample images show the expression pattern of hα-syn (green) in the sagittal sections of 1-month-old *tetO-SNCA* mice. DA neurons were marked by TH staining (red). Topro3 was used for counter-staining (blue). CX; cerebral cortex; HIP: hippocampus; CB: cerebellum; STR: striatum; SNc: *substantia nigra pars compacta*. Scale bar: 1 mm. **b** Sample images show the staining of hα-syn (green) and TH (red) in the SNc of 1- and 18-month-old *tetO-SNCA* mice. Insets highlight the boxed area. Arrowheads point to the hα-syn-positive puncta. SNr: *substantia nigra pars reticulata*. Scale bar: 100 μm. **c** Sample images show the staining of m/hα-syn (green) and TH (red) in the SNc of 18-month-old *tetO-SNCA* single transgenic and *Pitx3-tTA* heterozygous knock-in mice. Arrowheads point to the hα-syn-positive puncta. Scale bar: 10 μm

Thus, to test whether hα–syn would induce the aggregation of endogenous mouse α–syn (mα–syn) in SNc DA neurons, we stained the midbrain sections of 18–month–old *tetO–SNCA* single transgenic and *Pitx3–tTA* heterozygous knock–in mice with an antibody that recognizes both mouse and human α–syn (m/hα–syn). We observed a similar number of small m/hα–syn–positive puncta in the SNc DA neurons of *tetO–SNCA* and control *Pitx3–tTA* mice (Fig. 1c), indicating a lack of recruitment of endogenous α–syn. Together, these observations suggest a lack of long–range transneuronal propagation of transgenic hα–syn into SNc DA neurons during aging.

α–synuclein is not transmitted from presynaptic terminals into SNc DA neurons

We next examined the transmission between anatomically connected brain regions, specifically the SNc and striatum in the basal ganglia. The majority of DA neurons in the SNc send projections to SPNs in the striatum [19]. SPNs comprise two main subpopulations that form direct and indirect pathways in the basal ganglia [19]. In the direct pathway, most SPNs that express dopamine receptor D1 (*Drd1*) send projections to neurons at *substantia nigra pars reticulata* (SNr), while some directly form synapses with SNc DA neurons [20, 21]. To further investigate propagation in the direct pathway, we used a line of mice that utilizes a *reverse tetracycline transactivator* (*rtTA*) and the *Drd1a* promoter, which directs transgene expression in the SPNs of direct pathway. When crossed with *tetO–SNCA* mice, we expect to see hα–syn expression along the direct pathway. Indeed at 1-month-old, *Drd1–rtTA/tetO–SNCA* mice showed strong hα–syn expression in the striatum and SNr, but no expression in the SNc (Fig. 2a). Once again, hα–syn expression at later ages would indicate that propagation is

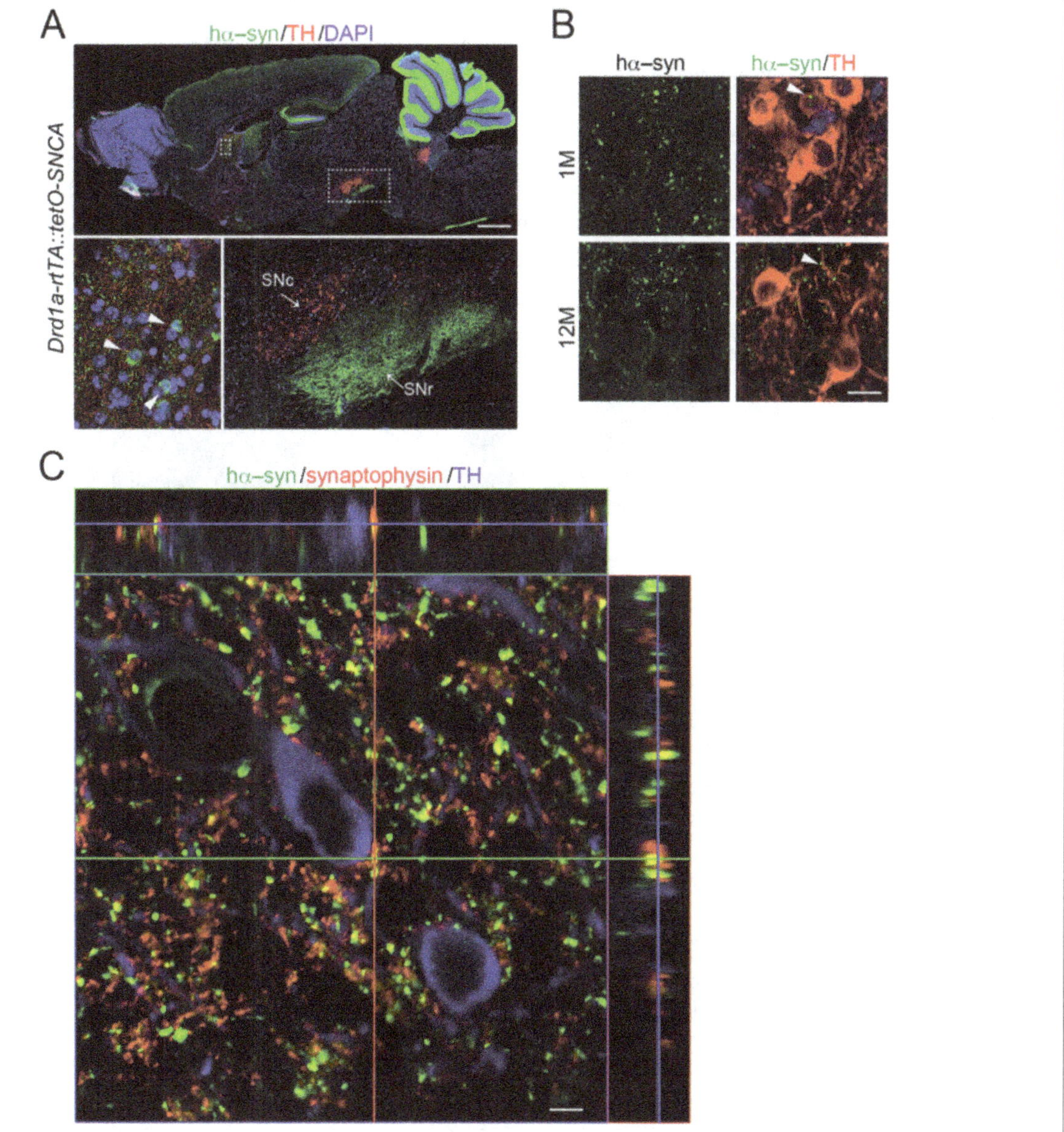

Fig. 2 α-synuclein is not transmitted in anatomically connected regions. **a** In the top panel, sample image shows the expression pattern of hα-syn (green) and TH (red) in the sagittal sections of 1-month-old *Drd1a-rtTA::tetO-SNCA* bigenic mice. Topro3 was used for counter-staining (blue). In the bottom left panel, arrowheads point to Drd1-type striatal neurons that express hα-syn. The bottom right panel highlights the boxed area in the top panel. Scale bar: 1 mm. **b** Sample images show the staining of hα-syn (green) and TH (red) in the SNc of 1- and 18-month-old *Drd1a-rtTA::-tetO-SNCA* bigenic mice. Arrowheads point to the hα-syn-positive puncta. Scale bar: 10 μm. **c** Sample image shows the staining of hα-syn (green), synaptophysin (red) and TH (blue) in the SNc of 18-month-old *Drd1a-rtTA::tetO-SNCA* bigenic transgenic mice. The panels at the top and right depict the distribution of different fluorophores along the Y- and X-axis. Scale bar: 10 μm

present. We then looked at 12–month-old mice and found that they too had no hα–syn–positive cells present in the SNc (Fig. 2b). As seen with the *tetO–SNCA* mice (Fig. 1b and c), small hα–syn–positive puncta were observed near or on top of SNc DA neurons (Fig. 2b). These puncta were also positive for synaptophysin, a marker for presynaptic terminals [22] (Fig. 2c), indicating a presynaptic enrichment of α–syn as previously documented [23]. The same as the previous experiments, we again found no indication that hα–syn possesses the ability to propagate across the synapses.

α-synuclein is unable to undergo cell-to-cell transmission between SNc DA neurons

We finally examined α–syn propagation within SNc DA neurons. To express *SNCA* in the midbrain, we cross-bred *Pitx3–tTA* heterozygous knock–in mice with *tetO–SNCA* heterozygous transgenic mice to generate

Pitx3–tTA::tetO–SNCA bigenic mice. The cells expressing hα–syn co–localize well with TH in the SNc in these mice (Fig. 3a). We subsequently examined co–localization patterns in the *Pitx–tTA::tetO–SNCA* bigenic mice that expressed hα–syn in midbrain DA neurons and (Fig. 3b-d). We looked at mice that were 1– and 16–18–month–old to determine how co–localization values changed with age. *Pitx3* is mainly expressed in the ventral SNc DA neurons, but not in the dorsal ones that account for about 20 % of total DA neuron population [24]. In our study, this translated to ~80 % of the TH–positive SNc cells expressing hα–syn under the control of the *Pitx3* promoter (Fig. 3d). We wanted to see if this percentage would increase with age, indicating the presence of cell–to–cell transmission of hα–syn in these cells. Contrary to what would

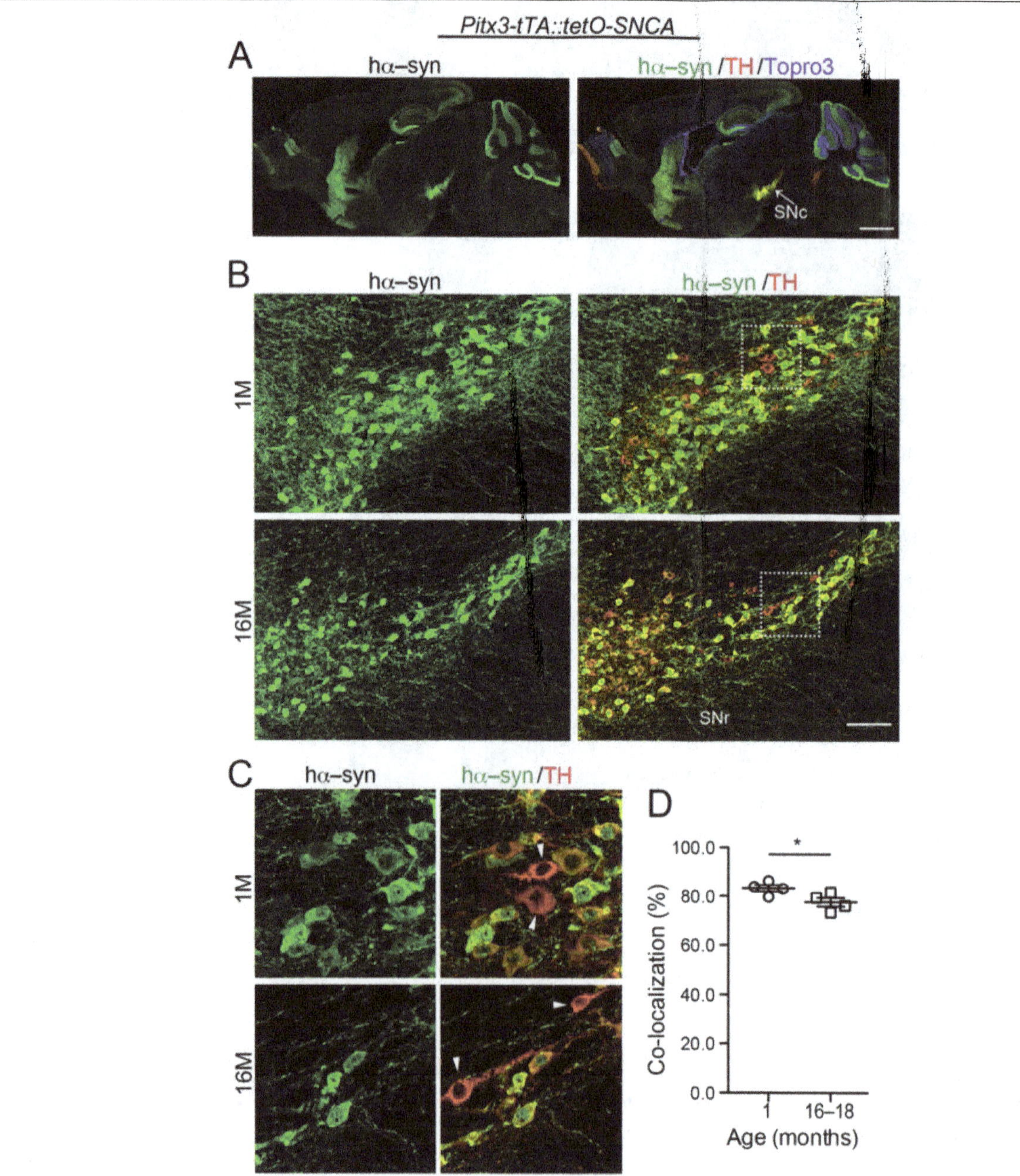

Fig. 3 α-syn is unable to undergo cell-to-cell transmission at SNc. **a** Sample images show the expression pattern of hα-syn (green) and TH (red) in the sagittal sections of 1-month-old *Pitx3-tTA::tetO-SNCA* bigenic mice. Topro3 was used for counter-staining (blue). Scale bar: 1 mm. **b** Sample images show the staining of hα-syn (green) and TH (red) in the SNc of 1- and 16-month-old *Pitx3–tTA::tetO-SNCA* bigenic mice. Scale bar: 100 μm. **c** Images highlight the boxed areas in **b**. Arrowheads point to the hα-syn-negative DA neurons. **d** Scatter plot depicts co-localization percentages at 1 month and 16 months. Data were presented as mean ± SEM. $*P < 0.05$

be expected for propagation, we found that the average percentage of co–localized cells at 1–month–old was 83.3 %, whereas the percentage at 16–18–month–old was 77.6 % (Fig. 3d). As we did not see the increase that indicates the presence of propagation, this experiment provided no evidence for local propagation between neighboring SNc DA neurons.

In addition to tissue staining, Western blotting revealed more than 5–fold increase of α–syn expression in cerebellum of *tetO-SNCA* single and *Pitx3–tTA::-tetO–SNCA* double transgenic mice (Fig. 4a). Furthermore, α–syn–positive high molecular weight (HMW) bands were also detected in the whole brain homogenates of *tetO-SNCA* single, *Pitx3–tTA::tetO–SNCA,* and *Drd1–rtTA::tetO-SNCA* double transgenic mice (Fig. 4b), suggesting the existence of α–syn aggregates in the mouse brains of all the transgenic lines. Western bolting also showed the hα–syn expression was substantially increased in the striatum of *Pitx3–tTA::-tetO–SNCA* double transgenic mice compared to the *tetO–SNCA* single animals (Fig. 4c), resulting from the projection of hα–syn–expressing DA axons at the striatum (Fig. 3a).

Discussion

We show here that transgenic hα–syn does not show detectable propagation to nigrostriatal DA neurons in various mouse models. We first used tetO–*SNCA* single transgenic mice to show that we could not observe long–range propagation of hα–syn into SNc DA

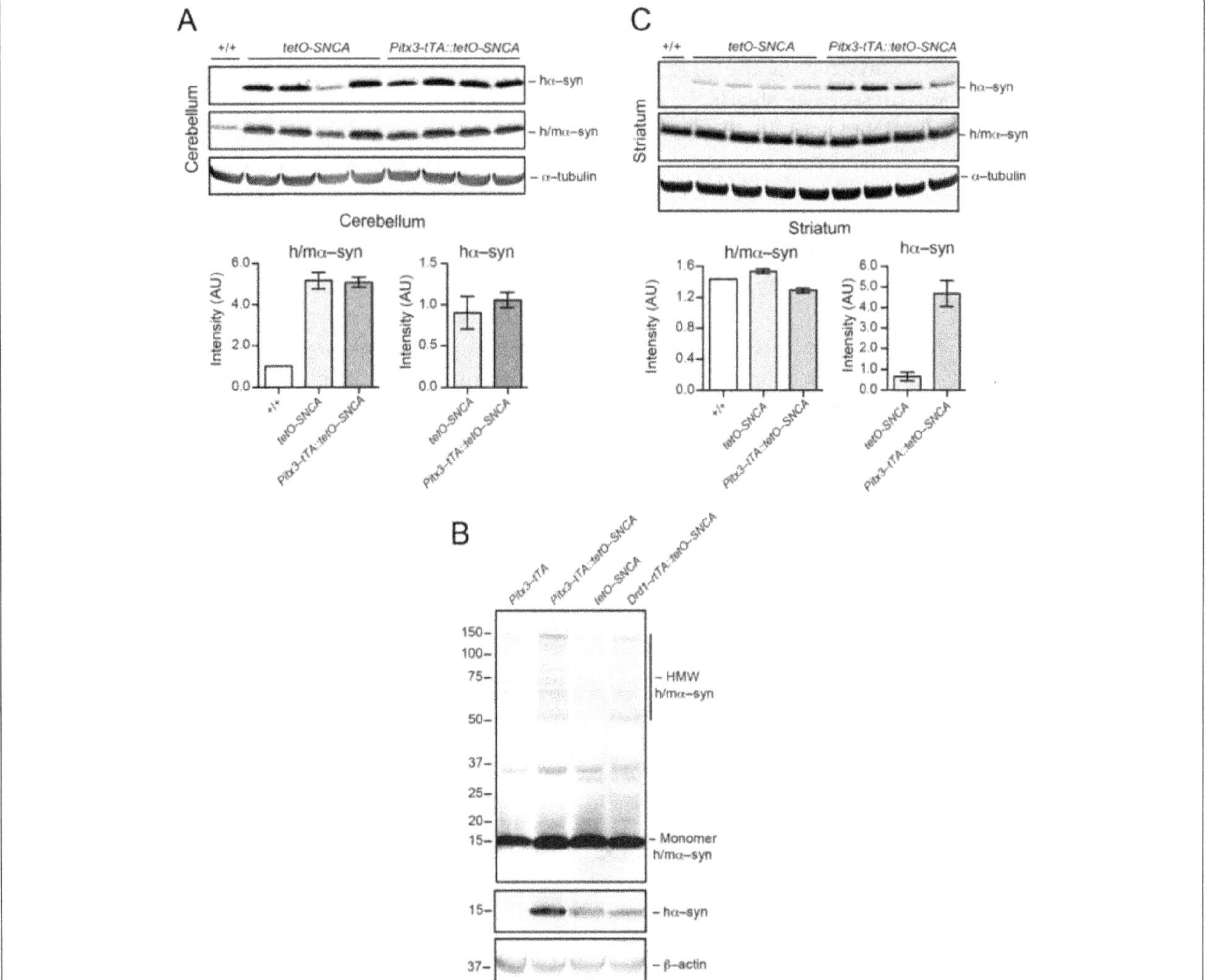

Fig. 4 Overexpression of hα-syn in *tetO-SNCA* single and *Pitx3–tTA::tetO–SNCA* bigenic mice. **a** Western blots show expression of hα-syn and m/hα-syn in the cerebellum of 1–month–old *tetO-SNCA* single and *Pitx3–tTA::tetO–SNCA* bigenic mice. α-tubulin was used as loading control. Bar graphs depict the signal intensity. Data were presented as mean ± SEM. **b** Western blot shows expression of hα-syn and m/hα-syn in the whole brain of 18–month–old *Pitx3–tTA, tetO-SNCA* single, *Drd1a–rtTA::tetO–SNCA* bigenic and *Pitx3–tTA::tetO–SNCA* bigenic mice. β-actin was used as loading control. **c** Western blots show expression of hα-syn and m/hα-syn in the striatum of 1–month–old *tetO-SNCA* single and *Pitx3–tTA::tetO–SNCA* bigenic mice. α-tubulin was used as loading control. Bar graphs depict the signal intensity. Data were presented as mean ± SEM

neurons. These mice have no transgenic hα–syn expression in the nigrostriatal pathway; however, they do have "leaky", non–specific hα–syn expression in other brain regions (i.e. hippocampus, cortex, and cerebellum). Any of these other regions could have played a role being a source of α–syn if the protein could indeed propagate. We performed immunohistochemical experiments on young and aged mice to see if we can observe hα–syn–positive staining anywhere in the SNc DA neurons of aged animals. However, these experiments gave no indication that long–range propagation was present in *SNCA* mice.

The following experiment tested propagation that may occur through neuronal projections from neighboring brain regions. For these experiments, we utilized a line of mice, *Drd1a–rtTA::tetO–SNCA*, which had hα–syn expression in the striatum and SNr, modeling the direct pathway of the basal ganglia. At 1–month of age, these mice exhibited no hα–syn expression in the SNc DA neurons. If propagation was present, we should be able to see hα–syn expression at later ages in these mice. This may have occurred as transmission directly to the SNc from the SPNs that form synapses onto SNc DA neurons [21]. However, as with the previous experiments, we found no evidence of hα–syn being present in the SNc, again showing that there was no evident propagation.

Finally, we looked at *Pitx3–tTA::tetO–SNCA* bigenic mice, which utilize the *Pitx3* driver to promote hα–syn expression along the nigrostriatal pathway, in addition to the leaky expression patterns seen in the *tetO–SNCA* single transgenic mice. Following the expression pattern of *Pitx3*, we found that ~80 % of cells were both hα–syn–positive and TH–positive in 1–month–old bigenic mice. An increase in this percentage in aged mice would indicate that more cells were becoming hα–syn–positive, thus giving evidence for cell–cell transmission of α–syn. While there was about 50 % loss of SNc DA neurons in *Pitx3–tTA::tetO–SNCA* bigenic mice compared to *Pitx3–tTA* knock-in mice, no further degeneration occurred between 1–month and 16–18–month–old bigenic mice (Fig. 5a–b). Thus any increase could be attributed to the spread of α–syn, as opposed to cell death that may have resulted from α–syn toxicity. Instead of seeing the increase that would indicate propagation, we actually saw a slight decrease. However, the lack of degeneration led us to conclude that this decrease likely has no actual significance in the pathogenesis.

Conclusion

Many studies have shown the ability of α–syn to propagate with the use of stereotaxic injections of preformed fibrils and have provided very convincing data for the ability of α–syn to behave as a prion, both in neurons and in glial cells [14]. However, these studies often take advantage of artificial injections or inoculations, which may not be as applicable in a clinical, physiological setting. Therefore, alternative explanations to the prion hypothesis cannot be dismissed, including oxidative stress, excitotoxicity, neuroinflammation, and loss of neurotrophic factor support.

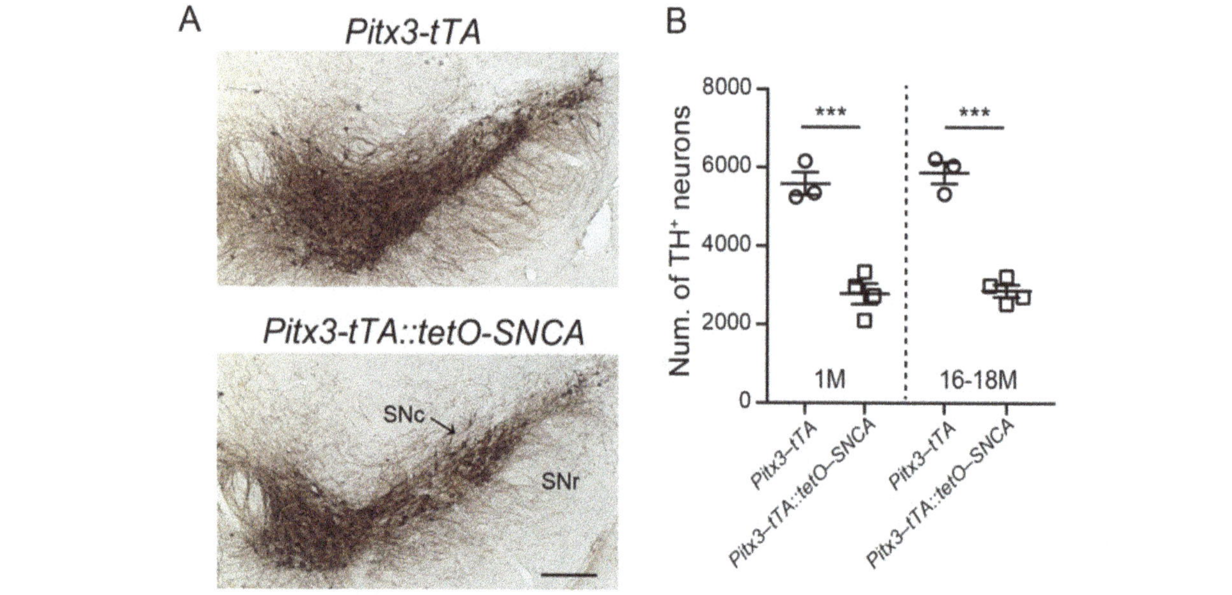

Fig. 5 Loss of DA neurons in the SNc of *Pitx3–tTA::tetO–SNCA* bigenic mice. **a** Sample images show the staining of TH (brown) in the SNc of 16–month–old *Pitx3–tTA* heterozygous knock-in and *Pitx3–tTA::tetO–SNCA* bigenic mice. Scale bar: 100 μm. **b** Scatter plot depicts the number of remaining TH–positive neurons in the SNc of 1 month and 16–18 months. Data were presented as mean ± SEM. ***$P < 0.001$

These alternative explanations are not mutually exclusive and may potentially induce pathogenesis in a synergistic manner. Future studies should focus on microglial activation and other inflammatory responses in the brain resulting from intracerebral injections and inoculations. In addition, further scrutiny into the effect of inflammation on α–syn expression can provide answers about the causes and mechanisms by which α–syn adopts its abnormal prion–like qualities.

Competing interests

The authors declare that they have no competing interests.

Authors' contributions

NS carried out immunostaining experiments and data analyses, drafted the manuscript. ZW provided additional immunostaining data. GL, CS, LS, and CX provided tetO-SNCA transgenic mice and initial characterization. HW, XC, MC, and PC performed Western blot. LS provided mice. HC designed the experiments and wrote the manuscript. All authors read and approved the final manuscript.

Acknowledgement

This work was supported by the intramural research program of National Institute on Aging (HC: AG-000928, 929). The authors would like to thank members of Cai lab for providing various supports.

Author details

[1]Transgenics Section, Laboratory of Neurogenetics, National Institute on Aging, National Institutes of Health, Building 35, Room 1A112, MSC 3707, 35 Convent Drive, Bethesda, MD 20892-3707, USA. [2]Unit on Synapse Development Plasticity, Clinical Brain Disorder Branch, National Institute of Mental Health, National Institutes of Health, Bethesda, MD 20892, USA. [3]Present addresses: Feinberg School of Medicine, Northwestern University, Chicago, IL 60611, USA. [4]Present addresses: Swarthmore College, Swarthmore, PA 19081, USA. [5]Present addresses: Centennial High School, Elicott City, MD 21042, USA. [6]Present addresses: George Washington University, Washington, DC 20052, USA.

References

1. Thomas B, Beal MF. Parkinson's disease. Hum Mol Genet. 2007;16(Spec No. 2):R183–94. doi:10.1093/hmg/ddm159.
2. Tolosa E, Pont-Sunyer C. Progress in defining the premotor phase of Parkinson's disease. J Neurol Sci. 2011;310(1–2):4–8. doi:10.1016/j.jns.2011.05.027.
3. Spillantini MG, Schmidt ML, Lee VM, Trojanowski JQ, Jakes R, Goedert M. Alpha-synuclein in Lewy bodies. Nature. 1997;388(6645):839–40. doi:10.1038/42166.
4. Picconi B, Piccoli G, Calabresi P. Synaptic dysfunction in Parkinson's disease. Adv Exp Med Biol. 2012;970:553–72. doi:10.1007/978-3-7091-0932-8_24.
5. Hardy J, Cai H, Cookson MR, Gwinn-Hardy K, Singleton A. Genetics of Parkinson's disease and parkinsonism. Ann Neurol. 2006;60(4):389–98. doi:10.1002/ana.21022.
6. Braak H, Del Tredici K, Rub U, de Vos RA, Jansen Steur EN, Braak E. Staging of brain pathology related to sporadic Parkinson's disease. Neurobiol Aging. 2003;24(2):197–211.
7. Volpicelli-Daley LA, Luk KC, Patel TP, Tanik SA, Riddle DM, Stieber A, et al. Exogenous alpha-synuclein fibrils induce Lewy body pathology leading to synaptic dysfunction and neuron death. Neuron. 2011;72(1):57–71. doi:10.1016/j.neuron.2011.08.033.
8. Aulic S, Le TT, Moda F, Abounit S, Corvaglia S, Casalis L, et al. Defined alpha-synuclein prion-like molecular assemblies spreading in cell culture. BMC Neurosci. 2014;15:69. doi:10.1186/1471-2202-15-69.
9. Luk KC, Kehm V, Carroll J, Zhang B, O'Brien P, Trojanowski JQ, et al. Pathological alpha-synuclein transmission initiates Parkinson-like neurodegeneration in nontransgenic mice. Science. 2012;338(6109):949–53. doi:10.1126/science.1227157.
10. Luk KC, Kehm VM, Zhang B, O'Brien P, Trojanowski JQ, Lee VM. Intracerebral inoculation of pathological alpha-synuclein initiates a rapidly progressive neurodegenerative alpha-synucleinopathy in mice. J Exp Med. 2012;209(5):975–86. doi:10.1084/jem.20112457.
11. Betemps D, Verchere J, Brot S, Morignat E, Bousset L, Gaillard D, et al. Alpha-synuclein spreading in M83 mice brain revealed by detection of pathological alpha-synuclein by enhanced ELISA. Acta Neuropathol Commun. 2014;2:29. doi:10.1186/2051-5960-2-29.
12. Watts JC, Giles K, Oehler A, Middleton L, Dexter DT, Gentleman SM, et al. Transmission of multiple system atrophy prions to transgenic mice. Proc Natl Acad Sci U S A. 2013;110(48):19555–60. doi:10.1073/pnas.1318268110.
13. Recasens A, Dehay B, Bove J, Carballo-Carbajal I, Dovero S, Perez-Villalba A, et al. Lewy body extracts from Parkinson disease brains trigger alpha-synuclein pathology and neurodegeneration in mice and monkeys. Ann Neurol. 2014;75(3):351–62. doi:10.1002/ana.24066.
14. Luk KC, Lee VM. Modeling Lewy pathology propagation in Parkinson's disease. Parkinsonism Relat Disord. 2014;20 Suppl 1:S85–7. doi:10.1016/S1353-8020(13)70022-1.
15. Jankowsky JL, Savonenko A, Schilling G, Wang J, Xu G, Borchelt DR. Transgenic mouse models of neurodegenerative disease: opportunities for therapeutic development. Curr Neurol Neurosci Rep. 2002;2(5):457–64.
16. Lin X, Parisiadou L, Sgobio C, Liu G, Yu J, Sun L, et al. Conditional expression of Parkinson's disease-related mutant alpha-synuclein in the midbrain dopaminergic neurons causes progressive neurodegeneration and degradation of transcription factor nuclear receptor related 1. J Neurosci. 2012;32(27):9248–64. doi:10.1523/JNEUROSCI.1731-12.2012.
17. Gossen M, Bujard H. Tight control of gene expression in mammalian cells by tetracycline-responsive promoters. Proc Natl Acad Sci U S A. 1992;89(12):5547–51.
18. Smidt MP, Smits SM, Bouwmeester H, Hamers FP, van der Linden AJ, Hellemons AJ, et al. Early developmental failure of substantia nigra dopamine neurons in mice lacking the homeodomain gene Pitx3. Development. 2004;131(5):1145–55. doi:10.1242/dev.01022.
19. Gerfen CR, Surmeier DJ. Modulation of striatal projection systems by dopamine. Annu Rev Neurosci. 2011;34:441–66. doi:10.1146/annurev-neuro-061010-113641.
20. Gerfen CR. The neostriatal mosaic: compartmentalization of corticostriatal input and striatonigral output systems. Nature. 1984;311(5985):461–4.
21. Watabe-Uchida M, Zhu L, Ogawa SK, Vamanrao A, Uchida N. Whole-brain mapping of direct inputs to midbrain dopamine neurons. Neuron. 2012;74(5):858–73. doi:10.1016/j.neuron.2012.03.017.
22. Wiedenmann B, Franke WW. Identification and localization of synaptophysin, an integral membrane glycoprotein of Mr 38,000 characteristic of presynaptic vesicles. Cell. 1985;41(3):1017–28.
23. Maroteaux L, Campanelli JT, Scheller RH. Synuclein: a neuron-specific protein localized to the nucleus and presynaptic nerve terminal. J Neurosci. 1988;8(8):2804–15.
24. Bifsha P, Yang J, Fisher RA, Drouin J. Rgs6 is required for adult maintenance of dopaminergic neurons in the ventral substantia nigra. PLoS Genet. 2014;10(12):e1004863. doi:10.1371/journal.pgen.1004863.

2

Rest tremor revisited: Parkinson's disease and other disorders

Wei Chen[1,2], Franziska Hopfner[2], Jos Steffen Becktepe[2] and Günther Deuschl[1,2*]

Abstract

Tremor is the most common movement disorder characterized by a rhythmical, involuntary oscillatory movement of a body part. Since distinct diseases can cause similar tremor manifestations and vice-versa, it is challenging to make an accurate diagnosis. This applies particularly for tremor at rest. This entity was only rarely studied in the past, although a multitude of clinical studies on prevalence and clinical features of tremor in Parkinson's disease (PD), essential tremor and dystonia, have been carried out. Monosymptomatic rest tremor has been further separated from tremor-dominated PD. Rest tremor is also found in dystonic tremor, essential tremor with a rest component, Holmes tremor and a few even rarer conditions. Dopamine transporter imaging and several electrophysiological methods provide additional clues for tremor differential diagnosis. New evidence from neuroimaging and electrophysiological studies has broadened our knowledge on the pathophysiology of Parkinsonian and non-Parkinsonian tremor. Large cohort studies are warranted in future to explore the nature course and biological basis of tremor in common tremor related disorders.

Keywords: Tremor, Parkinson's disease, Essential tremor, Dystonia, Pathophysiology

Background

Tremor is defined as a rhythmical, involuntary oscillatory movement of a body part [1]. Making an accurate diagnosis of tremor disorders is challenging, since similar clinical entities may be caused by different diseases. Due to the lack of biomarkers, misdiagnoses among parkinsonian tremor, essential tremor (ET) and dystonic tremor are not uncommon [2]. Generally, tremor may be evaluated by features of medical history (family history, onset age, and temporal evolution), tremor characteristics (topography, activation condition, frequency and amplitude) and associated systemic or neurological signs. Besides, ancillary tests (dopamine transporter imaging, electrophysiological evaluation, response to levodopa etc.) are needed for patients with undetermined tremor entities (Table 1).

The consensus statement of Movement Disorder Society (MDS) on tremor in 1998 constitutes the main clinical classification system for tremor, is widely accepted and has been followed in the past two decades [1]. Many studies have been conducted to explore the prevalence and clinical correlates of tremor in common tremor related disorders. Some practical clinical cues and ancillary tests for clinical distinction are found [3]. Besides, accumulating structural and functional neuroimaging, as well as electrophysiological studies broaden our understanding on the pathophysiology of tremor in different kinds of movement disorders.

Therefore, the present review will mainly revisit the progress on prevalence and clinical features of rest tremor in Parkinson's disease (PD), ET and dystonia. For patients with monosymptomatic tremor at rest, the possible clinical outcomes are discussed. Also, the potential ancillary tests for tremor differential diagnosis and underlying pathophysiological basis of tremor in common tremor related disorders are debated.

Tremor in Parkinson's disease

Prevalence

The epidemiology of tremor in PD has not yet been deeply studied. A case series of 100 pathologically proven PD revealed tremor in 68% of cases at disease onset, in 75% during the course of the disease, and in 9%, tremor disappeared late in the course of the illness [4]. Rest tremor was noted at least during one evaluation among 47 pathologically verified Parkinsonian patients [5]. Action tremor

* Correspondence: g.deuschl@neurologie.uni-kiel.de
[1]Department of Neurology, Shanghai Ninth People's Hospital affiliated to Shanghai Jiao Tong University School of Medicine, 200011 Shanghai, China
[2]Department of Neurology, Universitätsklinikum Schleswig-Holstein, Kiel Campus, Christian-Albrechts-University, Rosalind Franklinstr.10, 24105 Kiel, Germany

Table 1 Key clinical features and pathophysiological basis of tremor in Parkinson's disease, essential tremor and dystonia

	Parkinsonian tremor	Essential tremor	Dystonic tremor
Key clinical features			
Topography	Hand > others	Hands > head > voice > others	head > Hands > others
Activation condition	Rest > postural/kinetic	Postural > kinetic > rest	Postural > kinetic > rest
Symmetry	Asymmetrical	Symmetrical	Asymmetrical
Suppression of tremor during movement onset	in most cases	not found	rare
Frequency	4-6Hz	4-8 Hz	7 Hz
Amplitude	Regular	Regular	Irregular
Potential accompanying signs	Bradykinesia, rigidity, etc	Impaired tandem gait	Dystonic posture
Possible pathophysiological basis			
Triggering factor	Dopaminergic dysfunction in nigrostriatal system	Reduced inhibition in cerebellum and brainstem	Reduced inhibitory reflex at multiple levels (spinal, brainstem, and cortical, etc.)
Activated circuit	Cerebello-thalamo-cortical circuit		

was reported in 46–93% of PD patients depending on the selected populations [6, 7].

Clinical features

All different forms of tremor i.e. rest, postural or kinetic tremor may occur in patients with PD. The most common form, classical Parkinsonian rest tremor, refers to a 4- to 6-Hz pill-rolling tremor in the fully resting limb, which is suppressed during movement initiation [8]. It can be provoked by stressful situations like backwards counting, tapping of the contralateral limb or by using the Stroop test. [9] The maximal amplitude is reached on average after 2–3 min [9]. As most motor symptoms of PD, rest tremor is often more pronounced unilaterally, and the upper limbs are usually more affected than the legs. Besides extremities, rest tremor also occurs in the tongue, lip or chin, but rarely involves the head. Other types like postural and kinetic tremor may also occur in PD. It is reported that action tremor is associated with rest tremor in PD, and appears more severely on the side of the body in which the rest tremor is predominant [6]. One of the most important diagnostic features is the suppression of rest tremor during movement onset [10]. Re-emergent tremor, defined as tremor slowly emerging when a new position of the extremity is acquired, is regarded as the same phenomenon when it is clinically more severely expressed [11].

Accumulating evidence indicates that tremor dominant PD is a distinct subtype from those with bradykinesia and rigidity. Clinically, tremor can even be worse on the opposite side of the more severe bradykinesia. Tremor dominant patients have higher dopamine transporter binding, compared to akinetic-rigid type [12], whereas tremor severity does not correlate with striatal dopamine deficits [13]. As demonstrated in DATATOP cohort, tremor dominant PD reported a less severe motor, cognition and functional disability than patients with postural instability and gait difficulty [14]. Prospective studies suggest that this subtype may predict a more favorable prognosis in terms of less mortality risk and lower probability of developing levodopa induced dyskinesia (LID) [15]. However, at later stages of the condition the course is similar for the akinetic-rigid variant and the tremor-dominant variant [16].

Essential tremor

Prevalence

The prevalence of ET ranges from 1% in the total population to 5% for those beyond the age of 60 years [17]. Regarding tremor localizations, arm tremor was reported in 90–100%, head tremor was reported in 21–44%; whereas voice tremor was found in 12–49% of ET. With respect to the conditions activating tremor, intention tremor (IT) occurs approximately in one third of ET cases [18]. Rest tremor was also noted in ET, its prevalence is highly dependent on the selected cohorts, ranging from as low as 2% in the population-based setting to 46% in the brain bank samples [19]. As a feature of ET, alcohol sensitivity was reported in at least 46% of the patients [20].

Clinical features

ET is a common movement disorder defined by sparse clinical criteria. The clinical hallmark of ET is an involuntary postural or kinetic tremor affecting mainly the hands and forearms in the absence of other neurological signs, in particular dystonia and clear-cut ataxia or bradykinesia [1]. In addition to classic postural tremor in ET, patients may also have IT and rest tremor. Head and voice tremor are regarded as the second and third common tremor localizations [21].

Accumulating evidence indicates that ET is not a single entity but a group of diseases with diverse etiologies most of which are currently unknown [22, 23]. However, it is unknown if there are clinical criteria which separate different conditions. One promising stratifying marker is age at onset. Most epidemiological studies of ET show two distinct age at onset peaks: early and late disease onset. Early-onset patients more frequently reported a positive family history and alcohol sensitivity of tremor [24], whereas late-onset patients have faster tremor progression, more frequent dementia and earlier mortality [25]. Another subgrouping may be possible on the basis of the topography of ET. Phenotypic differences were found among patients stratified by head and voice tremor condition [21]. Female gender is associated with head tremor in ET as shown in our latest meta-analysis [21]. Both female and severe hand tremor may increase the risk of head and/or voice tremor in ET [21]. Activation conditions may also be phenotypical features separating different entities [26, 27]. It has been reported that ET patients with IT were older and had more frequent head and trunk involvement [26]; whereas patients with rest tremor were also older and have longer disease duration and greater tremor severity [19]. Neuroimaging studies reported that ET with head tremor had more cerebellar atrophy, especially in the vermis of the anterior lobe [28, 29]. Also, a recent pathological study found that patients with head and voice tremors had more Purkinje cell axonal swellings with torpedoes in the cerebellar vermis [30].

Tremor in dystonia

Tremor has been recognized as an important clinical feature in dystonia. According to the consensus classification of tremor in 1998, tremor in dystonia may be classified into 1): dystonic tremor (DT), with tremor in the same body parts by dystonia, 2) tremor associated with dystonia (TAWD), with tremor in the unaffected regions of dystonia, and 3) dystonia gene-associated tremor [1].

Prevalence

There is a wide variability of tremor prevalence in dystonia, ranging from 14 to 87%, due to selected cases and the sample size [31, 32]. So far, the largest case series found that 262 (55%) out of 473 adult-onset primary dystonia showed tremor as a main symptom, with head tremor being the most common affected location ($n = 196$, 41%), followed by hand tremor ($n = 140$, 30%) [33]. Among 140 patients with arm tremor, all presented postural tremor, 103 patients (73.6%) presented a kinetic component, whereas 57 patients (40.7%) also had rest tremor [33].

Clinical features

Tremor occurs at, before or after the onset of dystonia. Tremor in dystonia is usually postural or kinetic but rest tremor can also be found [33]. Topographically, most studies reported a greater occurrence for head tremor than for upper limb tremor, whereas voice and leg tremor were considerably rare [31].

Accumulating observational studies indicated that some phenotypic parameters including gender, age at onset, localizations of dystonia, may influence the status of tremor in dystonia. Data on gender distribution in tremor of dystonia indicated a female to male predominance ranging from 1.2:1 to 3.7:1 [31]. Rest tremor was noted more frequent in patients with late-onset dystonia than in those with early-onset dystonia [34]. Based on two large cohorts with dystonia [33, 35], patients with segmental, multifocal and generalized dystonia had a higher proportion of tremor relative to focal dystonia. Among subgroups patients with focal dystonia, both studies showed a greater tremor occurrence in patients with cervical dystonia than in those with blepharospasm and task-specific upper limb dystonia.

Apart from the clinical characteristics, genetic factors may also contribute to the occurrence of tremor in dystonia. Pathogenic mutations in the anoctamin 3 gene (*ANO3*) were identified to cause autosomal dominant craniocervical dystonia and have been assigned to the dystonia locus dystonia-24 (DYT24) [36]. It was reported the presence of tremor was the characteristic feature in all affected individuals. In some individuals with *ANO3* mutations, tremor was the sole initial manifestation leading to the misdiagnosis of ET [37, 38]. Head tremor was also noted in DYT25 patients with guanine nucleotide-binding protein(*GNAL*) mutation [39].

Monosymptomatic rest tremor (mRT)

A diagnostic challenge comes from patients presenting with predominant rest tremor without unequivocal bradykinesia or rigidity. According to MDS consensus statement on tremor in 1998, 'monosymptomatic rest tremor'(mRT) was used if these patients had a tremor duration of at least 2 years [1]. Since rest tremor is a classic sign of PD, this entity of patients was also labelled as 'benign tremulous Parkinsonism'(BTP) in some previous clinical studies [40, 41].

There is still a debate on the etiology of mRT and its relation to PD. An early study indicated that patients with mRT had a nearly identical striatal dopaminergic deficit as in PD [42]. The majority of these patients with mRT will develop PD after a decade or more [43]. But they can also have ET with a rest component, dystonic tremor, Holmes tremor or a few even rarer conditions [43] (Fig. 1). If PD is the cause of mRT patients, this can be proven in-vivo with dopamine transporter (DAT)

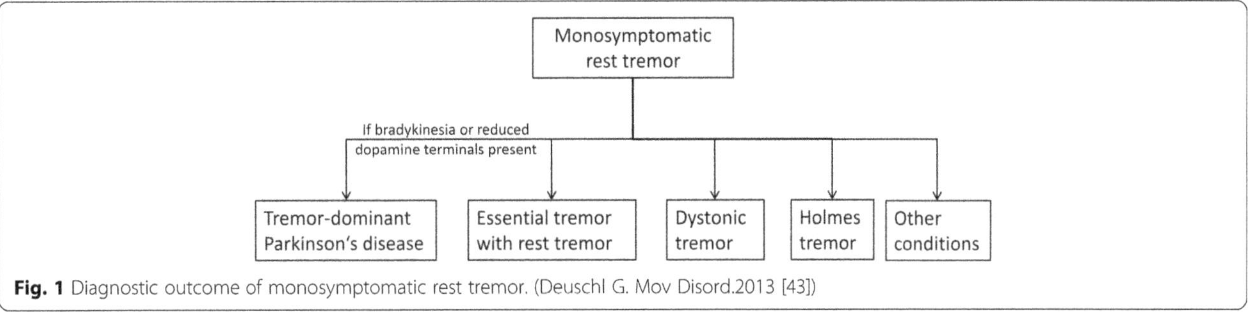

Fig. 1 Diagnostic outcome of monosymptomatic rest tremor. (Deuschl G. Mov Disord.2013 [43])

imaging. A recent prospective study found that 28 out of 33 patients with mRT developed PD verified by DAT positron emission tomography (DAT-PET), whereas 5 cases (15%) have scans without evidence of dopaminergic deficits (SWEDDs) [44]. An important pathological study came from 21 patients with the initial presentation of mRT (labeled by the authors as BTP). At postmortem, 16 of them fulfilled the neuropathological criteria of PD, 5 cases (24%) didn't have nigral impairment and were diagnosed as ET with associated rest tremor or dystonic tremor [45]. These reports also provide a good argument for replacing the term 'BTP' by 'mRT" in the literature, as some of these cases never develop PD and if they do, the course is not benign [43].

Ancillary tests for tremor differential diagnoses

The overlap among tremor disorders is wide and complex. ET patients may present postural tremor coexisting with resting tremor, while postural tremor may coexist with resting tremor in PD and tremor in dystonia is often mixed including a rest tremor component. For the most complicated tremor patients, Dopamine transporter imaging (DATScan) can provide objective evidence to demonstrate presynaptic nigrostriatal dopaminergic deficit in PD, whereas, it is normal in essential, dystonic and psychogenic tremor.

Several electrophysiological tests also showed the potential value for the clinical distinction [46] (Table 2). One method is based on quantified analysis of forearm electromyography (EMG) and accelerometry. Advanced mathematical techniques, in this case the 'mean harmonic power', using these data have shown to be a useful measure to separate clinically difficult cases of advanced ET from tremulous PD, and the accuracy is up to 94% [47]. As one of the most common functional movement disorders, psychogenic tremor (PT) can present with all kinds of tremor type with variable tremor frequency and severity. The key clinical features that help to differentiate psychogenic from organic tremor are a sudden tremor onset, unusual disease course, often with fluctuations or remissions, distractibility of the tremor if attention is removed from the affected body part, tremor entrainment, tremor variability, and a coactivation sign [48]. In cases where the clinical diagnosis remains challenging, providing a "laboratory-supported" level of certainty aids an early positive diagnosis [49]. Due to the inability of a patient with PT to generate voluntary tapping oscillations independent of their ongoing tremor oscillation, coherence entrainment test (CET) was used as a sensitive and specific means to distinguish PT from dystonic and other organic tremors, with nearly 100% concordance with clinical diagnosis [50]. Another method is blink reflex technique reflecting the brainstem excitability. Increased R2 recovery index was found in dystonic tremor, whereas it is within the normal range in ET, with 100% accuracy [51]. Regarding the interstimulus intervals (ISI) of 100 ms, this method also seems to be reliable (100% accuracy) for the distinction of Parkinsonian from essential tremor [52]. The third promising technique comes from sensory function tests. It is reported that temporal discrimination movement threshold (TDMT) is higher in ET, in contrast to dystonic tremor with increased somatosensory temporal discrimination threshold (TDT) [53]. Reduced reciprocal inhibition (RI) of arm muscles assessed with an H-reflex technique was found to be abnormal in patients with early onset of arm tremor and later development of torticollis, but ET had normal presynaptic inhibition [54]. Patients with a late and simultaneous onset of arm tremor and torticollis had normal RI [54]. This is put forward as an argument that dystonic tremor and tremor in dystonia do not necessarily share the same pathophysiological mechanism.

Pathophysiology of Parkinsonian and non-Parkinsonian tremor

It is assumed that tremor networks within the brain are responsible for the different tremors. These circuits are not yet precisely known. Some nodes seem to play an important role. Ventral intermediate nucleus (Vim) of the thalamus is the relay site in cerebellar outflow pathway where deep brain stimulation (DBS) can improve almost all tremors (PD, ET and dystonia) indicating that cerebellum and its outflow pathway may involve in tremor genesis [55] (Table 1).

Table 2 Potential neurophysiological tests for tremor differential diagnosis

Techniques	Diagnostic reliability	Design	Parkinsonian tremor	Essential tremor	Dystonic tremor	Psychogenic tremor	References
Mean hormonic peak power	Accuracy 94%	Tremulous PD($n = 39$) vs. ET($n = 41$)	Tremulous PD > ET		-	-	Muthuraman M. Mov Disord. 2011 [47]
Coherence entrainment test (CET)	Accuracy 100%	Psychogenic trmeor ($n = 10$) vs. DT ($n = 11$) vs. HC($n = 10$)	-	-	negative	positive	McAuley J. Mov Disord. 2004 [50]
Blink reflex recovery curve (BRrc)	Accuracy 100%	DT($n = 10$) vs. ET($n = 10$) vs. HC($n = 12$)	-	Normal	Increased R2 recovery index	-	Nistico R. Neurology. 2012 [51]
	Accuracy 100%	tPD($n = 11$) vs. ET with rest tremor($n = 10$) vs. HC($n = 20$)	Incresed R2 component	Normal at ISI 100	-	-	Nistico R. Parkinsonism Relat. Disord. 2014 [52]
Temporal discrimination movement threshold (TDMT)	PPV 86.7%, NPV 70.8%	ET($n = 19$) vs. TAD($n = 20$) VS. HC($n = 25$)	-	Higher	Normal	-	Tinazzi M. Neurology. 2013 [53]
Somatosensory Temporal discrimination threshold (TDT)	PPV 100.0%, NPV 74.1%	TAD ($n = 20$) vs. ET($n = 19$) VS. HC($n = 25$)	-	Normal	Higher	-	Tinazzi M. Neurology. 2013 [53]
Reciprocal inhibition (RI)	Not given	CD with arm tremor($n = 13$) vs. ET($n = 8$)	-	Normal	Partially reduced	-	Munchau L. Brain. 2001 [54]

TAD Tremor associated with dystonia, *DT* dystonic tremor, *CD* cervical dystonia, *tPD* tremor dominant PD, *PPV* positive predictive value, *NPV* negative predictive value, *ISI* interstimulus intervals, -, not given

Emerging neuroimaging evidence showed that both the basal ganglia and the cerebellum are involved in Parkinsonian tremor [56]. It was reported that PD with rest tremor had more grey matter volume decrease in the right quadrangular lobe and declive of the cerebellum [57] and more iron accumulation in dentate nucleus, relative to those with akinetic-rigid type [58]. Data from functional neuroimaging indicates that dopaminergic dysfunction in pallidum triggers the onset of tremor, whereas, the tremor amplitude is regulated within the cerebello-thalamo-cortical circuit [59].

Theories on the pathophysiology of ET include the neurodegenerative, GABAergic and oscillatory network hypotheses [60]. For patients with ET, there is no post-mortem gold standard for histopathological confirmation of the diagnosis, as it is in PD [61]. Limited pathological and neurochemical studies point to cerebellum and brainstem abnormalities in ET, including cerebellar Purkinje cell loss, axonal swellings (torpedoes) [62], as well as GABAergic dysfunction of the dentate nucleus in the cerebellum [63] and locus coeruleus in the brainstem [64]. The methodology beetwen different reseach groups investigating the pathology of ET diverge Torpedo cells, so-called Torpedoes were found only by one rearch group [62]. Other features like Purkinje cell loss in one study [65] cannot be confirmed by others [66]. Advanced neuroimaging provides an alternative way to understand the mechanism and networks involved in ET. A PET study indicated that ET is associated with reduced GABAergic function and increased binding of GABA receptor sites in brain regions implicated specifically in tremor genesis [67]. A recent study combining voxel-based morphometry, tractography and resting-state functional MRI suggests that a primary cerebellar defect leads to the emergence of a pathological oscillation which sets the tremor frequency, but the clinical manifestation of tremor is dependent on the cortical output [68].

Available electrophysiological studies demonstrate that patients with dystonia and tremor had reduced reciprocal inhibition between agonist and antagonist of upper limb muscles, a lack of brainstem interneuronal inhibition (BRrc), and abnormal sensory integration (TDT), indicating a lack of inhibitory mechanism at multiple levels (spinal, brainstem, and cortical) [31]. The neurophysiologic abnormalities in patients with dystonia and tremor resemble those in dystonia but differ from those described in ET, indicating tremor as phenotypic feature of dystonia. It has further been hypothesized that tremor in dystonia was caused by distorted cerebellar output due to abnormal burst firing pattern in Purkinje cells [31]. Structural MRI found that 27 (14%) of 188 dystonia cases had cerebellar atrophy or cerebellar lesions [69] whereas functional neuroimaging studies on tremor in dystonia are lacking.

Conclusions

A series of epidemiological studies have yielded variable tremor prevalence among PD, ET and dystonia. These discrepancies may be partly due to sample selection as well as different definitions for rest tremor in parkinsonian tremor, ET and dystonic tremor and their subtypes. A diagnostic challenge comes from patients with mRT. Besides key clinical phenotypic differences and DAT scan, several transducer-based techniques like accelerometry, gyroscopy, EMG, and digitizing tablet-based meaures may provide extra clues for the distinction [70]. Compared to rating scales, these transducers are far more sensitive to changes in tremor amplitude and frequency. However, due to the natural variability of tremor, they are not more sensitive in defining the minimal detectable change than rating scales [70]. Also, their potential diagnostic values (sensitivity and specificity) still merit further validation in larger cohort studies. More studies on the pathophysiology of the different tremor entities are needed, which may help to develop new diagnostic markers and hence a more tailored therapeutic strategy. Studies on the natural course and biological basis of tremor are still warranted with standardized terminology, diagnostic criteria, validated evaluation tools and research protocols.

Abbreviations

ANO3: Anoctamin 3 gene; BRrc: Brainstem interneuronal inhibition; BTP: Benign tremulous Parkinsonism; CET: Coherence entrainment test; DAT: Dopamine transporter; DBS: Deep brain stimulation; DT: Dystonic tremor; DYT24: Dystonia locus dystonia-24; EMG: Electromyography; ET: Essential tremor; *GNAL*: Guanine nucleotide-binding protein; IT: Intention tremor; LID: Levodopa induced dyskinesia; MDS: Movement disorder society; mRT: Monosymptomatic rest tremor; PD: Parkinson's disease; PT: Psychogenic tremor; SWEDDs: Scans without evidence of dopaminergic deficits; TAWD: Tremor associated with dystonia; TDMT: Temporal discrimination movement threshold; TDT: Temporal discrimination threshold; Vim: Ventral intermediate nucleus

Acknowledgements

Not applicable.

Funding

Wei Chen received grants from Youth Fund of Shanghai Ninth People's Hospital, K.C.Wong Medical Fund of Shanghai Jiao Tong University, and National Natural Science Fund of China (81401039). Franziska Hopfner received grants from the German Research Council (DFG), the International Essential Tremor Foundation (IETF) and the medical faculty of the Christian-Albrechts-University Kiel. Günther Deuschl received grants from the German Research Council (DFG), the German Ministry of Education and Health. Jos Steffen Becktepe reports no disclosures.

Authors' contributions

GD conceived the study, gave suggestions on writing and revised the article. WC acquired the data, drafted the review. FH gave suggestions on organizing the materials and revised the manuscript. JSB gave comments on the content of the manuscript. All authors read and approved the final manuscript.

Competing interests

The authors declare that they have no competing interests.

References

1. Deuschl G, Bain P, Brin M. Consensus statement of the movement disorder society on tremor. Ad Hoc Sci Committee Mov Disord. 1998;13 Suppl 3:2–23.
2. Jain S, Lo SE, Louis ED. Common misdiagnosis of a common neurological disorder: how are we misdiagnosing essential tremor? Arch Neurol. 2006;63:1100–4.
3. Gövert F, Deuschl G. Tremor entities and their classification: an update. Curr Opin Neurol. 2015;28:393–9.
4. Hughes AJ, Daniel SE, Blankson S, Lees AJ. A clinicopathologic study of 100 cases of Parkinson's disease. Arch Neurol. 1993;50:140–8.
5. Rajput AH, Rozdilsky B, Ang L. Occurrence of resting tremor in Parkinson's disease. Neurology. 1991;41:1298–9.
6. Louis ED, Levy G, Côte LJ, Mejia H, Fahn S, Marder K. Clinical correlates of action tremor in Parkinson disease. Arch Neurol. 2001;58:1630–4.
7. Gigante AF, Bruno G, Iliceto G, Guido M, Liuzzi D, Mancino PV, et al. Action tremor in Parkinson's disease: frequency and relationship to motor and non-motor signs. Eur J Neurol. 2015;22:223–8.
8. Deuschl G, Papengut F, Hellriegel H. The phenomenology of parkinsonian tremor. Parkinsonism Relat Disord. 2012;18 Suppl 1:S87–89.
9. Raethjen J, Austermann K, Witt K, Zeuner KE, Papengut F, Deuschl G. Provocation of Parkinsonian tremor. Mov Disord. 2008;23:1019–23.
10. Papengut F, Raethjen J, Binder A, Deuschl G. Rest tremor suppression may separate essential from parkinsonian rest tremor. Parkinsonism Relat Disord. 2013;19:693–7.
11. Jankovic J, Schwartz KS, Ondo W. Re-emergent tremor of Parkinson's disease. J Neurol Neurosurg Psychiatry. 1999;67:646–50.
12. Spiegel J, Hellwig D, Samnick S, Jost W, Möllers M-O, Fassbender K, et al. Striatal FP-CIT uptake differs in the subtypes of early Parkinson's disease. J Neural Transm. 2007;114:331–5. 1996.
13. Rossi C, Frosini D, Volterrani D, De Feo P, Unti E, Nicoletti V, et al. Differences in nigro-striatal impairment in clinical variants of early Parkinson's disease: evidence from a FP-CIT SPECT study. Eur J Neurol. 2010;17:626–30.
14. Jankovic J, McDermott M, Carter J, Gauthier S, Goetz C, Golbe L, et al. Variable expression of Parkinson's disease: a base-line analysis of the DATATOP cohort. The Parkinson study group. Neurology. 1990;40:1529–34.
15. Kipfer S, Stephan MA, Schüpbach WMM, Ballinari P, Kaelin-Lang A. Resting tremor in Parkinson disease: a negative predictor of levodopa-induced dyskinesia. Arch Neurol. 2011;68:1037–9.
16. Selikhova M, Williams DR, Kempster PA, Holton JL, Revesz T, Lees AJ. A clinico-pathological study of subtypes in Parkinson's disease. Brain. 2009;132:2947–57.
17. Louis ED, Ottman R, Hauser WA. How common is the most common adult movement disorder? estimates of the prevalence of essential tremor throughout the world. Mov Disord. 1998;13:5–10.
18. Louis ED, Frucht SJ, Rios E. Intention tremor in essential tremor: Prevalence and association with disease duration. Mov Disord. 2009;24:626–7.
19. Louis ED, Hernandez N, Michalec M. Prevalence and correlates of rest tremor in essential tremor: cross-sectional survey of 831 patients across four distinct cohorts. Eur J Neurol. 2015;22:927–32.
20. Hopfner F, Erhart T, Knudsen K, Lorenz D, Schneider SA, Zeuner KE, et al. Testing for alcohol sensitivity of tremor amplitude in a large cohort with essential tremor. Parkinsonism Relat Disord. 2015;21:848–51.
21. Chen W, Hopfner F, Szymczak S, Granert O, Müller SH, Kuhlenbäumer G, et al. Topography of essential tremor. Parkinsonism Relat. Disord. 2017. doi: 10.1016/j.parkreldis.2017.04.012.
22. Marsden C, Obeso J, Rothwell J. Benign essential tremor is not a single entity. In: Yahr MD, editor. Curr. Concepts park. Dis. Relat. Disord. Amsterdam: Excerpta Medica; 1983. p. 31–46.
23. Louis ED. "Essential tremor" or "the essential tremors": is this one disease or a family of diseases? Neuroepidemiology. 2014;42:81–9.
24. Hopfner F, Ahlf A, Lorenz D, Klebe S, Zeuner KE, Kuhlenbäumer G, et al. Early- and late-onset essential tremor patients represent clinically distinct subgroups. Mov Disord. 2016;31:1560–6.
25. Deuschl G, Petersen I, Lorenz D, Christensen K. Tremor in the elderly: essential and aging-related tremor. Mov Disord. 2015;30:1327–34.
26. Deuschl G, Wenzelburger R, Löffler K, Raethjen J, Stolze H. Essential tremor and cerebellar dysfunction clinical and kinematic analysis of intention tremor. Brain. 2000;123(Pt 8):1568–80.
27. Cohen O, Pullman S, Jurewicz E, Watner D, Louis ED. Rest tremor in patients with essential tremor: prevalence, clinical correlates, and electrophysiologic characteristics. Arch. Neurol. 2003;60:405–10.
28. Quattrone A, Cerasa A, Messina D, Nicoletti G, Hagberg GE, Lemieux L, et al. Essential head tremor is associated with cerebellar vermis atrophy: a volumetric and voxel-based morphometry MR imaging study. AJNR. 2008;29:1692–7.
29. Cerasa A, Messina D, Nicoletti G, Novellino F, Lanza P, Condino F, et al. Cerebellar atrophy in essential tremor using an automated segmentation method. AJNR. 2009;30:1240–3.
30. Louis ED, Faust PL, Ma KJ, Yu M, Cortes E, Vonsattel J-PG. Torpedoes in the cerebellar vermis in essential tremor cases vs. controls. Cerebellum. 2011;10:812–9.
31. Defazio G, Conte A, Gigante AF, Fabbrini G, Berardelli A. Is tremor in dystonia a phenotypic feature of dystonia? Neurology. 2015;84:1053–9.
32. Pandey S, Sarma N. Tremor in dystonia. Parkinsonism Relat Disord. 2016;29:3–9.
33. Erro R, Rubio-Agusti I, Saifee TA, Cordivari C, Ganos C, Batla A, et al. Rest and other types of tremor in adult-onset primary dystonia. J Neurol Neurosurg Psychiatry. 2014;85:965–8.
34. Gigante AF, Berardelli A, Defazio G. Rest tremor in idiopathic adult-onset dystonia. Eur J Neurol. 2016;23:935–9.
35. Defazio G, Gigante AF, Abbruzzese G, Bentivoglio AR, Colosimo C, Esposito M, et al. Tremor in primary adult-onset dystonia: prevalence and associated clinical features. J Neurol Neurosurg Psychiatry. 2013;84:404–8.
36. Charlesworth G, Plagnol V, Holmström KM, Bras J, Sheerin U-M, Preza E, et al. Mutations in ANO3 cause dominant craniocervical dystonia: ion channel implicated in pathogenesis. Am J Hum Genet. 2012;91:1041–50.
37. Hopfner F, Bungeroth M, Pendziwiat M, Tittmann L, Deuschl G, Schneider SA, et al. Rare variants in ANO3 are not a susceptibility factor in essential tremor. Parkinsonism Relat Disord. 2014;20:134–5.
38. Stamelou M, Charlesworth G, Cordivari C, Schneider SA, Kägi G, Sheerin U-M, et al. The phenotypic spectrum of DYT24 due to ANO3 mutations. Mov Disord. 2014;29:928–34.
39. Fuchs T, Saunders-Pullman R, Masuho I, Luciano MS, Raymond D, Factor S, et al. Mutations in GNAL cause primary torsion dystonia. Nat Genet. 2013;45:88–92.
40. Josephs KA, Matsumoto JY, Ahlskog JE. Benign tremulous parkinsonism. Arch Neurol. 2006;63:354–7.
41. Deeb W, Hu W, Almeida L, Patterson A, Martinez-Ramirez D, Wagle SA. Benign tremulous Parkinsonism: a unique entity or another facet of Parkinson's disease? Transl Neurodegener. 2016;5:10.
42. Ghaemi M, Raethjen J, Hilker R, Rudolf J, Sobesky J, Deuschl G, et al. Monosymptomatic resting tremor and Parkinson's disease: a multitracer positron emission tomographic study. Mov Disord. 2002;17:782–8.
43. Deuschl G. Benign tremulous Parkinson's disease: a misnomer? Mov Disord. 2013;28:117–9.
44. Zheng H-G, Zhang R, Li X, Li F-F, Wang Y-C, Wang X-M, et al. Heterogeneity of monosymptomatic resting tremor in a prospective study: clinical features, electrophysiological test, and dopamine transporter positron emission tomography. Chin Med J (Engl). 2015;128:1765–71.
45. Selikhova M, Kempster PA, Revesz T, Holton JL, Lees AJ. Neuropathological findings in benign tremulous parkinsonism. Mov Disord. 2013;28:145–52.
46. van der Stouwe AMM, Elting JW, van der Hoeven JH, van Laar T, Leenders KL, Maurits NM, et al. How typical are "typical" tremor characteristics? sensitivity and specificity of five tremor phenomena. Parkinsonism Relat Disord. 2016;30:23–8.
47. Muthuraman M, Hossen A, Heute U, Deuschl G, Raethjen J. A new diagnostic test to distinguish tremulous Parkinson's disease from advanced essential tremor. Mov Disord. 2011;26:1548–52.
48. Schwingenschuh P, Deuschl G. Functional tremor. Handb Clin Neurol. 2016;139:229–33.
49. Schwingenschuh P, Saifee TA, Katschnig-Winter P, Macerollo A, Koegl-Wallner M, Culea V, et al. Validation of "laboratory-supported" criteria for functional (psychogenic) tremor. Mov Disord. 2016;31:555–62.
50. McAuley J, Rothwell J. Identification of psychogenic, dystonic, and other organic tremors by a coherence entrainment test. Mov Disord. 2004;19:253–67.
51. Nisticò R, Pirritano D, Salsone M, Valentino P, Novellino F, Condino F, et al. Blink reflex recovery cycle in patients with dystonic tremor: a cross-sectional study. Neurology. 2012;78:1363–5.

52. Nisticò R, Salsone M, Vescio B, Morelli M, Trotta M, Barbagallo G, et al. Blink reflex recovery cycle distinguishes essential tremor with resting tremor from de novo Parkinson's disease: an exploratory study. Parkinsonism Relat Disord. 2014;20:153–6.
53. Tinazzi M, Fasano A, Di Matteo A, Conte A, Bove F, Bovi T, et al. Temporal discrimination in patients with dystonia and tremor and patients with essential tremor. Neurology. 2013;80:76–84.
54. Münchau A, Schrag A, Chuang C, MacKinnon CD, Bhatia KP, Quinn NP, et al. Arm tremor in cervical dystonia differs from essential tremor and can be classified by onset age and spread of symptoms. Brain. 2001;124:1765–76.
55. Hallett M. Tremor: pathophysiology. Parkinsonism relat. Disord. 2014;20 Suppl 1:S118–122.
56. Hallett M. Parkinson's disease tremor: pathophysiology. Parkinsonism relat. Disord. 2012;18 Suppl 1:S85–86.
57. Benninger DH, Thees S, Kollias SS, Bassetti CL, Waldvogel D. Morphological differences in Parkinson's disease with and without rest tremor. J Neurol. 2009;256:256–63.
58. He N, Huang P, Ling H, Langley J, Liu C, Ding B, et al. Dentate nucleus iron deposition is a potential biomarker for tremor-dominant Parkinson's disease. NMR Biomed. 2017. doi:10.1002/nbm.3554.
59. Helmich RC, Janssen MJR, Oyen WJG, Bloem BR, Toni I. Pallidal dysfunction drives a cerebellothalamic circuit into Parkinson tremor. Ann Neurol. 2011;69:269–81.
60. Gövert F, Becktepe JS, Deuschl G. Current concepts of essential tremor. Rev Neurol. 2016;172:416–22.
61. Braak H, Del Tredici K, Rüb U, de Vos RAI, Jansen Steur ENH, Braak E. Staging of brain pathology related to sporadic Parkinson's disease. Neurobiol Aging. 2003;24:197–211.
62. Louis ED, Faust PL, Vonsattel J-PG, Honig LS, Rajput A, Robinson CA, et al. Neuropathological changes in essential tremor: 33 cases compared with 21 controls. Brain. 2007;130:3297–307.
63. Paris-Robidas S, Brochu E, Sintes M, Emond V, Bousquet M, Vandal M, et al. Defective dentate nucleus GABA receptors in essential tremor. Brain. 2012;135:105–16.
64. Shill HA, Adler CH, Beach TG, Lue L-F, Caviness JN, Sabbagh MN, et al. Brain biochemistry in autopsied patients with essential tremor. Mov Disord. 2012;27:113–7.
65. Louis ED, Lee M, Babij R, Ma K, Cortés E, Vonsattel J-PG, et al. Reduced Purkinje cell dendritic arborization and loss of dendritic spines in essential tremor. Brain. 2014;137:3142–8.
66. Rajput AH, Robinson CA, Rajput ML, Robinson SL, Rajput A. Essential tremor is not dependent upon cerebellar Purkinje cell loss. Parkinsonism Relat Disord. 2012;18:626–8.
67. Boecker H, Weindl A, Brooks DJ, Ceballos-Baumann AO, Liedtke C, Miederer M, et al. GABAergic dysfunction in essential tremor: an 11C-flumazenil PET study. J Nucl Med. 2010;51:1030–5.
68. Gallea C, Popa T, García-Lorenzo D, Valabregue R, Legrand A-P, Marais L, et al. Intrinsic signature of essential tremor in the cerebello-frontal network. Brain. 2015;138:2920–33.
69. Batla A, Sánchez MC, Erro R, Ganos C, Stamelou M, Balint B, et al. The role of cerebellum in patients with late onset cervical/segmental dystonia?–evidence from the clinic. Parkinsonism Relat Disord. 2015;21:1317–22.
70. Haubenberger D, Abbruzzese G, Bain PG, Bajaj N, Benito-León J, Bhatia KP, et al. Transducer-based evaluation of tremor. Mov Disord. 2016;31:1327–36.

3

Clinicians' prescription preferences for treating patients with Alzheimer's disease in Shanghai

Chun-Xia Ban[1,2], Shi-Fu Xiao[1], Xiang Lin[1], Tao Wang[1], Qi Qiu[1], Min-Jie Zhu[1] and Xia Li[1*]

Abstract

Background: China has more cases of Alzheimer's disease (AD) than any other country in the world. As training to recognize and manage dementia is in its early stage, it is important to study clinicians' current prescription preferences for treating patients with AD.

Methods: This study surveyed neurologists, psychiatrists, and general physicians (GPs) in Shanghai who had outpatients with AD, using a questionnaire asking about their prescription preferences for these patients.

Results: Among the 148 clinicians in the study, 26.4 % were psychiatrists, 44.6 % were neurologists, and 29.1 % were GPs. The groups did not differ significantly in age, gender, or their monthly cases of new patients with mild or moderate AD ($P > 0.05$). Most clinicians prescribed Cholinesterase inhibitors (ChEIs), including Huperzine A, but there were significant group-differences in prescribing specific ChEIs ($P < 0.05$). The daily dosages of ChEI and Memantine prescribed by all three groups were small ($P > 0.05$), and all three groups prescribed piracetam, ergot, and ginkgo biloba drugs. All three groups also tended to treat AD patients with a combination of antidepressants and anxiolytics, although psychiatrists were significantly more likely than neurologists to combine antipsychotics with other drugs ($P < 0.05$).

Conclusion: Clinicians in Shanghai prescribed low doses of ChEIs and Memantine for patients with AD. A relatively high proportion also prescribed cognitive enhancers, which lack evidence-based support of their use, and antipsychotics. There is a need for more training about treating patients with AD and for clinicians to standardize their clinical practice.

Keyword: Alzheimer's disease, Clinicians, Cognitive enhancers, Prescriptions, Survey research

Background

Alzheimer's disease (AD) is a chronic neurodegenerative disease that has become one of the largest public health problems. Over 25 % of all people with AD are living in China [1]. In 2010, China had 5.69 million cases of AD, which was more than any other country in the world [2]. With the accelerated growth of the older population, the number of people with AD is estimated to triple by 2050 [3]. Although there is no current cure for AD, appropriate treatment can benefit the elderly with AD and improve their quality of life. Medication is one of the most important interventions [4].

Worldwide, only three cholinesterase inhibitors (ChEIs)—Donepezil, Rivastigmine, and Galantamine—and the NMDA-receptor antagonist Memantine are recommended for managing AD. Compared to other developing countries, these medicines were approved later by the Chinese government, so they became available later for Chinese patients. Nevertheless, another ChEI, Huperzine A, which was developed by Chinese scientists, has been used for treating AD in clinical practice for over thirty years [5]. In the USA, Huperzine A is a nutritional supplement for enhancing memory.

In China, training for the recognition and management of dementia is in the early stage [6]. The Chinese

* Correspondence: ja_1023@hotmail.com
[1]Alzheimer's Disease and Related Disorders Center, Department of Geriatric Psychiatry, Shanghai Mental Health Center, Shanghai Jiao Tong University School of Medicine, Shanghai, China
Full list of author information is available at the end of the article

guidelines for the treatment of AD are not necessarily taught to clinicians. Furthermore, memory clinics have been developed only in recent years. Given this background, it is worthwhile to examine how clinicians in China prescribe medications for patients with AD.

In many countries, such as the USA, Australia, Canada or European countries, patients with AD are usually treated first by family doctors—general physicians (GPs); 39 % of all patients with AD are treated by the departments of neurology, psychiatry, and other departments [7]. Because the Chinese medical system has its own characteristics, such as the lack of referrals between general and specialized departments, the clinical treatment of patients with AD is mainly done by the department of neurology, the department of psychiatry, and the general department (including internists at district hospitals and community physicians) without referrals. There has been no investigation, to date, on how clinicians prescribe medications for patients with AD, to see if there are similarities and differences in the medications prescribed by neurologists, GPs, and psychiatrists, and whether the medication principles of these three groups are in accordance with popular diagnostic and management manuals, such as EFNS guidelines for the diagnosis and management of Alzheimer's Disease (EFNS, 2010) [8]; Current pharmacologic treatment of dementia: a clinical practice guideline from the American College of Physicians and the American Academy of Family Physicians (2008) [9]; Practice Guideline for the Treatment of Patients With Alzheimer's Disease and Other Dementias (APA,2007) [10].

Shanghai, which is the largest city in China, has had rapid cultural and economic development. Moreover, the increase in Shanghai's aging population has been ahead of that in other cities. We developed a questionnaire to ask clinicians in Shanghai, who have outpatients with AD or cognitive disabilities, about their prescription preferences and the characteristics of their patients with AD in order to understand the current status of the diagnosis and treatment of patients with AD. The results can provide useful insights for developing relevant training and public health policies for the future.

Methods

Subjects

All the psychiatrists, neurologists, and GPs from community hospitals, second-tier hospitals, and tertiary hospitals who had patients with dementia in Shanghai were enrolled in the study from September 2012 to March 2013. The inclusion criteria were: (1) physicians who specialized in the diagnosis and treatment of AD; and (2) held a professional clinical position of attending doctor or above. The exclusion criteria were: (1) clinicians who did not have independent medicine prescriptive authority; (2) clinicians who treated less than five AD patients each month; (3) clinicians who did not complete half of the items on the questionnaire; and (4) clinicians who did not sign the consent form. This research was approved by the Ethical Review Board of the Shanghai Mental Health Center of Shanghai Jiaotong University.

The nature and aim of the study were explained to the potential participants. Clinicians who agreed to participate signed the informed consent form, and then they were instructed to complete an 18-item self-administered questionnaire. In total, 172 questionnaires were collected. We excluded 7 clinicians who never diagnosed or treated patients with AD, and 17 clinicians who did not complete the survey. leaving 148 physicians who were included in the analyses. There were 74 males (50.0 %) and 74 females (50.0 %), ranging in age from 26 to 60 years. Their mean age was 42.01 ± 7.936 years. The percentages of psychiatrists, neurologists, and GPs were 26.4 % (39/148), 44.6 % (66/148), and 29.1 % (43/148), respectively.

Measures

We developed a questionnaire that included three sections of questions. The three sections were: (1) prescription preferences for ChEIs and Memantine; (2) other prescription preferences for cognitive enhancers; and (3) prescription preferences for antidepressants and anxiolytics. The other types of information collected by the questionnaire were: age, gender, the clinician's department and hospital; the number of new cases each month involving the diagnosis and treatment of patients with AD; the proportion of treated patients with mild, moderate, or severe AD; the proportion of patients with AD using antidepressants, antipsychotics, anxiolytics, or sedative-hypnotic drugs; the proportion of agreement on using one type of ChEIs; preferences and reasons for patients with AD using a certain type of ChEI; reasons why patients with AD did not use a certain type of ChEI; the proportion and daily doses of patients with AD using Donepezil, Rivastigmine, Galantamine, and Huperzine A; the proportion and daily doses of patients with AD using Memantine, and the reasons for using it; the proportion of, and the daily doses, of patients with AD using combination of ChEIs and Memantine, and the reasons for using them in combination; the proportion of patients with AD using Qxiracetam/Aniracetam, ginkgo biloba extract (EGB), ergot alkaloids, vitamin E, nutritional supplements, herbs/traditional Chinese medicine (TCM); and, whether clinicians prescribed the medications described above for patients with AD. The questionnaire generally took 10 to 20 min to complete.

Statistical analysis

We checked and proofread the collected data and analyzed the data using SPSS software. Continuous data with normal distributions, including age, the number of new cases diagnosed per month, and the percentage of patients with different mild, moderate, and severe AD were expressed as the mean ± the standard deviation, and analyzed by one-way analysis of variance. Categorical data were expressed as percentages, including gender, the proportion of prescriptions for ChEIs, Donepezil, Rivastigmine, Galanthamine, Huperzine A, and Memantine, the reasons for choosing ChEIs and Memantine, and the prescription rates of other drugs. The comparison of the proportion of prescriptions of ChEIs was analyzed by Fisher's exact test and other comparisons of proportions were analyzed by the chi-square test. The proportion of prescriptions of anti-psychotics, antidepressants, and anxiolytics among the three groups of clinicians were expressed as the median (interquartile range); their distributions were assessed for normality by the Shapiro-Wilk test and their homogeneity of variance was assessed by Levene's test. If the data were not normally distributed, the non-parametric Kruskal-Wallis test for comparing medians was used, and the Mann–Whitney U-test was used for multiple comparisons among the different groups. The significant level was set at $\alpha = 0.05$, using two-tailed tests. Results that showed $P < 0.05$ were considered to be statistically significant.

Results

Characteristics of study participants

The characteristics of the clinicians who completed the survey are shown in Table 1. There was no statistical difference among the psychiatrists, neurologists, and GPs with respect to age, gender, the numbers of new cases diagnosed per month, or the proportion of cases with different levels of AD severity (the percentage of patients with mild, moderate, and severe AD) ($P > 0.05$).

Rates of prescribing ChEIs and Memantine

Most psychiatrists, neurologists, and GPs prescribed ChEIs to treat patients with AD (see Table 2). The three most commonly used ChEIs were, respectively: Donepezil (90.9 %), Huperzine A (68.2 %), and Rivastigmine (27.3 %) by neurologists; Huperzine A (87.2 %), Donepezil (51.3 %), and Galantamine (17.9 %) by psychiatrists; and Huperzine A (65.1 %), Donepezil (48.8 %), Rivastigmine (9.3 %) by GPs. There were significant differences in the percentages of psychiatrists, neurologists, and GPs choosing ChEIs agents ($P < 0.05$, see Table 2).

Memantine was used by 20.5 % of psychiatrists, 59.1 % of neurologists, and 20.9 % of GPs for treating AD. The rate of neurologists who prescribed Memantine was higher than the rate among psychiatrists and GPs ($P < 0.01$, see Table 2). There was no statistically significant difference among psychiatrists, neurologists, and GPs in their daily prescribed dosages of ChEIs and Memantine ($P > 0.05$, see Table 2).

Reasons for choosing ChEIs and Memantine

Regarding the reasons why clinicians prescribed ChEIs: 71.9 % of physicians agreed that ChEIs were effective, 35.9 % considered them safe, 10.9 % thought they were familiar with ChEIs, and 9.4 % of them used ChEIs based on support for ChEIs from evidence-based research. Other reasons for choosing ChEIs included convenience for patients to take them orally (once per day), the guidelines' recommendations, ChEIs being the only available AD medication in the hospital, and their ability to control behavioral and psychological symptoms of dementia (BPSD). In all, 37.8 % of physicians prescribed Memantine for treating patients with AD; 47.8 % prescribed Memantine for patients with moderate or severe AD; 19.6 % chose Memantine to control BPSD, and 13.0 % used Memantine when ChEIs had an inadequate effect on patients. Other reasons why physicians prescribed Memantine included fewer side-effects, patients having contraindications to ChEIs, combined use with ChEIs, and support from evidence-based research (see Table 3).

Table 1 Characteristics of the Study Participants

Characteristic	Psychiatrists ($n = 39$)	Neurologists ($n = 66$)	General Physicians ($n = 43$)	F/X^2	P value
Age,mean(SD)	41.87(8.36)	41.17 (7.38)	43.44 (8.34)	1.080	0.342
Gender,n (%)					
Male	22 (56.40)	32 (48.50)	20 (46.50)	0.911	0.634
Female	17 (43.60)	34 (51.50)	23 (53.50)		
Numbers of new cases which are diagnosed per month, mean(SD)	14.74(14.90)	13.26(16.04)	13.67(17.20)	0.105	0.900
Severity of AD (%)					
Mild, mean(SD)	31.95(20.60)	34.60(22.64)	37.09(23.48)	0.541	0.584
Moderate, mean(SD)	39.62(16.50)	40.17(20.46)	36.05(13.95)	0.753	0.473
Severe, mean(SD)	28.44(18.35)	25.24(18.09)	26.63(17.24)	0.391	0.677

Table 2 Rates of Prescribing ChEIs and Memantine

Drug Characteristics	Psychiatrists ($n = 39$)	Neurologists ($n = 66$)	General physicians ($n = 43$)	F/X^2	P value
ChEIs, n (%)	37(94.9)	65(98.5)	41(95.2)	1.605	0.601
Donepezil, n (%)	20(51.3)	60(90.9)	21(48.8)	28.295	0.000
Dose (mg/day), mean(SD)	5.75 ± 1.832	5.67 ± 1.714	5.24 ± 1.091	0.651	0.524
Rivastigmine, n (%)	1(2.6)	18(27.3)	4(9.3)	13.200	0.001
Dose (mg/day), mean(SD)	6.00 ± 0.000	5.83 ± 2.515	5.25 ± 2.872	0.090	0.915
Galanthamine, n (%)	7(17.9)	11(16.7)	1(2.3)	6.022	0.049
Dose (mg/day), mean(SD)	15.43 ± 2.760	14.91 ± 4.764	12.00 ± 0.000	0.303	0.743
Huperzine A, n (%)	34(87.2)	45(68.2)	28(65.1)	5.978	0.050
Dose (ug/day), mean(SD)	280.88 ± 81.66	263.33 ± 89.443	278.57 ± 95.674	0.456	0.635
Memantine, n(%)	8(20.5)	39(59.1)	9(20.9)	22.878	0.000
Dose (mg/day), mean(SD)	11.88 ± 4.581	11.15 ± 4.209	11.67 ± 2.500	0.140	0.870

Rates of prescribing other drugs

When diagnosing and treating patients with AD, 56.4 % of psychiatrists, 65.2 % of neurologists, and 69.8 % of GPs prescribed Oxiracetam/Aniracetam; 71.8 % of psychiatrists, 72.7 % of neurologists, and 79.9 % of GPs prescribed ginkgo biloba extract; 46.2 % of psychiatrists, 57.6 % of neurologists, and 41.9 % of GPs prescribed ergot alkaloid; 10.3 % of psychiatrists, 37.9 % of neurologists, and 53.5 % of GPs prescribed vitamin E; 17.9 % of psychiatrists, 60.6 % of neurologists, and 58.1 % of GPs prescribed nutritional supplements; and 28.2 % of psychiatrists, 50.0 % of neurologists, and 53.5 % of GPs prescribed herbs/traditional Chinese medicine.

There were significant differences in the percentages of the psychiatrists, neurologists, and GPs prescribing vitamin E, nutritional supplements, and herbs/traditional Chinese medicine ($P < 0.05$, see Table 4).

Rates of prescribing antipsychotics, antidepressants, and anxiolytics

There was a significant difference among the groups in terms of prescribing antipsychotics. A higher proportion of psychiatrists prescribed antipsychotics for patients with AD than neurologists or GPs. This difference was statistically significant between psychiatrists and neurologists ($P < 0.05$, see Fig. 1).

There was no significant difference among the three groups of clinicians with respect to the proportion who prescribed antidepressants or anxiolytics for patients with AD ($P > 0.05$, see Fig. 1).

Discussion

Alzheimer's disease (AD) is a disease with high rates of disability that have a great burden. There are nearly 44 million patients with AD worldwide, and it is estimated that the number will increase to 135 million by 2050 [11]. The number of patients with AD in China was 3.71 million in 2000, and 5.69 million in 2010 [2], and it is estimated that the number of patients with AD in China will increase to 27 million in 2050 [12]. All these numbers show rising trends. Because of the one-child policy and the internal migration policy in China, patients with dementia lack caregivers and will have serious economic burdens [12].

The EFNS and APA guidelines all suggest that clinicians use ChEIs (Donepezil, Rivastigmine, and Galantamine)

Table 3 Reasons for Choosing ChEIs and Memantine

Reasons for choosing ChEIs	Proportions of clinicians ($n = 64$)	Reasons for choosing memantine	Proportions of clinicians ($n = 64$)
Effectiveness	46 (71.9 %)	moderate or severe AD	22 (47.8 %)
Safety	23 (35.9 %)	controlling BPSD	9 (19.6 %)
Familiar with ChEIs	7 (10.9 %)	poor response to ChEIs	6 (13.0 %)
Support of evidence-based research	6 (9.4 %)	effectiveness	6 (13.0 %)
Convenience for patients oral taking	5 (7.8 %)	fewer side-effect	3 (6.5 %)
Guidelines' recommendation	4 (6.3 %)	Patients had contraindications to ChEIs	2 (4.3 %)
The only available AD medication in the hospital	3 (4.7 %)	combination use with ChEIs	1 (2.2 %)
Controlling BPSD	1 (1.6 %)	support of evidence-based research	1 (2.2 %)

Table 4 Percent of Clinicians Prescribing Other Drugs

	Psychiatrists ($n = 39$)	Neurologists ($n = 66$)	General physicians ($n = 43$)
Oxiracetam/aniracetam n (%)	22(56.4)	43(65.2)	30(69.8)
Ginkgo Biloba extract n (%)	28(71.8)	48(72.7)	34(79.1)
Ergot alkaloid n (%)	18(46.2)	38(57.6)	18(41.9)
Vitamin E n (%)**	4(10.3)	5(37.9)	223(53.5)
Nutrition supplements n (%)**	7(17.9)	40(60.6)	25(58.1)
Herbs/traditional Chinese medicine n (%)*	11(28.2)	33(50.0)	3(53.5)

Notes: *$P < 0.05$, **$P < 0.01$

and Memantine as first-line medications for treating patients with AD [10, 8]. Clinicians, today, still mainly use ChEIs to treat symptoms of patients with AD [13], and those medications have been shown to be clinically effective and safe [14]. Clinical practice guidelines published by the APA, the American College of Physicians (ACP), and the American Academy of Family Physicians (AAFP) all have noted the effectiveness and safety of using ChEIs [10, 9]. Memantine is a NMDA receptor antagonist that is approved for treating patients with moderate or severe AD [10]. Our results showed that over 94 % of clinicians in each group considered using ChEIs because of its effectiveness and safety. There were low proportions of clinicians in the three groups who chose Memantine, some of whom chose it because patients had moderate or severe AD. Therefore, the study's results are in line with the prescription recommendations given by clinical guidelines.

We should mention that there are special characteristics and circumstances in China. First, Chinese patients who follow clinicians' prescriptions mostly obtain their medications at the dispensary of the clinician's hospital, and every hospital's dispensary provides different kinds of medications. Dispensaries in tertiary hospitals have a relatively comprehensive range of medications, and they accept relatively new kinds of drugs. The dispensaries of community hospitals have the fewest kinds of drugs and provide relatively basic and inexpensive medications. The situation of second-tier hospitals is between that of the community hospitals and the tertiary hospitals. Second, Donepezil was approved by the FDA for use in public clinical practice in 1996, and it has been used in clinical practice in Shanghai since 2000. However, it was not until recently that Donepezil has been included in medicare reimbursement in Shanghai and other regions. Furthermore, Donepezil and Memantine are only available at some hospitals' dispensaries. The last characteristics is that Huperzine A, which is extracted from Huperzia serrata (a traditional Chinese medicine), is a new type of sesquiterpene alkaloid compound [5].

Huperzine A was independently developed by Chinese scientists, and it appeared on the Chinese market for treating patients with AD in 1995. Huperzine A was marketed much earlier than Donepezil and Memantine, and the price of Huperzine A is cheaper than these two drugs. If we calculate the daily dose of Huperzine A as 300 μg, the price of it is approximately 15 % of a 5 mg dose of Donepezil. Huperzine A is available in nearly every hospital in China. Because of the characteristics described above, the present study included neurologists, who were mostly from tertiary hospitals, psychiatrists, who were mainly from second-tier hospitals—a few were from tertiary hospitals (such as Shanghai Mental Health Center), and GPs, who were mainly from community hospitals (see Appendix). Thus, the results showed that most neurologists chose Donepezil and Memantine, and most psychiatrists and GPs chose Huperzine A. These findings may be related to the availability of different medications in different kinds of hospitals. The low prescription rates of Memantine may be that it was marketed in China late in 2006 and lack of availability at hospitals. In the near future, when patients in China could choose their medicine allocation, a further investigation on clinicians' prescription would be updated.

A previous study showed that the ChEIs dosage is related to its effects [15], and another study indicated that the administration of Memantine should be given in adequate doses [16]. The present study found that the medication doses of Memantine and ChEIs were both low. One reason for this may be that clinicians and patients did not have enough knowledge about AD. Li and her colleagues [17] investigated community residents in Shanghai and found that people had little understanding about the early phase of AD and the benefits of treatment. Under these circumstances, clinicians might not

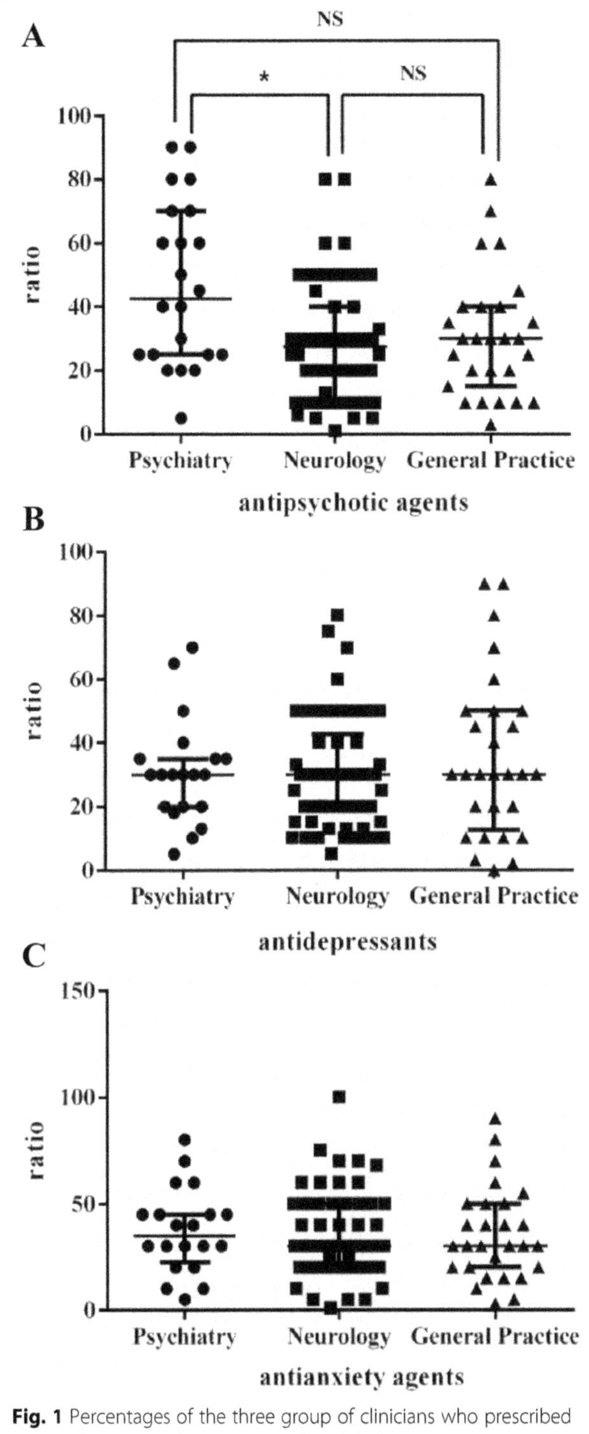

Fig. 1 Percentages of the three group of clinicians who prescribed antipsychotics, antidepressants, and anxiolytics

be very positive about treatment, thus, leading to low doses of medications. A second reason may be that clinicians did not have ready access to new theories and medications in their specialties. Some clinicians were not familiar with cognitive enhancers and had little knowledge about related theories and medications. The last reason might be the price of the drugs. Patients with AD have a huge economic burden, and medicine costs are one part of this burden. Most ChEIs and Memantine, which are approved by the FDA, are all expensive at present. Hence, patients who use their own money to buy drugs may choose lower doses or even stop treatment because of the price. Besides, medicare reimbursement in China has regulations that prevent clinicians from prescribing high priced medications. Therefore, even for patients who have medicare reimbursement, their clinicians may prescribe relatively low doses of ChEIs and Memantine.

The study showed that relatively high proportions of the three groups of clinicians used Oxiracetam/Aniracetam, ginkgo biloba extract, and ergot alkaloid. These medications do not have sufficient support from evidence-based research, which leaves their treatment effects unclear. Some of them may be ineffective, and the overuse of these medications may not only increase a patient's burden and obscure the effectiveness of other medications but may be potentially harmful. The reasons why these drugs have been used for treating patients with AD in China are complicated. Instruction manuals mostly claim that they can treat memory disabilities, thus, confusing clinicians about whether to choose them or not. Additionally, such medications are listed as alternatives for treating AD in many textbooks, and only a few medical textbooks express objective opinions toward them. Thus, clinicians prescribe such medications for patients with AD who have memory disabilities, which does not compromise their medical principles. These medications are also easy to explain to patients and their family members. We think this is the main reason why many clinicians used such medications.

BPSD are common in patients with AD, and their incidence can be as high as 90 %[18]. The main symptoms are hallucinations, delusions, apathy, depression, agitation, and irritability [19]. The APA stated that "antipsychotic medications are recommended for the treatment of psychosis in patients with dementia"[10]. Apart from psychiatrists, other clinicians in different departments also are faced with patients with BPSD. Without a medical referral system in China, neurologists and GPs must prescribe these drugs themselves. That is the reason the results showed that all clinicians prescribed antipsychotic, antidepressant, and antianxiety agents. The results also showed there was a higher proportion of psychiatrists who combined the use of antipsychotics with other drugs than the proportions of neurologists and GPs that did so. The main reason may be that patients with BPSD might receive treatment at a psychiatric department, and psychiatrists have a better attitude toward antipsychotics than do neurologists and GPs.

Although typical and atypical antipsychotics are commonly used to treat dementia, the treatment effects of atypical antipsychotics are obviously better than the typical antipsychotics [20]. The FDA has warned against initially using Olanzapine and Risperidone with patients because of concerns about increased fatality rates while using them [21]. The present study showed that the three groups of clinicians mostly chose atypical antipsychotics, which were mainly Olanzapine and Risperidone. The reason may be that, although atypical antipsychotics have the same treatment effects as atypical antipsychotics, the atypical antipsychotics have fewer side-effects than the latter [22].

Due to restrictions on time, regions, and related resources, the present study has some limitations. First, the sample consisted of clinicians in Shanghai, so the sample is not representative of other regions of China. In addition, the questionnaire was completed based on the clinicians' subjective memory recall, which may lead to certain recall biases. Future studies should be based on clinicians' actual prescriptions in order to investigate these questions further.

Conclusions

In conclusion, our study is the first study to report clinicians' prescription preferences for treating patients with AD in China. Most clinicians had their own prescription preferences. For example, Huperzine A was widely used as a ChEI, however, the doses of ChEIs as well as Memantine were relatively small. Clinicians also tended to use cognitive enhancers and herbal medicines; yet there is not enough information about these agents from evidence-based research. Antipsychotics were mainly used by psychiatrists although they may have been beneficial for some patients who were treated by other clinicians. More regulations and training are needed for clinicians treating patients with AD.

Appendix

Table 5 Hospital Distribution of the Clinicians in the Study

Hospital types	Psychiatrists (*n* = 39)	Neurologists (*n* = 66)	GP (*n* = 43)
Community hospitals, n (%)	7 (17.9 %)	0 (0)	21 (48.8)
Second-tier hospitals, n (%)	21(53.8 %)	18 (27.3 %)	8 (18.6 %)
Tertiary hospitals, n (%)	11 (28.2 %)	48 (72.7 %)	14 (32.6 %)

Competing interests

None of the authors received financial support or remuneration for, or have any conflict of interest related tothis manuscript. In the past five years, Xia Li has received honoraria for continuing medical educational lectures at conferences and meetings from Lundbeck, Eisa, and Novartis. Shifu Xiao has received honoraria for continuing medical educational lectures at conferences, meetings, and medical advisory boards from Eisa, Lundbeck, Novaritis, and Pfizer.

Authors' contributions

XL, TW, QQ, MJZ, XL and CXB were responsible for acquisition of data. CXB performed the statistical analysis and drafted the manuscript. XL conceived of the study, and participated in its design and coordination and helped to draft the manuscript. SFX was responsible for critical revision and supervision. All authors read and approved the final manuscript.

Acknowledgments

This study was supported by grants for National Key Clinical Disciplines to the Shanghai Mental Health Center (Office of Medical Affairs, Ministry of Health, 2011-873; OMA-MH, 2011-873) and the Shanghai Clinical Center for Mental Disorders (2014), Shanghai Science & Technology Committee (No. 15411961400).

Author details

[1]Alzheimer's Disease and Related Disorders Center, Department of Geriatric Psychiatry, Shanghai Mental Health Center, Shanghai Jiao Tong University School of Medicine, Shanghai, China. [2]Mental Health Center of Jiading District in Shanghai, Shanghai, China.

References

1. Prince M, Bryce R, Albanese E, Wimo A, Ribeiro W, Ferri CP. The global prevalence of dementia: a systematic review and metaanalysis. Alzheimers Dement. 2013;9(1):63–75. e62.
2. Chan KY, Wang W, Wu JJ, Liu L, Theodoratou E, Car J, Middleton L, Russ TC, Deary IJ, Campbell H. Epidemiology of Alzheimer's disease and other forms of dementia in China, 1990–2010: a systematic review and analysis. Lancet. 2013;381(9882):2016–23.
3. World Health Organization. Dementia: a public health priority. Perspect Public Health. 2012;5(3):123–5.
4. OECD: Dementia prevalence: OECD Publishing. Health at a Glance. Paris: OECD Indicators, OECD Publishing; 2013. doi:10.1787/health_glance-2013-74-en.
5. Jia-Sen Liu Y-LZ, Chao-Mei Y, You-Zuo Z, Yan-Yi H, Feng-Wu W, Bao-Feng Q. The structures of huperzine A and B, two new alkaloids exhibiting marked anticholinesterase activity. Can J Chem. 2011;64(4):837–9.
6. World Health Organization. Neurological disorders: public health challenges, Neurological Disorders Public Health Challenges. 2006.
7. Galvin JE, Sadowsky CH. Practical guidelines for the recognition and diagnosis of dementia. J Am Board Fam Med. 2012;25(3):367–82.
8. Hort J, O'Brien JT, Gainotti G, Pirttila T, Popescu BO, Rektorova I, Sorbi S, Scheltens P. EFNS guidelines for the diagnosis and management of Alzheimer's disease. Eur J Neurol. 2010;17(10):1236–48.
9. Amir Q, Vincenza S, J Thomas C, Mary Ann F, Robert H, Paul S, Alan A, David M, Kenneth S, Doug CO. Current Pharmacologic Treatment of Dementia: A Clinical Practice Guideline from the American College of Physicians and the American Academy of Family Physicians. Ann Intern Med. 2008;148(5):370–8.
10. Rabins PV, Deborah B, Rovner BW, Teresa R, Schneider LS, Tariot PN, Blass DM, Mcintyre JS, Charles SC, Anzia DJ. American Psychiatric Association practice guideline for the treatment of patients with Alzheimer's disease and other dementias. Second edition. Am J Psychiatr. 2007;12:5–56.
11. Egan KJ, Vesterinen HM, Mccann SK, Sena ES, Macleod MR. The development of an online database for interventions tested in transgenic mouse models of Alzheimer's disease. Evid-Based Preclinical Med. 2015;2(1):20–6.
12. Liu P, Kong M, Yuan S, Liu J, Wang P. History and experience: a survey of traditional chinese medicine treatment for Alzheimer's disease. Evid Based Complement Alternat Med. 2014;2014:642128.
13. Giancarlo P, Maria Grazia G, Laura B. Effect of cholinesterase inhibitors on attention. Chem Biol Interact. 2012;203(1):361–4.

14. Takashi O, Yojiro S, Yuichi O, Yuji K, Nami S, Takayuki S, Masayoshi T, Takumi K. The prediction of response to Galantamine treatment in Patients with mild to moderate Alzheimer's Disease. Curr Alzheimer Res. 2014;11(2):110–8.
15. Sabbagh M, Cummings J. Progressive cholinergic decline in Alzheimer's Disease: consideration for treatment with donepezil 23 mg in patients with moderate to severe symptomatology. BMC Neurol. 2011;11(1):1–6.
16. Shin K, Akira H, Nakamura Y. Late phase 2 study of memantine hydrochloride, a new NMDA receptor antagonist, in patients with moderate to severe Alzheimer's disease: efficacy, safety and recommended dose. Japanese J Geriatr Psychiatry. 2011;22:453–63.
17. Xia LI, Fang W, Ning SU, Liu Y, Xiao S, Xiao Z. Survey in Shanghai communities: the public awareness of and attitude towards dementia. Psychogeriatrics. 2011;11(2):83–9.
18. Fernández M, Gobartt AL, Balañá M. Behavioural symptoms in patients with Alzheimer's disease and their association with cognitive impairment. BMC Neurol. 2010;10(1):1–9.
19. Hishikawa N, Takahashi Y, Amakusa Y, Tanno Y, Tuji Y, Niwa H, Murakami N, Krishna UK. Effects of turmeric on Alzheimer's disease with behavioral and psychological symptoms of dementia. Ayu. 2013;33(4):499–504.
20. Lopez OL, Becker JT, Yue-Fang C, Sweet RA, Howard A, Beth S, Judith S, Eric D, M Ilyas K, Dekosky ST. The long-term effects of conventional and atypical antipsychotics in patients with probable Alzheimer's disease. Am J Psychiatr. 2013;170(9):1051–8.
21. Gallini A, Andrieu S, Donohue JM, Oumouhou N, Lapeyre-Mestre M, Gardette V. Trends in use of antipsychotics in elderly patients with dementia: Impact of national safety warnings. Eur Neuropsychopharmacol. 2014;24(1):95–104.
22. Liperoti R, Pedone C, Corsonello A. Antipsychotics for the treatment of behavioral and psychological symptoms of dementia (BPSD). Curr Neuropharmacol. 2008;6(2):117–24.

4

The role of exosomes in the pathogenesis of Alzheimer' disease

Tingting Xiao[1], Weiwei Zhang[1], Bin Jiao[1], Chu-Zheng Pan[1], Xixi Liu[1] and Lu Shen[1,2,3*]

Abstract

Exosomes are small vesicles secreted by most cell types including neurons that function in intercellular communication through transfer of their cargo or encapsulate and eliminate unnecessary cellular components and therefore have a broad impact on nerve development, activation and regeneration. In addition, exosomes have been observed to be involved in spreading pathological misfolded proteins, thereby leading to the onset and propagation of disease. Alzheimer disease (AD) is the most common form of dementia and characterized by two types of lesions: amyloid plaques and neurofibrillary tangles. Accumulating evidence has demonstrated that exosomes are associated with amyloid precursor (APP) and Tau proteins and play a controversial role in Alzheimer's disease process. In this review, we will discuss the role of exosomes in the metabolism and secretion of APP and Tau proteins and their subsequent impact on AD pathogenesis.

Background

According to the 2016 World Alzheimer Report, there are 47 million people living with dementia worldwide [1]. It is estimated that the total worldwide cost of dementia is $818 billion (USD) and is expected to reach $1 trillion (USD) by 2018, thus placing a huge burden on individuals, families, and societies [1]. As the leading cause of dementia, Alzheimer's disease (AD) accounts for an estimated 60 to 80% of all cases [2]. It is clinically characterized by cognitive impairment, a variety of neuropsychiatric symptoms and the restriction of daily life activities [3]. AD is pathologically defined by the deposits of the protein fragment beta-amyloid (Aβ plaques) outside neurons and twisted fibers of the protein tau that build up inside neurons (NFTs). The cause for most AD cases is still uncovered except for 1 to 5% of cases which develop as a result of mutations in the presenilin1 (*PSEN1*), presenilin2 (*PSEN2*), or amyloid precursor protein (*APP*) genes [4].

Recently, the role of "Prion-like mechanisms" in the pathogenesis of neurodegenerative diseases has attracted more and more attention. It has been suggested that pathologically misfolded proteins can transfer their conformation to properly folded proteins, thus resulting in the propagation of disease [5]. For instance, plaques and tangles tend to spread through the cortex in a predictable pattern as Alzheimer's disease progresses [6]. While, the mechanisms underlying the spread of misfolded proteins still poorly understood. There are several pathways for signal delivery and material communication between cells, such as synaptic transmission, direct communication trough gap junction and paracrine signaling [7]. Among these hypotheses, accumulating evidence supports the idea that exosomes may play as a messenger to participate in cell communication and contribute to this lesions spreading [8, 9].

Exosomes were first reported in reticulocytes and considered to function in the disposal of unnecessary cellular components [10, 11]. Exosomes are nanosized extracellular vesicles (generally 50-100 nm diameter) that can be released by nearly all cell types, including neuronal cells [12]. The exosomes' molecular contents include proteins, lipids and genetic material. Exosomes are released in bodily fluids and shuttle molecules for long distances for the purpose of intercellular communication. Exosomes have been reported to implicate in the spread of pathological proteins involved in neurodegenerative diseases, such as AD, Parkinson's disease (PD) and the prion diseases. APP, β- secretase, γ- secretase has been detected in exosomes, what's more, exosomal

* Correspondence: shenlu2505@126.com
[1]Department of Neurology, Xiangya Hospital, Central South University, Changsha, China
[2]State Key Laboratory of Medical Genetics, Changsha, China
Full list of author information is available at the end of the article

proteins such as Alix and Flotillin were also found to be accumulated in the plaques of AD patient brains [13].

In this review, we will discuss role of exosomes in the metabolism and secretion of APP and Tau proteins and the subsequent impact on AD pathogenesis.

Biogenesis of exosomes

Exosomes are small membrane vesicles that are generated via endocytic pathways [14, 15]. Inward budding of the plasma membrane forms small vesicles, which undergo fused together to form the early endosome. Intraluminal vesicles (ILVs) begin to compose through invagination of the limiting endosomal membrane during the maturation process of early endosome. Upon creation, cytoplasmic molecules such as proteins, lipids, and RNAs are encapsuled into the lumen and accumulated within the late endosome, thus forming multivesicular bodies (MVBs). There are two fates for MVBs, some of which transport to lysosomes for degradation (dMVBs), while others fuse with the plasma membrane and release ILVs into the extracellular space as exosomes (sMVBs). Compared with the dMVBs which are enriched in bismonoacylglycerophoshate (BMP, LBPA), the sMVBs contain more of ceramides [16, 17]. ILV formation is the key step in exosome biogenesis [18]. The formation of ILVs is mainly regulated by the complex of multi-molecular machinery named Endosomal Sorting Complex Required for Transport (ESCRT) [19, 20]. However, studies have shown that depletion of ESCRT subunits does not totally impair the composition of MVBs, which indicate that other mechanisms may exist in the process of ILVs formation [21]. It suggested that proper level of lipids and tetraspanin-enriched micro-domains is needed for MVBs formation [22–25]. Exosome secretion is also regulated by membrane depolarization.

Molecular contents of exosomes

The molecules within exosomes can be divided into two types: constitutive molecules and cargo molecules. Constitutive molecules are unique to exosomes regardless of the cell type from which they are derived and play an essential role in keeping fundamental structures and functions of exosomes. Cargo molecules, on the other hand, are proteins, lipids and genetic material which are sorted, encapsulated and transported by exosomes. The cargo molecules are variable according to cell origin and the physiological or pathological conditions when exosomes generate. In addition, sorting of molecules into exosomes is thought to be a selective process, since some accumulated factors observed in exosomes are barely detectable in parental cells.

The protein composition of exosomes has been analyzed extensively. Since exosomes are released through the endosome pathway, proteins such as tetraspanins (CD9, CD63, CD81 and CD82), Rab GTPases, flotillin, Alix, TSG101and heat shock proteins (Hsc70, Hsp90) have been all identified in exosomes [26–29]. In addition to constitutive molecules, exosomes with different cell origin carry specific proteins. For example, major histocompatibility complex class II (MHCII) is mainly present on exosomes derived from antigen presenting cells [30]. Cells can also release prions, beta-amyloid peptides, tau protein, misfolded superoxide dismutase-1(SOD1) and alpha-synuclein through exosomes in different pathological and physiological conditions [13, 31–34]. Lipids in exosomes mainly work as regulating exosomal sorting of small RNAs and proteins [35, 36].

In addition to proteins and lipids, genetic materials are also found in exosomes, such as DNA, mRNA, miRNA, ribosomal RNA (rRNA), circular RNA, and long noncoding RNA (lnRNA) [37–42]. Among them, small RNA (<30 nucleotides) account for a large proportion, making up >50% of all exosomal RNA species [38, 40, 43]. However, a few studies have shown different results in which ribosomal RNA, in particular 28S and 18S rRNA subunits, were found to be the major class of RNA in exosomes [39]. These conflicting results may be due to the purity of the exosome preparation and differences in cell origin. It has been shown that exosome RNA is functional. Valadi and colleagues detected the expression of mouse proteins after transfer of mouse exosomal RNA to human mast cells [43]. What' more previous studies showed that miR-222 transferred through exosome was able to increase tumor malignancy in melanoma through suppression of p27Kip1 expression and induction of the PI3K/AKT pathway [44].

Function of exosomes in the central nervous system (CNS)

Exosomes can be released by most cell types in the CNS, such as neurons, astrocytes, oligodendrocytes and microglia, and participate in regulating neuronal development, regeneration, and modulation of synaptic functions [45–47]. The main physiological roles of exosomes include eliminating cellular waste, regulating immune response and communicating between neural cells [20, 48, 49]. Once released into extracellular space, exosomes act as messengers, can be captured by neighboring cells or internalized by cells with a certain distance, or enter body fluids and taken up by different tissues [50]. There are several ways for signal transduction mediated by exosomes, such as receptor-ligand pathway, endocytosis and phagocytosis [51]. Because of the double membrane structure, exosomes pathway may have a higher efficiency in transfer substance.

In CNS, both glia and neuron secrete exosomes is regulated by glutamate in a certain degree. It has been hypothesized that exosomes can be served as messenger to mediate the communication between neuron and glia. While, as the reported, exosomes derived from neurons can only be captured by neurons, but not glia. It is interesting to note exosomes secreted by neuroblastoma cells can bind with both of neurons and glial cells. It demonstrate that cell communication mediated by exosomes has cell- selectivity [52].

In addition, the function of exosomes may be variable among different cell origins. Evidence shows that exosomes derived from N2a cells or isolated from human cerebrospinal fluid can abolish the synaptic plasticity disruption caused by both synthetic and AD brain-derived Aβ [53]. However, Asai and colleagues observed that exosomes derived from microglia can spread tau protein, and inhibiting exosome synthesis significantly reduced tau propagation in vitro and in vivo [47].

Except the physiological function, the role of exosomes in spreading toxic proteins and inducing the propagation of diseases such as AD has been discussed extensively.

Impact of exosomes on amyloidogenic processing of APP

The major component of amyloid deposits is small peptides, 39–43 amino acids in length named Aβ, which is derived from a sequence of successive cleavages of APP [54]. APP is a type-I transmembrane glycoproteins. Three secretases termed α, β and γ-secretases are involved in the metabolism of APP. In the amyloidogenic pathway, upon cleavage by β-secretase (BACE-1) and γ-secretase, a large soluble ectodomain fragment (sAPP-β), membrane-bound C-terminal fragment (β-CTF), a small APP intracellular fragment (AICD) and Aβ peptides are produced [55, 56]. In the non-amyloidogenic pathway, APP is initially cleaved at the α-secretase site, generating sAPP-α and α-CTF. The latter is further processed by the γ-secretase complex, releasing AICD and a p3 peptide [57]. β-cleavage of APP mainly occurs in early endosomes [51, 54]. Immunofluorescence experiments in HeLa cells (APP mutant) observed the colocalization of sAPPβ, APP and BACE with early endosomal markers (Rab5) and early endosomal antigen-1 [51]. It has been found that Aβ is accumulated in MVBs and can be released into extracellular space through exosomes [13, 58]. Although only a very small portion of Aβ (<1%) is associated with exosomes, APP, β- and γ-secretase have been detected in exosomes, suggesting that except transport Aβ peptide in the extracellular space, cleavage of APP to generate Aβ could be the main mechanism of spreading lesions [8, 48, 59].

However, the exact role of exosomes in AD progress is still controversial. Several studies have observed that exosomes play a harmful role. A unique Aβ species, tightly binding with GM1, was found in brains of early pathological stage of AD [60]. Endocytic pathway impairment in neurons, including the enlargement of early endosomes and the up-regulation of Rab5 was observed in the brain of a patient with sporadic AD. This impairment significantly accelerated the release of GM1-associated exosomes and induced amyloid fibril formation [61]. Furthermore, exosomes mediate the apoptosis of astrocytes caused by Aβ exposure. Wang and colleagues found that amyloid peptides could activate neutral sphingomyelinase 2 (nSMase2) and induce an increase of PAR-4 and ceramide-containing exosomes secretion in astrocytes. The exosomes were able to be captured by astrocytes and cause apoptosis [62]. Alternatively, fewer amyloid plaques were observed in a mouse model of AD after injection of GW4869, an inhibitor of nSMase2, through prevention of the secretion of exosomes [63]. The protective function of exosomes was also found in various studies. Neuronal exosomes rich in glycosphingolipids could capture Aβ and promote uptake of Aβ by microglia, thus decreasing Aβ and amyloid deposition in APP transgenic mice [64–66]. The cellular prion protein (PrP^C), a glycosylphosphatidylinositol (GPI)-anchored surface glycoprotein highly expressed on exosomes, was shown to bind oligomeric Aβ42 with high affinity via its flexible N-terminus and accelerate fibrillization of amyloid beta, thereby reducing the neurotoxic effects imparted by oligomeric Aβ [53, 67]. It should be noted that exosomes utilized as protective agents in recent studies almost always come from healthy cells.

In brief, exosomes may serve as a double-edged sword in Aβ metabolism. The imbalanced metabolism of APP may cause accumulation of intracellular Aβ. When beyond the clearance capacity of lysosomes or glial cells, the toxic protein will be released into extracellular space and spread through the brain via the exosome pathway.

Impact of exosomes on tau pathology

Hyperphosphorylated tau proteins are the major components of NFTs [68]. Tau protein is a member of the family of microtubule-associated proteins encoded by the *MAPT* gene. Because of the alternative splicing of exon 10, there are two major tau isoforms in the adult brain, denoted as 3R and 4R [5, 69]. An abnormal 3R/4R balance is thought to impair the function of tau in keeping stabilization of microtubule structure and material transport [70]. Differences in 3R/4R expression also exist among different diseases. For instance, 3R is the main tau isoform in Pick's disease, while the 4R tau isoform is a significant component of inclusions in progressive supranuclear palsy (PSP) and corticobasal degeneration (CBD) [71, 72]. In AD, two major tau isoforms are present in the filaments [73]. Tau pathology developed within a definite pattern in AD. The first involved region is entorhinal cortex (Braak stages I-II), then developed to limbic areas (Braak stages III-IV), finally reaches neocortical areas (Braak stages V and IV) [6]. The mechanism of this spreading characteristic of tauopathy throughout human brain has been discussed many years. There is accumulating evidence that tau aggregates spread and replicate in a prion-like manner, with the uptake of pathological tau causing misfolded aggregations of monomeric tau in recipient cells [74, 75]. Exosome-mediated secretion pathways may play an important role in this progress. Studies showed that tau can be exported via an exosome-mediated mechanism in the M1C neuroblastoma tauopathy model, where it is enriched in a phospho-tau biomarker for early AD (AT270). In addition, exosome-associated tau is also present in human CSF samples [76]. Previous studies discovered that propagation of mutant tau between brain regions depended on the presence of microglia, the resident phagocytes of the brain. Microglia spread tau via exosome secretion and depletion of microglia or inhibition of exosome synthesis significantly reduced tau propagation in vitro and in vivo [47]. Polanco and colleagues detected tau in exosomes from tau transgenic rTg4510 mice, and these vesicles were capable of seeding tau aggregation in a threshold-dependent manner [32].

Conclusions

Increased attention has been paid to the prion-like mechanism involved in the propagation of AD. In this review, we have illustrated the biogenesis and function of exosomes and their impact on amyloidogenic processing and tau pathology. The exosomes pathway may have a "double-edged sword" effect on the process of AD. And the effect is dependent on the cell origins of exosomes and the conditions when exosomes formed. The identification of exosomal pathways could provide not only important insights in the pathogenesis of AD, but due to the tissue-specificity and non-immunogenicity of exosomes, could also serve as an ideal platform for delivery of therapeutic drugs. Furthermore, the molecules packaged in exosomes can be secreted into a variety of bodily fluids, which may serve as biomarkers of disease. Despite the potential benefits of exosomes in diagnosis and therapy, there are some remaining issues, such as making improvements in exosomal isolation techniques and developing a more thorough understanding of the role of exosomes from different cell types under different conditions, which should be the focus of future studies.

Acknowledgements
Not applicable.

Funding
This study was supported through the National Natural Science Foundation of China (No.8167051815 to Lu Shen).

Authors' contributions
TX: Study conception; acquisition of data; drafting of the manuscript; critical revision of the manuscript for important intellectual content. BJ, WZ, C-ZP and XL: critical revision of the manuscript for important intellectual content. LS: Study conception, design, and organization; critical revision of the manuscript for important intellectual content; study supervision. All authors read and approved the final manuscript.

Competing interests
The authors declare that they have no competing interests.

Author details
[1]Department of Neurology, Xiangya Hospital, Central South University, Changsha, China. [2]State Key Laboratory of Medical Genetics, Changsha, China. [3]Key Laboratory of Hunan Province in Neurodegenerative Disorders, Central South University, Changsha, China.

References

1. Tian JY, Tang BS, Shi CH, Lv ZY, Li K, Yu RL, et al. Analysis of PLA2G6 gene mutation in sporadic early-onset parkinsonism patients from Chinese population. Neurosci Lett. 2012;514(2):156–8. doi:10.1016/j.neulet.2012.02.078.
2. Alzheimer's A. Alzheimer's disease facts and figures. Alzheimers Dement. 2015;11(3):332–84.
3. Sperling RA, Aisen PS, Beckett LA, Bennett DA, Craft S, Fagan AM, et al. Toward defining the preclinical stages of Alzheimer's disease: recommendations from the National Institute on Aging-Alzheimer's Association workgroups on diagnostic guidelines for Alzheimer's disease. Alzheimers Dement. 2011;7(3):280–92. doi:10.1016/j.jalz.2011.03.003.
4. Bekris LM, Yu CE, Bird TD, Tsuang DW. Genetics of Alzheimer disease. J Geriatr Psychiatry Neurol. 2010;23(4):213–27. doi:10.1177/0891988710383571.
5. Vingtdeux V, Sergeant N, Buee L. Potential contribution of exosomes to the prion-like propagation of lesions in Alzheimer's disease. Front Physiol. 2012; 3:229. doi:10.3389/fphys.2012.00229.
6. Braak H, Braak E. Neuropathological stageing of Alzheimer-related changes. Acta Neuropathol. 1991;82(4):239–59.
7. Schiera G, Di Liegro CM, Di Liegro I. Extracellular membrane vesicles as vehicles for brain cell-to-cell interactions in physiological as well as pathological conditions. Biomed Res Int. 2015;2015:152926. doi:10.1155/2015/152926.
8. Rajendran L, Honsho M, Zahn TR, Keller P, Geiger KD, Verkade P, et al. Alzheimer's disease beta-amyloid peptides are released in association with exosomes. Proc Natl Acad Sci U S A. 2006;103(30):11172–7. doi:10.1073/pnas.0603838103.
9. Eitan E, Suire C, Zhang S, Mattson MP. Impact of lysosome status on extracellular vesicle content and release. Ageing Res Rev. 2016. doi:10.1016/j.arr.2016.05.001.
10. Harding C, Heuser J, Stahl P. Receptor-mediated endocytosis of transferrin and recycling of the transferrin receptor in rat reticulocytes. J Cell Biol. 1983; 97(2):329–39.
11. Pan BT, Johnstone RM. Fate of the transferrin receptor during maturation of sheep reticulocytes in vitro: selective externalization of the receptor. Cell. 1983;33(3):967–78.
12. Pan BT, Teng K, Wu C, Adam M, Johnstone RM. Electron microscopic evidence for externalization of the transferrin receptor in vesicular form in sheep reticulocytes. J Cell Biol. 1985;101(3):942–8.
13. Takahashi RH, Milner TA, Li F, Nam EE, Edgar MA, Yamaguchi H, et al. Intraneuronal Alzheimer abeta42 accumulates in multivesicular bodies and is associated with synaptic pathology. Am J Pathol. 2002;161(5):1869–79.

14. Abels ER, Breakefield XO. Introduction to extracellular vesicles: biogenesis, RNA cargo selection, content, release, and uptake. Cell Mol Neurobiol. 2016; 36(3):301–12. doi:10.1007/s10571-016-0366-z.
15. Colombo M, Raposo G, Thery C. Biogenesis, secretion, and intercellular interactions of exosomes and other extracellular vesicles. Annu Rev Cell Dev Biol. 2014;30:255–89. doi:10.1146/annurev-cellbio-101512-122326.
16. Janas AM, Sapon K, Janas T, Stowell MH, Janas T. Exosomes and other extracellular vesicles in neural cells and neurodegenerative diseases. Biochim Biophys Acta. 2016;1858(6):1139–51. doi:10.1016/j.bbamem.2016.02.011.
17. Record M, Carayon K, Poirot M, Silvente-Poirot S. Exosomes as new vesicular lipid transporters involved in cell-cell communication and various pathophysiologies. Biochim Biophys Acta. 2014;1841(1):108–20. doi:10.1016/j.bbalip.2013.10.004.
18. Minciacchi VR, Freeman MR, Di Vizio D. Extracellular vesicles in cancer: exosomes, microvesicles and the emerging role of large oncosomes. Semin Cell Dev Biol. 2015;40:41–51. doi:10.1016/j.semcdb.2015.02.010.
19. Gibbings DJ, Ciaudo C, Erhardt M, Voinnet O. Multivesicular bodies associate with components of miRNA effector complexes and modulate miRNA activity. Nat Cell Biol. 2009;11(9):1143–9. doi:10.1038/ncb1929.
20. Kosaka N, Iguchi H, Yoshioka Y, Takeshita F, Matsuki Y, Ochiya T. Secretory mechanisms and intercellular transfer of microRNAs in living cells. J Biol Chem. 2010;285(23):17442–52. doi:10.1074/jbc.M110.107821.
21. Stuffers S, Sem Wegner C, Stenmark H, Brech A. Multivesicular endosome biogenesis in the absence of ESCRTs. Traffic. 2009;10(7):925–37. doi:10.1111/j.1600-0854.2009.00920.x.
22. Dinkins MB, Dasgupta S, Wang G, Zhu G, He Q, Kong JN, et al. The 5XFAD mouse model of alzheimer's disease exhibits an age-dependent increase in anti-ceramide igg and exogenous administration of ceramide further increases anti-ceramide titers and amyloid plaque burden. J Alzheimer's Dis. 2015;46(1):55–61. doi:10.3233/JAD-150088.
23. Guo BB, Bellingham SA, Hill AF. The neutral sphingomyelinase pathway regulates packaging of the prion protein into exosomes. J Biol Chem. 2015; 290(6):3455–67. doi:10.1074/jbc.M114.605253.
24. Kobuna H, Inoue T, Shibata M, Gengyo-Ando K, Yamamoto A, Mitani S et al. Multivesicular body formation requires OSBP-related proteins and cholesterol. PLoS genetics. 2010;6(8). doi:10.1371/journal.pgen.1001055.
25. Miwako I, Yamamoto A, Kitamura T, Nagayama K, Ohashi M. Cholesterol requirement for cation-independent mannose 6-phosphate receptor exit from multivesicular late endosomes to the Golgi. J Cell Sci. 2001;114(Pt 9): 1765–76.
26. Colombo M, Moita C, van Niel G, Kowal J, Vigneron J, Benaroch P, et al. Analysis of ESCRT functions in exosome biogenesis, composition and secretion highlights the heterogeneity of extracellular vesicles. J Cell Sci. 2013;126(Pt 24):5553–65. doi:10.1242/jcs.128868.
27. Stenmark H. Rab GTPases as coordinators of vesicle traffic. Nat Rev Mol Cell Biol. 2009;10(8):513–25. doi:10.1038/nrm2728.
28. Hsu C, Morohashi Y, Yoshimura S, Manrique-Hoyos N, Jung S, Lauterbach MA, et al. Regulation of exosome secretion by Rab35 and its GTPase-activating proteins TBC1D10A-C. J Cell Biol. 2010;189(2):223–32. doi:10.1083/jcb.200911018.
29. Tytell M, Lasek RJ, Gainer H. Axonal maintenance, glia, exosomes, and heat shock proteins. F1000Research. 2016;5. doi: 10.12688/f1000research.7247.1.
30. De Toro J, Herschlik L, Waldner C, Mongini C. Emerging roles of exosomes in normal and pathological conditions: new insights for diagnosis and therapeutic applications. Front Immunol. 2015;6:203. doi:10.3389/fimmu.2015.00203.
31. Arellano-Anaya ZE, Huor A, Leblanc P, Lehmann S, Provansal M, Raposo G, et al. Prion strains are differentially released through the exosomal pathway. Cell Mol Life Sci. 2015;72(6):1185–96. doi:10.1007/s00018-014-1735-8.
32. Polanco JC, Scicluna BJ, Hill AF, Gotz J. Extracellular vesicles isolated from the brains of rTg4510 mice seed Tau protein aggregation in a threshold-dependent manner. J Biol Chem. 2016;291(24):12445–66. doi:10.1074/jbc.M115.709485.
33. Loov C, Scherzer CR, Hyman BT, Breakefield XO, Ingelsson M. alpha-Synuclein in extracellular vesicles: functional implications and diagnostic opportunities. Cell Mol Neurobiol. 2016;36(3):437–48. doi:10.1007/s10571-015-0317-0.
34. Ding X, Ma M, Teng J, Teng RK, Zhou S, Yin J, et al. Exposure to ALS-FTD-CSF generates TDP-43 aggregates in glioblastoma cells through exosomes and TNTs-like structure. Oncotarget. 2015;6(27):24178–91. doi:10.18632/oncotarget.4680.
35. Llorente A, Skotland T, Sylvanne T, Kauhanen D, Rog T, Orlowski A, et al. Molecular lipidomics of exosomes released by PC-3 prostate cancer cells. Biochim Biophys Acta. 2013;1831(7):1302–9.
36. Yuyama K, Igarashi Y. Physiological and pathological roles of exosomes in the nervous system. Biomol Concepts. 2016;7(1):53–68. doi:10.1515/bmc-2015-0033.
37. Lamichhane TN, Raiker RS, Jay SM. Exogenous DNA loading into extracellular vesicles via electroporation is size-dependent and enables limited gene delivery. Mol Pharm. 2015;12(10):3650–7. doi:10.1021/acs.molpharmaceut.5b00364.
38. Huang X, Yuan T, Tschannen M, Sun Z, Jacob H, Du M, et al. Characterization of human plasma-derived exosomal RNAs by deep sequencing. BMC Genomics. 2013;14:319. doi:10.1186/1471-2164-14-319.
39. Jenjaroenpun P, Kremenska Y, Nair VM, Kremenskoy M, Joseph B, Kurochkin IV. Characterization of RNA in exosomes secreted by human breast cancer cell lines using next-generation sequencing. PeerJ. 2013;1:e201. doi:10.7717/peerj.201.
40. Crescitelli R, Lasser C, Szabo TG, Kittel A, Eldh M, Dianzani I et al. Distinct RNA profiles in subpopulations of extracellular vesicles: apoptotic bodies, microvesicles and exosomes. J Extracell Vesicles. 2013;2. doi:10.3402/jev.v2i0.20677.
41. Li Y, Zheng Q, Bao C, Li S, Guo W, Zhao J, et al. Circular RNA is enriched and stable in exosomes: a promising biomarker for cancer diagnosis. Cell Res. 2015;25(8):981–4. doi:10.1038/cr.2015.82.
42. Dong L, Lin W, Qi P, Xu MD, Wu X, Ni S, et al. Circulating long RNAs in serum extracellular vesicles: their characterization and potential application as biomarkers for diagnosis of colorectal cancer. Cancer Epidemiol Biomarkers Prev. 2016;25(7):1158–66. doi:10.1158/1055-9965.EPI-16-0006.
43. Valadi H, Ekstrom K, Bossios A, Sjostrand M, Lee JJ, Lotvall JO. Exosome-mediated transfer of mRNAs and microRNAs is a novel mechanism of genetic exchange between cells. Nat Cell Biol. 2007;9(6):654–9. doi:10.1038/ncb1596.
44. Felicetti F, De Feo A, Coscia C, Puglisi R, Pedini F, Pasquini L, et al. Exosome-mediated transfer of miR-222 is sufficient to increase tumor malignancy in melanoma. J Transl Med. 2016;14:56. doi:10.1186/s12967-016-0811-2.
45. Guitart K, Loers G, Buck F, Bork U, Schachner M, Kleene R. Improvement of neuronal cell survival by astrocyte-derived exosomes under hypoxic and ischemic conditions depends on prion protein. Glia. 2016;64(6):896–910. doi: 10.1002/glia.22963.
46. Frohlich D, Kuo WP, Fruhbeis C, Sun JJ, Zehendner CM, Luhmann HJ et al. Multifaceted effects of oligodendroglial exosomes on neurons: impact on neuronal firing rate, signal transduction and gene regulation. Philos Trans R Soc Lond B Biol Sci. 2014;369(1652). doi: 10.1098/rstb.2013.0510.
47. Asai H, Ikezu S, Tsunoda S, Medalla M, Luebke J, Haydar T, et al. Depletion of microglia and inhibition of exosome synthesis halt tau propagation. Nat Neurosci. 2015;18(11):1584–93. doi:10.1038/nn.4132.
48. Sharples RA, Vella LJ, Nisbet RM, Naylor R, Perez K, Barnham KJ, et al. Inhibition of gamma-secretase causes increased secretion of amyloid precursor protein C-terminal fragments in association with exosomes. FASEB J. 2008;22(5):1469–78. doi:10.1096/fj.07-9357com.
49. Gupta A, Pulliam L. Exosomes as mediators of neuroinflammation. J Neuroinflammation. 2014;11:68. doi:10.1186/1742-2094-11-68.
50. Dreyer F, Baur A. Biogenesis and functions of exosomes and extracellular vesicles. Methods Mol Biol. 2016;1448:201–16. doi:10.1007/978-1-4939-3753-0_15.
51. Tkach M, Thery C. Communication by extracellular vesicles: where we are and where we need to go. Cell. 2016;164(6):1226–32. doi:10.1016/j.cell.2016.01.043.
52. Chivet M, Javalet C, Laulagnier K, Blot B, Hemming FJ, Sadoul R. Exosomes secreted by cortical neurons upon glutamatergic synapse activation specifically interact with neurons. J Extracell Vesicles. 2014;3:24722.
53. An K, Klyubin I, Kim Y, Jung JH, Mably AJ, O'Dowd ST, et al. Exosomes neutralize synaptic-plasticity-disrupting activity of Abeta assemblies in vivo. Mol Brain. 2013;6:47. doi:10.1186/1756-6606-6-47.
54. Bibl M, Esselmann H, Wiltfang J. Neurochemical biomarkers in Alzheimer's disease and related disorders. Ther Adv Neurol Disord. 2012;5(6):335–48. doi: 10.1177/1756285612455367.
55. Palmert MR, Podlisny MB, Witker DS, Oltersdorf T, Younkin LH, Selkoe DJ, et al. The beta-amyloid protein precursor of Alzheimer disease has soluble derivatives found in human brain and cerebrospinal fluid. Proc Natl Acad Sci U S A. 1989;86(16):6338–42.
56. Rose C, Peoc'h K, Chasseigneaux S, Paquet C, Dumurgier J, Bourasset F, et al. New highly sensitive rodent and human tests for soluble amyloid precursor protein alpha quantification: preclinical and clinical applications in Alzheimer's disease. BMC Neurosci. 2012;13:84. doi:10.1186/1471-2202-13-84.

57. Cuchillo-Ibanez I, Lopez-Font I, Boix-Amoros A, Brinkmalm G, Blennow K, Molinuevo JL, et al. Heteromers of amyloid precursor protein in cerebrospinal fluid. Mol Neurodegener. 2015;10:2. doi:10.1186/1750-1326-10-2.
58. Vingtdeux V, Hamdane M, Loyens A, Gele P, Drobeck H, Begard S, et al. Alkalizing drugs induce accumulation of amyloid precursor protein by-products in luminal vesicles of multivesicular bodies. J Biol Chem. 2007; 282(25):18197–205. doi:10.1074/jbc.M609475200.
59. Coleman BM, Hill AF. Extracellular vesicles–Their role in the packaging and spread of misfolded proteins associated with neurodegenerative diseases. Semin Cell Dev Biol. 2015;40:89–96. doi:10.1016/j.semcdb.2015.02.007.
60. Kimura N, Yanagisawa K. Endosomal accumulation of GM1 ganglioside-bound amyloid beta-protein in neurons of aged monkey brains. Neuroreport. 2007;18(16):1669–73. doi:10.1097/WNR.0b013e3282f0d2ab.
61. Yuyama K, Yamamoto N, Yanagisawa K. Accelerated release of exosome-associated GM1 ganglioside (GM1) by endocytic pathway abnormality: another putative pathway for GM1-induced amyloid fibril formation. J Neurochem. 2008;105(1):217–24. doi:10.1111/j.1471-4159.2007.05128.x.
62. Wang G, Dinkins M, He Q, Zhu G, Poirier C, Campbell A, et al. Astrocytes secrete exosomes enriched with proapoptotic ceramide and prostate apoptosis response 4 (PAR-4): potential mechanism of apoptosis induction in Alzheimer disease (AD). J Biol Chem. 2012;287(25):21384–95. doi:10.1074/jbc.M112.340513.
63. Dinkins MB, Dasgupta S, Wang G, Zhu G, Bieberich E. Exosome reduction in vivo is associated with lower amyloid plaque load in the 5XFAD mouse model of Alzheimer's disease. Neurobiol Aging. 2014;35(8):1792–800. doi:10.1016/j.neurobiolaging.2014.02.012.
64. Yuyama K, Sun H, Sakai S, Mitsutake S, Okada M, Tahara H, et al. Decreased amyloid-beta pathologies by intracerebral loading of glycosphingolipid-enriched exosomes in Alzheimer model mice. J Biol Chem. 2014;289(35): 24488–98. doi:10.1074/jbc.M114.577213.
65. Yuyama K, Sun H, Usuki S, Sakai S, Hanamatsu H, Mioka T, et al. A potential function for neuronal exosomes: sequestering intracerebral amyloid-beta peptide. FEBS Lett. 2015;589(1):84–8. doi:10.1016/j.febslet.2014.11.027.
66. Yuyama K, Sun H, Mitsutake S, Igarashi Y. Sphingolipid-modulated exosome secretion promotes clearance of amyloid-beta by microglia. J Biol Chem. 2012;287(14):10977–89. doi:10.1074/jbc.M111.324616.
67. Falker C, Hartmann A, Guett I, Dohler F, Altmeppen H, Betzel C, et al. Exosomal cellular prion protein drives fibrillization of amyloid beta and counteracts amyloid beta-mediated neurotoxicity. J Neurochem. 2016; 137(1):88–100. doi:10.1111/jnc.13514.
68. Kopeikina KJ, Carlson GA, Pitstick R, Ludvigson AE, Peters A, Luebke JI, et al. Tau accumulation causes mitochondrial distribution deficits in neurons in a mouse model of tauopathy and in human Alzheimer's disease brain. Am J Pathol. 2011;179(4):2071–82. doi:10.1016/j.ajpath.2011.07.004.
69. Crespo-Biel N, Theunis C, Van Leuven F. Protein tau: prime cause of synaptic and neuronal degeneration in Alzheimer's disease. Int J Alzheimers Dis. 2012;2012:251426. doi:10.1155/2012/251426.
70. Goedert M, Jakes R. Expression of separate isoforms of human tau protein: correlation with the tau pattern in brain and effects on tubulin polymerization. EMBO J. 1990;9(13):4225–30.
71. Dickson DW, Kouri N, Murray ME, Josephs KA. Neuropathology of frontotemporal lobar degeneration-tau (FTLD-tau). J Mol Neurosci. 2011; 45(3):384–9. doi:10.1007/s12031-011-9589-0.
72. Katsuse O, Iseki E, Arai T, Akiyama H, Togo T, Uchikado H, et al. 4-repeat tauopathy sharing pathological and biochemical features of corticobasal degeneration and progressive supranuclear palsy. Acta Neuropathol. 2003; 106(3):251–60. doi:10.1007/s00401-003-0728-8.
73. Siddiqua A, Margittai M. Three- and four-repeat Tau coassemble into heterogeneous filaments: an implication for Alzheimer disease. J Biol Chem. 2010;285(48):37920–6. doi:10.1074/jbc.M110.185728.
74. Guo JL, Lee VM. Seeding of normal Tau by pathological Tau conformers drives pathogenesis of Alzheimer-like tangles. J Biol Chem. 2011;286(17): 15317–31. doi:10.1074/jbc.M110.209296.
75. Stancu IC, Vasconcelos B, Ris L, Wang P, Villers A, Peeraer E, et al. Templated misfolding of Tau by prion-like seeding along neuronal connections impairs neuronal network function and associated behavioral outcomes in Tau transgenic mice. Acta Neuropathol. 2015;129(6):875–94. doi:10.1007/s00401-015-1413-4.
76. Saman S, Kim W, Raya M, Visnick Y, Miro S, Saman S, et al. Exosome-associated tau is secreted in tauopathy models and is selectively phosphorylated in cerebrospinal fluid in early Alzheimer disease. J Biol Chem. 2012;287(6):3842–9. doi:10.1074/jbc.M111.277061.

5

Protein misfolding in neurodegenerative diseases: implications and strategies

Patrick Sweeney[1,2*], Hyunsun Park[3], Marc Baumann[4], John Dunlop[5], Judith Frydman[6], Ron Kopito[6], Alexander McCampbell[7], Gabrielle Leblanc[8], Anjli Venkateswaran[1], Antti Nurmi[1] and Robert Hodgson[1]

Abstract

A hallmark of neurodegenerative proteinopathies is the formation of misfolded protein aggregates that cause cellular toxicity and contribute to cellular proteostatic collapse. Therapeutic options are currently being explored that target different steps in the production and processing of proteins implicated in neurodegenerative disease, including synthesis, chaperone-assisted folding and trafficking, and degradation via the proteasome and autophagy pathways. Other therapies, like mTOR inhibitors and activators of the heat shock response, can rebalance the entire proteostatic network. However, there are major challenges that impact the development of novel therapies, including incomplete knowledge of druggable disease targets and their mechanism of action as well as a lack of biomarkers to monitor disease progression and therapeutic response. A notable development is the creation of collaborative ecosystems that include patients, clinicians, basic and translational researchers, foundations and regulatory agencies to promote scientific rigor and clinical data to accelerate the development of therapies that prevent, reverse or delay the progression of neurodegenerative proteinopathies.

Keywords: Neurodegeneration, Proteostasis, Mouse models, Biomarkers, Chaperones, Drug discovery

Background

Many neurodegenerative diseases involve the misfolding and aggregation of specific proteins into abnormal, toxic species. Therapeutic targeting of protein misfolding has generated unique challenges for drug discovery and development for several reasons, including 1) the dynamic nature of the protein species involved, 2) uncertainty about which forms of a given disease protein (monomers, oligomers, or insoluble aggregates) are primarily responsible for cellular toxicity, 3) our still limited understanding about which components of the cellular proteostatic machinery these disease proteins interact with and 4) lack of well-validated biomarkers for clinical trials. However, as we continue to gain knowledge of disease mechanisms, improve our abilities to model disease states in vitro and in vivo, and identify new biomarkers, there is increasing optimism that we will discover novel therapeutics that prevent, reverse, or delay the progression of neurodegenerative diseases. In concert with the scientific advances in the past several decades, the field of neurodegenerative disease research is undergoing significant change with respect to how various stakeholders engage each other and share information with the entire community. Increasing collaboration between scientists from the pharmaceutical industry disease foundations, academic researchers, contract research organizations, and patient advocacy group, and increasing communication between groups studying different diseases, has spurred promising initiatives in basic, translational, and clinical research in neurodegenerative disease.

There are multiple steps in the production and processing of disease proteins that could be targeted therapeutically, from initial synthesis to degradation and extracellular clearance (Fig. 1). This review discusses the advantages and potential problems associated with targeting different pathways involved in the production and processing of misfolded proteins, and highlights new candidate therapeutics that have been developed by targeting specific steps in the life cycles of disease proteins. It also discusses some key issues involved in translating preclinical findings to successful clinical trials[1].

* Correspondence: patrick.sweeney@crl.com
[1]Discovery Services, Charles Rivers Laboratories, Wilmington, MA, USA
[2]Royal Veterinary College, University of London, London, UK
Full list of author information is available at the end of the article

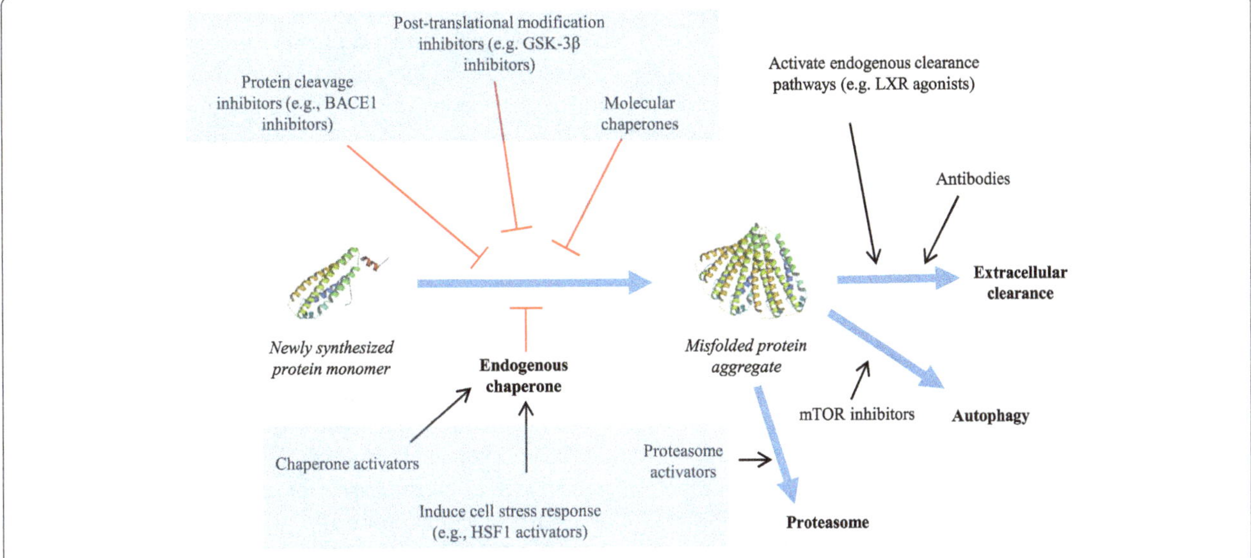

Fig. 1 Mechanisms involved in protein misfolding & therapeutic targets. A newly synthesized protein is stabilized by endogenous chaperone proteins. Under normal conditions abnormal protein aggregates (misfolded proteins) are degraded and/or cleared extracellularly, undergo autophagy or are degraded with the aid of the cellular proteasome. In cases of abnormality and misfolding of proteins (such as those present in many neurological diseases) post translational modification inhibitors, protein cleavage inhibitors and extrinsic molecular chaperones have been used in attempts to curtail or correct protein misfolding. In addition, post translational approaches to address and combat the presence of misfolded proteins include agonists that attempt to activate endogenous clearance pathways as well as the introduction of recombinant antibodies to work against the rogue protein

Roles of misfolded proteins and aggregates in proteinopathies

Misfolded proteins exist in cells together with unfolded, intermediately folded, and correctly folded species [1]. In healthy cells, misfolded proteins are either degraded or refolded correctly by chaperone proteins that are involved in protein folding and trafficking as well as intermediate stabilization [1]. Indeed, it is now believed that many, if not all, proteins can form amyloid fibrils under appropriate biochemical conditions [2, 3]. However, many disease-associated amyloidogenic proteins have extensive regions of intrinsic disorder in their free soluble forms [4] and have specific, often short, internal amino acid sequences that are necessary and sufficient to support aggregation [3, 5]. These same motifs can be found in other non-disease proteins, and when liberated from rest of protein these fragments will aggregate into cytotoxic amyloid fibrils [2, 5].

Once formed, higher order amyloid aggregates are highly resistant to degradation. Proteasomes can degrade only single chain polypeptides, and also require the proteins to be partially or fully (in the case of proteasomes) unfolded [6]. In addition, the amyloid state is extremely stable thermodynamically, because of the extensive contacts made between the protein chains of the polymer. The thermodynamic stability of amyloid aggregates also contributes to their ability to convert native proteins into amyloid forms (i.e., to seed prion-like propagation) [7].

Under conditions of proteotoxic stress, cellular aging, or the presence of disease mutations, proteins can escape a cell's quality control system and begin to aggregate into non-native structures, which range from oligomers and amorphous assemblies to highly ordered amyloid fibrils and plaques.

Cells are normally faced with a continuous stream of misfolded proteins arising from mistakes in biogenesis, disease-causing mutations, and physiological stressors (Table 1 lists misfolded proteins associated with neurodegenerative disease). They deal with misfolded proteins by refolding, degrading, or sequestering them in specific intracellular compartments, such as aggresomes or other types of inclusion bodies. Chaperone proteins bind to nascent polypeptides as they emerge from ribosomes

Table 1 Misfolded proteins associated with neurodegenerative diseases

Proteinopathy	Aggregating protein(s)
Alzheimer's disease	Amyloid beta (Ab) peptide; Tau
Parkinson's disease	α-synuclein
Multiple tauopathies	Tau protein (microtubule associated)
Huntington's disease	Huntingtin with tandem glutamine repeats
Amyotrophic lateral sclerosis	Superoxide dismutase 1
Spongiform encephalopathies	Prion proteins
Familial amyloidotic polyneuropathy	Transthyretin (mutant forms)

and assist in their folding, and oversee and participate in every step in the handling of misfolded proteins. Chaperones also monitor the quality of the folded chains and can in some cases unfold and refold misfolded proteins. Alternatively, chaperones target the misfolded proteins for degradation via the ubiquitin proteasome system or autophagy pathway, or for sequestration in various cellular compartments [8, 9].

Studies in yeast have revealed two overlapping but functionally distinct networks of chaperones [10, 11]. CLIPs (chaperones linked to protein synthesis) are physically associated with the translational machinery and oversee quality control of newly translated proteins. CLIPs comprise a large family of proteins, and evidence suggests that different CLIPs associate with different classes of proteins [12]. The second set of chaperones, heat shock proteins (HSPs), protects the proteome from denaturing environmental stressors, including thermal, oxidative, and hypoxic stresses. CLIPs and HSPs have different modes of transcriptional regulation in yeast: CLIPs are generally down-regulated under conditions of proteotoxic stress, whereas HSPs are up-regulated [9, 10]. Subnetworks of differentially regulated chaperones and co-chaperones have also been identified in *C. elegans* and in the human brain [13]. In addition, it has been found that as the human brain ages, a subset of chaperones consisting primarily of CLIPs are repressed, and chaperones that help protect the proteome against misfolded protein toxicity are induced mimicking proteotoxic stress; these differences are even more pronounced in the brains of people with Alzheimer's, Huntington's, or Parkinson's disease [13]. Misfolded proteins that are not immediately refolded are actively sequestered in spatially and functionally segregated quality control compartments [8, 14]. In yeast, the juxtanuclear quality control (JUNQ) compartment concentrates soluble misfolded proteins that are either later refolded by chaperones or degraded by the ubiquitin proteasome system (UPS). The insoluble protein deposit (IPOD) compartment, which may be equivalent to the aggresomes found in mammalian cells, sequesters insoluble aggregates. The sequestration of aggregated misfolded proteins may in many cases serve a beneficial role – by preventing misfolded proteins from saturating chaperones and proteasomes, facilitating their clearance via the UPS or through autophagy, or by preserving them for subsequent refolding and return to use in the cell [15, 16].

Proteostasis

The term "proteostasis" refers to the integrated activity of cellular mechanisms that regulate protein production, folding, trafficking, degradation, and clearance. Cellular responses to proteotoxic stress, like the heat shock response and the unfolded protein response (UPR) involve large-scale rebalancing of the proteostatic network via transcriptional regulation of both chaperones (e.g., Hsp70, Hsp90) and non-chaperone proteins (including transcription factors, signaling proteins and receptors, and cell cycle regulators [17]. Post-translational modifications can also radically change the activity of some chaperones [18], and likely also play a key role in proteostasis, although this area remains largely unexplored. During the ageing process, or in diseases associated with misfolded proteins, cells may experience "proteostatic collapse." Proteostatic collapse is associated with the accumulation of ubiquitinated inclusion bodies (IBs), which are seen in many neurodegenerative diseases [9]. It has been suggested that ubiquitinated aggregates can directly inhibit or clog proteasomes [19, 20]. However, in the case of ubiquitinated Huntingtin (Htt), this does not appear to be the case, nor is ubiquitination required for Htt to accumulate in IBs [21]. Rather, the accumulation of ubiquitinated species in misfolded protein diseases may reflect a global perturbation of proteostasis, in which chaperones and proteasomes are simply overwhelmed with client proteins.

Propagation

A key feature of misfolded protein diseases is the ability of the pathogenic protein species to propagate in a prion-like manner by recruiting normally folded counterparts to adopt pathogenic conformations. Pathogenic amyloids can also spread from neurons to other neurons and neighboring glia to initiate new pathology after injection into the brains of normal animals [22, 23]. Both in vivo and in vitro studies have shown that misfolding of one disease causing protein can induce misfolding of other aggregation-prone proteins [23], and aggregates of different disease proteins may be found in the same patient [24]. Moreover, the accumulation of one species of misfolded proteins can impair the entire proteostatic network, thereby triggering the misfolding of unrelated proteins that would otherwise fold normally [25, 26]. The mechanisms by which misfolded proteins spread from one neuron to another are currently an area of active investigation. New evidence suggests that interneuronal spread of misfolded proteins involves 1) activity-dependent secretion by exosomes ([27] and/or 2) chaperone-mediated pathways [28, 29].

Mechanisms of misfolded protein toxicity

In the long term, all neurodegenerative disease proteins produce synaptic dysfunction and loss and, ultimately, neuronal cell death. The precise upstream mechanisms by which different misfolded disease proteins cause neurotoxicity are still unclear, and appear to differ depending on the protein species involved. Misfolded disease proteins appear to act primarily by toxic gain-of-function and/or dominant-negative effects, although loss-of-function effects have also been observed. Direct, acute effects of misfolded proteins on neuronal function have been observed after treating neurons with purified oligomers or transfecting them with expression vectors. To give just a few examples, amyloid-beta, tau, and alpha-synuclein all interfere with synaptic signaling [30–32]; mutant tau disrupts microtubule function and neuronal transport mechanisms [32, 33]; and alpha-synuclein disrupts mitochondrial protein import [32, 34]. In addition, larger aggregates of misfolded proteins may exert toxic effects by binding to and sequestering other cytosolic proteins. For example, proteomic studies of artificial proteins designed to form amyloid-like fibrils showed that the toxicity of these proteins correlated with the ability of their aggregates to engage in aberrant protein interactions and disrupt the cytosolic stress response [35]. Notably, the endogenous cellular proteins sequestered by the amyloid aggregates tended to be relatively large in size and enriched in intrinsically unstructured regions, and many play key roles in essential cellular activities such as transcription, translation and protein quality control. Indeed, another emerging common feature among misfolded disease proteins is their ability to disrupt proteostasis (see more below). More recently, cytosolic aggregates of several different proteins, including artificial β-sheets, fragments of mutant huntingtin, and TAR DNA binding protein-43 (TDP-43) have also been shown to disrupt nucleocytoplasmic transport of both proteins and RNA [36].

In addition to synaptic dysfunction, other cellular changes common to the major neurodegenerative diseases include calcium signaling abnormalities, mitochondrial dysfunction, oxidative stress, and neuroinflammation. These symptoms of cellular distress often occur early in the disease process, and are believed to be a cause as well as a consequence of neurodegeneration. That is, the relationship between the accumulation of misfolded disease proteins and other signs of cellular distress is bidirectional, and in many cases mutually exacerbating. For example, amyloid-β, a-synuclein, and mHtt all cause acute oxidative stress in neurons and/or astrocytes, and impair astroglial anti-oxidant responses [37–40]. Conversely, oxidative stress promotes the aggregation of disease proteins, and contributes to age- and disease-related proteostatic collapse [41, 42]. Similarly, there appearaas a downward spiralling cycle of interactions between protein misfolding and neuroinflammation, which has been most extensively studied for AD. Soluble Aβ oligomers and insoluble Aβ aggregates have been shown to bind to and activate and microglia and astrocytes, stimulating a chronic low level state of neuroinflammation [43]. Several lines of evidence suggest that the pro-inflammatory effects of Aβ, while perhaps helpful in the short-term, ultimately impair the microglial and astroglial function, including their ability to dispose of Aβ and other misfolded proteins [38, 43–45]. The destructive consequences of the neuroinflammation provoked by misfolded disease proteins are likely exacerbated by ongoing, age-related senescence of the immune system senescence [46, 47].

Therapeutic targets

Targeting production, misfolding and aggregation

The development of drugs targeting protein misfolding or aggregation has been challenging due to the lack of certainty about which form/s of a given disease protein is primarily responsible for the disease. In the case of amyloid-β (Aβ), it was originally thought that fibrils and plaques were the pathogenic species in Alzheimer's disease, but more recent studies point to aggregation intermediates (oligomers and soluble protofibrils) as the primary culprits; similar findings have emerged with respect to different species of α-synuclein in Parkinson's disease [4, 48]. The situation is further complicated by the existence of the variety of intermediate species that exist during the folding and oligomerization processes. Recent studies have demonstrated that aggregated fibrils of tau, α-synuclein, and Aβ exist in different conformational variants, or 'strains', that have different propagation properties and different levels of neurotoxicity [49–51].

Identifying key toxic species of misfolded proteins has been challenged the inability of conventional biochemical analytic methods to detect and characterize intermediate species. For example, denaturing gel electrophoresis (SDS-PAGE) has been shown to alter the oligomerization state of Aβ42 oligomers [52]. Recently, ion mobility spectrometry-mass spectrometry (IMS-MS) and nuclear magnetic resonance (NMR) spectroscopy have been used to analyze the folding and aggregation of amyloid proteins in solution and to identify inhibitors of these processes [53–55]. As an alternative to preventing the initial misfolding and aggregation of amyloids, another approach now being explored is to stabilize mature fibrils to prevent their prion-like propagation [48, 56].

In cases where the relative pathogenicity of various misfolded protein species is unknown, one strategy would be to intervene therapeutically as far upstream as possible in the protein synthesis pathway: i.e., at the level of protein translation, cleavage, or post-translational modification. In theory, targeting early steps in the processing pathway would provide the highest degree of therapeutic specificity and eliminate toxic gains or losses of function caused by misfolded or aggregated forms of the protein, while preventing the propagation of abnormal folding and aggregation. Protein cleavage and post-translational modification targets are being actively explored for Aβ using Beta Amyloid Cleaving Enzyme (BACE) inhibitors (some of which are now in clinical trials) and for tau using inhibitors of tau phosphorylation (e.g., glycogen synthase 3β inhibitors) and acetylation [57–60].

Targeting chaperones

Chaperones are another possible target class for therapeutic intervention in protein misfolding disease states. As chaperones are involved in all aspects of proteostasis, they offer potential therapeutic entry points to each step in the processing of a pathogenic protein. There are over 200 different chaperone proteins expressed in the mammalian brain [61], and different cell types express different sets of chaperones and co-chaperones [62, 63]. Cell type-specific expression of chaperone subsets may help to explain why some misfolded proteins are toxic in one cell type and not in others, and also presents opportunities to develop drugs targeting neuron- or glial cell-specific chaperones. However, the sheer number of chaperones and the diversity in their mechanisms of action also presents challenge to therapeutics development; we still have limited knowledge of which chaperones interact with which disease proteins and how. Some clues have been offered by links between mutations in specific chaperones and hereditary forms of certain neurodegenerative diseases. For example, mutations in Hsp70 and Hsp40 have been linked to Parkinson's disease [64, 65], and mutations in the co-chaperone valosin-containing protein (VCP) have been found in ALS [66]. In addition, to date over 20 different chaperones have been found to confer neuroprotection when over-expressed in cell or animal models of various neurodegenerative diseases, and in many cases individual chaperones appear to protect against several different disease proteins [67].

One approach to therapeutically targeting the chaperone system has been to develop small molecule inhibitors or activators of specific chaperones. Among chaperones relevant to neurodegeneration, Hsp70 and Hsp90 have been the most intensely studied. Hsp70 and Hsp90 have opposing effects on client protein stability: Hsp70 promotes their degradation via the UPS system, whereas Hsp90 stabilizes client proteins and inhibits their ubiquitination. The activities of Hsp90 and Hsp70 are tightly linked via HSF1. Hsp90 inhibitors typically activate HSF1, which in turn induces Hsp70 [68]. A variety of small molecule drugs have been developed that inhibit Hsp90, activate Hsp70, or both, and have been shown to reduce the formation of disease protein aggregates, reduce cellular toxicity, and improve neurological phenotypes in cellular and animal models of SBMA, HD, PD, and AD [62, 67, 69–71]. None of these drugs have yet entered clinical trials for use in neurodegenerative diseases, due to issues of low brain penetration and/or peripheral cytotoxicity, but active effort in this area is continuing [70, 72–74].

A second approach to developing chaperone-based therapeutics has been through protein engineering. For example, it was discovered that the yeast disaggregate Hsp104 has the ability to dissolve in vitro fibrils formed from a variety of neurodegenerative disease proteins, including tau, polyglutamine, Aβ42, α-synuclein and prion protein [75, 76]. However, relatively high concentrations of Hsp104 are needed to dissolve these proteins. Making small changes in Hsp104's sequence yielded proteins with much higher dissaggregase activity and lower toxicity, including variants that reduced neurodegeneration in a *C. elegans* model of PD [77]. Other chaperones to which this approach might be applied include the yeast chaperonin Tric, which has the unusual ability to cross cell membranes and has been shown to protect against Htt toxicity [16], and metazoan chaperones known to have disaggregase activity (e.g., Hsp110, Hsp70, and Hsp40) [78].

Targeting degradation

Defects in both the UPS and autophagy pathways of protein degradation are often seen in neurodegenerative diseases [79, 80]. For example, many of the gene mutations that cause familial PD encode proteins involved in the UPS and/or autophagy, including PINK-1, Parkin (a ubiquitin ligase), UCH-L1 (Ub carboxy terminal hydrolase L1), DJ-1 (PARK7), and LRRK2/PRAK8 [79, 81, 82]. As with the chaperone system, choosing promising drug targets from the UPS or autophagy pathways is challenging because of the number of proteins involved (there are ~ 500 to 1000 associated just with the UPS system). In addition, for most diseases it isn't known which form/s of the disease protein are primarily responsible for cellular toxicity. This issue is critical when targeting protein degradation, because the pathway by which a given protein is degraded (e.g., UPS versus autophagy) can vary depending on whether the protein is in the soluble or fibrillar state, and on what specific post-translational modifications it bears [83, 84].

A number of small molecules have been identified that upregulate components of the UPS, promote the degradation of disease proteins and in vitro, and (in some cases) have neuroprotective effects on cultured cells [84–86], but few have yet been shown to be effective in vivo. One interesting exception is rolipram, an agent that stimulates the phosphorylation and activity of the 26S proteasome. Myeku and colleagues [21] showed that 26S proteasome function is impaired in a mouse tauopathy model, and that treating the mice with rolipram treatment improved 26S proteasome function, decreased tau aggregation, and improved cognition.

Inhibition of the mammalian target of rapamycin (mTOR) pathway has proven to be an exceptionally effective approach for stimulating the degradation of neurodegenerative disease proteins. mTOR, a serine/threonine kinase, is a signaling nexus that collects information about ambient levels of resources necessary for cell growth (e.g., nutrients, ATP, growth factors, and oxygen) and up- or downregulates protein synthesis and degradation accordingly. When growth conditions are favorable, mTOR inhibits autophagy by inhibiting the ULK1 complex, which is required for the biogenesis of autophagosomes. Thus, mTOR inhibitors typically have the net effect of stimulating autophagy [87, 88].

Rapamycin and other mTOR inhibitors increase the clearance of abnormal protein aggregates and slow neurodegeneration in both cell and animal models of a variety of neurodegenerative diseases, including AD, PD, spinocerebellar ataxia type 3, and frontotemporal dementia [87, 88]. In most of these cases, mTOR inhibitors have been shown to act at least in part via stimulation of autophagy. A recent study showed that in yeast, inhibiting mTOR also produces a rapid, coordinated upregulation of proteasomes and their 19S regulatory chaperones [89]. Thus, the efficacy of mTOR inhibitors in clearing a variety of neurodegenerative disease proteins may be due to the ability of these drugs to upregulate both the proteasomal and autophagic routes of protein degradation.

Several mTOR-dependent activators of autophagy, including the natural compounds curcurmin and resveratrol, are currently in clinical trials for treating neurodegenerative diseases. However, mTOR is a multifarious protein that regulates many cellular processes in addition to protein degradation, and in clinical trials to date wmTOR inhibitors have caused unpredictable and undesirable side effects. Autophagy can be stimulated mTOR-independent mechanisms [79, 87, 88], and a number of compounds, including FDA-approved drugs, have now been shown to stimulate clearance of abnormal proteins and confer protective effects in cell or animal models of neurodegenerative disease [87, 88, 90, 91]. It has been suggested that these compounds might be used in conjuction with mTOR inhibitors to maximize therapeutic benefit and minimize side effects [87, 90].

Targeting extracellular clearance

One of the best-explored examples of targeting clearance of misfolded proteins has been the use of antibodies to promote clearance of Aβ. These antibodies are thought to operate by either or both of two mechanisms: 1) by penetrating the blood brain barrier (BBB) to bind Aβ in the extracellular space, and 2) through a"peripheral sink" effect [92]. Almost all misfolded proteins show some extracellular leakage [93], and an advantage of targeting extracellular misfolded proteins is that it can theoretically be accomplished by highly selective antibodies. For example, monoclonal antibodies have been developed to Aβ and α-synuclein that show >1000-fold higher affinities for the oligomeric versus monomeric forms of the proteins [94–96].

Current challenges in the use of Aβ antibodies include low rates of BBB penetration [97], nonspecific engagement of Aβ and uncertainty as to which antibodies engage clinically relevant forms of Aβ [98–100]. Detailed structural studies of how different antibodies interact with specific epitopes in the Aβ molecule are now underway [101] and help inform antibody design and epitope-targeting in the future. An alternative method of improving the clearance of toxic misfolded species is to harness endogenous mechanisms of protein clearance into the extracellular space. For example, LXR beta receptor agonists, which promote clearance of Aβ into the extracellular space by the ABCA1 transporter, have shown therapeutic effects in AD mouse models [102, 103]. Yet another potential avenue for new therapies targeting extracellular clearance of disease proteins is the use of non-antibody scaffold drugs [104].

Rebalancing the proteostatic network

The ability of the cell's proteostatic machinery to counter proteotoxic stressors deteriorates with age, and is further compromised by mutations and other disease conditions that lead to the accumulation of misfolded proteins [16]. Thus, another potential approach to the development of therapeutics would involve large-scale rebalancing of the proteostatic network. Indeed, the efficacy of mTOR inhibitors may reflect their ability to provoke large-scale rebalancing of protein synthesis and degradation pathways. Another attractive target in this regard is heat shock factor 1 (HSF1), a transcriptional activator that helps coordinate the heat shock response. The heat shock response (and other proteotoxic stress responses) diminish with age and in neurodegenerative disease [105]. In addition, it was recently shown that HSF1 degradation is abnormally elevated in mouse and human α-synucleinopathy [106]. Over-expression of human HSF1 has been shown to be neuroprotective in cell models of neurodegenerative diseases [107, 108], to reduce polyglutamine aggregate formation and prolong lifespan in a mouse model of HD [17] and to reduce pathogenic androgen receptor accumulation and neurotoxicity in a mouse model of spinobulbar muscular atrophy [109]. Small molecule activators of HSF1 have now been identified and shown to have neuroprotective effects in cell or animal models of neurodegenerative diseases [107, 108].

Agents targeting HSF1 or other master regulators of the proteostatic network have the advantages of being fast-acting and relatively agnostic to the identities of the misfolded proteins involved in a given neurodegenerative disease and to their mechanisms of aggregation and toxicity. The effects of such drugs are hard to predict, however. For example, the induction of the heat shock response actually exacerbates Htt IB formation in a cellular model of HD [110]. In addition, it has been pointed out that, under normal physiological conditions, the heat shock response and other proteotoxic stress response pathways are activated only transiently, and that multiple cellular mechanisms are in place to limit and down-regulate these responses [111]. Consistent with those facts, an Hsp90 inhibitor that induces the heat shock response in HD model mice was found to provide short-term beneficial effects, but those benefits proved transient [112]. Yet another potential issue with HSF1 activators is that HSF1 promotes tumorigenesis and is activated in a broad range of highly malignant human cancers [113, 114]. This issue is not necessarily unsurmountable, however, as it has also been shown that the HSF1 drives a different transcriptional program and stimulates different sets of cellular processes in cancer cells (including proliferation, invasion, and metastasis) than it does in normal cells [113]. The ability of HSF1 to activate distinct transcriptional programs in cancer cells versus normal cells is thought to result in part from differences in post-transcriptional modifications to HSF1 in the different cell types [113, 114], which in turn raises the possibility that the neuroprotective effects of HSF1 could be harnessed separately from its tumorigenic ones.

Challenges in translating preclinical findings to clinical trials for diseases associated with misfolded proteins

The misfolded protein neuropathies have proven an exceptionally challenging arena for therapeutics development. Promising candidates for Alzheimer's disease, Parkinson's disease, ALS, and Huntington's disease have been identified in preclinical studies, but very few have shown significant benefits in clinical trials (Table 2 lists known drug-target interactions for neurodegenerative diseases associated with misfolded proteins). This "failure to translate" has plagued the development of therapeutics for neurological diseases in general, and likely reasons for it have been discussed in detail elsewhere [115–117]. A leading cause is the lack of robust targets whose modulation results in a therapeutic benefit. The uncertainties about which process or protein to target, and resulting failures to demonstrate target engagement, result in preclinical studies in animal models that do not have predictive validity. Additionally, there is a strong need to identify translatable biomarkers in animal models for clinical studies. Finally, pharmacokinetics and drug safety pose significant challenges to successful drug development for misfolded protein diseases. Recently, however, strides have been made in the area of Alzheimer's disease with structural studies of how antibodies interact with specific epitopes on the amyloid-β molecule, and how these interactions correlate with clinical outcomes [101].

Another area of opportunity is the identification of novel targets. For example, the area of cell type-specific targets has been relatively unexplored. A key feature of the proteinopathies is that the proteins involved are typically expressed in many or all cell types, but cause pathological phenotypes only in specific sets of neurons. Thus, informed development of therapeutics should include understanding not only of the species of misfolded proteins involved, but also of how they affect different populations of neurons. A recent genomic/proteomic study in HD model mice identified striatum- and cortex-specific transcription modules whose expression correlated strongly with both CAG repeat length and age [118]. Interestingly, striatal modules included genes involved in establishing and maintaining medium spiny neuron identity. Another study showed that the degeneration of different subtypes of neurons (e.g. striatal versus motor

Table 2 Drug-target pairs for neurodegenerative diseases associated with misfolded proteins

Compound name	Company	Disease indication	Mechanism of action	Status
TRx0237	TauRx Therapeutics	Alzheimer's disease	Tau aggregation inhibitor	Phase II clinical trials completed
AADvac1	Axon Neuroscience SE	Alzheimer's disease	Active tau based immunotherapy	Phase I clinical trials completed
ACI-35	AC Immune AG	Alzheimer's disease	Phospho-tau vaccine	Phase I trial active
Arimoclomol	Orphazyme ApS	Amyotrophic Lateral Sclerosis	HSP activation	Phase II/III active
Nuedexta	Avanir Pharmaceuticals	Amyotrophic Lateral Sclerosis – PBA symptom treatment	Unknown for PBA treatment; NMDA receptor antagonist	FDA approved
Deferiprone	Generic	Parkinson's disease	Iron chelator	Phase II recruiting
Istradefylline	Kyowa Hakko Kirin	Parkinson's disease	Adenosine A2A receptor antagonist	Approved in Japan; no FDA approval

neurons) is mediated by down-regulation of different sets of ER chaperones [119].

The use of transgenic rodent models to study pathogenic mechanisms presents more challenges in the case of the proteinopathies than in other diseases. The selection of the correct transgenic protein target is essential to develop a useful rodent model of overexpression. Transgenic models of disease are developed on the assumption that increased production of a particular protein drives disease development. When the correct protein target is not selected, the model does not accurately represent the pathogenic mechanism. Rodents differ from humans with respect to basic biology (i.e., glia to neuron ratio, anatomy of the brain vasculature) and the biochemical properties of misfolded disease protein aggregates [120]. A potential solution to the latter issue would be the use of human/mouse chimeras. For example, it has been shown that mutant huntingtin-expressing human glial precursor cells can impart the HD disease phenotype when grafted into the striata of normal mice, and that normal glial precursors can rescue certain phenotypes and slow disease progression when grafted into R6/2 HD mice [121].

Finally, there is a need for translatable biomarkers that robustly track the progression and severity of the disease for successful clinical trial. One approach has been to measure amounts of soluble disease protein in the cerebrospinal fluid (CSF). When analyzing soluble proteins, the stability and kinetics of protein turnover in the CSF must be established, along with inter- and intra-subject variability. A challenge with the use of soluble proteins as CSF biomarkers is their low concentrations in the CSF, which in turn produces a low signal-to-noise ratio. A new approach has been to study other components of the CSF, such as exosomes. Exosomes are released by most cell types, and carry cargoes of proteins that include misfolded disease proteins [122]. For chaperone or proteasome targets, which are intracellular, it may be necessary to develop surrogate markers to assess target engagement.

Molecular imaging approaches (e.g., positron emission tomography, or PET) are an alternate approach to assessing target distribution and engagement. Currently, direct imaging of neurodegenerative disease proteins in vivo is possible in humans only for amyloid and tau [123–125]. Most of the currently available amyloid PET ligands are limited in their utility because they bind only to insoluble fibrillar amyloid. Similarly, the development of tau tracers has challenged by the biochemical complexity and heterogeneity of tau deposits. Several promising tau tracers are now available for use in humans, but remain to be fully characterized with respect to their binding to specific isoforms and conformations of tau; in addition, all show significant off-target binding. The recent development of antibody-based PET ligands offers a potential solution to these issues. Such ligands have now been used to detect oligomeric Aβ in the mouse brain and this approach might also be used for α-synuclein and other neurodegenerative disease proteins for which no ligands are currently available [126].

A key issue that has arisen with respect to translatable biomarkers is lack of correlation between levels of disease proteins and functional outcomes in rodent models. For example, unlike humans, mouse AD models and some mouse HD models do not show neuronal cell death. However, even models that don't show cell death do typically show neuronal dysfunction and synaptic loss. Imaging ligands that demonstrate synaptic loss are now being developed in humans, and could be reverse-translated for use in rodent studies [127]. Alternative translatable measures of neuronal function currently being explored include EEG [128] and functional imaging markers [129].

Collaborating to accelerate therapeutic development

Until recently, drug discovery was the almost exclusive domain of biotechnology and pharmaceutical companies. Today, a new model for drug discovery has evolved, spurred in large part by initiatives led by patient advocacy groups, philanthropic organizations, the National Institutes of Health and other international funding agencies. This new model involves coordinated collaborations between academia, industry, private foundations, and government funding agencies, and incorporates patients and caregivers as key collaborators, knowledge resources, and decision-makers. Private foundations are increasingly taking on leadership roles that used to be handled primarily by government agencies, including the facilitation and scientific management of focused research initiatives, large-scale research consortia, and partnerships between academia, industry, and CROs.

Team approaches are particularly critical for the proteinopathies because of the heterogeneity and/or rarity of these conditions and the difficulty of recruiting sufficiently large patient cohorts for clinical trials for genetic disease. Patient advocacy groups and foundations are now playing critical roles in forcing some degree of standardization and scientific rigor, and providing critical natural history data for disease progression markers. Examples of such efforts include the Michael J. Fox Foundation Parkinson's Progression Markers Initiative, the Target ALS drug discovery program, the Alzheimer's disease Drug Discovery Foundation Access program, and the CHDI Foundation Preclinical Research program. Another key role for both governmental agencies and private foundations in supporting collaborations is through the development of public databases and "knowledge centers," such as the National Alzheimer's Coordinating Center and the Academic Drug Discovery Consortium. Recent national and international government initiatives supporting early drug discovery include the NIH Blueprint Neurotherapeutics Network and the European Innovative Medicines Initiative.

Conclusion

There is active research ongoing to uncover the mechanisms by which disease-associated proteins misfold, aggregate, and cause cellular toxicity. Continued progress in our ability to interrogate amyloid-forming proteins and their interactions with other cellular proteins provide confidence that novel therapies will be identified for multiple disease states. Therapeutic options now being explored include targeting misfolded protein-chaperone interactions at various points in the proteostatic pathway, promoting protein clearance, and large-scale rebalancing of proteostatic network. However, the identification and in vivo validation of new therapeutic compounds is impeded by the shortage of known disease drivers and the lack of reliable biomarkers for monitoring therapeutic responses in relevant animal models. However, the increase in cooperative research and collaboration among the drug discovery community (pharmaceutical companies, foundations, academia, contract research organizations, clinicians, regulatory agencies, advocacy groups and patients) is a positive shift that can help accelerate the identification of novel therapeutic modalities.

Endnotes

[1]This review is based in part on an open scientific satellite symposium entitled "Protein Misfolding – Implications and Strategies" held in conjunction with the 45th Annual Society for Neuroscience meeting in 2015, sponsored and organized by Charles River Laboratories. The meeting panelists included: Hyunsun Park (Health & Life Science Consulting), Judith Frydman (Stanford University), John Dunlop (Astra Zeneca), Marc Baumann (University of Helsinki), Alexander McCampbell (Biogen), Ron Kopito (Stanford University), Patrick Sweeney (Royal Veterinary College, University of London, Charles River Laboratories) and Robert Hodgson (Charles River Laboratories).

Abbreviations

AD: Alzheimer's disease; ALS: Amyotrophic lateral sclerosis; Aβ: Beta amyloid; BACE: Beta amyloid cleaving enzyme; BBB: Blood brain barrier; CLIP: Chaperones linked to protein synthesis; CRO: Contract research organization; CSF: Cerebrospinal fluid; DNA: Deoxyribonucleic acid; GFP: Green fluorescent protein; HSP: Heat shock proteins; Htt: Ubiquitinated Huntingtin; IMS: Ion mobility spectrometry; IMS-MS: Ion mobility spectrometry-mass spectrometry; IPOD: Insoluble protein deposit; JUNQ: Juxtanuclear quality control; MS: Mass spectrometry; mTOR: Mammalian target of rapamycin; NIH: National Institutes of Health; NMR: Nuclear magnetic resonance; SDS-PAGE: Denaturing gel electrophoresis; TDP-43: TAR DNA binding protein-43; UPR: Unfolded protein response; UPS: Ubiquitin proteasome system; VCP: Valosin-containing protein VCP

Acknowledgements

Not applicable.

Funding

The consortium of thought leaders from industry and academia that was the primary content source for the manuscript was funded by Charles River Laboratories. G. Leblanc (Bioscience Consulting, Berkeley, CA) is a paid consultant of Charles River Laboratories to provide scientific and writing assistance.

Authors' contributions

PS conceived of the study, organized the consortium and revised the manuscript. HP moderated the consortium and reviewed the manuscript. MB, JD, JF, RK and AM presented at the consortium and reviewed the manuscript. GL and AV drafted and reviewed the manuscript. RH co-organized the consortium and reviewed the manuscript. AN reviewed the manuscript. All authors read and approved the final manuscript.

Competing interests

The authors declare that they have no competing interests.

Author details

[1]Discovery Services, Charles Rivers Laboratories, Wilmington, MA, USA. [2]Royal Veterinary College, University of London, London, UK. [3]Health & Life Science Consulting, Los Angeles, CA, USA. [4]Biochemistry and Developmental Biology, University of Helsinki, Helsinki, Finland. [5]Neuroscience Innovation Medicines, Astra Zeneca, Cambridge, MA, USA. [6]Stanford University, Stanford, CA, USA. [7]Neurology, Biogen Idec, Cambridge, MA, USA. [8]Leblanc Bioscience Consulting, Berkeley, CA, USA.

References

1. Hartl FU, Hayer-Hartl M. Converging concepts of protein folding in vitro and in vivo. Nat Struct Mol Biol. 2009;16:574–81. doi:10.1038/nsmb.1591.
2. Guijarro JI, Sunde M, Jones JA, Campbell ID, Dobson CM. Amyloid fibril formation by an SH3 domain. Proc Natl Acad Sci U S A. 1998;95:4224–8.
3. Tzotzos S, Doig AJ. Amyloidogenic sequences in native protein structures. Protein Sci. 2010;19:327–48. doi:10.1002/pro.314.
4. Knowles TP, Vendruscolo M, Dobson CM. The amyloid state and its association with protein misfolding diseases. Nature reviews. Mol Cell Biol. 2014;15:384–96. doi:10.1038/nrm3810.
5. Kallijarvi J, Haltia M, Baumann MH. Amphoterin includes a sequence motif which is homologous to the Alzheimer's beta-amyloid peptide (Abeta), forms amyloid fibrils in vitro, and binds avidly to Abeta. Biochemistry. 2001; 40:10032–7.
6. Finley D. Recognition and processing of ubiquitin-protein conjugates by the proteasome. Annu Rev Biochem. 2009;78:477–513.
7. Brundin P, Melki R, Kopito R. Prion-like transmission of protein aggregates in neurodegenerative diseases. Nat Rev Mol Cell Biol. 2010;11(4):301–7. doi:10.1038/nrm2873.

8. Chen B, Retzlaff M, Roos T, Frydman J. Cellular strategies of protein quality control. Cold Spring Harb Perspect Biol. 2011;3:a004374. doi:10.1101/cshperspect.a004374.
9. Hipp MS, Park SH, Hartl FU. Proteostasis impairment in protein-misfolding and -aggregation diseases. Trends Cell Biol. 2014;24:506–14. doi:10.1016/j.tcb.2014.05.003.
10. Albanese V, Yam AY, Baughman J, Parnot C, Frydman J. Systems analyses reveal two chaperone networks with distinct functions in eukaryotic cells. Cell. 2006;124:75–88. doi:10.1016/j.cell.2005.11.039.
11. Albanese V, Reissmann S, Frydman J. A ribosome-anchored chaperone network that facilitates eukaryotic ribosome biogenesis. J Cell Biol. 2010;189: 69–81. doi:10.1083/jcb.201001054.
12. del Alamo M, Hogan DJ, Pechmann S, Albanese V, Brown PO, Frydman J. Defining the specificity of cotranslationally acting chaperones by systematic analysis of mRNAs associated with ribosome-nascent chain complexes. PLoS Biol. 2011;9, e1001100. doi:10.1371/journal.pbio.1001100.
13. Brehme M, Voisine C, Rolland T, Wachi S, Soper JH, Zhu Y, Orton K, Villella A, Garza D, Vidal M, Ge H, Morimoto RI. A chaperome subnetwork safeguards proteostasis in aging and neurodegenerative disease. Cell Rep. 2014;9:1135–50. doi:10.1016/j.celrep.2014.09.042.
14. Kaganovich D, Kopito R, Frydman J. Misfolded proteins partition between two distinct quality control compartments. Nature. 2008;454:1088–95. doi:10.1038/nature07195.
15. Escusa-Toret S, Vonk WI, Frydman J. Spatial sequestration of misfolded proteins by a dynamic chaperone pathway enhances cellular fitness during stress. Nat Cell Biol. 2013;15:1231–43. doi:10.1038/ncb2838.
16. Sontag EM, Vonk WI, Frydman J. Sorting out the trash: the spatial nature of eukaryotic protein quality control. Curr Opin Cell Biol. 2014;26:139–46. doi:10.1016/j.ceb.2013.12.006.
17. Hayashida N, Fujimoto M, Tan K, Prakasam R, Shinkawa T, Li L, Ichikawa H, Takii R, Nakai A. Heat shock factor 1 ameliorates proteotoxicity in cooperation with the transcription factor NFAT. EMBO J. 2010;29(20):3459–69. doi:10.1038/emboj.2010.225.
18. Mollapour M, Neckers L. Post-translational modifications of Hsp90 and their contributions to chaperone regulation. Biochim Biophys Acta. 1823;2012: 648–55. doi:10.1016/j.bbamcr.2011.07.018.
19. Hipp MS, Patel CN, Bersuker K, Riley BE, Kaiser SE, Shaler TA, Brandeis M, Kopito RR. Indirect inhibition of 26S proteasome activity in a cellular model of Huntington's disease. J Cell Biol. 2012;196:573–87. doi:10.1083/jcb.201110093.
20. Nonaka T, Hasegawa M. A cellular model to monitor proteasome dysfunction by alpha-synuclein. Biochemistry. 2009;48(33):8014–22. doi:10.1021/bi900619j.
21. Myeku N, Clelland CL, Emrani S, Kukushkin NV, Yu WH, Goldberg AL, Duff KE. Tau-driven 26S proteasome impairment and cognitive dysfunction can be prevented early in disease by activating cAMP-PKA signaling. Nat Med. 2016;22:46–53. doi:10.1038/nm.4011.
22. Pearce MM, Spartz EJ, Hong W, Luo L, Kopito RR. Prion-like transmission of neuronal huntingtin aggregates to phagocytic glia in the Drosophila brain. Nat Commun. 2015;6:6768. doi:10.1038/ncomms7768.
23. Brettschneider J, Del Tredici K, Lee VM, Trojanowski JQ. Spreading of pathology in neurodegenerative diseases: a focus on human studies. Nat Rev Neurosci. 2015;16:109–20. doi:10.1038/nrn3887.
24. Galpern WR, Lang AE. Interface between tauopathies and synucleinopathies: a tale of two proteins. Ann Neurol. 2006;59(3):449–58. doi:10.1002/ana.20819.
25. Gidalevitz T, Ben-Zvi A, Ho KH, Brignull HR, Morimoto RI. Progressive disruption of cellular protein folding in models of polyglutamine diseases. Science. 2006;311:1471–4. doi:10.1126/science.1124514.
26. Gidalevitz T, Krupinski T, Garcia S, Morimoto RI. Destabilizing protein polymorphisms in the genetic background direct phenotypic expression of mutant SOD1 toxicity. PLoS Genet. 2009;5, e1000399. doi:10.1371/journal.pgen.1000399.
27. Wu JW, Hussaini SA, Bastille IM, Rodriguez GA, Mrejeru A, Rilett K, Sanders DW, Cook C, Fu H, Boonen RA, Herman M, Nahmani E, Emrani S, Figueroa YH, Diamond MI, Clelland CL, Wray S, Duff KE. Neuronal activity enhances tau propagation and tau pathology in vivo. Nat Neurosci. 2016;19(8):1085–92. doi:10.1038/nn.4328.
28. Fontaine SN, Zheng D, Sabbagh JJ, Martin MD, Chaput D, Darling A, Trotter JH, Stothert AR, Nordhues BA, Lussier A, Baker J, Shelton L, Kahn M, Blair LJ, Stevens Jr SM, Dickey CA. DnaJ/Hsc70 chaperone complexes control the extracellular release of neurodegenerative-associated proteins. EMBO J. 2016;35(14):1537–49. doi:10.15252/embj.201593489.
29. Lee JG, Takahama S, Zhang G, Tomarev SI, Ye Y. Unconventional secretion of misfolded proteins promotes adaptation to proteasome dysfunction in mammalian cells. Nat Cell Biol. 2016;18(7):765–76. doi:10.1038/ncb3372.
30. Shankar GM, Li S, Mehta TH, Garcia-Munoz A, Shepardson NE, Smith I, Brett FM, Farrell MA, Rowan MJ, Lemere CA, Regan CM, Walsh DM, Sabatini BL, Selkoe DJ. Amyloid-beta protein dimers isolated directly from Alzheimer's brains impair synaptic plasticity and memory. Nat Med. 2008;14(8):837–42. doi:10.1038/nm1782.
31. Kopeikina KJ, Hyman BT, Spires-Jones TL. Soluble forms of tau are toxic in Alzheimer's disease. Transl Neurosci. 2012;3(3):223–33.
32. Ingelsson M. Alpha-Synuclein Oligomers-Neurotoxic Molecules in Parkinson's Disease and Other Lewy Body Disorders. Front Neurosci. 2016; 10:408. doi:10.3389/fnins.2016.00408.
33. Thies E, Mandelkow EM. Missorting of tau in neurons causes degeneration of synapses that can be rescued by the kinase MARK2/Par-1. J Neurosci. 2007;27(11):2896–907.
34. Di Maio R, Barrett PJ, Hoffman EK, Barrett CW, Zharikov A, Borah A, Hu X, McCoy J, Chu CT, Burton EA, Hastings TG, Greenamyre JT. α-Synuclein binds to TOM20 and inhibits mitochondrial protein import in Parkinson's disease. Sci Transl Med. 2016;8(342):342ra78. doi:10.1126/scitranslmed.aaf3634.
35. Olzscha H, Schermann SM, Woerner AC, Pinkert S, Hecht MH, Tartaglia GG, Vendruscolo M, Hayer-Hartl M, Hartl FU, Vabular RM. Amyloid-like aggregates sequester numerous metastable proteins with essential cellular functions. Cell. 2011;144:67–78. doi:10.1016/j.cell.2010.11.050.
36. Woerner AC, Frottin F, Hornburg D, Feng LR, Meissner F, Patra M, Tatzelt J, Mann M, Winklhofer KF, Hartl FU, Hipp MS. Cytoplasmic protein aggregates interfere with nucleocytoplasmic transport of protein and RNA. Science. 2016;351(6269):173–6. doi:10.1126/science.aad2033.
37. Majd S, Power JH, Grantham HJ. Neuronal response in Alzheimer's and Parkinson's disease: the effect of toxic proteins on intracellular pathways. BMC Neurosci. 2015;16:69. doi:10.1186/s12868-015-0211-1.
38. Ben Haim L, Carrillo-de Sauvage MA, Ceyzériat K. Escartin C Elusive roles for reactive astrocytes in neurodegenerative diseases. Front Cell Neurosci. 2015; 9:278. doi:10.3389/fncel.2015.00278.
39. Jiang T, Sun Q, Chen S. Oxidative stress: A major pathogenesis and potential therapeutic target of antioxidative agents in Parkinson's disease and Alzheimer's disease. Prog Neurobiol. 2016;147:1–19. doi:10.1016/j.pneurobio.2016.07.005.
40. Angelova PR, Abramov AY. Alpha-synuclein and beta-amyloid - different targets, same players: calcium, free radicals and mitochondria in the mechanism of neurodegeneration. Biochem Biophys Res Commun. 2017; 483(4):1110–5. doi:10.1016/j.bbrc.2016.07.103.
41. Taylor RC, Dillin A. Aging as an Event of Proteostasis Collapse. Cold Spring Harb Perspect Biol. 2011;3(5):a004440. doi:10.1101/cshperspect.a004440.
42. Höhn A, Weber D, Jung T, Ott C, Hugo M, Kochlik B, Kehm R, König J, Grune T, Castro JP. Happily (n)ever after: Aging in the context of oxidative stress, proteostasis loss and cellular senescence. Redox Biol. 2016;11:482–501. doi:10.1016/j.redox.2016.12.001.
43. Heppner FL, Ransohoff RM, Becher B. Immune attack: the role of inflammation in Alzheimer disease. Nat Rev Neurosci. 2015;16(6):358–72. doi:10.1038/nrn3880.
44. Chakrabarty P, Li A, Ceballos-Diaz C, Eddy JA, Funk CC, Moore B, DiNunno N, Rosario AM, Cruz PE, Verbeeck C, Sacino A, Nix S, Janus C, Price ND, Das P, Golde TE. IL-10 alters immunoproteostasis in APP mice, increasing plaque burden and worsening cognitive behavior. Neuron. 2015;85(3):519–33. doi:10.1016/j.neuron.2014.11.020.
45. Guillot-Sestier MV, Doty KR, Gate D, Rodriguez Jr J, Leung BP, Rezai-Zadeh K, Town T. Il10 deficiency rebalances innate immunity to mitigate Alzheimer-like pathology. Neuron. 2015;85(3):534–48. doi:10.1016/j.neuron.2014.12.068.
46. Deleidi M, Jäggle M, Rubino G. Immune aging, dysmetabolism, and inflammation in neurological diseases. Front Neurosci. 2015;9:172. doi:10.3389/fnins.2015.00172.
47. Currais A, Fischer W, Maher P, Schubert D. Intraneuronal protein aggregation as a trigger for inflammation and neurodegeneration in the aging brain. FASEB J. 2017;31(1):5–10. doi:10.1096/fj.201601184.
48. Lam HT, Graber MC, Gentry KA, Bieschke J. Stabilization of alpha-Synuclein Fibril Clusters Prevents Fragmentation and Reduces Seeding Activity and Toxicity. Biochemistry. 2016;55(5):675–85. doi:10.1021/acs.biochem.5b01168.

49. Guo JL, Covell DJ, Daniels JP, Iba M, Stieber A, Zhang B, Riddle DM, Kwong LK, Xu Y, Trojanowski JQ, Lee VM. Distinct alpha-synuclein strains differentially promote tau inclusions in neurons. Cell. 2013;154:103–17. doi: 10.1016/j.cell.2013.05.057.
50. Sanders DW, Kaufman SK, DeVos SL, Sharma AM, Mirbaha H, Li A, Barker SJ, Foley AC, Thorpe JR, Serpell LC, Miller TM, Grinberg LT, Seeley WW, Diamond MI. Distinct tau prion strains propagate in cells and mice and define different tauopathies. Neuron. 2014;82:1271–88. doi:10.1016/j.neuron.2014.04.047.
51. Heilbronner G, Eisele YS, Langer F, Kaeser SA, Novotny R, Nagaratinam A, Aslund A, Hammarstrom P, Nilsson KP, Jucker M. Seeded strain-like transmission of beta-amyloid morphotypes in APP transgenic mice. EMBO Rep. 2013;14:1017–22. doi:10.1038/embor.2013.137.
52. Pujol-Pina R, Vilaprinyo-Pascual S, Mazzucato R, Arcella A, Vilaseca M, Orozco M, Carulla N. SDS-PAGE analysis of Abeta oligomers is disserving research into Alzheimer s disease: appealing for ESI-IM-MS. Scientific reports. 2015;5: 14809. doi:10.1038/srep14809.
53. Woods LA, Platt GW, Hellewell AL, Hewitt EW, Homans SW, Ashcroft AE, Radford SE. Ligand binding to distinct states diverts aggregation of an amyloid-forming protein. Nat Chem Biol. 2011;7:730–9. doi:10.1038/ nchembio.635.
54. Bleiholder C, Do TD, Wu C, Economou NJ, Bernstein SS, BUratto SK, Shea JE, Bowers MT. Ion mobility spectrometry reveals the mechanism of amyloid formation of Abeta (25-35) and its modulation by inhibitors at the molecular level: epigallocatechin gallate and scyllo-inositol. J Am Chem Soc. 2013;135:16926–37. doi:10.1021/ja406197f.
55. Neudecker P, Robustelli P, Cavalli A, Walsh P, Lundstrom P, Zarrine-Afsar A, Sharpe S, Vendruscolo M, Kay LE. Structure of an intermediate state in protein folding and aggregation. Science. 2012;336:362–6. doi:10.1126/ science.1214203.
56. Bieschke J. Natural compounds may open new routes to treatment of amyloid diseases. Neurotherapeutics. 2013;10:429–39. doi:10.1007/s13311-013-0192-7.
57. Kennedy ME, Stamford AW, Chen X, Cox K, Cumming JN, Dockendorf MF, Egan M, Ereshefsky L, Hodgson RA, Hyde LA, Jhee S, Kleijn HJ, Kuvelkar R, Li W, Mattson BA, Mei H, Palcza J, Scott JD, Tanen M, Troyer MD, Tseng JL, Stone JA, Parker EM, Forman MS. The BACE1 inhibitor verubecestat (MK-8931) reduces CNS β-amyloid in animal models and in Alzheimer's disease patients. Sci Transl Med. 2016;8(363):363ra. 150.
58. Llorens-Marítin M, Jurado J, Hernández F, Avila J. GSK-3β, a pivotal kinase in Alzheimer disease. Front Mol Neurosci. 2014;7:46.
59. Roy SM, Grum-Tokars VL, Schavocky JP, Saeed F, Staniszewski A, Teich AF, Arancio O, Bachstetter AD, Webster SJ, Van Eldik LJ, Minasov G, Anderson WF, Pelletier JC, Watterson DM. Targeting human central nervous system protein kinases: An isoform selective p38αMAPK inhibitor that attenuates disease progression in Alzheimer's disease mouse models. ACS Chem Neurosci. 2015;6(4):666–80. Epub 2015 Feb 23.
60. Min SW, Chen X, Tracy TE, Li Y, Zhou Y, Wang C, Shirakawa K, Minami SS, Defensor E, Mok SA, Sohn PD, Schilling B, Cong X, Ellerby L, Gibson BW, Johnson J, Krogan N, Shamloo M, Gestwicki J, Masliah E, Verdin E, Gan L. Critical role of acetylation in tau-mediated neurodegeneration and cognitive deficits. Nat Med. 2015;21(10):1154–62. doi:10.1038/nm.3951.
61. Tebbenkamp AT, Borchelt DR. Analysis of chaperone mRNA expression in the adult mouse brain by meta analysis of the Allen Brain Atlas. PLoS One. 2010;5(10), e13675. doi:10.1371/journal.pone.0013675.
62. Lindberg I, Shorter J, Wiseman RL, Chiti F, Dickey CA, McLean PJ. Chaperones in Neurodegeneration. J Neurosci. 2015;35:13853–9. doi:10. 1523/JNEUROSCI.2600-15.2015.
63. Carnemolla A, Lazell H, Moussaoui S, Bates GP. In Vivo Profiling Reveals a Competent Heat Shock Response in Adult Neurons: Implications for Neurodegenerative Disorders. PLoS One. 2015;10, e0131985. doi:10.1371/ journal.pone.0131985.
64. Vilarino-Guell C, Rajput A, Milnerwood AJ, Shah B, Szu-Tu C, Trinh J, Yu I, Encarnacion M, Munsie LN, Tapia L, Gustavsson EK, Chou P, Tatarnikov I, Evans DM, Pishotta FT, Volta M, Beccano-Kelly D, Thompson C, Lin MK, Sherman HE, Han HJ, Guenther BL, Wasserman WW, Bernard V, Ross CJ, Appel-Cresswell S, Stoessl AJ, Robinson CA, Dickson DW, Ross OA, Wszolek ZK, Aasly JO, Wu RM, Hentati F, Gibson RA, McPherson PS, Girard M, Rajput M, Rajput AH, Farrer MJ. DNAJC13 mutations in Parkinson disease. Hum Mol Genet. 2014;23:1794–801. doi:10.1093/hmg/ddt570.
65. Wadhwa R, Ryu J, Ahn HM, Saxena N, Chaudhary A, Yun CO, Kaul SC. Functional significance of point mutations in stress chaperone mortalin and their relevance to Parkinson disease. J Biol Chem. 2015;290:8447–56. doi:10. 1074/jbc.M114.627463.
66. Johnson JO, Mandrioli J, Benatar M, Abramzon Y, Van Deerlin VM, Trojanowski JQ, Gibbs JR, Brunetti M, Gronka S, Wuu J, Ding J, McCluskey L, Martinez-Lage M, Falcone D, Hernandez DG, Arepalli S, Chong S, Schymick JC, Rothstein J, Landi F, Wang YD, Calvo A, Mora G, Sabatelli M, Monsurrò MR, Battistini S, Salvi F, Spataro R, Sola P, Borghero G, Consortium ITALSGEN, Galassi G, Scholz SW, Taylor JP, Restagno G, Chiò A, Traynor BJ. Exome sequencing reveals VCP mutations as a cause of familial ALS. Neuron. 2010; 68:857–64. doi:10.1016/j.neuron.2010.11.036.
67. Smith HL, Li W, Cheetham ME. Molecular chaperones and neuronal proteostasis. Semin Cell Dev Biol. 2015;40:142–52. doi:10.1016/j.semcdb.2015.03.003.
68. Thirstrup K, Sotty F, Montezinho LC, Badolo L, Thougaard A, Kristjánsson M, Jensen T, Watson S, Nielsen SM. Linking HSP90 target occupancy to HSP70 induction and efficacy in mouse brain. Pharmacol Res. 2016;104:197–205. doi:10.1016/j.phrs.2015.12.028.
69. Brandvold KR, Morimoto RI. The Chemical Biology of Molecular Chaperones–Implications for Modulation of Proteostasis. J Mol Biol. 2015; 427:2931–47. doi:10.1016/j.jmb.2015.05.010.
70. Pratt WB, Gestwicki JE, Osawa Y, Lieberman AP. Targeting Hsp90/ Hsp70-based protein quality control for treatment of adult onset neurodegenerative diseases. Annu Rev Pharmacol Toxicol. 2015;55: 353–71. doi:10.1146/annurev-pharmtox-010814-124332. Epub 2014 Sep 25.
71. Bose S, Cho J. Targeting chaperones, heat shock factor-1, and unfolded protein response: Promising therapeutic approaches for neurodegenerative disorders. Mol Psychiatry. 2016. doi:10.1038/mp.2016.104.
72. Fontaine SN, Martin MD, Dickey CA. Neurodegeneration and the Heat Shock Protein 70 Machinery: Implications for Therapeutic Development. Curr Top Med Chem. 2016;16(25):2741–52.
73. Wang B, Liu Y, Huang L, Chen J, Li JJ, Wang R, Kim E, Chen Y, Justicia C, Sakata K, Chen H, Planas A, Ostrom RS, Li W, Yang G, McDonald MP, Chen R, Heck DH, Liao FF. A CNS-permeable Hsp90 inhibitor rescues synaptic dysfunction and memory loss in APP-overexpressing Alzheimer's mouse model via an HSF1-mediated mechanism. Ageing Res Rev. 2016. doi:10. 1016/j.arr.2016.09.004.
74. Martin MD, Baker JD, Suntharalingam A, Nordhues BA, Shelton LB, Zheng D, Sabbagh JJ, Haystead TA, Gestwicki JE, Dickey CA. Inhibition of Both Hsp70 Activity and Tau Aggregation in Vitro Best Predicts Tau Lowering Activity of Small Molecules. ACS Chem Biol. 2016;11(7):2041–8. doi:10.1021/ acschembio.6b00223.
75. DeSantis ME, Leung EH, Sweeny EA, Jackrel ME, Cushman-Nick M, Neuhaus-Follini A, Vashist S, Sochor MA, Knight MN, Shorter J. Operational plasticity enables hsp104 to disaggregate diverse amyloid and nonamyloid clients. Cell. 2012;151(4):778–93. doi:10.1016/j.cell.2012.09.038.
76. Liu YH, Han YL, Song J, Wang Y, Jing YY, Shi Q, Tian C, Zang ZY, Li CP, Han J, Dong XP. Heat shock protein 104 inhibited the fibrillization of prion peptide 106-126 and disassembled prion peptide 106-126 fibrils in vitro. Int J Biochem Cell Biol. 2011;43(5):768–74. doi:10.1016/j.biocel.2011.01.022.
77. Jackrel ME, DeSantis ME, Martinez BA, Castellano LM, Stewart RM, Caldwell KA, Caldwell GA, Shorter J. Potentiated Hsp104 variants antagonize diverse proteotoxic misfolding events. Cell. 2014;156(1–2):170–82. doi:10.1016/j.cell. 2013.11.047.
78. Mack KL, Shorter J. Engineering and Evolution of Molecular Chaperones and Protein Disaggregases with Enhanced Activity. Front Mol Biosci. 2016;3:8. doi:10.3389/fmolb.2016.00008. eCollection 2016.
79. Ciechanover A, Kwon YT. Degradation of misfolded proteins in neurodegenerative diseases: therapeutic targets and strategies. Exp Mol Med. 2015;47, e147. doi:10.1038/emm.2014.117.
80. Dantuma NP, Bott LC. The ubiquitin-proteasome system in neurodegenerative diseases: precipitating factor, yet part of the solution. Front Mol Neurosci. 2014; 7:70. doi:10.3389/fnmol.2014.00070. eCollection 2014.
81. Cook C, Stetler C, Petrucelli L. Disruption of protein quality control in Parkinson's disease. Cold Spring Harb Perspect Med. 2012;2(5):a009423. doi:10.1101/cshperspect.a009423.
82. Moscovitz O, Ben-Nissan G, Fainer I, Pollack D, Mizrachi L, Sharon M. The Parkinson's-associated protein DJ-1 regulates the 20S proteasome. Nat Commun. 2015;6:6609. doi:10.1038/ncomms7609.
83. Ebrahimi-Fakhari D, Cantuti-Castelvetri I, Fan Z, Rockenstein E, Masliah E, Hyman BT, McLean PJ, Unni VK. Distinct roles in vivo for the ubiquitin-proteasome system and the autophagy-lysosomal pathway in the

degradation of α-synuclein. J Neurosci. 2011;31(41):14508–20. doi:10.1523/JNEUROSCI.1560-11.2011.
84. Opattova A, Cente M, Novak M, Filipcik P. The ubiquitin proteasome system as a potential therapeutic target for treatment of neurodegenerative diseases. Gen Physiol Biophys. 2015;34(4):337–52.
85. Lee JH, Shin SK, Jiang Y, Choi WH, Hong C, Kim DE, Lee MJ. Facilitated Tau Degradation by USP14 Aptamers via Enhanced Proteasome Activity. Sci Rep. 2015;5:10757. doi:10.1038/srep10757.
86. Rao G, Croft B, Teng C, Awasthi V. Ubiquitin-Proteasome System in Neurodegenerative Disorders. J Drug Metab Toxicol. 2015;6:187. doi:10.4172/2157-7609.1000187.
87. Harris H, Rubinsztein DC. Control of autophagy as a therapy for neurodegenerative disease. Nat Rev Neurol. 2011;8(2):108–17. doi:10.1038/nrneurol.2011.200.
88. Martinez-Vicente M. Autophagy in neurodegenerative diseases: From pathogenic dysfunction to therapeutic modulation. Semin Cell Dev Biol. 2015;40:115–26. doi:10.1016/j.semcdb.2015.03.005.
89. Rousseau A, Bertolotti A. An evolutionarily conserved pathway controls proteasome homeostasis. Nature. 2016;536(7615):184–9.
90. Sasazawa Y, Sato N, Umezawa K, Simizu S. Conophylline protects cells in cellular models of neurodegenerative diseases by inducing mammalian target of rapamycin (mTOR)-independent autophagy. J Biol Chem. 2015; 290(10):6168–78. doi:10.1074/jbc.M114.606293.
91. Manzoni C, Mamais A, Roosen DA, Dihanich S, Soutar MP, Plun-Favreau H, Bandopadhyay R, Hardy J, Tooze SA, Cookson MR, Lewis PA. mTOR independent regulation of macroautophagy by Leucine Rich Repeat Kinase 2 via Beclin-1. Sci Rep. 2016;6:35106. doi:10.1038/srep35106.
92. Wisniewski T, Goni F. Immunotherapeutic approaches for Alzheimer's disease. Neuron. 2015;85(6):1162–76. doi:10.1016/j.neuron.2014.12.064.
93. Genereux JC, Wiseman RL. Regulating extracellular proteostasis capacity through the unfolded protein response. Prion. 2015;9(1):10–21. doi:10.1080/19336896.2015.1011887.
94. Savage MJ, Kalinina J, Wolfe A, Tugusheva K, Korn R, Cash-Mason T, Maxwell JW, Hatcher NG, Haugabook SJ, Wu G, Howell BJ, Renger JJ, Shughrue PJ, McCampbell A. A sensitive abeta oligomer assay discriminates Alzheimer's and aged control cerebrospinal fluid. J Neurosci. 2014;34:2884–97. doi:10.1523/JNEUROSCI.1675-13.2014.
95. De Genst E, Messer A, Dobson CM. Antibodies and protein misfolding: From structural research tools to therapeutic strategies. Biochim Biophys Acta. 1844;2014:1907–19. doi:10.1016/j.bbapap.2014.08.016.
96. Vaikath NN, Majbour NK, Paleologou KE, Ardah MT, van Dam E, van de Berg WD, Forrest SL, Parkkinen L, Gai WP, Hattori N, Takanashi M, Lee SJ, Mann DM, Imai Y, Halliday GM, Li JY, El-Agnaf OM. Generation and characterization of novel conformation-specific monoclonal antibodies for alpha-synuclein pathology. Neurobiol Dis. 2015;79:81–99. doi:10.1016/j.nbd.2015.04.009.
97. Deane R, Bell RD, Sagare R, Zlokovic BV. Clearance of amyloid-beta peptide across the blood-brain barrier: implication for therapies in Alzheimer's disease. CNS Neurol Disord Drug Targets. 2009;8(1):16–30.
98. Watt AD, Crespi GA, Down RA, Ascher DB, Gunn A, Perez KA, McLean CA, Villemagne VL, Parker MW, Barnham KJ, Miles LA. Do current therapeutic anti-Aβ antibodies for Alzheimer's disease engage the target? Acta Neuropathol. 2014;127(6):803–10. doi:10.1007/s00401-014-1290-2.
99. Bouter Y, Lopez Noguerola JS, Tucholla P, Crespi GA, Parker MW, Wiltfang J, Miles LA, Bayer TA. Abeta targets of the biosimilar antibodies of Bapineuzumab, Crenezumab, Solanezumab in comparison to an antibody against N-truncated Abeta in sporadic Alzheimer disease cases and mouse models. Acta Neuropathol. 2015;130(5):713–29.
100. Fuller JP, Stavenhagen JB, Christensen S, Kartberg F, Glennie MJ, Teeling JL. Comparing the efficacy and neuroinflammatory potential of three anti-abeta antibodies. Acta Neuropathol. 2015;130(5):699–711. doi:10.1007/s00401-015-1484-2.
101. Crespi GA, Hermans SJ, Parker MW, Miles LA. Molecular basis for mid-region amyloid-β capture by leading Alzheimer's disease immunotherapies. Sci Rep. 2015;5:9649. doi:10.1038/srep09649.
102. Cramer PE, Cirrito JR, Wesson DW, Lee CY, Karlo JC, Zinn AE, Casali BT, Restivo JL, Goebel WD, James MJ, Brunden KR, Wilson DA, Landreth GE. ApoE-directed therapeutics rapidly clear beta-amyloid and reverse deficits in AD mouse models. Science. 2012;335:1503–6. doi:10.1126/science.1217697.
103. Boehm-Cagan A, Michaelson D. M. Reversal of apoE4-driven brain pathology and behavioral deficits by bexarotene. J Neurosci. 2014;34:7293–301. doi:10.1523/JNEUROSCI.5198-13.2014.
104. Vazquez-Lombardi R, Phan TG, Zimmermann C, Lowe D, Jermutus L, Christ D. Challenges and opportunities for non-antibody scaffold drugs. Drug Discov Today. 2015;20(10):1271–83. doi:10.1016/j.drudis.2015.09.004.
105. Iba M, Guo JL, McBride JD, Zhang B, Trojanowski JQ, Lee VM. Synthetic tau fibrils mediate transmission of neurofibrillary tangles in a transgenic mouse model of Alzheimer's-like tauopathy. J Neurosci. 2013;33:1024–37. doi:10.1523/JNEUROSCI.2642-12.2013.
106. Kim E, Wang B, Sastry N, Masliah E, Nelson PT, Cai H, Liao FF. NEDD4-mediated HSF1 degradation underlies α-synucleinopathy. Hum Mol Genet. 2016;25(2):211–22. doi:10.1093/hmg/ddv445.
107. Neef DW, Jaeger AM, Thiele DJ. Heat shock transcription factor 1 as a therapeutic target in neurodegenerative diseases. Nat Rev Drug Discov. 2011;10(12):930–44.
108. Verma P, Pfister JA, Mallick S, D'Mello SR. HSF1 protects neurons through a novel trimerization- and HSP-independent mechanism. J Neurosci. 2014; 34(5):1599–612. doi:10.1523/JNEUROSCI.3039-13.2014.
109. Kondo N, Katsuno M, Adachi H, Minamiyama M, Doi H, Matsumoto S, Miyazaki Y, Iida M, Tohnai G, Nakatsuji H, Ishigaki S, Fujioka Y, Watanabe H, Tanaka F, Nakai A, Sobue G. Heat shock factor-1 influences pathological lesion distribution of polyglutamine-induced neurodegeneration. Nat Commun. 2013;4:1405. doi:10.1038/ncomms2417.
110. Bersuker K, Hipp MS, Calamini B, Morimoto RI, Kopito RR. Heat shock response activation exacerbates inclusion body formation in a cellular model of Huntington disease. J Biol Chem. 2013;288:23633–8. doi:10.1074/jbc.C113.481945.
111. Lamech LT, Haynes CM. The unpredictability of prolonged activation of stress response pathways. J Cell Biol. 2015;209(6):781–7. doi:10.1083/jcb.201503107.
112. Labbadia J, Cunliffe H, Weiss A, Katsyuba E, Sathasivam K, Seredenina T, Woodman B, Moussaoui S, Frentzel S, Luthi-Carter R, Paganetti P, Bates GP. Altered chromatin architecture underlies progressive impairment of the heat shock response in mouse models of Huntington disease. J Clin Invest. 2011;121:3306–19. doi:10.1172/JCI57413.
113. Mendillo ML, Santagata S, Koeva M, Bell GW, Hu R, Tamimi RM, Fraenkel E, Ince TA, Whitesell L, Lindquist S. HSF1 drives a transcriptional program distinct from heat shock to support highly malignant human cancers. Cell. 2012;150(3):549–62. doi:10.1016/j.cell.2012.06.031.
114. Jaeger AM, Pemble CW, Sistoen L, Thiele DJ. Structures of HSF2 Reveal Mechanisms for Differential Regulation of Human Heat Shock Factors. Nat Struct Mol Biol. 2016;23(2):147–54. doi:10.1038/nsmb.3150.
115. Shineman DW, Basi GS, Bizon JL, Colton CA, Greenberg BD, Hollister BA, Lincecum J, Leblanc GG, Lee LB, Luo F, Morgan D, Morse I, Refolo LM, Riddell DR, Scearce-Levie K, Sweeney P, Yrjänheikki J, Fillit HM. Accelerating drug discovery for Alzheimer's disease: best practices for preclinical animal studies. Alzheimers Res Ther. 2011;3:28. doi:10.1186/alzrt90.
116. Karran E, Hardy J. A critique of the drug discovery and phase 3 clinical programs targeting the amyloid hypothesis for Alzheimer disease. Ann Neurol. 2014;76:185–205. doi:10.1002/ana.24188.
117. Sperling R, Mormino E, Johnson K. The evolution of preclinical Alzheimer's disease: implications for prevention trials. Neuron. 2014;84:608–22. doi:10.1016/j.neuron.2014.10.038.
118. Langfelder P, Cantle JP, Chatzopoulou D, Wang N, Gao F, Al-Ramahi I, Lu XH, Ramos EM, El-Zein K, Zhao Y, Deverasetty S, Tebbe A, Schaab C, Lavery DJ, Howland D, Kwak S, Botas J, Aaronson JS, Rosinski J, Coppola G, Horvath S, Yang XW. Integrated genomics and proteomics define huntingtin CAG length-dependent networks in mice. Nat Neurosci. 2016;19(4):623–33. doi:10.1038/nn.4256.
119. Yamanaka T, Tosaki A, Miyazaki H, Kurosawa M, Koike M, Uchiyama Y, Maity SN, Misawa H, Takahashi R, Shimogori T, Hattori N, Nukina N. Differential roles of NF-Y transcription factor in ER chaperone expression and neuronal maintenance in the CNS. Sci Rep. 2016;6:34575. doi:10.1038/srep34575.
120. Cavanaugh SE, Pippin JJ, Barnard ND. Animal models of Alzheimer disease: historical pitfalls and a path forward. ALTEX. 2014;31(3):279–302. http://dx.doi.org/10.14573/altex.1310071.
121. Benraiss A, Wang S, Herrlinger S, Li X, Chandler-Militello D, Mauceri J, Burm HB, Toner M, Osipovitch M, Jim Xu Q, Ding F, Wang F, Kang N, Kang J, Curtin PC, Brunner D, Windrem MS, Munoz-Sanjuan I, Nedergaard M,

Goldman SA. Human glia can both induce and rescue aspects of disease phenotype in Huntington disease. Nat Commun. 2016;7:11758. doi:10.1038/ncomms11758.

122. Thompson AG, Gray E, Heman-Ackah SM, Mäger I, Talbot K, Andaloussi SE, Wood MJ, Turner MR. Extracellular vesicles in neurodegenerative disease - pathogenesis to biomarkers. Nat Rev Neurol. 2016;12(6):346–57. doi:10.1038/nrneurol.2016.68.
123. Catafau AM, Bullich S. Non-amyloid PET imaging biomarkers for neurodegeneration: Focus on tau, alpha-synuclein and neuroinflamation. Curr Alzheimer Res. 2016. [Epub ahead of print].
124. Saint-Aubert L, Lemoine L, Chiotis K, Leuzy A, Rodriguez-Vieitez E, Nordberg A. Tau PET imaging: present and future directions. Mol Neurodegener. 2017; 12(1):19. doi:10.1186/s13024-017-0162-3.
125. Villemagne VL, Doré V, Bourgeat P, Burnham SC, Laws S, Salvado O, Masters CL, Rowe CC. Aβ-amyloid and Tau Imaging in Dementia. Semin Nucl Med. 2017; 47(1):75–88. doi:10.1053/j.semnuclmed.2016.09.006.
126. Sehlin D, Fang XT, Cato L, Antoni G, Lannfelt L, Syvänen S. Antibody-based PET imaging of amyloid beta in mouse models of Alzheimer's disease. Nat Commun. 2016;7:10759. doi:10.1038/ncomms10759.
127. Finneman SJ, Nabulsi NB, Eid T, Detyniecki K, Lin S, Chen M, Dhaher R, Matuskey D, Baum E, Holden D, Spencer DD, Mercier K, Hannestad J, Huang Y, Carson RE. Imaging synaptic density in the living human brain. Sci Transl Med. 2016;8(348):348ra96. doi:10.1126/scitranslmed.aaf6667.
128. Morris M, Sanchez PE, Verret L, Beagle AJ, Guo W, Dubal D, Ranasinghe KG, Koyama A, Ho K, Yu GQ, Vossel KA, Mucke L. Network dysfunction in α-synuclein transgenic mice and human Lewy body dementia. Ann Clin Transl Neurol. 2015;2(11):1012–28. doi:10.1002/acn3.257.
129. Sorg C, Göttler J, Zimmer C. Imaging Neurodegeneration: Steps Toward Brain Network-Based Pathophysiology and Its Potential for Multi-modal Imaging Diagnostics. Clin Neuroradiol. 2015;25 Suppl 2:177–81. doi:10.1007/s00062-015-0438-3.

6

Genotype-phenotype correlations of amyotrophic lateral sclerosis

Hong-Fu Li and Zhi-Ying Wu*

Abstract

Amyotrophic lateral sclerosis (ALS) is a devastating neurodegenerative disease characterized by progressive neuronal loss and degeneration of upper motor neuron (UMN) and lower motor neuron (LMN). The clinical presentations of ALS are heterogeneous and there is no single test or procedure to establish the diagnosis of ALS. Most cases are diagnosed based on symptoms, physical signs, progression, EMG, and tests to exclude the overlapping conditions. Familial ALS represents about 5 ~ 10 % of ALS cases, whereas the vast majority of patients are sporadic. To date, more than 20 causative genes have been identified in hereditary ALS. Detecting the pathogenic mutations or risk variants for each ALS individual is challenging. However, ALS patients carrying some specific mutations or variant may exhibit subtly distinct clinical features. Unraveling the respective genotype-phenotype correlation has important implications for the genetic explanations. In this review, we will delineate the clinical features of ALS, outline the major ALS-related genes, and summarize the possible genotype-phenotype correlations of ALS.

Keywords: Amyotrophic lateral sclerosis, Diagnosis of ALS, Causative genes, Genetic explanations, Genotype-phenotype correlations

Background

Amyotrophic lateral sclerosis (ALS) is a devastating and inexorable neurodegenerative disease characterized by progressive neuronal loss and degeneration of upper motor neuron (UMN) and lower motor neuron (LMN) [1]. It is the most widespread type of motor neuron disease and has become the third most common neurodegenerative disease in the world [2]. Patients affected with ALS typically suffer from progressive muscle weakness and atrophy and usually die from respiratory failure 2 to 3 years after the onset [3]. ALS is a relentless and incurable disease. There has been no effective therapeutic approach to halt the progression so far. ALS is heterogeneous in its presentation, course, and progression. No single test for diagnosing ALS exists; most cases are diagnosed based on symptoms, physical signs, progression, EMG, and tests to exclude the overlapping conditions.

The etiology of ALS is not fully understood. Appropriate 5 ~ 10 % of ALS is familial (FALS) with a Mendelian pattern of inheritance, suggesting that genetic factors play important roles in the pathogenesis of ALS [4]. To date, more than 20 causative genes have been identified in hereditary ALS. In addition, about 30 potential causative or disease-modifying genes have also been identified. Detecting the pathogenic mutations or risk variants for each ALS individual is therefore challenging. Clinical features do not reliably separate the hereditary ALS from sporadic ALS (SALS) due to phenotypic overlap. However, ALS patients carrying some specific mutations may exhibit subtly distinct clinical features. Unraveling the genotype-phenotype correlations has important implications for the genetic explanations. In this review, we will delineate the clinical features of ALS, outline the major ALS-related genes, and review the possible genotype-phenotype correlations. We hope this review will be in favor of improving the accuracy of genetic screenings.

Clinical features of ALS

ALS usually commences in later life, with a mean age at onset (AAO) of 65 year. The onset for FALS tends to be earlier than that of SALS. A small proportion of patients may developed juvenile ALS (JALS), in which onset occurs in the first two decades [5]. Symptoms usually begin

* Correspondence: zhiyingwu@zju.edu.cn
Department of Neurology and Research Center of Neurology in Second Affiliated Hospital, and the Collaborative Innovation Center for Brain Science, Zhejiang University School of Medicine, 88 Jiefang Rd, Hangzhou 310009, China

in the limbs (termed limb onset), although approximate 25 % of ALS patients have bulbar onset. Associated with poorer prognosis, bulbar onset is more common in elderly patients and women [6]. Upper limb weakness and atrophy at onset are most common, subsequently spreading to involve bulbar, trunk, or respiratory muscle [7]. After initial presentation of symptoms, the disease progresses to include both UMN and LMN symptoms and signs. The UMN disturbance involving limbs leads to spasticity, weakness, and brisk reflexes. The LMN features of limbs comprise muscle atrophy, weakness, fasciculation, and decreased reflexes. As limb function deteriorates, patients gradually lose their ability to walk. Bulbar UMN dysfunction includes spastic dysarthria and brisk jerk of gag and jaw, while bulbar LMN dysfunction includes tongue wasting, weakness, and fasciculation. In the later stage of ALS, most cases develop dysphagia, which are associated with weight loss and malnutrition.

Sensory loss is usually absent, but cognitive impairment is common in ALS cases. A significant proportion of ALS cases develop cognitive dysfunction, and in a minority, overt dementia [7]. With appropriate cognitive assessment, 20 ~ 50 % of patients with ALS fulfill the consensus criteria for probable or definite frontal temporal dementia (FTD) [8]. In addition, about 30 % of FTD patients manifest signs of motor system dysfunction [9]. The occurrence of ALS, FTD, or ALS with FTD in intra-familial members discloses a considerable overlap between ALS and FTD.

Causative genes

Since the identification of first causative gene in 1993, a growing number of ALS-causing genes associated with Mendelian inheritance have been identified. Although FALS represents only 5 ~ 10 % of ALS cases, investigations of the causative genes have greatly increased our understanding of the etiology of ALS. FALS is generally inherited in an autosomal dominant pattern and rarely inherited as an autosomal recessive or X-linked trait [10]. Adult onset autosomal dominant inheritance is more common than juvenile onset which is usually caused by recessive transmission.

To date, at least 21 chromosomal regions containing 19 identified genes have been linked to ALS, termed as ALS 1–21 respectively (Table 1). In 2011, the *chromosome 9 open reading frame 72* (*C9ORF72*) repeat expansions were identified in a significant proportion of ALS and FTD patients, becoming the most common genetic cause of ALS in the Caucasian population. There has been strong evidence to support the pathogenic role for mutations in *Cu/Zn superoxide dismutase 1* (*SOD1*), *Fused in sarcoma* (*FUS*), *TAR DNA-binding protein* (*TARDBP*), and *C9ORF72*. However, mutations in other genes are not common or even rarely seen in ALS cases. In addition to the aforementioned ALS genes, a constellation of other genes have also been implicated in ALS [11]. But mutations in these genes are only identified in a small fraction of ALS patients, indicating that these mutated genes have little contribution to the development of ALS.

Genotype-phenotype correlations

ALS1: SOD1

The first causative gene of ALS was identified as *SOD1* in 1993 [12]. Mutations in *SOD1* are very common, accounting for about 20 % of FALS and 1 ~ 2 % SALS cases [13]. To date, more than 185 disease-associated mutations have been described, spread throughout all the 5 exons of *SOD1* [14]. The majority of *SOD1* mutations are missense mutations, while small deletions or insertions are also described [15]. The pattern of inheritance is autosomal dominant except for the p.D90A mutation which is recessive in the Scandinavian population and dominant in others [16]. Among the *SOD1* mutations, p.D90A is the most common worldwide. However, regional disparity of *SOD1* mutations also exists. For example, the most frequent *SOD1* mutation in North America is p.A4V [17], but in the UK and Japan, the most common mutations are p.I113T, and p.H46R, respectively [18].

Overall, most patients with *SOD1* mutations develop a rapidly progressive ALS, although some cases show a diverse phenotype. AAO and severity may vary significantly depending on the variants involved. Patients with p.A4V, p.H43R, p.L84V, p.G85R, p.N86S, or p.G93A mutations exhibit an aggressive form of ALS with survival shorter than 3 years, while cases with p.G93C, p.D90A, or p.H46R mutations show longer life expectancies [18]. Cognitive impairment is very rare and bulbar onset is less frequent than in other FALS types [19]. Some cases with *SOD1* mutations have distinct clinical features. Patients carrying homozygous p.D90A mutation manifest insidious onset and a slow progression of ALS, with bladder involvement at the later stage [20]. In contrast, heterozygous p.D90A mutation is associated with various forms of ALS, including bulbar onset, upper-limb onset and fast progression, and lower-limb onset with fast progression [21, 22]. The p.A4V mutation causes a limb-onset aggressive form of ALS, with survival less than 2 years after the onset [23]. Cases with p.A4T mutation have a similar phenotype to that seen in p.A4V mutation [24]. We previously reported *SOD1* p.C111Y and p.G147D mutations in 3 Chinese ALS families. The p.C111Y mutation led to a relatively mild ALS phenotype, while the p.G147D was associated with a rapid progressive ALS [25]. The recently reported novel p.R115C mutation was identified in an ALS patient who had an extremely rapid progression and aggressive phenotype

Table 1 Different subtypes of familial ALS and their genotype–phenotype correlations

ALS type (chromosome)	Gene	Inheritance	ALS features	FTD	Other features/disorders
ALS 1 (21q22.1)	*SOD1*	AD; AR; De novo	AAO: adult > juvenile; Onset: LL > UL > bulbar; Progression: rapid > slow; UMN + LMN > LMN dominant	Rare	PMA, PBP, BFA, cerebellar ataxia, autonomic dysfunction
ALS 2 (2q33.2)	*ALSIN*	AR	AAO: juvenile; Onset: LL, UL; Progression: slow; UMN dominant > UMN + LMN	None	PLS, IAHSP
ALS 3 (18q21)	UN	AD	N/A	N/A	N/A
ALS 4 (9q34)	*SETX*	AD	AAO: juvenile > adult; Onset: LL > UL; Progression: slow; UMN + LMN > LMN dominant	None	AOA2, cerebellar ataxia, motor neuropathy
ALS 5 (15q21.1)	*SPG11*	AR	AAO: juvenile > adult; Onset: bulbar, limb; Progression: slow; UMN dominant > UMN + LMN	Rare	HSP, autonomic dysfunction, mental retardation
ALS 6 (16q11.2)	*FUS*	AD; AR; De novo	AAO: adult > juvenile; Onset: UL, bulbar > LL; Progression: rapid > slow; UMN + LMN > LMN dominant	Rare	PMA, Parkinsonism, essential tremor, mental retardation
ALS 7 (20p13)	UN	AD	N/A	N/A	N/A
ALS 8 (20q13.3)	*VAPB*	AD	AAO: adult > juvenile; Onset: limb; Progression: slow; LMN dominant	None	SMA, motor neuropathy, autonomic dysfunction
ALS 9 (14q11.2)	*ANG*	AD	AAO: adult > juvenile; Onset: limb, bulbar; Progression: N/A; UMN + LMN	Yes	PBP, PD
ALS 10 (1p36.22)	*TARDBP*	AD; AR	AAO: adult; Onset: limb, bulbar; Progression: variable; UMN + LMN	Yes	PSP, FTD with Parkinsonism, PD, chorea
ALS 11 (6q21)	*FIG4*	AD	AAO: adult; Onset: bulbar > limb; Progression: variable; UMN + LMN > UMN dominant	None	CMT4J, HSP, PLS, Yunis–Varon syndrome, epilepsy with polymicrogyria
ALS 12 (10p13)	*OPTN*	AD; AR	AAO: adult; Onset: bulbar, limb; Progression: slow; UMN + LMN	Yes	POAG, Parkinsonism, aphasia
ALS 13 (12q24)	*ATXN2*	AD	AAO: adult > juvenile; Onset: UL, LL; Progression: variable; UMN + LMN	None	SCA2, Parkinsonism
ALS 14 (9p13)	*VCP*	AD	AAO: adult > juvenile; Onset: limb > bulbar; Progression: variable; UMN + LMN	Yes	IBMPFD
ALS 15 (Xp11.21)	*UBQLN2*	XD	AAO: adult > juvenile; Onset: limb, bulbar; Progression: variable; UMN + LMN > UMN dominant	Yes	PLS
ALS 16 (9p13.3)	*SIGMAR1*	AD	AAO: juvenile; Onset: LL > UL; Progression: N/A; UMN + LMN	Rare	motor neuropathy
ALS 17 (3p12.1)	*CHMP2B*	AD	AAO: adult; Onset: bulbar, limb; Progression: N/A; UMN + LMN > LMN dominant	Yes	PMA; Parkinsonism
ALS 18 (17p13.2)	*PFN1*	AD	AAO: adult; Onset: limb; Progression: N/A; UMN + LMN	None	N/A
ALS 19 (2q33.3-q34)	*ERBB4*	AD	AAO: adult; Onset: UL, bulbar; Progression: slow; UMN + LMN	None	N/A
ALS 20 (12q13.1)	*hnRNPA1*	AD	AAO: adult; Onset: N/A; Progression: N/A; UMN + LMN > LMN dominant	Yes	multisystem proteinopathy
ALS 21	*MATR3*	AD	AAO: adult; Onset: bulbar, limb;	Yes	distal myopathy

Table 1 Different subtypes of familial ALS and their genotype–phenotype correlations *(Continued)*

(5q31.3)			Progression: slow; UMN + LMN > LMN dominant		
ALS-FTD	*C9ORF72*	AD	AAO: adult; Onset: bulbar, limb;	Yes	Parkinsonism, cerebellar ataxia
(9p21.2)			Progression: rapid > slow; UMN + LMN		

Abbreviations: AAO age at onset, *AD* autosomal dominant, *ALS* amyotrophic lateral sclerosis, *AOA2* ataxia and oculomotor apraxia type 2, *AR* autosomal recessive, *BFA* benign focal amyotrophy, *CMT4J* Charcot-Marie-Tooth disease, *FTD* frontotemporal dementia, *HSP* hereditary spastic paraplegia, *IAHSP* infantile-onset ascending hereditary spastic paralysis, *IBMPFD* inclusion body myopathy with Paget's disease and frontotemporal dementia, *LL* lower limb, *LMN* lower motor neuron, *N/A* not available, *PBP* progressive bulbar palsy, *PD* Parkinson's disease, *PLS* primary lateral sclerosis, *PMA* progressive muscular atrophy, *POAG* primary open angle glaucoma, *PSP* progressive supranuclear palsy, *SCA2* spinocerebellar ataxia 2, *UL* upper limb, *UMN* upper motor neuron; *UN* unknown, *XD* X-linked dominant

[14]. Another novel p.T137A mutation identified in two unrelated Italian families, however, causes a very slow progression of ALS [26, 27].

ALS2: Alsin

Mutations in *ALS2* are responsible for autosomal recessive, early-onset forms of upper motor neuron diseases, such as infantile ascending hereditary spastic paraplegia (IAHSP) and juvenile primary lateral sclerosis (PLS) [28, 29]. To date, more than 50 patients with early onset (~1 year) of the disease have been reported to harbor *Alsin* mutations [18]. In the typical adult onset ALS, *Alsin* gene is rarely mutated [30]. Recently, a novel splice-site mutation (c.3512 + 1G > A) in *Alsin* was identified in a consanguineous JALS family with early onset anarthria and generalized dystonia [31].

ALS4: senataxin (SETX)

ALS4 is a rare autosomal dominant form of juvenile-onset ALS due to mutations in *SETX* [32]. It is characterized by slowly evolving distal muscle weakness and atrophy, pyramidal signs, and sparing of bulbar and respiratory muscles [33]. In some cases, normal lifespan or atypical features are also described [34, 35]. A patient with *SETX* p.R2136C mutation presented with coexistence of ALS and inflammatory radiculoneuropathy [36]. We previously reported a missense mutation p.T1118I in a sporadic Chinese ALS patient who developed bulbar symptoms 3 years after the onset, and respiratory failure 2 years later [37]. In addition, recessive *SETX* mutations are reported to cause ataxia and oculomotor apraxia type 2 (AOA2) [38, 39].

ALS5: spatacsin (SPG11)

SPG11 mutations were recently identified in several juvenile-onset ALS cases, with autosomal recessive inheritance and AAO ranging from 7 to 23 years [18, 40]. Generally, the *SPG11*-associated ALS showed a slow progression and in some cases apparent UMN involvement [41]. In addition to ALS phenotype, mutations in *SPG11* also cause hereditary spastic paraplegia (HSP) with thin corpus callosum [42].

ALS6: FUS

Mutations in *FUS* gene have emerged as the second most common cause of ALS, accounting for about 3 ~ 5 % FALS and ~1 % SALS [43, 44]. Up to now, more than 60 mutations in *FUS* have been identified in ALS cases (http://www.hgmd.org, accessed in March, 2015). Among these mutations, the majority are clustered in exon 15 which encode the C-terminus of the protein, and the most common one is p.R521C [15]. The inheritance is autosomal dominant aside from an autosomal recessive p.H517Q mutation and several *de novo* mutations [44].

The phenotypes associated with *FUS* mutations include adult-onset ALS, JALS, ALS-FTD, and rarely pure FTD [45]. Although most patients carrying *FUS* mutations exhibit a classical ALS phenotype without cognitive impairment, the clinical course of these ALS cases are diverse, even among carriers of the same mutations. Compared to *SOD1* patients, *FUS*-related ALS have an earlier AAO, more frequent bulbar disease, and a more rapid progression [46]. Some *FUS* mutations are also observed in patients with juvenile-onset ALS with AAO younger than 25 years [47, 48]. Atypical features such as ALS with mental retardation, ALS with parkinsonism and dementia [46], and essential tremor were seen in some patients with *FUS* mutations [49].

ALS8: vesicle associated membrane protein B (VAPB)

VAPB mutation was firstly described in several Brazilian families with motor neuron degeneration of various patterns: late-onset spinal muscular atrophy, atypical ALS, or typical ALS [50]. Subsequently, five other point mutations and a small deletion were described. Overall, *VAPB* mutations are extremely rare in FALS. The phenotype-genotype correlation remains largely undetermined so far.

ALS9: angiogenin (ANG)

The role of *ANG* mutations in ALS remains ambiguous. Approximate 30 *ANG* mutations have been reported in ALS, but only the p.K17II mutation is shown to co-segregate with the disease [51]. Mutations in *ANG* account for a small fraction of ALS cases. A few FALS cases are identified to have concomitant *ANG* mutations with *FUS* [52] or *SOD1* [53] mutations. In addition, some *ANG* mutations are detected in healthy controls [54]. A subset of *ANG* mutation carriers showed cognitive impairment suggestive of FTD [55], or Parkinson's disease (PD) [56].

ALS10: TARDBP

Mutations in *TARDBP* encoding TDP-43 account for 4 % of FALS cases and ~1 % of SALS [57, 58]. More than 50 mutations have been identified so far (http://www.hgmd.org, accessed in March, 2015), mostly clustered in the C-terminal region encoded by exon 6 of *TARDBP*. Mutations in *TARDBP* are predominantly missense with an autosomal dominant inheritance. Although *TARDBP* mutations are detected in ALS cases worldwide, some regional diversity does exist. For instance, the p.A382T mutation has been found in 28.7 % of all ALS cases in Sardinia [59].

Patients with *TARDBP* mutations usually exhibit a typical ALS phenotype, with limb or bulbar onset, variable disease course, and no overt dementia [60]. It is reported that the *TARDBP*–linked ALS has a trend for earlier AAO, more upper limb onset, and a longer duration, compared to SALS patients [52, 61]. However, we previously reported a *TARDBP* p.S292N mutation in a FALS case who developed dysarthria, dysphagia, and atrophy of lingual muscle at the age of 64 years [62]. The progression of ALS in this case seemed to be rapid. Other phenotypes associated with T*ARDBP* mutations include FTD [63], ALS-FTD [64], ALS with extrapyramidal signs [65], FTD with parkinsonism [66], and PD [67].

ALS11: factor induced gene 4 (FIG4)

FIG4 was previously implicated in Charcot-Marie-Tooth disease type 4J (CMT4J) [68]. Later, *FIG4* mutations were found in autosomal dominant FALS and SALS cases [69]. However, ALS was a rare phenotype of *FIG4* gene. The other phenotypes associated with *FIG4* mutations include PLS [69], Yunis–Varon syndrome [70], and familial epilepsy with polymicrogyria [71].

ALS12: optineurin (OPTN)

Previously identified as the cause of primary open angle glaucoma (POAG) [72], mutations in *OPTN* have been found in both FALS and SALS cases in either a dominant or recessive manner [73]. Although *OPTN* mutations are relatively common in Japan ALS cases [73, 74], they are rare in Caucasian patients [75, 76]. The *OPTN*-related ALS showed relatively slow progression and long duration before respiratory dysfunction [73]. In addition to ALS phenotype, some patients with *OPTN* mutations present with extrapyramidal symptoms, aphasia, or FTD [77, 78].

ALS13: Ataxin-2 (ATXN2)

Long (more than 33) CAG repeat expansion in *ATXN2* gene has been identified as a cause of spinocerebellar ataxia type 2 (SCA2) [79]. Recent studies demonstrated that intermediate expansion (27 ~ 33 repeats) of *ATXN2* was a significant risk factor for ALS [80–82]. However, whether the clinical features of ALS can be affected by *ATXN2* intermediate repeats is still controversial, because no correlation between *ATXN2* repeat length and AAO or survival was observed [83]. A few case reports have described motor neuron degeneration in SCA2 families, raising the possibility that motor neuron involvement is part of SCA2 [84, 85].

ALS14: Valosin-containing protein (VCP)

The gene of *VCP* is known to be mutated in inclusion body myopathy with Paget disease of bone and frontotemporal dementia (IBMPFD) [86]. Recently, mutations in *VCP* were identified in patients with FALS or SALS [87]. Actually, *VCP* mutations are not a major cause of ALS. Although more than 38 mutations in *VCP* have been discovered (http://www.hgmd.org, accessed in March, 2015), only a few of them are responsible for ALS. The phenotype of patients with *VCP* mutations shows intra-familial variations from IBMPFD to FALS [88], or from ALS to FTD or ALS-FTD [87].

ALS15: ubiquilin 2 (UBQLN2)

Mutations in *UBQLN2* were recently identified in X-linked dominant FALS [89]. However, *UBQLN2* mutations are not a frequent cause of ALS [90]. In the affected cases, incomplete penetrance has been noted in females [89]. The predominant phenotype associated with *UBQLN2* mutations is ALS, although several patients have concomitant symptoms of FTD [10]. The AAO has been reported to be significantly younger in males than in females, presumably because males are hemizygous but females are heterozygous for the mutation [89].

ALS16: sigma non-opioid intracellular receptor 1 (SIGMAR1)

SIGMAR1 mutations were recently identified in families affected with juvenile ALS [91] or ALS with dementia [92]. However, these findings have not been replicated by other groups, suggesting that *SIGMAR1* is a rare causative gene of ALS. Recently a splice-site mutation (c.151 + 1G > T) in *SIGMAR1* was reported to cause autosomal recessive distal hereditary motor neuropathy in a consanguineous Chinese family [93].

ALS17: chromatin modifying protein 2B (CHMP2B)

Mutations in the *CHMP2B* gene were initially identified in patients with FTD [94] and then identified in patients with ALS [95, 96]. Since only several ALS cases with *CHMP2B* mutations were reported, there was no characteristic ALS clinical subtype associated with these patients. In addition, *CHMP2B* mutation (p.R69Q) was also identified in progressive muscular atrophy (PMA) [96].

ALS18: profilin 1 (PFN1)

Missense mutations in *PFN1* are firstly reported in two large ALS families and 7 FALS patients [97]. Later, screenings of sizeable ALS and FTD cohorts from diverse populations demonstrated that *PFN1* mutations are a rare cause of ALS [98–100]. The reported cases with *PFN1* mutations seem to present classical ALS with limb onset and no evidence of FTD [97, 99, 101].

ALS19: erb-b2 receptor tyrosine kinase 4 (ERBB4)

Recently, *ERBB4* was identified a causative gene of FALS19, which was characterized by typical, slowly progressive ALS and a lack of obvious cognitive dysfunction [102]. However, this finding has not been replicated by other groups. The genotype-phenotype correlations are thus not determined.

ALS20: heterogeneous nuclear ribonucleoprotein A1 (hnRNPA1)

Mutations in *hnRNPA1* gene were recently identified in patients presenting with ALS and/or multisystem proteinopathy (MSP) [103]. However, subsequent studies failed to identify *hnRNPA1* mutations in patients with ALS, FTD, or MSP [103–105]. The associations of ALS with *hnRNPA1* mutations are still controversial.

ALS21: matrin-3 (MATR3)

Several mutations in *MATR3* were recently reported to cause ALS [106]. Later, a heterozygous *MATR3* p.A72T mutation was identified in a sporadic ALS patient with bulbar onset [107]. In another study, 2 splicing variants and a missense mutation were identified in 3 ALS cases with AAO ranging from 58 to 79 years, and bulbar onset in 2 cases [108].

ALS-FTD: C9ORF72

In 2011, two independent groups reported that the massive GGGGCC hexanucleotide repeat expansion in the non-coding regions of *C9ORF72* gene caused chromosome 9p-linked ALS and FTD [109, 110]. Currently, *C9ORF72* repeat expansions have become the most frequently genetic cause of FALS and familial FTD, accounting for about 40 and 25 % of the cases, respectively [13]. In families with ALS-FTD, the frequency reaches to 50–72 % [19]. Notwithstanding, the mutations seem to be geographically clustered, accounting for one third of FALS cases in Europe and North America, but a small percentage in Asian populations. Haplotype analysis indicates that a common European founder appears to be responsible for all cases [111].

The *C9ORF72* repeat expansions are associated with various phenotypes, including typical ALS, PMA, PLS, ALS-FTD, and pure FTD [44]. In patients with *C9ORF72* mutations, bulbar onset and cognitive impairment seems to be more frequent, and median survival is relatively lower than in patients carrying *TARDBP* or *SOD1* mutations [19]. However, there is no association between the repeat length and disease phenotype or AAO in *C9ORF72* mutation carriers [112]. In addition, the *C9ORF72* expansions also underlie a small portion of other neurological diseases, such as Alzheimer's disease (AD) [113], Huntington's disease (HD) [114], and PD [115].

Other genes implicated in ALS

Several other genes are also implicated in ALS. *DCTN1* mutations were first identified in a family affected with LMN disease [116] and soon identified in several ALS families [117, 118]. Subsequently, a cluster of *DCTN1* mutations were identified in pedigrees with Perry syndrome [119], PD [120] or progressive supranuclear paralysis (PSP) [121], suggestive of phenotypic variability of *DCTN1* mutations. Mutations in *SQSTM1* were initially identified as a cause of Paget disease of bone (PDB) [122]. Recently, *SQSTM1* mutations were identified in ALS [123, 124] as well as FTD [125]. It is speculated that *SQSTM1* mutations are mainly associated with late-onset SALS, because the number of early-onset patients with *SQSTM1* mutations is much less than that of late-onset patients with *SQSTM1* mutations [126].

In addition, mutations in several other genes such as *DAO*, *UNC13A*, *NEFH*, *PRPH*, *TAF15*, and *ELP3*, have been reported as rare causes of ALS. For some genes, there are no additional reports about the mutations as a cause of ALS since the initial publications. Therefore, the evidence supporting a causative role of ALS is not fully convincing.

Implication of the genotype-phenotype correlations

There is no a standard procedure to test the causative mutation in cases with ALS. Many factors should be considered, such as AAO, clinical features, progression, FTD involvement, inheritance manner, and even ethnicity. In this review, we summarized the possible genotype-phenotype correlations of ALS with the aim of providing some clue to improve the clinical decision. Here, we provided a flow diagram of genetic screening strategy in cases diagnosed with ALS (Fig. 1). AAO is an importance factor for the genetic investigations and can be divided into juvenile onset and adult onset. Juvenile

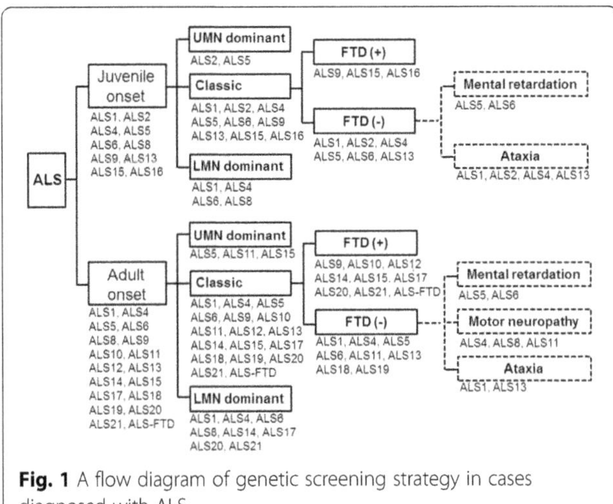

Fig. 1 A flow diagram of genetic screening strategy in cases diagnosed with ALS

onset is usually present in ALS1, ALS2, ALS4, ALS5, ALS6, ALS8, ALS9, ALS13, ALS15, and ALS16. For these cases with juvenile onset and UMN dominant symptoms, *Alsin*, *SPG11*, *SIGMAR1*, or *UBQLN2* might be a causative gene. In contrast, *FUS*, *VAPB*, *SOD1*, and *SETX* should be considered in cases with juvenile onset and LMN dominant phenotype. For these cases with juvenile onset and FTD symptoms, *ANG*, *UBQLN2*, and *SIGMAR1* can be investigated. In addition, *SPG11* and *FUS* can be sequenced in cases who also present mental retardation, while *SOD1*, *Alsin*, *SETX*, *ATXN2* can be considered in those cases with coexistence of cerebellar ataxia.

In cases with adult-onset ALS, many genes should be considered. Although the majority exhibit typical ALS features with both UMN and LMN symptoms, a fraction of cases present either UMN dominant symptoms or LMN dominant symptoms. *SPG11*, *FIG4*, *UBQLN2* may be mutated in cases with UMN dominant symptoms. In these cases with LMN dominant symptoms, mutations in *SOD1*, *SETX*, *FUS*, VAPB, *VCP*, *CHMP2B*, *hnRNPA1*, or *MATR3* might be identified. Presence of FTD hints possible mutations in *ANG*, *TARDBP*, *OPTN*, *VCP*, *UBQLN2*, *CHMP2B*, *hnRNPA1*, *MATR3*, or *C9ORF72*. Motor neuropathy involvement might occur in cases with mutations in *SETX*, *VAPB*, or *FIG4*. Complications of ataxia may be seen in cases with *SOD1* or *ATXN2* mutations.

Inheritance pattern also provides critical information as to the potential involvement of one or other specific genes in ALS. However, the diverse clinical features between intra-familial cases or a deceased parent at a young age may results in the appearance of "lack of familial history" in some cases. The presentation of ALS or FTD in first-degree relatives and the co-occurrence of ALS with FTD in some patients with ALS supported a positive family history. In addition, ethnic background should be considered when determining which genes are most likely. For example, *C9ORF72* has been regarded as the most common cause of ALS in Caucasians, but very rare in Asian population.

Conclusions

Here, we outline the genotype-phenotype correlations of ALS. We hope this review is helpful for detecting the causative mutation in cases with ALS. Although a number of genes have been reported, many ALS cases still do not carry any mutation in the aforementioned genes. Other more genes might be identified as causative genes of ALS in the future.

Abbreviations

AAO: age at onset; AD: Alzheimer's disease; ALS: amyotrophic lateral sclerosis; ANG: angiogenin; AOA2: oculomotor apraxia type 2; ATXN2: ataxin-2; C9ORF72: chromosome 9 open reading frame 72; CMT4J: Charcot-Marie-Tooth disease; DCTN1: dynactin; ERBB4: erb-b2 receptor tyrosine kinase 4; FALS: familial amyotrophic lateral sclerosis; FIG4: factor induced gene 4; FTD: frontal temporal dementia; FUS: fused in sarcoma; HD: Huntington's disease; hnRNPA1: heterogeneous nuclear ribonucleoprotein A1; HSP: hereditary spastic paraplegia; IAHSP: infantile-onset ascending hereditary spastic paralysis; IBMPFD: inclusion body myopathy with Paget disease of bone and frontotemporal dementia; JALS: juvenile amyotrophic lateral sclerosis; LMN: lower motor neuron; MATR3: matrin-3; MSP: multisystem proteinopathy; OPTN: optineurin; PD: Parkinson's disease; PDB: Paget disease of bone; PFN1: profilin 1; PLS: juvenile primary lateral sclerosis; PMA: progressive muscular atrophy; PSP: progressive supranuclear paralysis; SALS: sporadic amyotrophic lateral sclerosis; SCA: spinocerebellar ataxia; SETX: senataxin; SIGMAR1: sigma non-opioid intracellular receptor 1; SOD1: superoxide dismutase 1; SPG11: spatacsin; SQSTM1: sequestosome 1; TARDBP: TAR DNA-binding protein; UBQLN2: ubiquilin 2; UMN: upper motor neuron; VAPB: vesicle associated membrane protein B.

Competing interests

The authors declare that they have no competing interests.

Authors' contributions

L-HF drafted and W-ZY critically revised the manuscript. Both authors read and approved the final manuscript.

Acknowledgements

This work was supported by grants from the National Natural Science Foundation to Zhi-Ying Wu (81125009, Beijing).

References

1. Logroscino G, Traynor BJ, Hardiman O, Chio A, Mitchell D, Swingler RJ, et al. Incidence of amyotrophic lateral sclerosis in Europe. J Neurol Neurosurg Psychiatry. 2010;81:385–90.
2. Sathasivam S. Motor neurone disease: clinical features, diagnosis, diagnostic pitfalls and prognostic markers. Singapore Med J. 2010;51:367–72. quiz 73.
3. Finsterer J, Burgunder JM. Recent progress in the genetics of motor neuron disease. Eur J Med Genet. 2014;57:103–12.
4. Forbes RB, Colville S, Swingler RJ. The epidemiology of amyotrophic lateral sclerosis (ALS/MND) in people aged 80 or over. Age Ageing. 2004;33:131–4.
5. Gouveia LO, de Carvalho M. Young-onset sporadic amyotrophic lateral sclerosis: a distinct nosological entity? Amyotroph Lateral Scler. 2007;8:323–7.
6. McCombe PA, Henderson RD. Effects of gender in amyotrophic lateral sclerosis. Gend Med. 2010;7:557–70.
7. Kiernan MC, Vucic S, Cheah BC, Turner MR, Eisen A, Hardiman O, et al. Amyotrophic lateral sclerosis. Lancet. 2011;377:942–55.

8. Ringholz GM, Appel SH, Bradshaw M, Cooke NA, Mosnik DM, Schulz PE. Prevalence and patterns of cognitive impairment in sporadic ALS. Neurology. 2005;65:586–90.
9. Burrell JR, Kiernan MC, Vucic S, Hodges JR. Motor neuron dysfunction in frontotemporal dementia. Brain. 2011;134:2582–94.
10. Renton AE, Chio A, Traynor BJ. State of play in amyotrophic lateral sclerosis genetics. Nat Neurosci. 2014;17:17–23.
11. Al-Chalabi A, Hardiman O. The epidemiology of ALS: a conspiracy of genes, environment and time. Nat Rev Neurol. 2013;9:617–28.
12. Deng HX, Hentati A, Tainer JA, Iqbal Z, Cayabyab A, Hung WY, et al. Amyotrophic lateral sclerosis and structural defects in Cu, Zn superoxide dismutase. Science. 1993;261:1047–51.
13. Baumer D, Talbot K, Turner MR. Advances in motor neurone disease. J R Soc Med. 2014;107:14–21.
14. Tortelli R, Conforti FL, Cortese R, D'Errico E, Distaso E, Mazzei R, et al. Amyotrophic lateral sclerosis: a new missense mutation in the SOD1 gene. Neurobiol Aging. 2013;1709(34):e3–5.
15. Andersen PM, Al-Chalabi A. Clinical genetics of amyotrophic lateral sclerosis: what do we really know? Nature reviews. Neurology. 2011;7:603–15.
16. Jonsson PA, Backstrand A, Andersen PM, Jacobsson J, Parton M, Shaw C, et al. CuZn-superoxide dismutase in D90A heterozygotes from recessive and dominant ALS pedigrees. Neurobiol Dis. 2002;10:327–33.
17. Saeed M, Yang Y, Deng HX, Hung WY, Siddique N, Dellefave L, et al. Age and founder effect of SOD1 A4V mutation causing ALS. Neurology. 2009;72:1634–9.
18. Yamashita S, Ando Y. Genotype-phenotype relationship in hereditary amyotrophic lateral sclerosis. Transl Neurodegener. 2015;4:13.
19. Sabatelli M, Conte A, Zollino M. Clinical and genetic heterogeneity of amyotrophic lateral sclerosis. Clin Genet. 2013;83:408–16.
20. Andersen PM, Forsgren L, Binzer M, Nilsson P, Ala-Hurula V, Keranen ML, et al. Autosomal recessive adult-onset amyotrophic lateral sclerosis associated with homozygosity for Asp90Ala CuZn-superoxide dismutase mutation. A clinical and genealogical study of 36 patients. Brain. 1996;119(Pt 4):1153–72.
21. Parton MJ, Broom W, Andersen PM, Al-Chalabi A, Nigel Leigh P, Powell JF, et al. D90A-SOD1 mediated amyotrophic lateral sclerosis: a single founder for all cases with evidence for a Cis-acting disease modifier in the recessive haplotype. Hum Mutat. 2002;20:473.
22. Robberecht W, Aguirre T, Van den Bosch L, Tilkin P, Cassiman JJ, Matthijs G. D90A heterozygosity in the SOD1 gene is associated with familial and apparently sporadic amyotrophic lateral sclerosis. Neurology. 1996;47:1336–9.
23. Juneja T, Pericak-Vance MA, Laing NG, Dave S, Siddique T. Prognosis in familial amyotrophic lateral sclerosis: progression and survival in patients with glu100gly and ala4val mutations in Cu, Zn superoxide dismutase. Neurology. 1997;48:55–7.
24. Aksoy H, Dean G, Elian M, Deng HX, Deng G, Juneja T, et al. A4T mutation in the SOD1 gene causing familial amyotrophic lateral sclerosis. Neuroepidemiology. 2003;22:235–8.
25. Niu YF, Xiong HL, Wu JJ, Chen Y, Qiao K, Wu ZY. [Screening of mutations in SOD1 gene and analysis of genotype-phenotype correlation in Chinese patients with amyotrophic lateral sclerosis]. Yi chuan = Hereditas / Zhongguo yi chuan xue hui bian ji. 2011;33:720–4.
26. Origone P, Caponnetto C, Verdiani S, Mantero V, Cichero E, Fossa P, et al. T137A variant is a pathogenetic SOD1 mutation associated with a slowly progressive ALS phenotype. Amyotroph Lateral Scler. 2012;13:398–9.
27. Visani M, de Biase D, Bartolomei I, Plasmati R, Morandi L, Cenacchi G, et al. A novel T137A SOD1 mutation in an Italian family with two subjects affected by amyotrophic lateral sclerosis. Amyotroph Lateral Scler. 2011;12:385–8.
28. Hadano S, Hand CK, Osuga H, Yanagisawa Y, Otomo A, Devon RS, et al. A gene encoding a putative GTPase regulator is mutated in familial amyotrophic lateral sclerosis 2. Nat Genet. 2001;29:166–73.
29. Eymard-Pierre E, Lesca G, Dollet S, Santorelli FM, di Capua M, Bertini E, et al. Infantile-onset ascending hereditary spastic paralysis is associated with mutations in the alsin gene. Am J Hum Genet. 2002;71:518–27.
30. Hand CK, Devon RS, Gros-Louis F, Rochefort D, Khoris J, Meininger V, et al. Mutation screening of the ALS2 gene in sporadic and familial amyotrophic lateral sclerosis. Arch Neurol. 2003;60:1768–71.
31. Siddiqi S, Foo JN, Vu A, Azim S, Silver DL, Mansoor A, et al. A novel splice-site mutation in ALS2 establishes the diagnosis of juvenile amyotrophic lateral sclerosis in a family with early onset anarthria and generalized dystonias. PLoS One. 2014;9:e113258.
32. Chen YZ, Bennett CL, Huynh HM, Blair IP, Puls I, Irobi J, et al. DNA/RNA helicase gene mutations in a form of juvenile amyotrophic lateral sclerosis (ALS4). Am J Hum Genet. 2004;74:1128–35.
33. Hirano M, Quinzii CM, Mitsumoto H, Hays AP, Roberts JK, Richard P, et al. Senataxin mutations and amyotrophic lateral sclerosis. Amyotroph Lateral Scler. 2011;12:223–7.
34. Pasinelli P, Brown RH. Molecular biology of amyotrophic lateral sclerosis: insights from genetics. Nat Rev Neurosci. 2006;7:710–23.
35. Rabin BA, Griffin JW, Crain BJ, Scavina M, Chance PF, Cornblath DR. Autosomal dominant juvenile amyotrophic lateral sclerosis. Brain. 1999;122(Pt 8):1539–50.
36. Saiga T, Tateishi T, Torii T, Kawamura N, Nagara Y, Shigeto H, et al. Inflammatory radiculoneuropathy in an ALS4 patient with a novel SETX mutation. J Neurol Neurosurg Psychiatry. 2012;83:763–4.
37. Zhao ZH, Chen WZ, Wu ZY, Wang N, Zhao GX, Chen WJ, et al. A novel mutation in the senataxin gene identified in a Chinese patient with sporadic amyotrophic lateral sclerosis. Amyotroph Lateral Scler. 2009;10:118–22.
38. Chen YZ, Hashemi SH, Anderson SK, Huang Y, Moreira MC, Lynch DR, et al. Senataxin, the yeast Sen1p orthologue: characterization of a unique protein in which recessive mutations cause ataxia and dominant mutations cause motor neuron disease. Neurobiol Dis. 2006;23:97–108.
39. Moreira MC, Klur S, Watanabe M, Nemeth AH, Le Ber I, Moniz JC, et al. Senataxin, the ortholog of a yeast RNA helicase, is mutant in ataxia-ocular apraxia 2. Nat Genet. 2004;36:225–7.
40. Orlacchio A, Babalini C, Borreca A, Patrono C, Massa R, Basaran S, et al. SPATACSIN mutations cause autosomal recessive juvenile amyotrophic lateral sclerosis. Brain. 2010;133:591–8.
41. Iguchi Y, Katsuno M, Ikenaka K, Ishigaki S, Sobue G. Amyotrophic lateral sclerosis: an update on recent genetic insights. J Neurol. 2013;260:2917–27.
42. Paisan-Ruiz C, Dogu O, Yilmaz A, Houlden H, Singleton A. SPG11 mutations are common in familial cases of complicated hereditary spastic paraplegia. Neurology. 2008;70:1384–9.
43. Polymenidou M, Lagier-Tourenne C, Hutt KR, Bennett CF, Cleveland DW, Yeo GW. Misregulated RNA processing in amyotrophic lateral sclerosis. Brain Res. 2012;1462:3–15.
44. Boylan K. Familial Amyotrophic Lateral Sclerosis. Neurol Clin. 2015;33:807–30.
45. Deng H, Gao K, Jankovic J. The role of FUS gene variants in neurodegenerative diseases. Nat Rev Neurol. 2014;10:337–48.
46. Yan J, Deng HX, Siddique N, Fecto F, Chen W, Yang Y, et al. Frameshift and novel mutations in FUS in familial amyotrophic lateral sclerosis and ALS/dementia. Neurology. 2010;75:807–14.
47. Baumer D, Hilton D, Paine SM, Turner MR, Lowe J, Talbot K, et al. Juvenile ALS with basophilic inclusions is a FUS proteinopathy with FUS mutations. Neurology. 2010;75:611–8.
48. Munoz DG. FUS mutations in sporadic juvenile ALS: another step toward understanding ALS pathogenesis. Neurology. 2010;75:584–5.
49. Merner ND, Girard SL, Catoire H, Bourassa CV, Belzil VV, Riviere JB, et al. Exome sequencing identifies FUS mutations as a cause of essential tremor. Am J Hum Genet. 2012;91:313–9.
50. Nishimura AL, Mitne-Neto M, Silva HC, Richieri-Costa A, Middleton S, Cascio D, et al. A mutation in the vesicle-trafficking protein VAPB causes late-onset spinal muscular atrophy and amyotrophic lateral sclerosis. Am J Hum Genet. 2004;75:822–31.
51. van Es MA, Diekstra FP, Veldink JH, Baas F, Bourque PR, Schelhaas HJ, et al. A case of ALS-FTD in a large FALS pedigree with a K17I ANG mutation. Neurology. 2009;72:287–8.
52. Millecamps S, Salachas F, Cazeneuve C, Gordon P, Bricka B, Camuzat A, et al. SOD1, ANG, VAPB, TARDBP, and FUS mutations in familial amyotrophic lateral sclerosis: genotype-phenotype correlations. J Med Genet. 2010;47: 554–60.
53. Luigetti M, Lattante S, Zollino M, Conte A, Marangi G, Del Grande A, et al. SOD1 G93D sporadic amyotrophic lateral sclerosis (SALS) patient with rapid progression and concomitant novel ANG variant. Neurobiol Aging. 2011;1924(32):e15–8.
54. Gellera C, Colombrita C, Ticozzi N, Castellotti B, Bragato C, Ratti A, et al. Identification of new ANG gene mutations in a large cohort of Italian patients with amyotrophic lateral sclerosis. Neurogenetics. 2008;9:33–40.
55. Seilhean D, Cazeneuve C, Thuries V, Russaouen O, Millecamps S, Salachas F, et al. Accumulation of TDP-43 and alpha-actin in an amyotrophic lateral sclerosis patient with the K17I ANG mutation. Acta Neuropathol. 2009;118:561–73.

56. van Es MA, Schelhaas HJ, van Vught PW, Ticozzi N, Andersen PM, Groen EJ, et al. Angiogenin variants in Parkinson disease and amyotrophic lateral sclerosis. Ann Neurol. 2011;70:964–73.
57. Millecamps S, Boillee S, Le Ber I, Seilhean D, Teyssou E, Giraudeau M, et al. Phenotype difference between ALS patients with expanded repeats in C9ORF72 and patients with mutations in other ALS-related genes. J Med Genet. 2012;49:258–63.
58. Mackenzie IR, Rademakers R, Neumann M. TDP-43 and FUS in amyotrophic lateral sclerosis and frontotemporal dementia. Lancet Neurol. 2010;9:995–1007.
59. Chio A, Borghero G, Pugliatti M, Ticca A, Calvo A, Moglia C, et al. Large proportion of amyotrophic lateral sclerosis cases in Sardinia due to a single founder mutation of the TARDBP gene. Arch Neurol. 2011;68:594–8.
60. Kirby J, Goodall EF, Smith W, Highley JR, Masanzu R, Hartley JA, et al. Broad clinical phenotypes associated with TAR-DNA binding protein (TARDBP) mutations in amyotrophic lateral sclerosis. Neurogenetics. 2010;11:217–25.
61. Corcia P, Valdmanis P, Millecamps S, Lionnet C, Blasco H, Mouzat K, et al. Phenotype and genotype analysis in amyotrophic lateral sclerosis with TARDBP gene mutations. Neurology. 2012;78:1519–26.
62. Xiong HL, Wang JY, Sun YM, Wu JJ, Chen Y, Qiao K, et al. Association between novel TARDBP mutations and Chinese patients with amyotrophic lateral sclerosis. BMC Med Genet. 2010;11:8.
63. Gitcho MA, Bigio EH, Mishra M, Johnson N, Weintraub S, Mesulam M, et al. TARDBP 3'-UTR variant in autopsy-confirmed frontotemporal lobar degeneration with TDP-43 proteinopathy. Acta Neuropathol. 2009;118:633–45.
64. Benajiba L, Le Ber I, Camuzat A, Lacoste M, Thomas-Anterion C, Couratier P, et al. TARDBP mutations in motoneuron disease with frontotemporal lobar degeneration. Ann Neurol. 2009;65:470–3.
65. Origone P, Caponnetto C, Bandettini Di Poggio M, Ghiglione E, Bellone E, Ferrandes G, et al. Enlarging clinical spectrum of FALS with TARDBP gene mutations: S393L variant in an Italian family showing phenotypic variability and relevance for genetic counselling. Amyotroph Lateral Scler. 2010;11:223–7.
66. Quadri M, Cossu G, Saddi V, Simons EJ, Murgia D, Melis M, et al. Broadening the phenotype of TARDBP mutations: the TARDBP Ala382Thr mutation and Parkinson's disease in Sardinia. Neurogenetics. 2011;12:203–9.
67. Rayaprolu S, Fujioka S, Traynor S, Soto-Ortolaza AI, Petrucelli L, Dickson DW, et al. TARDBP mutations in Parkinson's disease. Parkinsonism Relat Disord. 2013;19:312–5.
68. Chow CY, Zhang Y, Dowling JJ, Jin N, Adamska M, Shiga K, et al. Mutation of FIG4 causes neurodegeneration in the pale tremor mouse and patients with CMT4J. Nature. 2007;448:68–72.
69. Chow CY, Landers JE, Bergren SK, Sapp PC, Grant AE, Jones JM, et al. Deleterious variants of FIG4, a phosphoinositide phosphatase, in patients with ALS. Am J Hum Genet. 2009;84:85–8.
70. Campeau PM, Lenk GM, Lu JT, Bae Y, Burrage L, Turnpenny P, et al. Yunis-Varon syndrome is caused by mutations in FIG4, encoding a phosphoinositide phosphatase. Am J Hum Genet. 2013;92:781–91.
71. Baulac S, Lenk GM, Dufresnois B, Ouled Amar Bencheikh B, Couarch P, Renard J, et al. Role of the phosphoinositide phosphatase FIG4 gene in familial epilepsy with polymicrogyria. Neurology. 2014;82:1068–75.
72. Rezaie T, Child A, Hitchings R, Brice G, Miller L, Coca-Prados M, et al. Adult-onset primary open-angle glaucoma caused by mutations in optineurin. Science. 2002;295:1077–9.
73. Maruyama H, Morino H, Ito H, Izumi Y, Kato H, Watanabe Y, et al. Mutations of optineurin in amyotrophic lateral sclerosis. Nature. 2010;465:223–6.
74. Iida A, Hosono N, Sano M, Kamei T, Oshima S, Tokuda T, et al. Novel deletion mutations of OPTN in amyotrophic lateral sclerosis in Japanese. Neurobiol Aging. 2012;1843(33):e19–24.
75. Johnson L, Miller JW, Gkazi AS, Vance C, Topp SD, Newhouse SJ, et al. Screening for OPTN mutations in a cohort of British amyotrophic lateral sclerosis patients. Neurobiol Aging. 2012;33:2948. e15-7.
76. Millecamps S, Boillee S, Chabrol E, Camu W, Cazeneuve C, Salachas F, et al. Screening of OPTN in French familial amyotrophic lateral sclerosis. Neurobiol Aging. 2011;32:557. e11-3.
77. Kamada M, Izumi Y, Ayaki T, Nakamura M, Kagawa S, Kudo E, et al. Clinicopathologic features of autosomal recessive amyotrophic lateral sclerosis associated with optineurin mutation. Neuropathology. 2014;34:64–70.
78. Weishaupt JH, Waibel S, Birve A, Volk AE, Mayer B, Meyer T, et al. A novel optineurin truncating mutation and three glaucoma-associated missense variants in patients with familial amyotrophic lateral sclerosis in Germany. Neurobiol Aging. 2013;34:1516. e9-15.
79. Imbert G, Saudou F, Yvert G, Devys D, Trottier Y, Garnier JM, et al. Cloning of the gene for spinocerebellar ataxia 2 reveals a locus with high sensitivity to expanded CAG/glutamine repeats. Nat Genet. 1996;14:285–91.
80. Elden AC, Kim HJ, Hart MP, Chen-Plotkin AS, Johnson BS, Fang X, et al. Ataxin-2 intermediate-length polyglutamine expansions are associated with increased risk for ALS. Nature. 2010;466:1069–75.
81. Liu X, Lu M, Tang L, Zhang N, Chui D, Fan D. ATXN2 CAG repeat expansions increase the risk for Chinese patients with amyotrophic lateral sclerosis. Neurobiol Aging. 2013;34:2236. e5-8.
82. Lu HP, Gan SR, Chen S, Li HF, Liu ZJ, Ni W, et al. Intermediate-length polyglutamine in ATXN2 is a possible risk factor among Eastern Chinese patients with amyotrophic lateral sclerosis. Neurobiol Aging. 2014;36:1603.
83. Van Damme P, Veldink JH, van Blitterswijk M, Corveleyn A, van Vught PW, Thijs V, et al. Expanded ATXN2 CAG repeat size in ALS identifies genetic overlap between ALS and SCA2. Neurology. 2011;76:2066–72.
84. Infante J, Berciano J, Volpini V, Corral J, Polo JM, Pascual J, et al. Spinocerebellar ataxia type 2 with Levodopa-responsive parkinsonism culminating in motor neuron disease. Mov Disord. 2004;19:848–52.
85. Nanetti L, Fancellu R, Tomasello C, Gellera C, Pareyson D, Mariotti C. Rare association of motor neuron disease and spinocerebellar ataxia type 2 (SCA2): a new case and review of the literature. J Neurol. 2009;256:1926–8.
86. Watts GD, Wymer J, Kovach MJ, Mehta SG, Mumm S, Darvish D, et al. Inclusion body myopathy associated with Paget disease of bone and frontotemporal dementia is caused by mutant valosin-containing protein. Nat Genet. 2004;36:377–81.
87. Johnson JO, Mandrioli J, Benatar M, Abramzon Y, Van Deerlin VM, Trojanowski JQ, et al. Exome sequencing reveals VCP mutations as a cause of familial ALS. Neuron. 2010;68:857–64.
88. Gonzalez-Perez P, Cirulli ET, Drory VE, Dabby R, Nisipeanu P, Carasso RL, et al. Novel mutation in VCP gene causes atypical amyotrophic lateral sclerosis. Neurology. 2012;79:2201–8.
89. Deng HX, Chen W, Hong ST, Boycott KM, Gorrie GH, Siddique N, et al. Mutations in UBQLN2 cause dominant X-linked juvenile and adult-onset ALS and ALS/dementia. Nature. 2011;477:211–5.
90. Millecamps S, Corcia P, Cazeneuve C, Boillee S, Seilhean D, Danel-Brunaud V, et al. Mutations in UBQLN2 are rare in French amyotrophic lateral sclerosis. Neurobiol Aging. 2012;33:839. e1-3.
91. Al-Saif A, Al-Mohanna F, Bohlega S. A mutation in sigma-1 receptor causes juvenile amyotrophic lateral sclerosis. Ann Neurol. 2011;70:913–9.
92. Belzil W, Daoud H, Camu W, Strong MJ, Dion PA, Rouleau GA. Genetic analysis of SIGMAR1 as a cause of familial ALS with dementia. Eur J Hum Genet. 2013;21:237–9.
93. Li X, Hu Z, Liu L, Xie Y, Zhan Y, Zi X, et al. A SIGMAR1 splice-site mutation causes distal hereditary motor neuropathy. Neurology. 2015;84:2430–7.
94. Skibinski G, Parkinson NJ, Brown JM, Chakrabarti L, Lloyd SL, Hummerich H, et al. Mutations in the endosomal ESCRTIII-complex subunit CHMP2B in frontotemporal dementia. Nat Genet. 2005;37:806–8.
95. Cox LE, Ferraiuolo L, Goodall EF, Heath PR, Higginbottom A, Mortiboys H, et al. Mutations in CHMP2B in lower motor neuron predominant amyotrophic lateral sclerosis (ALS). PLoS One. 2010;5:e9872.
96. van Blitterswijk M, Vlam L, van Es MA, van der Pol WL, Hennekam EA, Dooijes D, et al. Genetic overlap between apparently sporadic motor neuron diseases. PLoS One. 2012;7:e48983.
97. Wu CH, Fallini C, Ticozzi N, Keagle PJ, Sapp PC, Piotrowska K, et al. Mutations in the profilin 1 gene cause familial amyotrophic lateral sclerosis. Nature. 2012;488:499–503.
98. Daoud H, Dobrzeniecka S, Camu W, Meininger V, Dupre N, Dion PA, et al. Mutation analysis of PFN1 in familial amyotrophic lateral sclerosis patients. Neurobiol Aging. 2013;34:1311. e1-2.
99. Ingre C, Landers JE, Rizik N, Volk AE, Akimoto C, Birve A, et al. A novel phosphorylation site mutation in profilin 1 revealed in a large screen of US, Nordic, and German amyotrophic lateral sclerosis/frontotemporal dementia cohorts. Neurobiol Aging. 2013;1708(34):e1–6.
100. Lattante S, Le Ber I, Camuzat A, Brice A, Kabashi E. Mutations in the PFN1 gene are not a common cause in patients with amyotrophic lateral sclerosis and frontotemporal lobar degeneration in France. Neurobiol Aging. 2013;1709(34):e1–2.
101. Smith BN, Vance C, Scotter EL, Troakes C, Wong CH, Topp S, et al. Novel mutations support a role for Profilin 1 in the pathogenesis of ALS. Neurobiol Aging. 2015;1602(36):e17–27.

102. Takahashi Y, Fukuda Y, Yoshimura J, Toyoda A, Kurppa K, Moritoyo H, et al. ERBB4 mutations that disrupt the neuregulin-ErbB4 pathway cause amyotrophic lateral sclerosis type 19. Am J Hum Genet. 2013;93:900–5.
103. Kim HJ, Kim NC, Wang YD, Scarborough EA, Moore J, Diaz Z, et al. Mutations in prion-like domains in hnRNPA2B1 and hnRNPA1 cause multisystem proteinopathy and ALS. Nature. 2013;495:467–73.
104. Seelen M, Visser AE, Overste DJ, Kim HJ, Palud A, Wong TH, et al. No mutations in hnRNPA1 and hnRNPA2B1 in Dutch patients with amyotrophic lateral sclerosis, frontotemporal dementia, and inclusion body myopathy. Neurobiol Aging. 2014;35:1956. e9-56 e11.
105. Le Ber I, Van Bortel I, Nicolas G, Bouya-Ahmed K, Camuzat A, Wallon D, et al. hnRNPA2B1 and hnRNPA1 mutations are rare in patients with "multisystem proteinopathy" and frontotemporal lobar degeneration phenotypes. Neurobiol Aging. 2014;35:934. e5-6.
106. Johnson JO, Pioro EP, Boehringer A, Chia R, Feit H, Renton AE, et al. Mutations in the Matrin 3 gene cause familial amyotrophic lateral sclerosis. Nat Neurosci. 2014;17:664–6.
107. Lin KP, Tsai PC, Liao YC, Chen WT, Tsai CP, Soong BW, et al. Mutational analysis of MATR3 in Taiwanese patients with amyotrophic lateral sclerosis. Neurobiol Aging. 2005;2015(36):e1–4.
108. Leblond CS, Gan-Or Z, Spiegelman D, Laurent SB, Szuto A, Hodgkinson A, et al. Replication study of MATR3 in familial and sporadic amyotrophic lateral sclerosis. Neurobiol Aging. 2015;37:209.
109. DeJesus-Hernandez M, Mackenzie IR, Boeve BF, Boxer AL, Baker M, Rutherford NJ, et al. Expanded GGGGCC hexanucleotide repeat in noncoding region of C9ORF72 causes chromosome 9p-linked FTD and ALS. Neuron. 2011;72:245–56.
110. Renton AE, Majounie E, Waite A, Simon-Sanchez J, Rollinson S, Gibbs JR, et al. A hexanucleotide repeat expansion in C9ORF72 is the cause of chromosome 9p21-linked ALS-FTD. Neuron. 2011;72:257–68.
111. Smith BN, Newhouse S, Shatunov A, Vance C, Topp S, Johnson L, et al. The C9ORF72 expansion mutation is a common cause of ALS+/−FTD in Europe and has a single founder. Eur J Hum Genet. 2013;21:102–8.
112. Rutherford NJ, Heckman MG, Dejesus-Hernandez M, Baker MC, Soto-Ortolaza AI, Rayaprolu S, et al. Length of normal alleles of C9ORF72 GGGGCC repeat do not influence disease phenotype. Neurobiol Aging. 2012;33:2950. e5-7.
113. Majounie E, Abramzon Y, Renton AE, Perry R, Bassett SS, Pletnikova O, et al. Repeat expansion in C9ORF72 in Alzheimer's disease. N Engl J Med. 2012;366:283–4.
114. Hensman Moss DJ, Poulter M, Beck J, Hehir J, Polke JM, Campbell T, et al. C9orf72 expansions are the most common genetic cause of Huntington disease phenocopies. Neurology. 2014;82:292–9.
115. Lesage S, Le Ber I, Condroyer C, Broussolle E, Gabelle A, Thobois S, et al. C9orf72 repeat expansions are a rare genetic cause of parkinsonism. Brain. 2013;136:385–91.
116. Puls I, Jonnakuty C, LaMonte BH, Holzbaur EL, Tokito M, Mann E, et al. Mutant dynactin in motor neuron disease. Nat Genet. 2003;33:455–6.
117. Liu ZJ, Li HF, Tan GH, Tao QQ, Ni W, Cheng XW, et al. Identify mutation in amyotrophic lateral sclerosis cases using HaloPlex target enrichment system. Neurobiol Aging. 2014;35:2881. e11-5.
118. Munch C, Rosenbohm A, Sperfeld AD, Uttner I, Reske S, Krause BJ, et al. Heterozygous R1101K mutation of the DCTN1 gene in a family with ALS and FTD. Ann Neurol. 2005;58:777–80.
119. Farrer MJ, Hulihan MM, Kachergus JM, Dachsel JC, Stoessl AJ, Grantier LL, et al. DCTN1 mutations in Perry syndrome. Nat Genet. 2009;41:163–5.
120. Araki E, Tsuboi Y, Daechsel J, Milnerwood A, Vilarino-Guell C, Fujii N, et al. A novel DCTN1 mutation with late-onset parkinsonism and frontotemporal atrophy. Mov Disord. 2014;29:1201–4.
121. Caroppo P, Le Ber I, Clot F, Rivaud-Pechoux S, Camuzat A, De Septenville A, et al. DCTN1 mutation analysis in families with progressive supranuclear palsy-like phenotypes. JAMA Neurol. 2014;71:208–15.
122. Laurin N, Brown JP, Morissette J, Raymond V. Recurrent mutation of the gene encoding sequestosome 1 (SQSTM1/p62) in Paget disease of bone. Am J Hum Genet. 2002;70:1582–8.
123. Fecto F, Yan J, Vemula SP, Liu E, Yang Y, Chen W, et al. SQSTM1 mutations in familial and sporadic amyotrophic lateral sclerosis. Arch Neurol. 2011;68:1440–6.
124. Hirano M, Nakamura Y, Saigoh K, Sakamoto H, Ueno S, Isono C, et al. Mutations in the gene encoding p62 in Japanese patients with amyotrophic lateral sclerosis. Neurology. 2013;80:458–63.
125. Rubino E, Rainero I, Chio A, Rogaeva E, Galimberti D, Fenoglio P, et al. SQSTM1 mutations in frontotemporal lobar degeneration and amyotrophic lateral sclerosis. Neurology. 2012;79:1556–62.
126. Chen Y, Zheng ZZ, Chen X, Huang R, Yang Y, Yuan L, et al. SQSTM1 mutations in Han Chinese populations with sporadic amyotrophic lateral sclerosis. Neurobiol Aging. 2014;35:726. e7-9.

7

Pathological correlations between traumatic brain injury and chronic neurodegenerative diseases

Marcela Cruz-Haces[1†], Jonathan Tang[1†], Glen Acosta[2†], Joseph Fernandez[1] and Riyi Shi[1,2*]

Abstract

Traumatic brain injury is among the most common causes of death and disability in youth and young adults. In addition to the acute risk of morbidity with moderate to severe injuries, traumatic brain injury is associated with a number of chronic neurological and neuropsychiatric sequelae including neurodegenerative diseases such as Alzheimer's disease and Parkinson's disease. However, despite the high incidence of traumatic brain injuries and the established clinical correlation with neurodegeneration, the causative factors linking these processes have not yet been fully elucidated. Apart from removal from activity, few, if any prophylactic treatments against post-traumatic brain injury neurodegeneration exist. Therefore, it is imperative to understand the pathophysiological mechanisms of traumatic brain injury and neurodegeneration in order to identify potential factors that initiate neurodegenerative processes. Oxidative stress, neuroinflammation, and glutamatergic excitotoxicity have previously been implicated in both secondary brain injury and neurodegeneration. In particular, reactive oxygen species appear to be key in mediating molecular insult in neuroinflammation and excitotoxicity. As such, it is likely that post injury oxidative stress is a key mechanism which links traumatic brain injury to increased risk of neurodegeneration. Consequently, reactive oxygen species and their subsequent byproducts may serve as novel fluid markers for identification and monitoring of cellular damage. Furthermore, these reactive species may further serve as a suitable therapeutic target to reduce the risk of post-injury neurodegeneration and provide long term quality of life improvements for those suffering from traumatic brain injury.

Keywords: Traumatic brain injury, Neurodegenerative diseases, Alzheimer's disease, Parkinson's disease, Amyotrophic lateral sclerosis, Oxidative stress, Reactive oxygen species

Background

Traumatic brain injury (TBI) represents one of the most common causes of death and disability in young people [1–3]. About 1.6 million people per year experience traumatic brain injuries in the USA [4, 5]. Besides the initial mechanical damage, TBI can induce a process of secondary injury [6, 7], which can lead to long term neurological and neuropsychiatric sequelae [8, 9], depicting a serious public health problem worldwide [10]. Some of the observed post-TBI sequelae include, but are not limited to, neurodegenerative diseases [11], such as Alzheimer's disease (AD) [12], Parkinson's disease (PD) [13], and amyotrophic lateral sclerosis (ALS) [14].

Importantly, the mechanisms underlying the pathogenesis that lead to such disabilities are still incompletely understood [15, 16]. Therefore, while the post-TBI central nervous system (CNS) illnesses have a high prevalence [17]; few, if any, treatments are available to deter and prevent the pathological progression thought to lead to chronic neurological diseases and conditions [18–21]. Thus, a better understanding of the molecular mechanisms underlying TBI and neurological diseases is crucial to uncover the potential link between these conditions to enable development of effective diagnostic and treatment strategies which could reduce the incidence of post-TBI neurological complications.

* Correspondence: riyi@purdue.edu
†Equal contributors
[1]Weldon School of Biomedical Engineering, Purdue University, West Lafayette, IN 47907, USA
[2]Department of Basic Medical Sciences, Purdue University, West Lafayette, USA

This review intends to present the analysis of the current related published literature, that could lead to a better understanding of the mechanisms underlying TBI and neurodegenerative diseases, that might be linked to the development of neurodegenerative diseases post-TBI.

Pathological mechanisms of TBI

In most cases, TBI results from a physical blow to the head during traumatic events such as falls [22], motor vehicle collisions [23], or sports related injuries [24], although these injuries can also be inflicted by exposure to explosive blasts [25]. TBI is currently classified as mild, moderate, or severe based on clinical observations and history such as duration of loss of consciousness and post traumatic amnesia [26, 27]. Mild TBI (mTBI) comprises the majority of cases [28]; however, diagnosis is primarily by exclusion of injuries requiring specific intervention [29]. Furthermore, inconsistent clinical definitions between governing organizations presents challenges in comparing incidence rates of mTBI [28, 30]. This difficulty in diagnosis can be a serious concern due to acute effects such as second impact syndrome [24] or through chronic effects arising from repetitive TBI [31].

Damage to nervous tissue can be classified as primary injury, which occurs as a direct result of the experienced physical forces [32]; and secondary injury, which arises from pathophysiological processes following the traumatic event [33]. The primary injury process consists of the rapid acceleration-deceleration applied to the head, which is thought to damage the brain by producing shear forces within nervous tissue resulting in axonal injury and impact with the cranial wall [34]. These injuries can be ipsilateral or contralateral to the blow, and have been described in literature as coup and contre-coup, respectively [35]. In more severe cases, injury can cause intracranial hemorrhage and subsequent intracranial hypertension [26]. This increase in pressure not only damages brain tissue by compression, but also by causing cerebral hypoperfusion and potential ischemic injury by decreasing cerebral perfusion pressure [36].

Secondary injury in TBI typically occurs in the days, weeks, and months following the traumatic event due to biochemical changes in nervous tissue [37, 38]. This damage is frequently mediated by free radicals and reactive oxygen species (ROS) produced from ischemia-reperfusion injury, glutamatergic excitotoxicity, or neuroinflammation [39–41]. Following the initial trauma, axonal damage from the shear forces of primary injury affects membrane permeability and ionic balance [42]. In particular, uptake of calcium through either membrane disruption or activation of NMDA and AMPA receptors by glutamate can result in mitochondrial dysfunction and overproduction of free radicals and activation of apoptotic caspase signaling [43–45]. Subsequent inflammatory processes such as activation of native microglia may also contribute to oxidative stress via oxidative burst or through secondary effects of inflammatory cytokines [46]. These reactive radicals can overwhelm endogenous antioxidant systems and inflict cellular damage via lipid peroxidation and protein modifications [47]. The secondary products of free radical mediated lipid peroxidation, such as reactive carbonyl species, are also electrophilic and can further propagate oxidative damage to biomacromolecules [48, 49].

Clinical and preclinical studies have demonstrated the presence of oxidative stress and its byproducts following TBI with both serological and histological methods [50–52]. In animal studies, these products have been shown to be elevated as early as one day [53] following a single traumatic event and to persist up to 42 days with repeated injury [50]. Furthermore, spectroscopic evaluation suggests that the major endogenous antioxidants glutathione and ascorbic acid may remain diminished for 3 and 14 days post injury, respectively [38]. Elevation of F_2-isoprostane, a lipid peroxidation byproduct, has been observed in the cerebrospinal fluid of human severe TBI patients with peak levels at 1 day post injury; however this was primarily an evaluation of hypothermia treatment and did not establish comparison with healthy controls [47]. Lipid peroxidation products such as 4-hydroxynoneal were also found to be elevated in the serum of severe TBI patients requiring long term care [54]. Although chronic oxidative stress has not currently been observed following single mild injuries in humans, it appears likely that oxidative stress and its associated processes may exacerbate or prolong post-concussive symptoms [55]. Given the common involvement of oxidative stress in excitotoxicity and reperfusion injury, it is likely that oxidative stress plays a central role in secondary neuronal injury following TBI.

The pathological mechanisms in secondary TBI are particularly interesting due to capacity to prolong cellular injury beyond the initial traumatic event. Some of these characteristic changes, such as oxidative stress and excitotoxicity, have also been observed in the pathophysiology of neurodegenerative diseases which suggests a potential pathological mechanistic link between TBI and neurodegenerative diseases. Therefore, review of the pathological mechanisms in neurodegenerative diseases and TBI may be helpful in elucidating the causative factors for development of neurodegenerative diseases after TBI.

Pathological mechanisms of neurodegenerative diseases

Despite divergent clinical presentation, AD, PD, and ALS have several common characteristics [56]. Each disease has identified genetic risk factors, although most cases are idiopathic [57–59]. Pathologically, these diseases are characterized by the degeneration of specific neuronal populations associated with the observed clinical symptoms [60, 61]. In addition, aggregation or dysfunction of amyloid-β (Aβ), α-synuclein, and superoxide dismutase (SOD1) are commonly found in AD, PD, and ALS, respectively [56, 62–65]. Although the exact mechanisms of pathogenesis have not been fully determined, it has been suggested that oxidative stress, glutamatergic excitotoxicity, and neuroinflammation play key roles in the pathophysiology of neurodegeneration, particularly in AD [66–71], PD [72–76], and ALS [56, 77–81].

Alzheimer's disease has an extraordinary high prevalence in the elderly population that greatly reduces the quality of life and the survival [82]. In 2008, as many people as 24 million had dementia world-wide, of whom most had AD; number which was expected to double every 20 years as the population aged [83]. Alzheimer's disease's pathology involves the presence of neuritic plaques and the loss of cholinergic neurons in the brain, but the underlying mechanisms leading to these events are still unclear [84]. Neurodegeneration in Alzheimer's disease is thought to occur due to the accumulation of amyloid β-peptide (Aβ) in plaques in the brain tissue, but the mechanisms underlying its aggregation and toxicity are still incompletely understood [85].

Specifically, studies have indicated that oxidative stress might play a major role in AD pathogenesis [86], due to direct evidence of increased neurotoxic markers of lipid peroxidation, such as 4-hydroxynonenal, in human subjects [87], excessive brain protein oxidation in AD [88], increased nuclear DNA oxidation in the brain of AD patients [89], 30% increased activity of the free radical scavenging enzyme SOD-1 in cell lines of AD patients [90], and significantly, direct evidence that beta amyloid generates free radical peptides [70, 91]. Additionally, it has been well documented that Aβ-induced free radicals and lipid peroxidation are major contributors to neuronal death in AD [92, 93]. Remarkably, in vitro and animal studies have shown that the antioxidant effect of cannabinoids was able to prevent the neurodegenerative process occurring in the disease [94], suggestive of the important role of oxidative stress in the neurodegenerative process of AD.

Another process that has been related to Aβ toxicity is inflammation, which has also been linked to oxidative stress by inflammatory cytokines' activity [95]. Under healthy conditions, inflammatory processes are expected to restore cellular homeostasis and rebalance redox equilibrium [96]; but in AD conditions, the inflammatory processes are altered with co-localized Aβ deposits, inflammatory related proteins, and activated microglia [97]. Microglia and astroglia recognize misfolded and aggregated proteins to trigger an innate immune response that contributes to the disease progression and severity [98]. In other words, microglia recruitment promotes Aβ clearance and is neuroprotective in early stages of AD, but as the disease progresses, inflammatory cytokines downregulate Aβ clearance genes, and promote Aβ accumulation, contributing to neurodegeneration [99]. Furthermore, cytokines can induce the production of arachidonic acid, which exacerbates neurodegenerative processes by increasing extracellular levels of glutamate, known to cause excitotoxicity in AD [100]; and can also lead to the formation of superoxide free radicals, which have a direct effect in cellular death [101]. Moreover, studies suggest that non-enzymatically glycated tau induces oxidative stress, which results in cytokine gene expression and release of Aβ-peptide in AD [102], indicating a vicious pathological mechanistic circle between cytokines and oxidative stress that contributes to the progression and severity of AD. Additionally, oxidative damage from reactive oxygen species and lipid peroxidation products, such as 4-hydroxy-2-nonenal (HNE), is capable of inhibiting glutamate transporters, causing a decreased glutamate uptake critical for neuronal survival, an increased glutamate concentration in the synaptic cleft, and subsequent excitotoxicity that leads to neurodegeneration in AD [103].

Chronic traumatic encephalopathy (CTE) is a progressive neurodegenerative syndrome associated with repeated blunt force impacts to the head with transfer of acceleration and deceleration forces to the brain [104]; in other words, caused by repetitive mild traumatic brain injuries [105], although the central pathological mechanism explaining the development of progressive degeneration in CTE has not been elucidated [106]. CTE has been clinically associated with behavioral and personality changes, parkinsonism and dementia [107, 108]. Original findings of CTE studies were similar to Alzheimer's disease, but different in the predominance of tau protein deposition over amyloid [109]. The tau protein deposition in CTE is interesting since it has been previously demonstrated that tau inhibits kinesin-dependent transport of peroxisomes, and that the loss of peroxisomes makes the cells vulnerable to oxidative stress, leading to degeneration [110]. This tau protein deposition, which also occurs in AD but less dramatically when compared to CTE, also inhibits the transport of amyloid precursor protein (APP) into axons or dendrites, causing its accumulation in the cell body [110]. Besides tau proteins, fragments of TDP43, a nuclear RNA/DNA binding protein that regulates the transcription of thousands of genes [111], have been identified in AD, PD, ALS, and CTE, which induce the misfolding of SOD1, predisposing the surrounding cells to free-radical damage [112, 113]. These observations indicate the relevance of oxidative stress also in CTE neurodegeneration.

Chronic inflammation has also been observed in CTE and AD, which is thought to exacerbate the neurodegenerative process [31], and as previously described, has a relationship with oxidative stress though inflammatory cytokines. Moreover, it has been previously described that after the initial head trauma in CTE, microglia get activated and release toxic levels of cytokines, excitotoxins like glutamate, etc.; the excitotoxins inhibit phosphatases, resulting in hyperphosphorylated tau, neurotubule dysfunction, and neurofibrillary tangle deposition, all being relevant components of the CTE syndrome; and besides, there appears to be a synergy between proinflammatory cytokines and glutamate receptors that increases reactive oxygen species and worsens neurodegeneration in the injured brain [106, 114].

Parkinson's disease is the second most prevalent neurodegenerative disease in industrialized countries with prevalence of approximately 0.3% of the adult population [59]. Histologically, PD is characterized by the formation of α-synuclein rich Lewy bodies and subsequent death of the dopaminergic neurons of the *substantia nigra* [63]. Several genetic risk factors have been identified including mutations to the ubiquitin proteasome system [59, 115]. Although the exact mechanisms which initiate dopaminergic degeneration in non-hereditary PD are still unclear, it has been suggested that oxidative modification or carbonylation of the lysine rich N-terminus and non-amyloid component of α-synuclein may contribute to α-synuclein aggregation [63, 116, 117].

Consistent with this notion, the reactive carbonyls produced as secondary products in oxidative stress have been shown to form lysine adducts and induce α-synuclein aggregation in vitro [118, 119]. In addition, animal models of PD using agents such as 1-methyl-4-phenyl-1,2,3,6-tetrahydropyridine have demonstrated increased production of superoxide in dopaminergic cells relative to cortex [120]. Furthermore, mitochondrial localization of α-synuclein has been shown to promote oxidative stress in vitro [121]. Neuroinflammation has been proposed as a partial contributor to the oxidative stress in PD [122] with activated microglia being observed in the *substantia nigra* and striatum of deceased PD patients [123, 124]. Similarly, activated microglia were seen in rhesus monkeys up to 14 years after model induction [125]. Additionally, glutamatergic excitotoxicity has been proposed to play a role in PD. Rotigotine, an FDA approved dopamine receptor agonist, has been suggested to improve the efficiency of glutamate transporter 1 [126] (GLT-1), and has been shown to offer neuroprotection against glutamatergic excitotoxicity in dopaminergic cell culture [127].

On the other hand, ALS is a fatal neurodegenerative disease characterized by the death of motor neurons in the central nervous system and is the most common motor neuron disease [128]. Approximately 10% of ALS cases have been attributed to genetic causes while the majority are idiopathic [57]. Mutations affecting superoxide dismutase (SOD1) account for nearly 20%, of familial cases; however, this accounts for only 2% of cases overall [58]. Despite identification of these mutations, the exact pathological mechanism is yet to be determined [129].

SOD1 mutant mouse models have demonstrated formation of SOD1 aggregates [64]. Given the role of SOD1 in detoxification of the superoxide radical [130], it was previously suggested that loss of function could cause increased cellular exposure to reactive oxygen species [131]; however, this hypothesis has been challenged by findings of normal development of SOD1 deficient mice in the absence of significant traumatic insult [132]. Furthermore, Bruijn et al. found that SOD1 mutant animals showed no significant improvement in symptomatic progression with knockout or coexpression of wild type SOD1 [64] which suggests that the mutation results not in loss of function, but rather a gain of toxic properties. Studies in rats and human patients suggest that, similar to α-synuclein and Aβ, SOD1 mutation results in formation of potentially cytotoxic protein aggregates even in patients lacking known mutations of SOD1 [62, 64, 133]. In addition, the altered catalysis performed by some mutant variants results in diminished astroglial reuptake of glutamate via inhibition of GLT-1 [134–137]. Indeed, Riluzole, an FDA approved treatment for ALS, has been suggested to alleviate glutamatergic excitotoxicity via a variety of mechanisms including increased glutamate uptake via GLT-1 [138] and blockade of sensitive channels [126]. Hence, it appears that oxidative stress is also involved in the processes of neuronal death and disease progression in ALS [139].

Given its role in mediating damage from neuroinflammation and excitotoxicity, it is likely that oxidative stress plays an important role in the pathophysiology of AD, PD, and ALS in a similar fashion to TBI. As such, addressing oxidative stress in neurodegeneration could serve as an effective strategy in neuroprotection.

Behavioral and molecular mechanisms linking TBI to neurodegenerative diseases

Several studies have reported an increased incidence of the development of neurodegenerative diseases after TBI events. Previous reports have indicated a three times higher incidence of PD among TBI victims, compared to overall cases [13]. Similarly, the incidence of AD has been reported to be higher for post-TBI cases [140, 141]. TBI has also been suggested to be a risk factor for ALS with repeated studies in professional Italian soccer players showing elevated risk of disease [142, 143]. A case control study of ALS patients in the United States also found a nearly 11-fold increase in ALS risk with repeated TBI [14]. However, at this time it appears unlikely that a single occurrence of TBI significantly affects risk of ALS [14, 144]. In addition, chronic traumatic encephalitis (CTE), a tau pathology, has drawn increasing attention due to presence in NFL players and professional athletes that suffer from repeated TBI [107, 145]. Because the incidence of neurodegenerative diseases and conditions appears to be increased after TBI, it is relevant to discuss the possible behavioral and molecular mechanisms linking TBI to neurodegeneration.

TBI victims and TBI animal models have been shown to present characteristic pathological changes in key proteins, reflecting the interruption of axonal transport due to axonal injury [146]. The accumulated proteins that induce protein neuropathy include Aβ [147], α-synuclein [148], and tau protein [149]. These protein changes are particularly interesting, since it is well-established that Aβ protein aggregation is an important pathological component of AD [150], α-synuclein protein aggregation is a critical characteristic of PD [151, 152], and tau protein aggregation is important in the pathogenesis of CTE [153] and AD [154]. Remarkably, these protein neuropathological changes can be promoted in all three proteins via oxidative stress related free radicals and reactive aldehydes which are commonly elevated following TBI [77, 118, 119, 155, 156]. In addition, the reactive aldehyde byproducts of lipid peroxidation have been shown to cause further lipid peroxidation [52]. Given that these pathological protein states can also induce production of free radicals through excitotoxicity [127, 128] or alteration of mitochondrial ion balance [92, 121] and that reactive aldehydes can induce further lipid peroxidation and protein carbonylation [48, 49, 157, 158], it is possible that oxidative stress holds a key role in a self-propagating cycle of lipid peroxidation, protein carbonylation, and neurodegenerative protein aggregation.

TBI patients and TBI animal models have shown behavioral signs such as post-TBI dementia that resembles AD [159]; post-TBI motor deficits that provide evidence of post-TBI brain tissue damage in the area of the hippocampus [160], resembling brain tissue damage in AD [161]; and damage in the basal ganglia [162], resembling the brain tissue damage that occurs in PD [163]. Functional magnetic resonance imaging (fMRI) studies have also indicated transient and persistent neuropathological functional changes in the brain of TBI victims that could contribute to the development of chronic neurodegenerative diseases [164]. These changes observed in post-injury patients suggest that TBI could inflict the initial tissue damage that resembles or promotes processes common in the pathophysiology of neurodegenerative diseases.

Based on the central role that oxidative stress plays in post-TBI secondary injury and in the pathophysiology of neurodegeneration, it is probable that oxidative stress is a key process in linking TBI to increased incidence of neurodegeneration. Therefore, oxidative stress may serve as a therapeutic, diagnostic, or prognostic marker in evaluating the risks of long term neurological consequences following TBI.

Effective diagnosis and treatment of post-TBI neurological sequelae

Considering the significant risks incurred by TBI, it is clear that there is an imminent need for effective methods of early diagnosis, management, and monitoring of TBI patients to curtail the incidence of post-TBI neurological sequelae. At this time, diagnosis of TBI is based primarily on patient provided history and clinical observations [165–167]. Several clinical workflows have been developed for evaluation of mTBI, which is the most prevalent form of clinical TBI, including the Sport Concussion Assessment Tool and Military Acute Concussion Evaluation; however, these assessments are designed for use shortly following injury and, as such, rapidly diminish in sensitivity with delayed evaluation [168]. As well, the Glasgow Coma Scale has been in use for decades and allows for both rapid and consistent communication of patient condition [169]; nevertheless, the currently accepted threshold score of 13 may not be adequate to exclude visible abnormalities on computed tomography imaging that require neurosurgical intervention [170]. Due to these shortcomings in current diagnostic methodologies, civilian and military work groups have recommended the development of fluid or imaging based biomarkers for identification of mTBI [166, 168].

Several compounds and proteins have been suggested to serve as fluid biomarkers including glial fibrillary acidic protein (GFAP), calcium binding protein S100B, and tau protein [171]. In most cases, presence of these biomarkers is partially indicative of blood brain barrier disruption as they are typically confined within the central nervous system [171]. These proteins have been shown to be acutely elevated following TBI in human patients [172–174], but currently face challenges of low specificity [175, 176], poor correlation with development of post-concussive symptoms [177], and poor correlation with imaging abnormalities [178, 179].

Given the key role of oxidative stress and neuroinflammation in secondary neuronal injury and neurodegeneration, it is likely that the products of these processes may also serve as suitable biomarkers. As previously discussed, plasma levels of several oxidative stress and inflammation related markers have been observed to be elevated in serum up to 42 days after multiple blast injuries [50] and as early as 1 day following a single injury [53]. Furthermore, lipid peroxidation products, such as acrolein and 4-hydroxynonenal, have also been shown to be involved not only in TBI secondary injury [50, 53], but also in other modes of neuronal insult such as spinal cord injury [51, 180] and ischemia-reperfusion injury [181]. Given that these peroxidation products are not only indicative of damage, but also capable of causing modification of biomacromolecules, it is possible that measured elevations may be indicative not only of present damage, but also of continued secondary injury [49, 52, 182, 183]. As such, alleviation of oxidative stress could serve as a viable prophylactic strategy to diminish the risk of post TBI neurodegeneration. Direct supplementation with endogenous antioxidants, such as glutathione and superoxide dismutase, has not shown significant benefits as they do not easily cross the blood brain barrier [184–186]. However, the glutathione precursor N-acetylcysteine has shown some acute benefits in both animal and human studies [55, 187]. In addition, targeting of downstream components of the oxidative cascade, such as reactive aldehydes, has been suggested as a potential strategy due to the more extended half-lives of these compounds when compared to ROS [180, 184, 185]. However, despite extended elevation of inflammatory and oxidative byproducts, trials of antioxidant therapies have typically favored acute treatment, often within hours of the traumatic event, suggesting that acute treatment and monitoring may be more appropriate [184].

Considering the crucial role of post-TBI oxidative stress in the development and progression of chronic neurological diseases, detection and therapeutic targeting of this process appears to be a promising strategy for assessment, treatment, and monitoring of neurodegeneration risk post TBI. Given their connection to oxidative stress, inflammatory markers and lipid peroxidation byproducts could serve as surrogate biofluid markers. In addition, antioxidant treatment strategies can help neutralize perpetuation of cellular and molecular damage and diminish risks of long term neurological sequelae.

Conclusion

Despite the prevalence of TBI in both civilian and military populations and the significant neurological sequelae incurred by such injuries, diagnosis and treatment of TBI remains poorly understood. Furthermore, the causative factors linking TBI to neurodegenerative diseases, such as AD, PD, ALS, and CTE, have not been fully elucidated. Several processes, including oxidative stress and neuroinflammation, have been found to be common between TBI secondary injury and several neurodegenerative diseases. In particular, oxidative stress appears to be the key mechanism linking neuroinflammation and glutamatergic excitotoxicity in both TBI and neurodegeneration. As such, it is probable that the oxidative cascade induced by TBI initiates and subsequently propagates the characteristic pathologies of neurodegeneration via oxidation or carbonylation of key proteins.

Due to the high prevalence of TBI and neurodegenerative diseases, the development of new effective strategies for early diagnosis and treatment for TBI is imperative. Given the key role that oxidative stress plays in linking secondary injury and neurodegeneration, detection of ROS and key byproducts could serve as a novel method for identification and monitoring of potential cellular damage. Furthermore, these reactive species may serve as a viable therapeutic target for reduction of long term neurodegeneration risk following TBI, having the potential to reduce the disability and death, and improve the quality of life in the long term of the civilian and military populations that suffer of TBI.

Abbreviations

AD: Alzheimer's disease; ALS: Amyotrophic lateral sclerosis; APP: Amyloid precursor protein; Aβ: Amyloid beta; CNS: Central nervous system; CTE: Chronic traumatic encephalopathy; GLT-1: Glutamate transporter 1; mTBI: Mild traumatic brain injury; PD: Parkinson's disease; ROS: Reactive Oxygen Species; SOD1: Superoxide dismutase; TBI: Traumatic brain injury

Acknowledgements

Research findings described here were partially supported by the Indiana State Department of Health, Indiana Clinical and Translational Science Institute, National Institutes of Health. All funding was used for the design, collection, analysis and interpretation of data and in the writing of the manuscript.

Funding

Indiana State Department of Health, Indiana Clinical and Translational Science Institute, National Institutes of Health.

Authors' contributions

All authors have contributed to all parts of the production of this manuscript. All authors have read and approved the final manuscript.

Competing interests

Riyi Shi is the co-founder of Neuro Vigor, a start-up company with business interests of developing effective therapies for CNS neurodegenerative diseases and trauma. The other authors declare they have no competing interest.

References

1. Ghajar J. Traumatic brain injury. Lancet. 2000;356:923–9.
2. Maas AI, Stocchetti N, Bullock R. Moderate and severe traumatic brain injury in adults. Lancet Neurol. 2008;7:728–41.
3. McIntosh TK, Smith DH, Meaney DF, Kotapka MJ, Gennarelli TA, Graham DI. Neuropathological sequelae of traumatic brain injury: relationship to neurochemical and biomechanical mechanisms. Lab Investig J Tech Methods Pathol. 1996;74:315–42.

4. Sosin DM, Sniezek JE, Thurman DJ. Incidence of mild and moderate brain injury in the United States, 1991. Brain Inj. 1996;10:47–54.
5. Faul M, Xu L, Wald MM, Coronado VG. Traumatic brain injury in the United States. Atlanta GA Natl. Cent. Inj. Prev. Control Cent. Dis. Control Prev. [Internet]. 2010 [cited 2016 Nov 12]; Available from: https://www.cdc.gov/traumaticbraininjury/pdf/blue_book.pdf
6. Bales JW, Kline AE, Wagner AK, Dixon CE. Targeting dopamine in acute traumatic brain injury. Open Drug Discov J. 2010;2:119–28.
7. Masel BE, DeWitt DS. Traumatic brain injury: a disease process. Not an Event J Neurotrauma. 2010;27:1529–40.
8. Rimel RW, Giordani B, Barth JT, Boll TJ, Jane JA. Disability caused by minor head injury. Neurosurgery. 1981;9:221–8.
9. Riggio S, Wong M. Neurobehavioral sequelae of traumatic brain injury. Mt. Sinai J. Med. J. Transl. Pers. Med. 2009;76:163–72.
10. Langlois JA, Rutland-Brown W, Wald MM. The epidemiology and impact of traumatic brain injury: a brief overview. J Head Trauma Rehabil. 2006;21:375–8.
11. Uryu K, Chen X-H, Martinez D, Browne KD, Johnson VE, Graham DI, et al. Multiple proteins implicated in neurodegenerative diseases accumulate in axons after brain trauma in humans. Exp Neurol. 2007;208:185–92.
12. Gardner RC, Yaffe K. Epidemiology of mild traumatic brain injury and neurodegenerative disease. Mol Cell Neurosci. 2015;66:75–80.
13. Goldman SM, Tanner CM, Oakes D, Bhudhikanok GS, Gupta A, Langston JW. Head injury and Parkinson's disease risk in twins. Ann Neurol. 2006;60:65–72.
14. Chen H, Richard M, Sandler DP, Umbach DM, Kamel F. Head injury and amyotrophic lateral sclerosis. Am J Epidemiol. 2007;166:810–6.
15. Kampfl A, Posmantur RM, Zhao X, Schmutzhard E, Clifton GL, Hayes RL. Mechanisms of Calpain proteolysis following traumatic brain injury: implications for pathology and therapy: a review and update. J Neurotrauma. 1997;14:121–34.
16. Johnson VE, Stewart W, Smith DH. Widespread tau and Amyloid-Beta pathology many years after a single traumatic brain injury in humans: long-term AD-like pathology after single TBI. Brain Pathol. 2012;22:142–9.
17. DeKosky ST, Ikonomovic MD, Gandy S. Traumatic brain injury — football, warfare, and long-term effects. N Engl J Med. 2010;363:1293–6.
18. Marion DW, Penrod LE, Kelsey SF, Obrist WD, Kochanek PM, Palmer AM, et al. Treatment of traumatic brain injury with moderate hypothermia. N Engl J Med. 1997;336:540–6.
19. Faden AL, Demediuk P, Panter SS, Vink R. The role of excitatory amino acids and NMDA receptors in traumatic brain injury. Science. 1989;244:798.
20. Khanna S, Davis D, Peterson B, Fisher B, Tung H, O'Quigley J, et al. Use of hypertonic saline in the treatment of severe refractory posttraumatic intracranial hypertension in pediatric traumatic brain injury: Crit. Care Med. 2000;28:1144–51.
21. Hoge CW, McGurk D, Thomas JL, Cox AL, Engel CC, Castro CA. Mild traumatic brain injury in U.S. soldiers returning from Iraq. N Engl J Med. 2008;358:453–63.
22. Rutland-Brown W, Langlois JA, Thomas KE, Xi YL, et al. Incidence of traumatic brain injury in the United States, 2003. J Head Trauma Rehabil. 2006;21:544.
23. Fu TS, Jing R, McFaull SR, Cusimano MD. Health & Economic Burden of traumatic brain injury in the emergency Department. Can J Neurol Sci. 2016;43:238–47.
24. Jordan BD. The clinical spectrum of sport-related traumatic brain injury. Nat Rev Neurol. 2013;9:222–30.
25. Cernak I, Noble-Haeusslein LJ. Traumatic brain injury: an overview of pathobiology with emphasis on military populations. J Cereb Blood Flow Metab. 2010;30:255–66.
26. Malec JF, Brown AW, Leibson CL, Flaada JT, Mandrekar JN, Diehl NN, et al. The Mayo classification system for traumatic brain injury severity. J Neurotrauma. 2007;24:1417–24.
27. Graham DI, Adams JH, Nicoll JAR, Maxwell WL, Gennarelli TA. The nature, distribution and causes of traumatic brain injury. Brain Pathol. 1995;5:397–406.
28. Faul M, Coronado V. Epidemiology of traumatic brain injury. Handb Clin Neurol. 2015;127:3–13.
29. Carroll L, Cassidy JD, Peloso P, Borg J, Von Holst H, Holm L, et al. Prognosis for mild traumatic brain injury: results of the WHO collaborating Centre task force on mild traumatic brain injury. J Rehabil Med. 2004;36:84–105.
30. Summers CR, Ivins B, Schwab KA. Traumatic brain injury in the United States: an epidemiologic overview. Mt. Sinai J. Med. J. Transl. Pers. Med. 2009;76:105–10.
31. Stern RA, Riley DO, Daneshvar DH, Nowinski CJ, Cantu RC, McKee AC. Long-term consequences of repetitive brain trauma: chronic traumatic encephalopathy. PM&R. 2011;3:S460–7.
32. Cernak I, Wang Z, Jiang J, Bian X, Savic J. Ultrastructural and functional characteristics of blast injury-induced neurotrauma. J Trauma Acute Care Surg. 2001;50:695–706.
33. Tator CH, Fehlings MG. Review of the secondary injury theory of acute spinal cord trauma with emphasis on vascular mechanisms. J Neurosurg. 1991;75:15–26.
34. Shaw NA. The neurophysiology of concussion. Prog Neurobiol. 2002;67:281–344.
35. Ommaya AK, Grubb RL Jr, Naumann RA. Coup and contre-coup injury: observations on the mechanics of visible brain injuries in the rhesus monkey. J Neurosurg. 1971;35:503–16.
36. Bratton SL, Chestnut RM, Ghajar J, McConnell Hammond FF, Harris OA, Hartl R, et al. Guidelines for the management of severe traumatic brain injury. VI. Indications for intracranial pressure monitoring. J Neurotrauma. 2007; 24(Suppl 1):S37–44.
37. Greve MW, Zink BJ. Pathophysiology of traumatic brain injury. Mt Sinai J Med J Transl Pers Med. 2009;76:97–104.
38. Harris JL, Yeh H-W, Choi I-Y, Lee P, Berman NE, Swerdlow RH, et al. Altered neurochemical profile after traumatic brain injury: 1H-MRS biomarkers of pathological mechanisms. J Cereb Blood Flow Metab. 2012;32:2122–34.
39. Bang SA, Song YS, Moon BS, Lee BC, Lee H, Kim J-M, et al. Neuropsychological, metabolic, and $GABA_A$ receptor studies in subjects with repetitive traumatic brain injury. J Neurotrauma. 2016;33:1005–14.
40. Bose R, Schnell CL, Pinsky C, Zitko V. Effects of excitotoxins on free radical indices in mouse brain. Toxicol Lett. 1992;60:211–9.
41. Cornelius C, Crupi R, Calabrese V, Graziano A, Milone P, Pennisi G, et al. Traumatic brain injury: oxidative stress and Neuroprotection. Antioxid Redox Signal. 2013;19:836–53.
42. Werner C, Engelhard K. Pathophysiology of traumatic brain injury. Br J Anaesth. 2007;99:4–9.
43. Globus MY-T, Alonso O, Dietrich WD, Busto R, Ginsberg MD. Glutamate release and free radical production following brain injury: effects of posttraumatic hypothermia. J Neurochem. 2002;65:1704–11.
44. Leist M, Volbracht C, Kühnle S, Fava E, Ferrando-May E, Nicotera P. Caspase-mediated apoptosis in neuronal excitotoxicity triggered by nitric oxide. Mol Med. 1997;3:750–64.
45. Zhang Y, Bhavnani BR. Glutamate-induced apoptosis in neuronal cells is mediated via caspase-dependent and independent mechanisms involving calpain and caspase-3 proteases as well as apoptosis inducing factor (AIF) and this process is inhibited by equine estrogens. BMC Neurosci. 2006;7:49.
46. DiSabato DJ, Quan N, Godbout JP. Neuroinflammation: the devil is in the details. J Neurochem. 139:136–53.
47. Bayir H, Marion DW, Puccio AM, Wisniewski SR, Janesko KL, Clark RSB, et al. Marked gender effect on lipid peroxidation after severe traumatic brain injury in adult patients. J Neurotrauma. 2004;21:1–8.
48. Negre-Salvayre A, Coatrieux C, Ingueneau C, Salvayre R. Advanced lipid peroxidation end products in oxidative damage to proteins. Potential role in diseases and therapeutic prospects for the inhibitors. Br J Pharmacol. 2008;153:6–20.
49. Stevens JF, Maier CS. Acrolein: sources, metabolism, and biomolecular interactions relevant to human health and disease. Mol Nutr Food Res. 2008;52:7–25.
50. Ahmed FA, Kamnaksh A, Kovesdi E, Long JB, Agoston DV. Long-term consequences of single and multiple mild blast exposure on select physiological parameters and blood-based biomarkers. Electrophoresis. 2013;34:2229–33.
51. Zheng L, Park J, Walls M, Tully M, Jannasch A, Cooper B, et al. Determination of urine 3-HPMA, a stable acrolein metabolite in a rat model of spinal cord injury. J Neurotrauma. 2013;30:1334–41.
52. Uchida K, Kanematsu M, Sakai K, Matsuda T, Hattori N, Mizuno Y, et al. Protein-bound acrolein: potential markers for oxidative stress. Proc Natl Acad Sci U A. 1998;95:4882–7.
53. Walls MK, Race N, Zheng L, Vega-Alvarez SM, Acosta G, Park J, et al. Structural and biochemical abnormalities in the absence of acute deficits in mild primary blast-induced head trauma. J Neurosurg. 2016;124:675–86.
54. Mackay GM, Forrest CM, Stoy N, Christofides J, Egerton M, Stone TW, et al. Tryptophan metabolism and oxidative stress in patients with chronic brain injury. Eur J Neurol. 2006;13:30–42.
55. Hoffer ME, Balaban C, Slade MD, Tsao JW, Hoffer B. Amelioration of acute Sequelae of blast induced mild traumatic brain injury by N-acetyl Cysteine: a double-blind, placebo controlled study. PLoS One. 2013;8

56. Ransohoff RM. How neuroinflammation contributes to neurodegeneration. Science. 2016;353:777–83.
57. Kwiatkowski TJ, Bosco DA, LeClerc AL, Tamrazian E, Vanderburg CR, Russ C, et al. Mutations in the FUS/TLS Gene on chromosome 16 cause familial amyotrophic lateral sclerosis. Science. 2009;323:1205–8.
58. Ajroud-Driss S, Siddique T. Sporadic and hereditary amyotrophic lateral sclerosis (ALS). Biochim. Biophys. Acta BBA-Mol. Basis Dis. 1852;2015: 679–84.
59. de Lau LML, Breteler MMB. Epidemiology of Parkinson's disease. Lancet Neurol. 2006;5:525–35.
60. Zarei S, Carr K, Reiley L, Diaz K, Guerra O, Altamirano PF, et al. A comprehensive review of amyotrophic lateral sclerosis. Surg Neurol Int. 2015;6:171.
61. Kalia LV, Lang AE. Parkinson's disease. Lancet. 2015;386:896–912.
62. Forsberg K, Andersen PM, Marklund SL, Brannstrom T. Glial nuclear aggregates of superoxide dismutase-1 are regularly present in patients with amyotrophic lateral sclerosis. Acta Neuropathol. 2011;121:623–34.
63. Stefanis L. Alpha-Synuclein in Parkinson's disease. Cold Spring Harb Perspect Med. 2012;2:a009399.
64. Bruijn LI. Aggregation and motor neuron toxicity of an ALS-linked SOD1 mutant independent from wild-type SOD1. Science. 1998;281:1851–4.
65. Petrov D, Daura X, Zagrovic B. Effect of oxidative damage on the stability and Dimerization of superoxide dismutase 1. Biophys J. 2016;110:1499–509.
66. Smith MA, Rottkamp CA, Nunomura A, Raina AK, Perry G. Oxidative stress in Alzheimer's disease. Biochim. Biophys. Acta BBA-Mol. Basis Dis. 2000;1502:139–44.
67. Barnham KJ, Masters CL, Bush AI. Neurodegenerative diseases and oxidative stress. Nat Rev Drug Discov. 2004;3:205–14.
68. Coyle J, Puttfarcken P. Oxidative stress, glutamate, and neurodegenerative disorders. Science. 1993;262:689–95.
69. Cutler RG, Kelly J, Storie K, Pedersen WA, Tammara A, Hatanpaa K, et al. Involvement of oxidative stress-induced abnormalities in ceramide and cholesterol metabolism in brain aging and Alzheimer's disease. Proc Natl Acad Sci. 2004;101:2070–5.
70. Butterfield DA, Lauderback CM. Lipid peroxidation and protein oxidation in Alzheimer's disease brain: potential causes and consequences involving amyloid β-peptide-associated free radical oxidative stress1,2 1Guest editors: mark a. Smith and George Perry 2This article is part of a series of reviews on "causes and consequences of oxidative stress in Alzheimer's disease." the full list of papers may be found on the homepage of the journal. Free Radic Biol Med. 2002;32:1050–60.
71. Akiyama H. Inflammation and Alzheimer's disease. Neurobiol Aging. 2000;21:383–421.
72. Ebadi M, Srinivasan SK, Baxi MD. Oxidative stress and antioxidant therapy in Parkinson's disease. Prog Neurobiol. 1996;48:1–19.
73. Jenner P, Dexter DT, Sian J, Schapira AHV, Marsden CD. The Royal Kings and Queens Parkinson's disease research group. Oxidative stress as a cause of nigral cell death in Parkinson's disease and incidental lewy body disease. Ann. Neurol. 1992;32:S82–7.
74. Jenner P, Olanow CW. Oxidative stress and the pathogenesis of Parkinson's disease. Neurology. 1996;47:161S–70S.
75. Jenner P. Oxidative stress in Parkinson's disease. Ann Neurol. 2003;53:S26–38.
76. Hald A, Lotharius J. Oxidative stress and inflammation in Parkinson's disease: is there a causal link? Exp Neurol. 2005;193:279–90.
77. Bizzozero OA. Protein carbonylation in neurodegenerative and demyelinating CNS diseases. Handb. Neurochem. Mol. Neurobiol. Brain spinal cord. Trauma. 2009:543–62.
78. Kabashi E, Valdmanis PN, Dion P, Rouleau GA. Oxidized/misfolded superoxide dismutase-1: the cause of all amyotrophic lateral sclerosis? Ann Neurol. 2007;62:553–9.
79. Barber SC, Mead RJ, Shaw PJ. Oxidative stress in ALS: a mechanism of neurodegeneration and a therapeutic target. Biochim Biophys Acta BBA-Mol Basis Dis. 2006;1762:1051–67.
80. Glass CK, Saijo K, Winner B, Marchetto MC, Gage FH. Mechanisms Underlying Inflammation in Neurodegeneration. Cell. 2010;140:918–34.
81. Beal MF. Aging, energy, and oxidative stress in neurodegenerative diseases. Ann Neurol. 1995;38:357–66.
82. Editorial KR. The prevalence and malignancy of Alzheimer disease. A major killer. Arch. Neurol. 1976;33:217–8.
83. Mayeux R. Alzheimer's disease: epidemiology. In: Neurology B-H of C, editor. Elsevier; 2008 [cited 2017 Apr 18]. p. 195–205. Available from: https://doi.org/10.1016/S0072-9752(07)01218-3
84. Wang H-Y. Beta -Amyloid1-42 binds to alpha 7 nicotinic acetylcholine receptor with high affinity. IMPLICATIONS FOR ALZHEIMER'S DISEASE PATHOLOGY. J Biol Chem. 2000;275:5626–32.
85. Hardy J. The Amyloid hypothesis of Alzheimer's disease: progress and problems on the road to therapeutics. Science. 2002;297:353–6.
86. Markesbery WR. Oxidative stress hypothesis in Alzheimer's disease. Free Radic Biol Med. 1997;23:134–47.
87. Williams TI, Lynn BC, Markesbery WR, Lovell MA. Increased levels of 4-hydroxynonenal and acrolein, neurotoxic markers of lipid peroxidation, in the brain in mild cognitive impairment and early Alzheimer's disease. Neurobiol Aging. 2006;27:1094–9.
88. Smith CD, Carney JM, Starke-Reed PE, Oliver CN, Stadtman ER, Floyd RA, et al. Excess brain protein oxidation and enzyme dysfunction in normal aging and in Alzheimer disease. Proc Natl Acad Sci. 1991;88:10540–3.
89. Gabbita SP, Lovell MA, Markesbery WR. Increased nuclear DNA oxidation in the brain in Alzheimer's disease. J Neurochem. 2002;71:2034–40.
90. Zemlan FP, Thienhaus OJ, Bosmann HB. Superoxide dismutase activity in Alzheimer's disease: possible mechanism for paired helical filament formation. Brain Res. 1989;476:160–2.
91. Hensley K, Carney JM, Mattson MP, Aksenova M, Harris M, Wu JF, et al. A model for beta-amyloid aggregation and neurotoxicity based on free radical generation by the peptide: relevance to Alzheimer disease. Proc Natl Acad Sci. 1994;91:3270–4.
92. Varadarajan S, Yatin S, Aksenova M, Butterfield DA. Review: Alzheimer's Amyloid β-peptide-associated free radical oxidative stress and neurotoxicity. J Struct Biol. 2000;130:184–208.
93. Allan BD. Amyloid β-peptide (1-42)-induced oxidative stress and neurotoxicity: implications for Neurodegeneration in Alzheimer's disease brain. A Review Free Radic Res. 2002;36:1307–13.
94. Ramirez BG. Prevention of Alzheimer's disease pathology by Cannabinoids: Neuroprotection mediated by blockade of Microglial activation. J Neurosci. 2005;25:1904–13.
95. Moneim AE. Oxidant/antioxidant imbalance and the risk of Alzheimer's disease. Curr Alzheimer Res. 2015;12:335–49.
96. Bona D, Scapagnini G, Candore G, Castiglia L, Colonna-Romano G, Duro G, et al. Immune-inflammatory responses and oxidative stress in Alzheimers disease: therapeutic implications. Curr Pharm Des. 2010;16:684–91.
97. Eikelenboom P, Bate C, Van Gool WA, Hoozemans JJM, Rozemuller JM, Veerhuis R, et al. Neuroinflammation in Alzheimer's disease and prion disease. Glia. 2002;40:232–9.
98. Heneka MT, Carson MJ, Khoury JE, Landreth GE, Brosseron F, Feinstein DL, et al. Neuroinflammation in Alzheimer's disease. Lancet Neurol. 2015;14:388–405.
99. Hickman SE, Allison EK, El Khoury J. Microglial dysfunction and defective-Amyloid clearance pathways in aging Alzheimer's disease mice. J Neurosci. 2008;28:8354–60.
100. Hynd M. Glutamate-mediated excitotoxicity and neurodegeneration in Alzheimer?S disease. Neurochem Int. 2004;45:583–95.
101. DeLeo JA, Yezierski RP. The role of neuroinflammation and neuroimmune activation in persistent pain. Pain. 2001;90:1–6.
102. Stern D. Non-enzymatically glycated tau in Alzheimer's disease induces neuronal oxidant stress resulting in cytokine gene expression and release of amyloid b-peptide. Nat Med. 1995;1:693–9.
103. Lauderback CM, Hackett JM, Huang FF, Keller JN, Szweda LI, Markesbery WR, et al. The glial glutamate transporter, GLT-1, is oxidatively modified by 4-hydroxy-2-nonenal in the Alzheimer's disease brain: the role of Aβ1-42: Aβ1-42 and HNE binding to GLT-1 in AD brain. J Neurochem. 2001;78:413–6.
104. Omalu B. Chronic Traumatic Encephalopathy. In: Niranjan A, Lunsford LD, editors. Prog. Neurol. Surg. [Internet]. Basel: S. KARGER AG; 2014 [cited 2017 Apr 18]. p. 38–49. Available from: http://www.karger.com?doi=10.1159/000358761
105. McKee AC, Stein TD, Nowinski CJ, Stern RA, Daneshvar DH, Alvarez VE, et al. The spectrum of disease in chronic traumatic encephalopathy. Brain. 2013;136:43–64.
106. Blaylock RL, Maroon J, et al. Immunoexcitotoxicity as a central mechanism in chronic traumatic encephalopathy-a unifying hypothesis. Surg Neurol Int. 2011;2:4103.
107. McKee AC, Cantu RC, Nowinski CJ, Hedley-Whyte ET, Gavett BE, Budson AE, et al. Chronic traumatic encephalopathy in athletes: progressive Tauopathy after repetitive head injury. J Neuropathol Exp Neurol. 2009;68:709–35.
108. McKee AC, Gavett BE, Stern RA, Nowinski CJ, Cantu RC, Kowall NW, et al. TDP-43 Proteinopathy and motor neuron disease in chronic traumatic encephalopathy. J Neuropathol Exp Neurol. 2010;69:918–29.

109. Yi J, Padalino DJ, Chin LS, Montenegro P, Cantu RC. Chronic traumatic encephalopathy: Curr. Sports Med Rep. 2013;12:28–32.
110. Stamer K, Vogel R, Thies E, Mandelkow E, Mandelkow E-M. Tau blocks traffic of organelles, neurofilaments, and APP vesicles in neurons and enhances oxidative stress. J Cell Biol. 2002;156:1051–63.
111. Hebron ML, Lonskaya I, Sharpe K, Weerasinghe PPK, Algarzae NK, Shekoyan AR, et al. Parkin Ubiquitinates tar-DNA binding protein-43 (TDP-43) and promotes its Cytosolic accumulation via interaction with Histone Deacetylase 6 (HDAC6). J Biol Chem. 2013;288:4103–15.
112. Bandyopadhyay U, Cotney J, Nagy M, Oh S, Leng J, Mahajan M, et al. RNA-Seq profiling of spinal cord motor neurons from a Presymptomatic SOD1 ALS mouse. PLoS One. 2013;8:e53575. Cai H, editor
113. Lucke-Wold BP, Turner RC, Logsdon AF, Bailes JE, Huber JD, Rosen CL. Linking traumatic brain injury to chronic traumatic encephalopathy: identification of potential mechanisms leading to Neurofibrillary tangle development. J Neurotrauma. 2014;31:1129–38.
114. Saulle M, Greenwald BD. Chronic traumatic encephalopathy: a review. Rehabil Res Pract. 2012;2012:1–9.
115. Zhang Y, Dawson VL, Dawson TM. Oxidative stress and genetics in the pathogenesis of Parkinson's disease. Neurobiol Dis. 2000;7:240–50.
116. Atsmon-Raz Y, Miller Y. Non-Amyloid-beta component of human alpha-Synuclein Oligomers induces formation of new Abeta Oligomers: insight into the mechanisms that link Parkinson's and Alzheimer's diseases. ACS Chem Neurosci. 2016;7:46–55.
117. Plotegher N, Bubacco L. Lysines, Achilles' heel in alpha-synuclein conversion to a deadly neuronal endotoxin. Ageing Res Rev. 2016;26:62–71.
118. Shamoto-Nagai M, Maruyama W, Hashizume Y, Yoshida M, Osawa T, Riederer P, et al. In parkinsonian substantia nigra, α-synuclein is modified by acrolein, a lipid-peroxidation product, and accumulates in the dopamine neurons with inhibition of proteasome activity. J Neural Transm. 2007;114:1559–67.
119. Qin Z, Hu D, Han S, Reaney SH, Di Monte DA, Fink AL. Effect of 4-Hydroxy-2-nonenal modification on -Synuclein aggregation. J Biol Chem. 2007;282:5862–70.
120. Zhelev Z, Bakalova R, Aoki I, Lazarova D, Saga T. Imaging of superoxide generation in the Dopaminergic area of the brain in Parkinson's disease, using Mito-TEMPO. ACS Chem Neurosci. 2013;4:1439–45.
121. Parihar MS, Parihar A, Fujita M, Hashimoto M, Ghafourifar P. Mitochondrial association of alpha-synuclein causes oxidative stress. Cell Mol Life Sci. 2008;65:1272–84.
122. McGeer PL, McGeer EG. Inflammation and neurodegeneration in Parkinson's disease. Parkinsonism Relat Disord. 2004;10:S3–7.
123. McGeer PL, Itagaki S, Boyes BE, McGeer EG. Reactive microglia are positive for HLA-DR in the substantia nigra of Parkinson's and Alzheimer's disease brains. Neurology. 1988;38:1285–91.
124. Yamada T, McGeer EG, Schelper RL, Wszolek ZK, McGeer PL, Pfeiffer RF, et al. Histological and biochemical pathology in a family with autosomal dominant parkinsonism and dementia. Neurol Psychiatry Brain Res. 1993;2
125. McGeer PL, Schwab C, Parent A, Doudet D. Presence of reactive microglia in monkey substantia nigra years after 1-methyl-4-phenyl-1,2,3,4-tetrahydropyridine administration. Ann Neurol. 2003;54:599–604.
126. Doble A. The pharmacology and mechanism of action of riluzole. Neurology. 1996;47:233S–41S.
127. Oster S, Radad K, Scheller D, Hesse M, Balanzew W, Reichmann H, et al. Rotigotine protects against glutamate toxicity in primary dopaminergic cell culture. Eur J Pharmacol. 2014;724:31–42.
128. Rowland LP, Shneider NA. Amyotrophic lateral sclerosis. N Engl J Med. 2001;344:1688–700.
129. Sreedharan J, Blair IP, Tripathi VB, Hu X, Vance C, Rogelj B, et al. TDP-43 mutations in familial and sporadic amyotrophic lateral sclerosis. Science. 2008;319:1668–72.
130. Zelko IN, Mariani TJ, Folz RJ. Superoxide dismutase multigene family: a comparison of the CuZn-SOD (SOD1), Mn-SOD (SOD2), and EC-SOD (SOD3) gene structures, evolution, and expression. Free Radic Biol Med. 2002;33:337–49.
131. Barber SC, Shaw PJ. Oxidative stress in ALS: key role in motor neuron injury and therapeutic target. Free Radic Biol Med. 2010;48:629–41.
132. Reaume AG, Elliott JL, Hoffman EK, Kowall NW, Ferrante RJ, Siwek DF, et al. Motor neurons in cu/Zn superoxide dismutase-deficient mice develop normally but exhibit enhanced cell death after axonal injury. Nat Genet. 1996;13:43–7.
133. Liu J, Lillo C, Jonsson PA, Vande Velde C, Ward CM, Miller TM, et al. Toxicity of familial ALS-linked SOD1 mutants from selective recruitment to spinal mitochondria. Neuron. 2004;43:5–17.
134. Trotti D, Rolfs A, Danbolt NC, Brown RH, Hediger MA. SOD1 mutants linked to amyotrophic lateral sclerosis selectively inactivate a glial glutamate transporter. Nat Neurosci. 1999;2:427–33.
135. Staats KA, Van Den Bosch L. Astrocytes in amyotrophic lateral sclerosis: direct effects on motor neuron survival. J Biol Phys. 2009;35:337–46.
136. Foran E, Trotti D. Glutamate transporters and the excitotoxic path to motor neuron degeneration in amyotrophic lateral sclerosis. Antioxid Redox Signal. 2009;11:1587–602.
137. McGeer PL, McGeer EG. Inflammatory processes in amyotrophic lateral sclerosis. Muscle Nerve. 2002;26:459–70.
138. Carbone M, Duty S, Rattray M. Riluzole elevates GLT-1 activity and levels in striatal astrocytes. Neurochem Int. 2012;60:31–8.
139. Wootz H, Hansson I, Korhonen L, Näpänkangas U, Lindholm D. Caspase-12 cleavage and increased oxidative stress during motoneuron degeneration in transgenic mouse model of ALS. Biochem Biophys Res Commun. 2004;322:281–6.
140. Roberts GW, Gentleman SM, Lynch A, Graham DI. βA4 amyloid protein deposition in brain after head trauma. Lancet. 1991;338:1422–3.
141. Lye TC, Shores EA. Traumatic brain injury as a risk factor for Alzheimer's disease: a review. Neuropsychol Rev. 2000;10:115–29.
142. Chiò A, Benzi G, Dossena M, Mutani R, Mora G. Severely increased risk of amyotrophic lateral sclerosis among Italian professional football players. Brain. 2005;128:472.
143. Chio A, Calvo A, Dossena M, Ghiglione P, Mutani R, Mora G. ALS in Italian professional soccer players: the risk is still present and could be soccer-specific. Amyotroph Lateral Scler. 2009;10:205–9.
144. Armon C, Nelson LM. Is head trauma a risk factor for amyotrophic lateral sclerosis? An evidence based review. Amyotroph Lateral Scler. 2012;13:351–6.
145. Omalu BI, DeKosky ST, Minster RL, Kamboh MI, Hamilton RL, Wecht CH. Chronic traumatic encephalopathy in a National Football League Player. Neurosurgery. 2005;57:128–34.
146. Smith DH, Uryu K, Saatman KE, Trojanowski JQ, McIntosh TK. Protein accumulation in traumatic brain injury. Neuro Molecular Med. 2003;4:59–72.
147. Bramlett HM, Kraydieh S, Green EJ, Dietrich WD. Temporal and regional patterns of axonal damage following traumatic brain injury: a Beta-amyloid precursor protein Immunocytochemical study in rats. J Neuropathol Exp Neurol. 1997;56:1132–41.
148. Goldman SM, Kamel F, Ross GW, Jewell SA, Bhudhikanok GS, Umbach D, et al. Head injury, alpha-synuclein Rep1, and Parkinson's disease. Ann Neurol. 2012;71:40–8.
149. Franz G, Beer R, Kampfl A, Engelhardt K, Schmutzhard E, Ulmer H, et al. Amyloid beta 1-42 and tau in cerebrospinal fluid after severe traumatic brain injury. Neurology. 2003;60:1457–61.
150. Tanzi R, Gusella J, Watkins P, Bruns G, St George-Hyslop P, Van Keuren M, et al. Amyloid beta protein gene: cDNA, mRNA distribution, and genetic linkage near the Alzheimer locus. Science. 1987;235:880–4.
151. Braak H, Del Tredici K, Bratzke H, Hamm-Clement J, Sandmann-Keil D, Rüb U. Staging of the intracerebral inclusion body pathology associated with idiopathic Parkinson's disease (preclinical and clinical stages). J Neurol. 2002;249:1–1.
152. Acosta SA, Tajiri N, de la Pena I, Bastawrous M, Sanberg PR, Kaneko Y, et al. Alpha-synuclein as a pathological link between chronic traumatic brain injury and Parkinson's disease. J Cell Physiol. 2015;230:1024–32.
153. Gavett BE, Stern RA, McKee AC. Chronic traumatic encephalopathy: a potential late effect of sport-related concussive and Subconcussive head trauma. Clin Sports Med. 2011;30:179–88.
154. Spillantini MG, Goedert M. Tau protein pathology in neurodegenerative diseases. Trends Neurosci. 1998;21:428–33.
155. Pappolla MA, Chyan YJ, Omar TR, Hsiao K, Perry G, Smith MA, et al. Evidence of oxidative stress and in vivo neurotoxicity of beta-amyloid in a transgenic mouse model of Alzheimer's disease: a chronic oxidative paradigm for testing antioxidant therapies in vivo. Am J Pathol. 1998;152:871.
156. Poppek D, Keck S, Ermak G, Jung T, Stolzing A, Ullrich O, et al. Phosphorylation inhibits turnover of the tau protein by the proteasome: influence of *RCAN1* and oxidative stress. Biochem J. 2006;400:511–20.
157. Moghe A, Ghare S, Lamoreau B, Mohammad M, Barve S, McClain C, et al. Molecular mechanisms of acrolein toxicity: relevance to human disease. Toxicol Sci. 2015;143:242–55.
158. Wood PL, Khan MA, Kulow SR, Mahmood SA, Moskal JR. Neurotoxicity of reactive aldehydes: the concept of "aldehyde load" as demonstrated by neuroprotection with hydroxylamines. Brain Res. 2006;1095:190–9.
159. Starkstein SE, Jorge R. Dementia after traumatic brain injury. Int Psychogeriatr. 2005;17:S93.

160. Hicks RR, Smith DH, Lowenstein DH, Marie RS, McINTOSH TK. Mild experimental brain injury in the rat induces cognitive deficits associated with regional neuronal loss in the hippocampus. J Neurotrauma. 1993;10:405–14.
161. Šimić G, Lucassen PJ, Krsnik Ž, Krušlin B, Kostović I, Winblad B, et al. nNOS expression in reactive Astrocytes correlates with increased cell death related DNA damage in the hippocampus and Entorhinal cortex in Alzheimer's disease. Exp Neurol. 2000;165:12–26.
162. Wilde EA, Bigler ED, Hunter JV, Fearing MA, Scheibel RS, Newsome MR, et al. Hippocampus, amygdala, and basal ganglia morphometrics in children after moderate-to-severe traumatic brain injury. Dev Med Child Neurol. 2007;49:294–9.
163. Carlsson M, Carlsson A. Interactions between glutamatergic and monoaminergic systems within the basal ganglia-implications for schizophrenia and Parkinson's disease. Trends Neurosci. 1990;13:272–6.
164. Baugh CM, Stamm JM, Riley DO, Gavett BE, Shenton ME, Lin A, et al. Chronic traumatic encephalopathy: neurodegeneration following repetitive concussive and subconcussive brain trauma. Brain Imaging Behav. 2012;6:244–54.
165. Brasure M, Lamberty GJ, Sayer NA, Nelson NW, MacDonald R, Ouellette J, et al. Multidisciplinary Postacute rehabilitation for moderate to severe traumatic brain injury in adults; 2012. p. ES1–ES20.
166. Centers for Disease Control and Prevention (CDC). Traumatic brain injury in the United States: epidemiology and rehabilitation. 2015.
167. Menon DK, Schwab K, Wright DW, Maas AI, Demographics, Clinical Assessment Working Group of the I, et al. Position statement: definition of traumatic brain injury. Arch Phys Med Rehabil. 2010;91:1637–40.
168. Marion DW, Curley KC, Schwab K, Hicks RR, mTBI Diagonstics Workgroup. Proceedings of the military mTBI diagnostics workshop, St. Pete Beach, august 2010. J Neurotrauma. 2011, 28:517–26.
169. Teasdale G, Maas A, Lecky F, Manley G, Stocchetti N, Murray G. The Glasgow coma scale at 40 years: standing the test of time. Lancet Neurol. 2014;13:844–54.
170. Stein SC. Minor head injury: 13 is an unlucky number. J Trauma. 2001;50:759–60.
171. Kulbe JR, Geddes JW. Current status of fluid biomarkers in mild traumatic brain injury. Exp Neurol. 2016;275:334–52.
172. Townend W, Dibble C, Abid K, Vail A, Sherwood R, Lecky F. Rapid elimination of protein S-100B from serum after minor head trauma. J Neurotrauma. 2006;23:149–55.
173. Gatson JW, Barillas J, Hynan LS, Diaz-Arrastia R, Wolf SE, Minei JP. Detection of neurofilament-H in serum as a diagnostic tool to predict injury severity in patients who have suffered mild traumatic brain injury. J Neurosurg. 2014;121:1232–8.
174. Papa L, Silvestri S, Brophy GM, Giordano P, Falk JL, Braga CF, et al. GFAP out-performs S100beta in detecting traumatic intracranial lesions on computed tomography in trauma patients with mild traumatic brain injury and those with extracranial lesions. J Neurotrauma. 2014;31:1815–22.
175. Biberthaler P, Linsenmeier U, Pfeifer KJ, Kroetz M, Mussack T, Kanz KG, et al. Serum S-100B concentration provides additional information fot the indication of computed tomography in patients after minor head injury: a prospective multicenter study. Shock. 2006;25:446–53.
176. Tenovuo O, Posti J, Hossain I, Takalak R, Liedes H, Newcombe V, et al. GFAP and UCH-L1 are not specific biomarkers for mild CT-negative traumatic brain injury. Abstr. 34th Annu. Natl. Neurotrauma Symp. 2016. p. A-20.
177. Bazarian JJ, Zemlan FP, Mookerjee S, Stigbrand T. Serum S-100B and cleaved-tau are poor predictors of long-term outcome after mild traumatic brain injury. Brain Inj. 2006;20:759–65.
178. Kou Z, Gattu R, Kobeissy F, Welch RD, O'Neil BJ, Woodard JL, et al. Combining biochemical and imaging markers to improve diagnosis and characterization of mild traumatic brain injury in the acute setting: results from a pilot study. PLoS One. 2013;8:e80296.
179. Kavalci C, Pekdemir M, Durukan P, Ilhan N, Yildiz M, Serhatlioglu S, et al. The value of serum tau protein for the diagnosis of intracranial injury in minor head trauma. Am J Emerg Med. 2007;25:391–5.
180. Luo J, Uchida K, Shi R. Accumulation of acrolein-protein adducts after traumatic spinal cord injury. Neurochem Res. 2005;30:291–5.
181. Wood PL, Khan MA, Moskal JR, Todd KG, Tanay VA, Baker G. Aldehyde load in ischemia-reperfusion brain injury: neuroprotection by neutralization of reactive aldehydes with phenelzine. Brain Res. 2006;1122:184–90.
182. Putiev YP, Tashpulatov YT, Gafurov TG, Usmanov KU. Infrared study of modified cellulose. Polym Sci USSR. 1964;6:1565–70.
183. Kaminskas LM, Pyke SM, Burcham PC. Strong protein adduct trapping accompanies abolition of acrolein-mediated hepatotoxicity by hydralazine in mice. J Pharmacol Exp Ther. 2004;310:1003–10.
184. Gilgun-Sherki Y, Rosenbaum Z, Melamed E, Offen D. Antioxidant therapy in acute central nervous system injury: current state. Pharmacol Rev. 2002;54:271–84.
185. Bains M, Hall ED. Antioxidant therapies in traumatic brain and spinal cord injury. Biochim Biophys Acta. 1822;2012:675–84.
186. Kochanek PM, Jackson TC, Ferguson NM, Carlson SW, Simon DW, Brockman EC, et al. Emerging therapies in traumatic brain injury. Semin Neurol. 2015;35:83–100.
187. Bavarsad Shahripour R, Harrigan MR, Alexandrov AV. N-acetylcysteine (NAC) in neurological disorders: mechanisms of action and therapeutic opportunities. Brain Behav. 2014;4:108–22.

8

Elevated axonal membrane permeability and its correlation with motor deficits in an animal model of multiple sclerosis

Gary Leung[1], Melissa Tully[2,3], Jonathan Tang[1,2], Shengxi Wu[4] and Riyi Shi[1,2*]

Abstract

Background: It is increasingly clear that in addition to myelin disruption, axonal degeneration may also represent a key pathology in multiple sclerosis (MS). Hence, elucidating the mechanisms of axonal degeneration may not only enhance our understanding of the overall MS pathology, but also elucidate additional therapeutic targets. The objective of this study is assess the degree of axonal membrane disruption and its significance in motor deficits in EAE mice.

Methods: Experimental Autoimmune Encephalomyelitis was induced in mice by subcutaneous injection of myelin oligodendrocyte glycoprotein/complete Freud's adjuvant emulsion, followed by two intraperitoneal injections of pertussis toxin. Behavioral assessment was performed using a 5-point scale. Horseradish Peroxidase Exclusion test was used to quantify the disruption of axonal membrane. Polyethylene glycol was prepared as a 30% (w/v) solution in phosphate buffered saline and injected intraperitoneally.

Results: We have found evidence of axonal membrane disruption in EAE mice when symptoms peak and to a lesser degree, in the pre-symptomatic stage of EAE mice. Furthermore, polyethylene glycol (PEG), a known membrane fusogen, significantly reduces axonal membrane disruption in EAE mice. Such PEG-mediated membrane repair was accompanied by significant amelioration of behavioral deficits, including a delay in the emergence of motor deficits, a delay of the emergence of peak symptom, and a reduction in the severity of peak symptom.

Conclusions: The current study is the first indication that axonal membrane disruption may be an important part of the pathology in EAE mice and may underlies behavioral deficits. Our study also presents the initial observation that PEG may be a therapeutic agent that can repair axolemma, arrest axonal degeneration and reduce motor deficits in EAE mice.

Keywords: Multiple sclerosis, EAE, Axonal membrane damage, Polyethylene glycol, Acrolein, Horseradish Peroxidase, Membrane permeability, Neurodegeneration

Background

Although inflammation is known to be the major pathology of multiple sclerosis (MS), the mechanisms underlying tissue damage and functional loss remain unclear [1, 2]. While myelin degeneration has long been considered the primary neuropathological characteristic for MS, recent studies indicate that axonal degeneration is also an important component of the pathology [3–5]. In fact, there is strong evidence suggesting that MS is a neurodegenerative diseases [3, 6–8]. Indeed, the integrities of both myelin and axons are indispensable for neuronal function and survival [9]. Therefore, either myelin or axonal damage could theoretically lead to axonal conduction loss and degeneration seen in MS [10–13]. Consistent with this notion, it has been suggested that axonal disruption may represent irreversible neurodegeneration in patients with MS [3]. This may in part explain why conventional strategies focusing solely on myelin protection have resulted in

* Correspondence: riyi@purdue.edu
[1]Department of Basic Medical Sciences, College of Veterinary Medicine, Purdue University, West Lafayette, IN 47907, USA
[2]Weldon School of Biomedical Engineering, Purdue University, West Lafayette, IN 47907, USA
Full list of author information is available at the end of the article

few effective treatments to slow or prevent MS progression [1].

Despite its potential importance in MS, axonal damage has attracted significantly less attention compared to myelin damage while both are known to lead to neurodegeneration in MS [6, 7, 14]. Consequently, the pathological role of axonal damage in MS remains insufficiently characterized. Specifically, the key cellular processes that trigger axonal degeneration remain unclear. We have previously shown that axonal membrane damage contributes to axonal degeneration observed in CNS trauma [11–13, 15–17]. We have also shown that acrolein, a pro-inflammatory aldehyde that is capable of inflicting axonal membrane damage and functional loss [18–24], is elevated and likely plays an important pathological role in MS [25]. In light of this evidence, we speculate that damage to the axonal membrane, or axolemma, likely leads to neuronal degeneration and loss of neurological function, and therefore contributes to the development and progression of symptoms observed in MS.

Polyethylene glycol (PEG), a hydrophilic polymer, is well known for its ability to seal neuronal membranes and consequently restore integrity and associated neuronal function [13, 26–29]. In particular, it has been shown that PEG is capable of repairing axolemmal damage and provide neuroprotection in traumatic spinal cord injury [19, 26–28, 30–40]. However, the therapeutic effect of PEG has not been examined in non-traumatic CNS illnesses, such as MS, in which axonal membrane damage likely plays a role leading to axonal degeneration. Therefore, the primary focus of this study was to determine whether axolemmal disruption can be detected and to examine its possible correlation with functional deficits associated with MS. Subsequently, we also aimed to confirm the pathological role of axolemmal disruption in MS and to assess the therapeutic efficacy of administering PEG as a membrane sealant.

Methods

Experimental autoimmune encephalomyelitis mice

We certify that all applicable institutional and governmental regulations concerning the ethical use of animals were followed during the course of this research. Female C57BL/6 mice were purchased from Harlan Laboratories (Indianapolis, IN, USA) and were housed in the Purdue University veterinary animal housing facilities. Ten to twelve week old mice received two subcutaneous injections of 0.1 mL myelin oligodendrocyte glycoprotein/complete Freud's adjuvant emulsion (EK-0115, Hooke Laboratories, Lawrence, MA, USA) into the upper and lower back. Immediately following the emulsion injections, 0.1 mL of pertussis toxin (EK-0115, Hook Laboratories) was administered intraperitoneally to the mice, and again 22–26 h later. Behavioral assessment was performed using a 5-point scale [41]. Animals were placed on a metal grate to record their walking ability and motor function. The behavioral scale used was as follows: 0 – no deficit; 1 – limp tail only; 2 – hind limb paresis without frank leg dragging; 3 – partial hind limb weakness with one or both legs dragging; 4 – complete hind limb paralysis; 5 – moribund, paralysis in hind limbs and forelimbs. These studies were approved by the Purdue Animal Care and Use Committee, Purdue University, West Lafayette, IN.

Horseradish peroxidase exclusion test

The mice were separated into 4 groups: healthy control mice, EAE mice before the onset of symptoms (pre-symptom), EAE mice at peak behavioral deficit (peak symptoms), and PEG-treated EAE mice. After confirmation of behavior at various pre-determined experimental end points (Fig. 1), each group of animals was anesthetized with Ketamine (90 mg/kg) and Xylazine (10 mg/kg) and perfused (intra-cardiac) with a cold, oxygenated Krebs solution. The spinal columns were quickly removed from the animal and a complete laminectomy was performed. The spinal cord was then excised from the vertebrae and placed in cold, oxygenated Krebs solution containing 0.015% horseradish peroxidase (Sigma

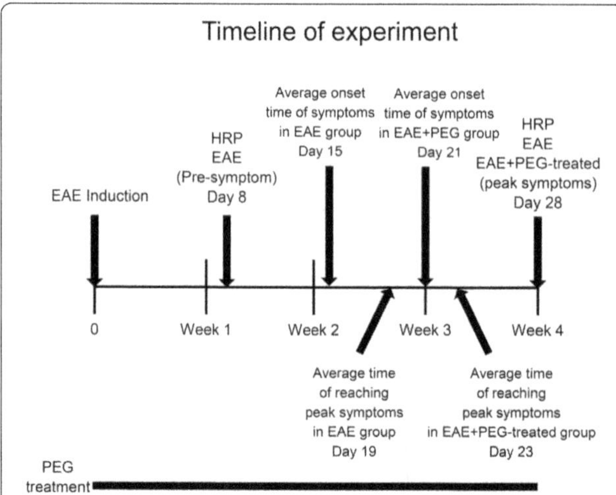

Fig. 1 Experimental design and time course. Diagram illustrates the time course of the overall experiment related to EAE, pre-symptom (EAE) and peak symptom (both EAE and EAE + PEG-treated) groups. In addition, the time points when the HRP-exclusion assay was conducted are illustrated: at pre-symptom (day 8 post-induction) and at peak symptom (Day 28 post-induction), with or without PEG treatment. Behavioral analysis was conducted daily and the average time of onset of symptoms, and the average time of reaching peak symptoms for both the EAE and the EAE + PEG group are illustrated. In the EAE + PEG group, PEG treatment was carried out for the entire period of study starting on the day of induction, as indicated in the diagram. Tissue samples for HRP testing were extracted for 4 different groups: healthy controls, pre-symptom EAE mice, peak symptom EAE mice and PEG-treated EAE mice

Type IV, Sigma Aldrich) for 2 h. The tissue was then fixed in 2.5% glutaraldehyde in phosphate buffer for 4 h at room temperature. After fixation, a Vibratome (Electron Microscopy Science, Hatfield, PA, USA) was used to cut 30 μm transverse sections of the tissue. Tissue was then processed in a diaminobenzidene solution to visualize HRP uptake by damaged. Digital images of HRP-stained spinal cord sections were obtained with an optical microscope connected to a computer. Stained axons were counted and expressed as density (axons/mm^2) using Image J analysis [15, 17, 30]. Animals were sacrificed for structural analysis at pre-induction (control), 8 days post-induction (pre-symptom), or 4 weeks post-induction (peak symptom).

Polyethylene glycol treatment

Polyethylene glycol (295906, Sigma Aldrich, St. Louis, MO, USA) was prepared as a 30% (w/v) solution in phosphate buffered saline. The solution was then filtered for sterilization and injected into each animal every day after induction for the whole study (4 weeks post-induction). A volume of 0.1 mL was administered intraperitoneally daily after induction for the duration of the study. EAE only animals were administered the same amount of saline rather than PEG.

Statistical analysis

Throughout the paper, Mann Whitney U test was used to compare the difference of the severity of motor defects, the onset of motor deficits, and the onset of peak symptoms between EAE and EAE + PEG-treated groups. Kruskal-Wallis test was used for comparison of membrane permeability assessed by HRP-exclusion test in various groups. The statistical significance level was set at $p < 0.05$. All data are expressed as mean ± standard error of the mean (SEM).

Results

Significant axonal membrane damage in EAE mouse and its reduction by Polyethylene glycol

Using an EAE mouse model, we first examined axonal membrane damage using a well-established HRP-exclusion assay. The integrity of axonal membrane from the spinal cord of control mice, EAE mice before the onset of symptoms (pre-symptom), and EAE mice at peak behavioral deficit (peak symptom) was examined (Fig. 1). We have found that the average HRP labeling for these conditions was 811 ± 130 axons/mm^2, 3293 ± 500 axons/mm^2, and 6147 ± 655 axons/mm^2 respectively (Fig. 2). EAE mice at peak deficit demonstrated significantly higher levels of HRP labeling compared to control mice ($P < 0.01$). Interestingly, pre-symptom EAE mice also displayed increased axonal membrane permeability compared to control mice ($P < 0.05$).

We further examined the possibility that PEG can reduce axonal membrane permeability. Specifically, EAE mice were given daily injections of 0.1 mL of either polyethylene glycol (30% w/v) (EAE + PEG), or saline (EAE only) beginning on the first day of induction and then daily for 4 weeks (Fig. 1). Axonal integrity based on the HRP exclusion assay was carried out at the end of the treatment period. We have found that the density of HRP-labeled axons in the EAE-PEG treated group was 1581 ± 247 axons/mm^2, which is significantly lower than that of the EAE only mice at peak deficit (6147 ± 655 axons/mm^2, $p < 0.01$) (Fig. 2).

Polyethylene glycol temporally ameliorates motor deficits in EAE mice

In addition to axonal membrane permeability examination, we also carried out behavioral analysis in two experimental groups, EAE and EAE + PEG mice. The behavioral observation for each animal was recorded daily on a 5-point scale immediately following induction and continuously for 4 weeks. The average behavioral score was calculated for each day in two groups and displayed over time in Fig. 3. The severity of behavioral deficit in the EAE/PEG-treated group was significantly lower than the EAE group during the period of day 16 to 25 days post EAE induction. When averaging the highest scores of each animal within each group, the PEG-treated EAE mice (1.91 ± 0.4) displayed a significantly lower score than the EAE mice (3.33 ± 0.3, $P < 0.05$) (Fig. 3 upper inset). In addition, PEG treatment also significantly delayed the time of reaching peak symptoms (23.1 ± 1.6 days for EAE-PEG, and 18.7 ± 0.8 days for EAE group, $P < 0.05$) (Fig. 3 lower inset).

In addition to decreased peak symptom severity and delayed time to reach the peak symptom, PEG treated animals also showed delayed symptom onset as depicted in Fig. 4. Specifically, in the EAE group, all mice began to display their behavioral deficit between days 13 and 18. In contrast, the EAE + PEG group revealed a more dispersed result with a trend of delayed onset. Specifically, five EAE + PEG animals began exhibiting symptoms at approximately the same time as the EAE group (13–18 days induction) while the others were later in time: three exhibited no observable behavioral deficit throughout the 4-week observation (counted as day 28 when averaging) while the remaining three mice showed their first motor defects at between day 20–26 post induction. Overall, the average day of onset for EAE mice that received PEG-treatment was 20.63 ± 1.8 days which is significantly delayed compared to EAE mice (15.42 ± 0.4 days, $P < 0.01$) (Fig. 4).

Discussion

Based on the current study using the HRP-exclusion assay, a well-established method of assessing axonal

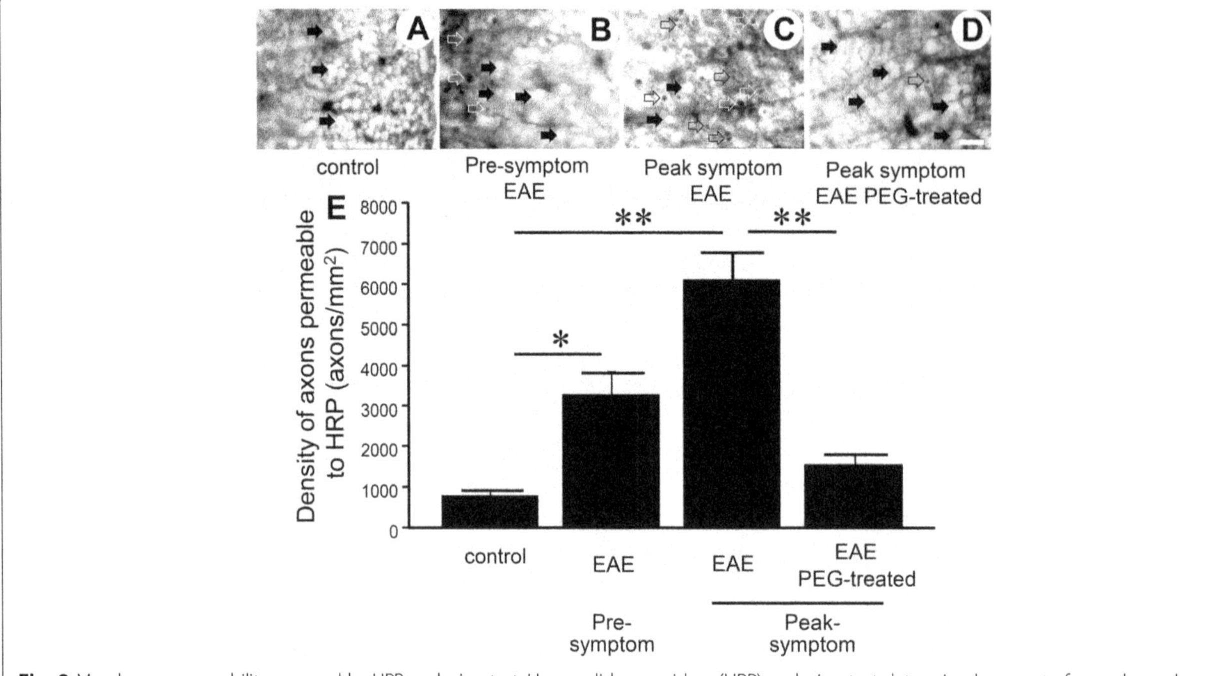

Fig. 2 Membrane permeability assessed by HRP-exclusion test. Horseradish peroxidase (HRP)-exclusion test determined amount of axonal membrane damage in healthy control mice ($n = 5$), pre-symptom EAE mice ($n = 7$), peak symptom EAE mice ($n = 6$), and peak symptom EAE + PEG-treated mice ($n = 7$). For pre-symptom EAE group, samples were taken at 8 days post-induction, before symptom emerges. The samples of peak symptom group (for both EAE and EAE + PEG-treated) were taken at 28 days post-induction. **a–d** The images represent HRP-stained sections of spinal cord tissue from the four groups. *Solid arrows* denote areas in which HRP did not penetrate the cell while the *open arrows* point to areas depicting HRP penetration revealing increased axonal membrane permeability. **e** The *bar graph* quantifies HRP uptake in each group. The average density for the control group was 811 ± 130 axons/mm^2. The peak symptom group had the highest levels of axonal damage (6147 ± 665 axons/mm^2, ** $P < 0.01$ compared to control) while the pre-symptom group exhibited increased levels compared to the control group (3293 ± 500 axons/mm^2, * $P < 0.05$ compared to control). In addition, HRP labeling in the EAE/PEG-treated group (1581 ± 247 axons/mm^2) is significantly lower than EAE group (** $p < 0.01$). Scale bar = 10 mm for **a**, **b**, **c** and **d**

membrane permeability [11, 13, 15–17, 30, 42], we have determined that there is a significant level of axonal membrane disruption in EAE mice when symptoms peak. In addition, we also noted a prominent increase, although at a lesser degree, of axonal membrane damage in the pre-symptom stage in EAE mice (Fig. 2). To our knowledge, this is the first evidence of axonal membrane damage in EAE mice, an animal model MS.

Furthermore, PEG, a known membrane repairing agent [28–31], when applied daily for 4 weeks after induction, can significantly reduce axonal membrane disruption in EAE mice (Fig. 2). The restoration of axonal membrane integrity by PEG was accompanied by significant amelioration of behavioral deficits, including a delay of the onset of motor deficits typical of EAE, a delay of emergence of peak symptom, and a reduction of peak symptom severity (Figs. 3 and 4). Taken together, we have presented initial evidence that axonal membrane disruption is an important feature of the overall pathology in EAE mice that is at least in part responsible for the behavioral deficits. Our study also presents the first indication that PEG could be used as a therapeutic agent to effectively repair axolemma, arrest axonal degeneration and reduce motor deficits in EAE mice.

Although not examined in this study, it is likely that PEG-mediated axonal membrane repair also leads to the reduction of axonal degeneration, a known pathology of MS [3, 4, 43]. It is well known that axonal membrane disruption, if not repaired, will lead to axonal degeneration, neuronal cell death and overall neuronal tissue degeneration [13, 17, 44–46]. It has also been demonstrated repeatedly that PEG-mediated neuronal membrane repair can lead to the reduction of oxidative stress and mitochondrial dysfunction which are known contributors to axonal degeneration and neuronal cell death [19, 26, 29, 35, 47]. As such, PEG may also provide neuroprotection by indirectly suppressing oxidative stress and inflammation. Therefore, we postulate that PEG-mediated membrane repair can mitigate axonal degeneration and could promote a range of cellular functions that lead to the improvement of motor function in EAE mice.

Although we did not confirm the presence of PEG inside the spinal cord in the current study following

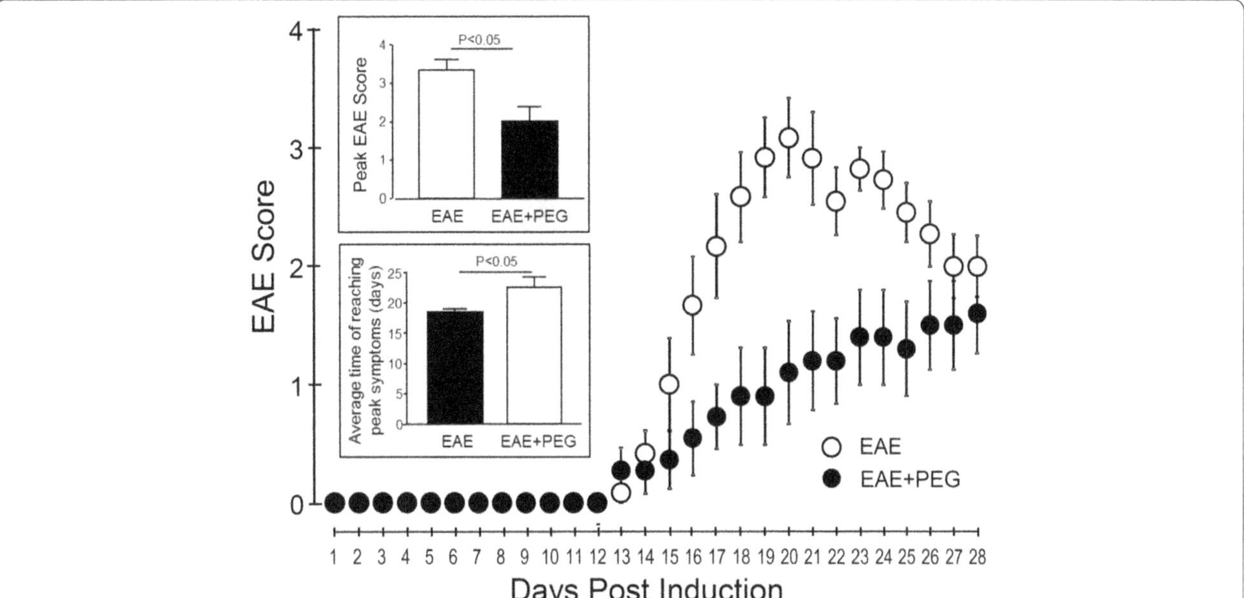

Fig. 3 PEG ameliorated the severity of motor defects and delayed the time of reaching peak motor deficits. Comparison of behavioral assessment each day between EAE (saline-treated, $n = 12$) and EAE + PEG (EAE-treated with PEG, $n = 11$) groups. The graph represents the average score for each group of animals throughout the study. The *upper inset* demonstrates that administration of PEG significantly decreased the peak symptom severity in EAE mice ($P < 0.05$). The highest score of each animal was recorded and averaged within each group to quantify the mean score of severity to be used for the *upper inset*. As indicated, the average of the peak EAE score in EAE + PEG group (1.91 ± 0.4) is significantly lower than that in EAE group (3.33 ± 0.3, $P < 0.05$). The *lower inset* describes the average time of reaching peak symptom of motor deficits in both EAE and EAE + PEG groups. For both EAE and EAE-PEG group, the time of reaching peak symptom is defined as the time that the most severe symptom, or the highest EAE score (≥2) first appears for each animal. If an EAE score of 2 is never reached during the experimental duration (28 days), then 28 day is used as the time of reaching peak symptom. As shown, the average time of reaching the peak EAE score in EAE + PEG group (23.1 ± 1.6) is significantly longer than that in EAE group (18.7 ± 0.8, $P < 0.05$)

systemic application, we believe the main location of PEG treatment is in the central nervous system (CNS), particularly in spinal cord. This is because we have detected significant membrane repair in spinal cord when PEG was applied comparing to no PEG (Fig. 2), and PEG is known to be able to reach spinal cord following systemic application [48]. It is unlikely that PEG-mediated neuroprotection is due to peripheral effects, considering the main pathology of EAE is in CNS [2].

Despite the strong evidence of severe axonal membrane damage in EAE, the mechanisms of such axolemmal damage remain to be elucidated. Based on the previous studies from our and other labs, we suggest that acrolein, a lipid peroxidation byproduct, may be one of the culprits. In a recent study from our lab it was shown that acrolein was increased significantly in EAE mice [25]. We have also shown that acrolein can cause membrane disruption in various preparations at levels that are likely achievable in in vivo pathological conditions [20–22, 49–51]. In fact, acrolein has been suggested to cause neuronal damage in trauma by disrupting neuronal membrane through a delayed mechanism [24, 49, 50, 52–54]. In light of this evidence, we hypothesize that acrolein may play a role in axonal membrane disruption in EAE mice. One critical piece of evidence supports this hypothesis is that hydralazine, an effective acrolein scavenger, can lower acrolein levels and reduce motor deficits in EAE mice [25]. In addition, a recent study from our group demonstrated that acrolein-mediated axonal conduction loss can be partially mitigated by a potassium channel blocker, indicating a concomitant acrolein-mediated myelin damage in addition to axonal lesions [24]. This is because augmented potassium channel activity is a known consequence of myelin damage in injured axons [55]. Consistent with such notion, we also have found that acrolein trapping treatment was associated with restoration of neuronal membrane integrity, reduced neurodegeneration and enhanced functional recovery in traumatic spinal cord injury [21, 22, 24, 50, 51, 53]. It will be interesting to confirm the likely scenario that anti-acrolein therapy alone could lead to the preservation or restoration of axonal membrane integrity in EAE.

In the current study, in addition to the severe membrane disruption observed when symptoms peak, we also noted a less severe, yet still significant level of membrane disruption, and therefore neurodegeneration, in the presymptom period defined as a week prior to the emergence of motor deficits (Figs. 1 and 2). Therefore, significant

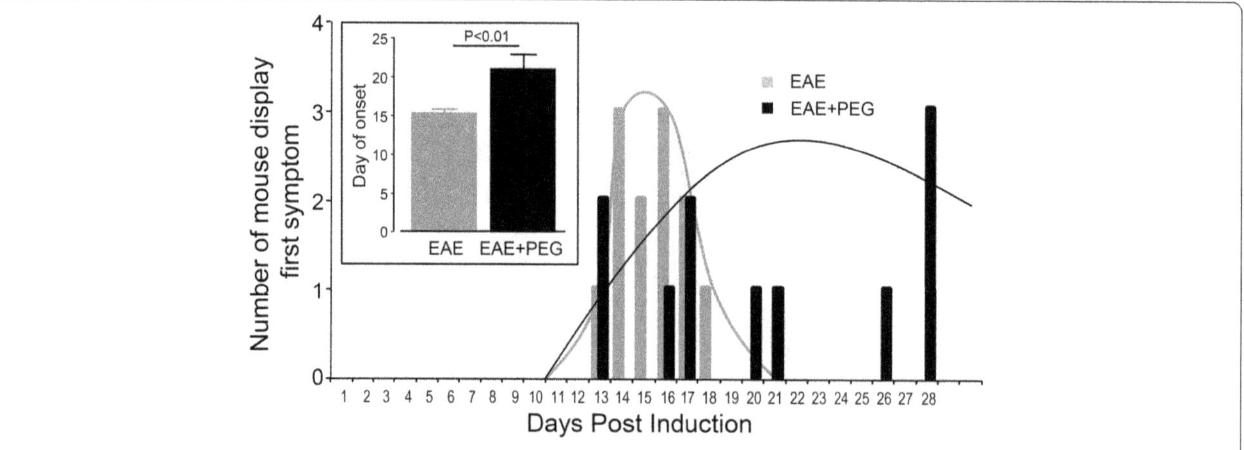

Fig. 4 PEG delayed the onset of motor deficits. Comparison of onset of symptoms between EAE (saline-treated, $n = 12$) and EAE + PEG (EAE-treated with PEG, $n = 11$) groups. The graph represents the temporal distribution or symptom onset for EAE and EAE + PEG mice. The number of mice showing initial symptoms was recorded daily for each group. Symptom onset for EAE mice was tightly clustered early in the study while onset for EAE + PEG mice was more dispersed. The *inset graph* represents the average day of onset for EAE and EAE + PEG groups. Animals in EAE + PEG group developed symptoms significantly later in the study compared to EAE mice ($P < 0.01$). Three mice in the EAE + PEG-group never developed symptoms and were counted as day 28 for both graphs

level of membrane damage and neurodegeneration appear to already exist in the pre-symptom period while no concomitant noticeable behavioral deficits were detected. This phenomenon may be explained by the fact that there is a significant amount of implicit redundancy of axons to support neuronal function. Therefore, there is likely a threshold level of axonal damage and neurodegeneration that must be reached before observing behavioral changes. This would justify the notion that membrane damage could start before the onset of behavioral deficits and that the emergence of behavioral deficits signifies a critical level of axonal damage and degeneration. Hence, the initial membrane damage could theoretically serve as an indication to predict the onset of behavioral deficits at a later date.

In light of these observations related to the relationship between axonal membrane damage and behavioral performance, we suggest that axonal membrane damage in MS could serve as an important diagnostic measurement. First, it can potentially be used as a biomarker for the detection of MS before the emergence of symptoms. This could help to institute earlier treatments to deter neurodegeneration for better therapeutic outcomes provided that the pre-symptomatic axonal membrane damage can be firmly identified. Second, axonal membrane integrity could also serve as an indication of the effectiveness of membrane repair therapy such as PEG. Such a strategy is understandably dependent on development of a reliable non-invasive imaging method to detect axonal membrane disruption or degeneration.

It has become increasingly clear that, in addition to myelin damage, axonal degeneration may also play a critical role in EAE pathology. From a basic cellular biology view, the integrity of both myelin and the axonal membrane are essential for axonal conduction. Therefore, axonal degeneration along with myelin damage, are likely to be equally important contributing factors in axonal conduction failure and behavioral deficits in EAE mice [5, 12, 15, 17, 54, 56, 57]. The current study further highlighted the critical role of axonal damage, and axolemmal disruption in particular, in neurodegeneration and the functional loss in MS. To further stress the importance of axonal degeneration in MS, there is evidence that axonal damage and neurodegeneration may be the main cause of functional loss without obvious myelin damage in some human case of MS. For example, based on a histopathologic investigation using autopsy tissue from MS patients, Trapp and his colleagues have shown compelling evidence of axonal degeneration in the absence of myelin loss [43]. Therefore, axonal damage, a key feature of neurodegeneration, may not just be one of the important compounding pathological factors, but rather it may be among the primary and critical factors that are sufficient to cause clinical functional deficits in MS. To further highlight the importance and causal role of axonal damage in MS pathology, we have noted a significantly higher susceptibility of acrolein-mediated axonal damage compared to acrolein-mediated myelin damage. Specifically, Shi and his colleagues have found that using an ex vivo preparation of extracted rodent spinal cord segment, the threshold of acrolein needed to inflict membrane damage is two magnitudes lower than that needed to cause significant myelin damage [10, 49]. This suggests that in MS patients, axonal degeneration may be, in some cases, the primary pathology that precedes myelin damage. Furthermore, due to the existing evidence of damaging both axon and myelin, acrolein may be a critical link for the damage of both myelin and axons, two known pathologies in EAE. This hypothesis is supported by the factor that acrolein scavenging could mitigate the damage of both myelin and axons [25, 26, 29].

The emergence of the importance of axonal damage as the critical pathology warrants closer examination of our existing therapeutic strategies as well as our efforts to establish new therapies. It appears reasonable to suggest that a treatment regimen should include axonal repair and protection in addition to myelin protection. This combination of treatments may be a synergistic treatment strategy and could result in increased efficacy. We have previously shown that both anti-acrolein (by hydralazine) and membrane repair (by PEG), when used alone, can offer significant, albeit partial alleviation of behavioral deficits [25] (Fig. 3). Furthermore, though PEG significantly delayed the onset and reduced severity in most of the symptomatic periods, such symptom reduction was temporary. PEG treatment did not lead to significant behavioral improvement beyond 26 days post induction, despite effective sealing of the axonal membrane. Therefore, it appears that PEG-mediated membrane repair alone cannot offer long-term symptom reduction. This could be the case for at least two reasons. First, this may indicate that membrane repair strategies need to be combined with approaches that remove causes of cellular damage, such as acrolein, to ultimately protect the cell. Second, although a proven axonal membrane repair agent, PEG has not been shown to also repair myelin damage.

Conclusions

Our findings demonstrate that there is significant axonal membrane damage in addition to myelin destruction and both likley contribute to neurodegeneration in EAE mice. Further, the impairment of axon and myelin may require distinct protective measures and both are critical for a normalization of neuronal function. Taken together, PEG-mediated membrane repair strategy may need to be combined with other measures designed to protect and repair myelin in order to maximize the therapeutic effect and ultimate functional preservation and recovery in MS.

Abbreviations

EAE: Experimental autoimmune encephalomyelitis; MS: Multiple sclerosis; PEG: Polyethylene glycol

Acknowledgements

Not applicable.

Funding

This work was supported by the State of Indiana and the Indiana Clinical and Translational Sciences Institute (PHS NCCR # TL1RR025759 and # RR025761).

Authors' contributions

GL, MT and RS conceived the experiments, GL, MT and JT, conducted the experiments, GL, MT, JT, SW and RS analyzed the results, all authors have read and approved the final manuscript.

Competing interests

Riyi Shi is the co-founder of Neuro Vigor, a start-up company with business interests of developing effective therapies for CNS neurodegenerative diseases and trauma. The authors declare that they have no competing interests.

Author details

[1]Department of Basic Medical Sciences, College of Veterinary Medicine, Purdue University, West Lafayette, IN 47907, USA. [2]Weldon School of Biomedical Engineering, Purdue University, West Lafayette, IN 47907, USA. [3]MSTP program, Indiana University School of Medicine, Indianapolis, IN, USA. [4]Department of Neurobiology, Fourth Military Medical University, Xi'an, China.

References

1. Compston A, Coles A. Multiple sclerosis. Lancet. 2008;372:1502–17.
2. Gold R, Linington C, Lassmann H. Understanding pathogenesis and therapy of multiple sclerosis via animal models: 70 years of merits and culprits in experimental autoimmune encephalomyelitis research. Brain. 2006;129:1953–71.
3. Trapp BD, Nave KA. Multiple sclerosis: an immune or neurodegenerative disorder? Annu Rev Neurosci. 2008;31:247–69.
4. Dutta R, Trapp BD. Pathogenesis of axonal and neuronal damage in multiple sclerosis. Neurology. 2007;68:S22–31. discussion S43-54.
5. Tully M, Shi R. New insights in the pathogenesis of multiple sclerosis—role of acrolein in neuronal and myelin damage. Int J Mol Sci. 2013;14:20037–47.
6. Stadelmann C. Multiple sclerosis as a neurodegenerative disease: pathology, mechanisms and therapeutic implications. Curr Opin Neurol. 2011;24:224–9.
7. Frischer JM, Bramow S, Dal-Bianco A, Lucchinetti CF, Rauschka H, Schmidbauer M, Laursen H, Sorensen PS, Lassmann H. The relation between inflammation and neurodegeneration in multiple sclerosis brains. Brain. 2009;132:1175–89.
8. Haider L, Simeonidou C, Steinberger G, Hametner S, Grigoriadis N, Deretzi G, Kovacs GG, Kutzelnigg A, Lassmann H, Frischer JM. Multiple sclerosis deep grey matter: the relation between demyelination, neurodegeneration, inflammation and iron. J Neurol Neurosurg Psychiatry. 2014;85:1386–95.
9. Kandel ER, Schwartz JH, Jessell TM. Principles of neural science. 4th ed. New York: McGraw-cbrhill; 2000.
10. Shi Y, Sun W, McBride JJ, Cheng JX, Shi R. Acrolein induces myelin damage in mammalian spinal cord. J Neurochem. 2011;117:554–64.
11. Shi R, Whitebone J. Conduction deficits and membrane disruption of spinal cord axons as a function of magnitude and rate of strain. J Neurophysiol. 2006;95:3384–90.
12. Ouyang H, Sun W, Fu Y, Li J, Cheng JX, Nauman E, Shi R. Compression induces acute demyelination and potassium channel exposure in spinal cord. J Neurotrauma. 2010;27:1109–20.
13. Hendricks BK, Shi R. Mechanisms of neuronal membrane sealing following mechanical trauma. Neurosci Bull. 2014;30:627–44.
14. Charil A, Filippi M. Inflammatory demyelination and neurodegeneration in early multiple sclerosis. J Neurol Sci. 2007;259:7–15.
15. Shi R. The dynamics of axolemmal disruption in guinea pig spinal cord following compression. J Neurocytol. 2004;33:203–11.
16. Shi R, Pryor JD. Pathological changes of isolated spinal cord axons in response to mechanical stretch. Neuroscience. 2002;110:765–77.
17. Shi R, Asano T, Vining NC, Blight AR. Control of membrane sealing in injured mammalian spinal cord axons. J Neurophysiol. 2000;84:1763–9.
18. Shi R, Luo J, Peasley MA. Acrolein inflicts axonal membrane disruption and conduction loss in isolated guinea pig spinal cord. Neuroscience. 2002;115:337–40.
19. Luo J, Shi R. Diffusive oxidative stress following acute spinal cord injury in guinea pigs and its inhibition by polyethylene glycol. Neurosci Lett. 2004;359:167–70.
20. Liu-Snyder P, McNally H, Shi R, Borgens RB. Acrolein-mediated mechanisms of neuronal death. J Neurosci Res. 2006;84:209–18.
21. Hamann K, Durkes A, Ouyang H, Uchida K, Pond A, Shi R. Critical role of acrolein in secondary injury following ex vivo spinal cord trauma. J Neurochem. 2008;107:712–21.

22. Hamann K, Nehrt G, Ouyang H, Duerstock B, Shi R. Hydralazine inhibits compression and acrolein-mediated injuries in ex vivo spinal cord. J Neurochem. 2008;104:708–18.
23. Shi R, Rickett T, Sun W. Acrolein-mediated injury in nervous system trauma and diseases. Mol Nutr Food Res. 2011;55:1320–31.
24. Yan R, Page JC, Shi R. Acrolein-mediated conduction loss is partially restored by K+ channel blockers. J Neurophysiol. 2016;115:701–10.
25. Leung G, Sun W, Zheng L, Brookes S, Tully M, Shi R. Anti-acrolein treatment improves behavioral outcome and alleviates myelin damage in experimental autoimmune enchephalomyelitis mouse. Neuroscience. 2011;173:150–5.
26. Luo J, Borgens R, Shi R. Polyethylene glycol immediately repairs neuronal membranes and inhibits free radical production after acute spinal cord injury. J Neurochem. 2002;83:471–80.
27. Luo J, Borgens R, Shi R. Polyethylene glycol improves function and reduces oxidative stress in synaptosomal preparations following spinal cord injury. J Neurotrauma. 2004;21:994–1007.
28. Shi R, Borgens RB. Acute repair of crushed guinea pig spinal cord by polyethylene glycol. J Neurophysiol. 1999;81:2406–14.
29. Nehrt A, Hamann K, Ouyang H, Shi R. Polyethylene glycol enhances axolemmal resealing following transection in cultured cells and in ex vivo spinal cord. J Neurotrauma. 2010;27:151–61.
30. Shi R, Borgens RB. Anatomical repair of nerve membranes in crushed mammalian spinal cord with polyethylene glycol. J Neurocytol. 2000;29:633–43.
31. Borgens RB, Shi R. Immediate recovery from spinal cord injury through molecular repair of nerve membranes with polyethylene glycol. Faseb J. 2000;14:27–35.
32. Shi R. Polyethylene glycol repairs membrane damage and enhances functional recovery: a tissue engineering approach to spinal cord injury. Neurosci Bull. 2013;29:460–6.
33. Shi Y, Kim S, Huff TB, Borgens RB, Park K, Shi R, Cheng JX. Effective repair of traumatically injured spinal cord by nanoscale block copolymer micelles. Nat Nanotechnol. 2010;5:80–7.
34. Baptiste DC, Austin JW, Zhao W, Nahirny A, Sugita S, Fehlings MG. Systemic polyethylene glycol promotes neurological recovery and tissue sparing in rats after cervical spinal cord injury. J Neuropathol Exp Neurol. 2009;68:661–76.
35. Luo J, Shi R. Polyethylene glycol inhibits apoptotic cell death following traumatic spinal cord injury. Brain Res. 2007;1155:10–6.
36. Liu-Snyder P, Logan MP, Shi R, Smith DT, Borgens RB. Neuroprotection from secondary injury by polyethylene glycol requires its internalization. J Exp Biol. 2007;210:1455–62.
37. Ditor DS, John SM, Roy J, Marx JC, Kittmer C, Weaver LC. Effects of polyethylene glycol and magnesium sulfate administration on clinically relevant neurological outcomes after spinal cord injury in the rat. J Neurosci Res. 2007;85:1458–67.
38. Detloff MR, Lavik E, Fisher LC, Langer R, Basso DM. Polyethylene glycol administration after moderate spinal cord injury decreases lesionsize and improves locomotor recovery. J Neurotrauma. 2005;22:1219.
39. Duerstock BS, Borgens RB. Three-dimentional morphometry of spinal cord injury follow polyethylene glycol treatment. J Exp Biol. 2002;205:13–24.
40. Borgens RB, Shi R, Bohnert D. Behavioral recovery from spinal cord injury following delayed application of polyethylene glycol. J Exp Biol. 2002;205:1–12.
41. Kalyvas A, David S. Cytosolic phospholipase A2 plays a key role in the pathogenesis of multiple sclerosis-like disease. Neuron. 2004;41:323–35.
42. Shi R, Pryor JD. Temperature dependence of membrane sealing following transection in mammalian spinal cord axons. Neuroscince. 2000;98:157–66.
43. Bjartmar C, Kinkel RP, Kidd G, Rudick RA, Trapp BD. Axonal loss in normal-appearing white matter in a patient with acute MS. Neurology. 2001;57: 1248–52.
44. Schanne FAX, Kane AB, Young EE, Farber JL. Calcium dependence of toxic cell death: a final common pathway. Science. 1979;206:700–2.
45. Xie X, Barrett JN. Membrane resealing in cultured rat septal neurons after neurite transection: evidence for enhancement by Ca2 + −triggered protease activity and cytoskeletal disassembly. J Neurosci. 1991;11:3257–67.
46. Schlaepfer WW, Bunge RP. Effects of calcium ion concentration on the degeneration of amputated axons in tissue culture. J Cell Biol. 1973;59:456–70.
47. Chen H, Quick E, Leung G, Hamann K, Fu Y, Cheng JX, Shi R. Polyethylene glycol protects injured neuronal mitochondria. Pathobiology. 2009;76:117–28.
48. Borgens RB, Bohnert D. Rapid recovery from spinal cord injury following subcutaneously administered polyethylene glycol. J Neurosci Res. 2001;66: 1179–86.
49. Luo J, Shi R. Acrolein induces axolemmal disruption, oxidative stress, and mitochondrial impairment in spinal cord tissue. Neurochem Int. 2004;44: 475–86.
50. Hamann K, Shi R. Acrolein scavenging: a potential novel mechanism of attenuating oxidative stress following spinal cord injury. J Neurochem. 2009;111:1348–56.
51. Liu-Snyder P, Borgens RB, Shi R. Hydralazine rescues PC12 cells from acrolein-mediated death. J Neurosci Res. 2006;84:219–27.
52. Shi R, Luo L. The role of acrolein in spinal cord injury. Appl Neurol. 2006;2:22–7.
53. Park J, Zheng L, Marquis A, Walls M, Duerstock B, Pond A, Vega-Alvarez S, Wang H, Ouyang Z, Shi R. Neuroprotective role of hydralazine in rat spinal cord injury-attenuation of acrolein-mediated damage. J Neurochem. 2014; 129:339–49.
54. Park J, Muratori B, Shi R. Acrolein as a novel therapeutic target for motor and sensory deficits in spinal cord injury. Neural Regen Res. 2014;9:677–83.
55. Shi R, Sun W. Potassium channel blockers as an effective treatment to restore impulse conduction in injured axons. Neurosci Bull. 2011;27:36–44.
56. Leung G, Sun W, Brookes S, Smith D, Shi R. Potassium channel blocker, 4-Aminopyridine-3-Methanol, restores axonal conduction in spinal cord of an animal model of multiple sclerosis. Exp Neurol. 2011;227:232–5.
57. Shi R, Page JC, Tully M. Molecular mechanisms of acrolein-mediated myelin destruction in CNS trauma and disease. Free Radic Res. 2015;49:888–95.

9

The development prospection of HDAC inhibitors as a potential therapeutic direction in Alzheimer's disease

Shuang-shuang Yang[1], Rui Zhang[1], Gang Wang[2*] and Yong-fang Zhang[1*]

Abstract

Alzheimer's disease (AD) is a chronic neurodegenerative disease, which is associated with learning and memory impairment in the elderly. Recent studies have found that treating AD in the way of chromatin remodeling via histone acetylation is a promising therapeutic regimen. In a number of recent studies, inhibitors of histone deacetylase (HDACs) have been found to be a novel promising therapeutic agents for neurological disorders, particularly for AD and other neurodegenerative diseases. Although HDAC inhibitors have the ability to ameliorate cognitive impairment, successful treatments in the classic AD animal model are rarely translated into clinical trials. As for the reduction of unwanted side effects, the development of HDAC inhibitors with increased isoform selectivity or seeking other directions is a key issue that needs to be addressed. The review focused on literatures on epigenetic mechanisms in recent years, especially on histone acetylation in terms of the enhancement of specificity, efficacy and avoiding side effects for treating AD.

Keywords: Histone deacetylase inhibitors, Alzheimer's disease, Side effects, Specificity, Efficacy

Background

Alzheimer's disease (AD) is a common form of chronic neurodegenerative dementia which is characterized by cognitive impairment and memory deficits [1]. At present, although AD is the most common type of brain disorder caused by multiple factors, its etiology and pathogenesis haven't been fully understood. The major hallmarks of AD pathogenesis, amyloid-β(Aβ) plaques and tau neurofibrillary tangles (NFTs), may cause synaptic loss [2]. The abnormal aggregation and deposition of Aβ are neurotoxic and further cause the pathological changes of the cerebral cortex and apoptosis of nerve cells. NFTs are composed of double helix fibers produced by abnormal phosphorylation of tau protein, which leads to cell death by disrupting transportation. As a complex and interactive relationship between genes and environment, it is believed that epigenetic mechanisms including histone acetylation, DNA methylation, and microRNA modification, are also vital factors to the pathology of AD [3].

Epigenetic modification has opened up a new way for the study of AD. DNA methylation and histone modification have become one of the most significant research hot spots. In previous studies, a great deal of evidence has indicated that histone acetylation plays a vital role in rescuing learning and memory impairment [4]. Histones are building blocks of the nucleosome which is the fundamental unit of chromatin. It is the joint action and dynamic equilibrium of histone-acetyltransferases (HATs) and histone-deacetylases (HDACs) that regulate histone acetylation properly [5]. In general, histone acetylation makes chromatin more loosely packed to activate transcription while histone-deacetylation represses gene transcription.

The state of chromatin structure depends largely on the chemical modification of histone protein complexes. In addition to methylation, phosphorylation, sulfonylation, and ADP ribosylation, histone acetylation

* Correspondence: wgneuron@hotmail.com; zhangyongfang1@yahoo.com
[2]Department of Neurology Ruijin Hospital, School of Medicine, Shanghai Jiao Tong University, Ruijin 2nd Road 197, Shanghai 200025, China
[1]Department of Pharmacology, Institute of Medical Sciences, School of Medicine, Shanghai Jiao Tong University, 280 South Chongqing Road, Shanghai 200025, China

serves as the essential role in transcriptional regulation [6]. In normal neurons, the protein levels of HAT and HDAC as well as their corresponding activities keep in a highly-harmonized balance state, which is conductive to regulate normal gene expression and neurophysiological outputs. However, the acetylation homeostasis is disturbed in neurodegenerative state [7]. Histone deacetylase inhibitors (HDACIs) have, therefore, gained increasing attention and interest as a promising treatment alternative for the field of neurodegenerative diseases [8, 9].

In AD animal models, HDAC inhibitors exhibit neuroprotective and neurodegenerative properties, and it is a promising strategy for brain diseases [10]. Most of the HDAC inhibitors that treat AD models are poorly selective and often cause some undesirable side effects. Therefore, comprehending the position of individual HDAC in AD pathogenesis is critical to the development of more selective HDAC inhibitors. Researchers are looking for various strategies to avoid side effects as much as possible.

Based on the findings in recent years, in this review, we summarized methods to reduce side effects and improve drug efficacy, and some issues remained to be addressed in the future.

Histone deacetylase inhibitors

Theoretically speaking, HDAC inhibitors were originally applied to the cancer therapy. In 2008, Hahnen and colleagues found that the histone deacetylase inhibitors were possible to be an effective strategy for neurodegenerative disorders and identified two major neuroprotective mechanisms including the transcriptional activation of disease-modifying genes and the rectification of destabilization in histone acetylation homeostasis [11].

Recently, many studies have proved that histone acetylation is reduced in various neurodegenerative disorders, such as AD [12]. For example, treatment of SH-SY5Y cells with trichostatin A, a HDAC inhibitor, resulted in a marked up-regulation of Aβ-degrading enzyme neprilysin (NEP) expression [13]. Administration of histone deacetylase inhibitor MS-275 in APP/PS1 models showed ameliorated microglial activation, decreased Aβ deposition, and attenuated inflammatory activation in vitro as well [14]. Therefore, the study of increasing histone acetylation to ameliorate the impairment of memory in AD patients may be a promising strategy. Generally, histone acetylation usually activates gene transcription, whereas histone deacetylation is closely associated with gene transcriptional repression [15]. Both of them alter chromatin structure and transcription factors for the regulation of gene expression.

Strategies to reduce side effects

Enhancing specificity of targeted HDAC isoforms to reduce side effects

Studies have shown that HDAC inhibitors exhibit neuroprotective properties in AD mouse models. Nevertheless, the action of specific HDACs in neurodegenerative disease remains poorly understood in detail and merely pan-HDAC inhibitors were tested in preclinical studies so far. Identifying the role of individual HDAC in AD is critical to the development of specific HDAC inhibitors in curing AD.

In mammals, HDAC enzymes are sorted out into four classes on the basis of their homology to yeast. Class I of HDACs is mainly located in the nucleus and, contains HDAC 1, 2, 3, and 8. Class II of HDACs is further separated into two subtypes: Class IIa includes HDAC4, 5, 7, 9; class IIb includes HDAC 6, 10. In general, class III of HDACs is called as "sirtuins". Class III of HDACs sharing homologous sequence with Sir2 protein contains SirT1-7. Class IV HDACs only has HDAC11 that possesses a catalytic domain at the N-terminus [1].

It is believed that unfavorable side effects are associated with pan-selective isoforms. Enhancing the specificity of isoforms of HDAC inhibitors may be more effective and beneficial to restore cognitive deficits in the AD models.

Targeting at class I of HDACs to enhance specificity

It is the isoform selectivity that determines the specific properties of class I HDAC inhibitors to ameliorate memory impairment. The location and levels of expression differ according to the individual form of different HDACs. Compared with HDAC2 and -3, HDAC1 were detected at relatively lower mRNA levels [16]. A novel selective HDAC2 inhibitor called as W2 was found to decrease Aβ levels and further ameliorate cognitive impairment via promoting the formation and growth of dendric spine density [8, 17].

It's known that amyloid-oligomer attenuates long-term potentiation (LTP), RGFP966 is a specific HDAC3 inhibitor that is a crucial epigenetic negative regulator of cognition. Kumar Krishna et al. provided the first evidence that inhibiting HDAC3 enzyme in single neuron or neuronal populations had the ability of preventing synaptic plasticity induced by amyloid-oligomer [18].

Furthermore, in terms of stimulating synaptogenesis, RGFP963 and RGFP968, acted more efficiently as the HDAC inhibitors comparing with RGFP966, a selective HDAC inhibitor with the ability of ameliorating cognition deficits. Additionally, RGFP963 was invalid in inhibiting HDAC3 while could increase hippocampal spine density. Subsequent research indicated that RGFP963 rather than RGFP966 induced a transcriptional mechanism that enhanced synaptic efficacy and finally rescued learning and memory abilities in AD mouse models [16]. Consistent with the results, researches indicated that inhibiting class I HDAC isoforms simultaneously could be an promising therapy, which might bring a transcriptional synergy and further increase efficacy of producing synapses and treating cognition impairment [16].

Targeting at class IIa of HDACs to enhance specificity

However, not every isoform can be the target to inhibit and ameliorate pathological state. Take HDAC5 for example, R. C. Agis-Balboa et al. tested the role of HDAC5 in AD pathogenesis. They observed the phenomenon that reduced HDAC5 could cause memory impairment and rarely affect the deposition of amyloid plaque [19]. This study elucidated a special function of HDAC5 and revealed HDAC5 isoform should be excluded when seeking for selective HDAC inhibitors in further approaches aiming at treating AD.

Targeting at class IIb of HDACs to enhance specificity

Reduction of HDAC6 is associated with the clearance of both tau and Aβ [20, 21]. HDAC6 is a vital regulator for mitochondrial transport and pharmacological inhibition of HDAC6 promotes the mitochondrial dynamics in Aβ-treated neurons, which can be identified as a new the therapeutic approach [22]. Most importantly, inhibition of HDAC6 is not harmful for cell survival [23]. Inhibiting HDAC6 via deacetylating α-tubulin significantly restored the length of the mitochondria shortened by Aβ to a normal level and rescued hippocampal neuron impairment induced by Aβ. Similarly, one study found that the loss of endogenous HDAC6 levels restored cognitive dysfunction and α-tubulin acetylation in AD mouse models [24]. The finding revealed the therapeutic effect was associated with reduction of HDAC6 rendered neurons against Aβ-mediated disorder of mitochondrial trafficking [24]. HDAC6 might be developed as a potential suitable target for treating AD.

Research found that two selective HDAC6 inhibitors, tubastatin A and ACY-1215, could improve microtubule stability and ameliorate cognitive impairment in AD mouse by promoting tubulin acetylation, reducing production of Aβ and hyper-phosphorylated tau and facilitating autophagic clearance of Aβ and hyper-phosphorylated tau [25]. Compared with SAHA, tubastatin A and ACY-1215 are less toxic indeed. These preclinical results offer prospective approaches for the application of tubastatin A/ACY-1215 to cure AD.

In addition, HDAC6 can drive the deacetylation of KXGS motifs, and further promotes hyper-phosphorylation and polymerization of tau. On the basis of this pathogenic mechanism, inhibiting HDAC6 selectively could improve acetylation and prevent tau accumulation. According to this finding, HDAC6 inhibitors have the ability of enhancing acetylation on KXGS motifs by shifting the ratio between acetylation and phosphorylation to alleviate tau burden. In brief, inhibitors that focus on HDAC6 alone might be a potential perspective for AD with less side effect [26].

Drug combination to reduce side effects

Pan-HDAC inhibitors usually contain unwanted off-target effects limiting the clinical application unavoidably. Drug combination is a feasible strategy that could utilize the compensatory mechanisms and overcome the disadvantages [27]. Indeed, simultaneously inhibiting different targets is possible to bring more efficient effects compared with only use of specific inhibitors [28]. Acting on several effective enzyme activities simultaneously is also a novel pattern of inhibitory action that can reduce side effect. Combining vorinostat (a pan-HDACI) with tadalafil (a phosphodiesterase-5 inhibitor), cognitive deficits, LTP as well as the amyloid and tau pathology were alleviated in AD mice. Remarkably, take curative effect and duration of drug action into account, combining vorinostat with tadalafil was much better than each drug alone [29].

Moreover, Suberoylanilide Hydroxamic Acid (SAHA) is a HDAC inhibitor that can improve cognition [30]. But SAHA is a non-selective inhibitor owing to extensive target at HDAC 1, 2, 3, 6, 8 [31]. Experiments showed that combination of low doses SAHA and curcumin could improve therapeutic selectivity and provide comprehensive protection against Aβ-induced neuronal deficits [32]. These synergisms may contribute to the realization of more optimal safety profiles for HDACIs in chronic treatments.

Balanced dual inhibitors to reduce side effects

To develop a selective and potent drug with minimal unwanted off-target effects, a new attempt is to design selective chemical probes possessing unequivocally validate targets. This method requires chemical probes with optimizing pharmacokinetics so that they could cross the blood brain barrier (BBB) and simultaneously meet the critical safety criteria. These probes will be essential pharmacological tools for in vivo target validation in the search for AD pharmacotherapies [33]. In 2017, Mar Cuadrado-Tejedor and colleagues discovered a new first-in-class small-molecule (CM-414) which is a dual inhibitor of PDE5 and HDACs [34]. CM-414 acts as a chemical probe to achieve both moderate class I HDAC inhibition and PDE5 inhibition that makes histone acetylation more efficient. CM-414 significantly ameliorated the impaired (LTP) and reduced the levels of brain Aβ and tau phosphorylation in Tg2576 mice. As a balanced dual inhibitor, CM-414 may offer an innovative originality to find methods that provided safe and effective treatment for AD patients.

Strategies to improve drug efficacy

Co-location to improve drug efficacy

Not only AD treatment, but the therapies of other aging disease are associated with HDACIs. To receive multiple effects, one study observed that HDAC2 was co-located with insulin signaling components in postsynaptic glutamatergic neurons (PSGNs) of the mouse hippocampus. This may be conductive to understand the roles of both HDAC2 and insulin on neurological deficits of diabetes mellitus, in relation to AD. Of course, it is also beneficial to treat insulin-related diseases when referring to the cognition [35]. This method is available for those patients who suffered from multi-aging diseases.

Increasing permeability to improve drug efficacy

Two novel HDAC inhibitors, mercaptoacetamide-based class II HDACI (represented by W2) and hydroxyamide-based class I and II HDACI (represented by I2), were developed recently and both could reduce Aβ levels obviously and restored cognitive impairment. Most significantly, both W2 and I2 could go through blood brain barrier (BBB) more easily and have a longer half-life [17]. Side effects could be reduced by prolonging half-life and increasing permeability to BBB, which are beneficial to extend plasma half-life of drugs, elevate plasma drug concentration, increase therapeutic effect and diminish baneful adverse reaction.

Stage treatment to improve drug efficacy

Additionally, HDAC inhibitors need to be considered in age-dependent and/or stage-dependent manner when representing as a therapeutic target for AD. The study by Noh H et al. classified the pathogenic process into three different disease stages and sought therapeutic regimen from various angles in detail. They found administration of valproic acid (VPA) to inhibit HDAC reduced cytokine expression levels, raised sAPP and nerve growth factor (NGF) and finally enhanced cognitive function in Tg6799 AD mice [36]. AD in different progress stages may produce specific markers and stage-intervention targeted therapy would be a optimal choice.

Drug administration routes to improve drug efficacy

In recent years, apart from the isoforms-specific of HDAC inhibitors have been significantly developed, what is the best dosing regimen for HDACI to produce neuroprotection, that is, long term treatment vs pulse treatment vs acute treatment is still unclear. Similar to broad-spectrum HDACIs, dose-dependent side effects in patients is the reason of the restriction for chronic disease. Pulse treatment with trichostatin-A (TSA) was shown histone hyperacetylation and neuroprotection in previous study. Post-occlusion administration of sodium butyrate (SB) ameliorates cognitive impairment in a rat model induced by chronic cerebral hypo-perfusion (CCH) [37]. To some extent, treatment strategies like these may get long term HDACI drug treatment away from toxicity and side effects. In addition, HDAC inhibitors combined with other neuroprotective agents may be a good treatment regimen. HDAC inhibitors perhaps could be considered as an ideal target in combination with other neuroprotectants.

Conclusions and perspective

Given the increasing AD patients due to the extension of life span, and the lack of effective treatments, it is urgent to develop novel potential drugs. Most HDAC inhibitors are pan-targeted and easily cause more off-targeted side effects. Successful treatments in the classic AD animal model are also rarely translated into clinical trials, therefore further work is required to validate the findings detailed above before clinical use. Accordingly, therapeutic specificity for neurodegenerative disease can be improved by increasing HDACI isoform selectivity that has the benefit to simultaneously decrease off-target effects [38]. Besides, most researchers have to explore the link between various HDAC isoforms and cognition, particularly the cognitive impairment in mouse models. Enhancing isoform selectivity of HDAC inhibitors is the congruence of goals shared by those who intend to reduce unwanted side effects.

Many research institutes are actively working on selective, specific and orally effective HDAC inhibitors. The inhibitors that are able to enhance HDAC isoform specificity and pharmaceutical potency are thought to possess new chemical scaffolds and have received extensive concern. Researchers have been paying closer attention to the emerging medicinal chemistry principles of HDAC inhibitors and shifting trial-and-error approaches to sophisticated strategies to promote the discovery of ideal-effective HDAC inhibitors [39]. The development of HDACIs with increased isoform selectivity or seeking other directions in order to reduce unwanted side effects is a key issue to be addressed. Based on the various issues that hinder the use of HDAC inhibitors in clinical setting, this review is to sum up the recent research based on the various issues of HDAC inhibitors for reducing defects and improvingspecificity/efficacy. However, current articles on selective HDAC inhibitors are not enough to address the clinical application and much work remains to be carried out in the future.

Abbreviations

AD: Alzheimer's disease; Aβ: amyloid-β; BBB: Blood brain barrier; CCH: Chronic cerebral hypo-perfusion; HATs: Histone acetyltransferases; HDACIs: Histone deacetylases inhibitors; HDACs: Histone deacetylases; LTP: Long-term potentiation; NEP: Neprilysin; NFTs: Neurofibrillary tangles; NGF: Nerve growth factor; SB: Sodium butyrate

Acknowledgements
Not applicable.

Funding
This work was supported by the National Natural Science Foundation of China (Grant No. 81573401).

Authors' contributions
SSY and RZ mainly designed and drafted the manuscript. YFZ and GW were involved in critically revising the manuscript and provided intellectual thoughts. All authors read and approved the final manuscript to be published.

Competing interests
The authors declare that they have no competing interests.

References
1. Xu K, Dai XL, Huang HC, Jiang ZF. Targeting HDACs: a promising therapy for Alzheimer's disease. Oxidative Med Cell Longev. 2011;2011:143269.
2. Zuo L, Hemmelgarn BT, Chuang CC, Best TM. The role of Oxidative stress-induced epigenetic alterations in Amyloid-beta production in Alzheimer's disease. Oxidative Med Cell Longev. 2015;2015:604658.
3. Li X, Bao X, Wang R. Neurogenesis-based epigenetic therapeutics for Alzheimer's disease (review). Mol Med Rep. 2016;14(2):1043–53.
4. Liu RT, Zou LB, Lu QJ. Liquiritigenin inhibits Abeta(25-35)-induced neurotoxicity and secretion of Abeta(1-40) in rat hippocampal neurons. Acta Pharmacol Sin. 2009;30(7):899–906.
5. Fischer A. Targeting histone-modifications in Alzheimer's disease. What is the evidence that this is a promising therapeutic avenue? Neuropharmacology. 2014;80:95–102.
6. Konsoula Z, Barile FA. Epigenetic histone acetylation and deacetylation mechanisms in experimental models of neurodegenerative disorders. J Pharmacol Toxicol Methods. 2012;66(3):215–20.
7. Mai A, Rotili D, Valente S, Kazantsev AG. Histone deacetylase inhibitors and neurodegenerative disorders: holding the promise. Curr Pharm Des. 2009;15(34):3940–57.
8. Song JM, Sung YM, Nam JH, Yoon H, Chung A, Moffat E, Jung M, Pak DTS, Kim J, Hoe HS. A Mercaptoacetamide-based class II Histone Deacetylase inhibitor increases Dendritic spine density via RasGRF1/ERK pathway. J Alzheimers Dis. 2016;51(2):591–604.
9. Benito E, Urbanke H, Ramachandran B, Barth J, Halder R, Awasthi A, Jain G, Capece V, Burkhardt S, Navarro-Sala M, et al. HDAC inhibitor-dependent transcriptome and memory reinstatement in cognitive decline models. J Clin Invest. 2015;125(9):3572–84.
10. Graeff J, Tsai L-H: The potential of HDAC inhibitors as cognitive enhancers. In: Annual review of pharmacology and toxicology, Vol 53, 2013. Volume 53, edn. Edited by Insel PA; 2013: 311-330.
11. Hahnen E, Hauke J, Trankle C, Eyupoglu IY, Wirth B, Blumcke I. Histone deacetylase inhibitors: possible implications for neurodegenerative disorders. Expert Opin Investig Drugs. 2008;17(2):169–84.
12. Lockett GA, Wilkes F, Maleszka R. Brain plasticity, memory and neurological disorders: an epigenetic perspective. Neuroreport. 2010;21(14):909–13.
13. Kerridge C, Belyaev ND, Nalivaeva NN, Turner AJ. The a beta-clearance protein transthyretin, like neprilysin, is epigenetically regulated by the amyloid precursor protein intracellular domain. J Neurochem. 2014;130(3):419–31.
14. Zhang ZY, Schluesener HJ. Oral administration of histone deacetylase inhibitor MS-275 ameliorates neuroinflammation and cerebral amyloidosis and improves behavior in a mouse model. J Neuropathol Exp Neurol. 2013;72(3):178–85.
15. Lu X, Wang L, Yu CJ, Yu DH, Yu G. Histone acetylation modifiers in the pathogenesis of Alzheimer's disease. Front Cell Neurosci. 2015;9:3.
16. Rumbaugh G, Sillivan SE, Ozkan ED, Rojas CS, Hubbs CR, Aceti M, Kilgore M, Kudugunti S, Puthanveettil SV, Sweatt JD, et al. Pharmacological selectivity within class I Histone Deacetylases predicts effects on synaptic function and memory rescue. Neuropsychopharmacology. 2015;40(10):2307–16.
17. Sung YM, Lee T, Yoon H, DiBattista AM, Song JM, Sohn Y, Moffat EI, Turner RS, Jung M, Kim J, et al. Mercaptoacetamide-based class II HDAC inhibitor lowers Abeta levels and improves learning and memory in a mouse model of Alzheimer's disease. Exp Neurol. 2013;239:192–201.
18. Krishna K, Behnisch T, Sajikumar S. Inhibition of Histone Deacetylase 3 restores Amyloid-beta Oligomer-induced plasticity deficit in Hippocampal CA1 pyramidal neurons. J Alzheimers Dis. 2016;51(3):783–91.
19. Agis-Balboa RC, Pavelka Z, Kerimoglu C, Fischer A. Loss of HDAC5 impairs memory function: implications for Alzheimer's disease. J Alzheimers Dis. 2013;33(1):35–44.
20. Zhang L, Liu C, Wu J, Tao JJ, Sui XL, Yao ZG, Xu YF, Huang L, Zhu H, Sheng SL, et al. Tubastatin a/ACY-1215 improves cognition in Alzheimer's disease transgenic mice. J Alzheimer's Dis. 2014;41(4):1193–205.
21. Cook C, Gendron TF, Scheffel K, Carlomagno Y, Dunmore J, DeTure M, Petrucelli L. Loss of HDAC6, a novel CHIP substrate, alleviates abnormal tau accumulation. Hum Mol Genet. 2012;21(13):2936–45.
22. Kim C, Choi H, Jung ES, Lee W, Oh S, Jeon NL, Mook-Jung I. HDAC6 inhibitor blocks Amyloid Beta-induced impairment of mitochondrial transport in Hippocampal neurons. PLoS One. 2012:7(8).
23. Robers MB, Dart ML, Woodroofe CC, Zimprich CA, Kirkland TA, Machleidt T, Kupcho KR, Levin S, Hartnett JR, Zimmerman K, et al. Target engagement and drug residence time can be observed in living cells with BRET. Nat Commun. 2015;6:10091.
24. Govindarajan N, Rao P, Burkhardt S, Sananbenesi F, Schluter OM, Bradke F, Lu J, Fischer A. Reducing HDAC6 ameliorates cognitive deficits in a mouse model for Alzheimer's disease. EMBO Mol Med. 2013;5(1):52–63.
25. Zhang L, Liu C, Wu J, Tao J-J, Sui X-L, Yao Z-G, Xu Y-F, Huang L, Zhu H, Sheng S-L, et al. Tubastatin a/ACY-1215 improves cognition in Alzheimer's disease transgenic mice. J Alzheimers Dis. 2014;41(4):1193–205.
26. Cook C, Carlomagno Y, Gendron TF, Dunmore J, Scheffel K, Stetler C, Davis M, Dickson D, Jarpe M, DeTure M, et al. Acetylation of the KXGS motifs in tau is a critical determinant in modulation of tau aggregation and clearance. Hum Mol Genet. 2014;23(1):104–16.
27. Lehar J, Krueger AS, Avery W, Heilbut AM, Johansen LM, Price ER, Rickles RJ, Short GF 3rd, Staunton JE, Jin X, et al. Synergistic drug combinations tend to improve therapeutically relevant selectivity. Nat Biotechnol. 2009;27(7):659–66.
28. Zheng H, Fridkin M, Youdim M. From single target to multitarget/network therapeutics in Alzheimer's therapy. Pharmaceuticals. 2014;7(2):113–35.
29. Cuadrado-Tejedor M, Garcia-Barroso C, Sanzhez-Arias J, Mederos S, Rabal O, Ugarte A, Franco R, Pascual-Lucas M, Segura V, Perea G, et al. Concomitant histone deacetylase and phosphodiesterase 5 inhibition synergistically prevents the disruption in synaptic plasticity and it reverses cognitive impairment in a mouse model of Alzheimer's disease. Clin Epigenetics. 2015;7.
30. Kilgore M, Miller CA, Fass DM, Hennig KM, Haggarty SJ, Sweatt JD, Rumbaugh G. Inhibitors of class 1 histone deacetylases reverse contextual memory deficits in a mouse model of Alzheimer's disease. Neuropsychopharmacology. 2010;35(4):870–80.
31. Xu WS, Parmigiani RB, Marks PA. Histone deacetylase inhibitors: molecular mechanisms of action. Oncogene. 2007;26(37):5541–52.
32. Meng J, Li Y, Camarillo C, Yao Y, Zhang Y, Xu C, Jiang L. The anti-tumor histone deacetylase inhibitor SAHA and the natural flavonoid curcumin exhibit synergistic neuroprotection against amyloid-beta toxicity. PLoS One. 2014;9(1):e85570.
33. Cuadrado-Tejedor M, Oyarzabal J, Lucas MP, Franco R, Garcia-Osta A. Epigenetic drugs in Alzheimer's disease. Biomol concepts. 2013;4(5):433–45.
34. Cuadrado-Tejedor M, Garcia-Barroso C, Sánchez-Arias JA, Rabal O, Pérez-González M, Mederos S, Ugarte A, Franco R, Segura V, Perea G, et al. A first-in-class small-molecule that acts as a dual inhibitor of HDAC and PDE5 and

that rescues Hippocampal synaptic impairment in Alzheimer's disease mice. Neuropsychopharmacology. 2017;42(2):524–39.
35. Yao Z-G, Liu Y, Zhang L, Huang L, Ma C-M, Xu Y-F, Zhu H, Qin C. Co-location of HDAC2 and insulin signaling components in the adult mouse hippocampus. Cell Mol Neurobiol. 2012;32(8):1337–42.
36. Noh H, Seo H. Age-dependent effects of valproic acid in Alzheimer's disease (AD) mice are associated with nerve grow factor (NGF) regulation. Neuroscience. 2014;266:255–65.
37. Liu H, Zhang JJ, Li X, Yang Y, Xie XF, Hu K. Post-occlusion administration of sodium butyrate attenuates cognitive impairment in a rat model of chronic cerebral hypoperfusion. Pharmacol Biochem Behav. 2015;135:53–9.
38. Graff J, Tsai LH. The potential of HDAC inhibitors as cognitive enhancers. Annu Rev Pharmacol Toxicol. 2013;53:311–30.
39. Zhan P, Wang X, Liu X, Suzuki T. Medicinal chemistry insights into novel HDAC inhibitors: an updated patent review (2012-2016). Recent Pat Anticancer Drug Discov. 2017;12(4):16–34.

10

The predictive value of SS-16 in clinically diagnosed Parkinson's disease patients: comparison with ^{99m}Tc-TRODAT-1 SPECT scans

Wenyan Kang[1,2†], Fangyi Dong[1†], Dunhui Li[1], Thomas J. Quinn[3], Shengdi Chen[1] and Jun Liu[1*]

Abstract

Background: Dopamine transporter based imaging has high diagnostic performance in distinguishing patients with Parkinson's disease (PD) from patients with non-Parkinsonian syndromes. Our previous study indicated that the "Sniffin' Sticks" odor identification test (SS-16) acts as a valid instrument for olfactory assessment in Chinese PD patients. The aim of the study was to compare the efficacy of the two methods in diagnosing PD.

Methods: Fifty-two PD patients were involved in this study and underwent single photon emission computed tomography (SPECT) imaging using the labeled dopamine transporter radiotracer ^{99m}Tc-TRODAT-1 to assess nigrostriatal dopaminergic function. Olfactory function was assessed with the "Sniffin' Sticks" odor identification test (SS-16) in all patients who received DAT-SPECT scanning. Statistical analysis (SPSS version 21) was carried out to determine the diagnostic accuracy of SS-16 as well as its correlation with ^{99m}Tc-TRODAT-1 SPECT, its positive predictive value (PPV), and negative predictive value (NPV).

Results: We identified a negative correlation between SS-16 and DAT SPECT (Kappa = 0.269, $p = 0.004$). By using the ^{99m}Tc-TRODAT-1 uptake results as the gold standard, the sensitivity and specificity of SS-16 was 56.8 and 37.5 %, respectively. Furthermore, the negative and positive predictive values were calculated as 13.6 and 83.3 %, respectively.

Conclusions: SS-16 would not be used as a diagnostic tool for early stage PD patients. Negative results of SS-16 would not exclude the diagnosis of PD. Further tests are needed for validation.

Keywords: Parkinson's disease, DAT-SPECT, SS-16

Background

At least 50 % of nigrostriatal neurons have already been lost at the time of clinical diagnosis for Parkinson's disease (PD), a diagnosis which significantly relies on the identification of classical motor symptoms. An early and precise diagnosis of PD is critical since early treatment with neuroprotective agents before most substantial neuronal loss has occurred is believed to be beneficial which could potentially slow or prevent the development of PD symptoms.

As one of the most common non-motor symptoms, a majority of PD patients are diagnosed with olfactory impairment, which may even appear before the development of motor symptoms. Therefore, analysis of olfaction may be a useful diagnostic tool for PD. There are two main olfactory tests available that can readily be utilized in PD patients, the University of Pennsylvania 40-item smell identification test (UPSIT-40) and the "Sniffin' Sticks" 16-item identification test SS-16 [1]. Tests of odor identification might help differentiate PD patients from healthy controls and have many advantages, including: low cost, ease of administration and rapid results. Therefore, olfactory tests are suited for routine use in daily clinical practice and are currently utilized in Europe. Our previous study indicated that SS-

* Correspondence: jly0520@hotmail.com
†Equal contributors
[1]Department of Neurology & Institute of Neurology, Ruijin Hospital affiliated to Shanghai Jiaotong University School of Medicine, Shanghai, China
Full list of author information is available at the end of the article

16 act as a valid instrument for olfactory assessment in Chinese PD patients, and hyposmia may correlate with autonomic dysfunction in patients with PD [2].

In recent years, studies have demonstrated that a steady degradation of striatal uptake was observed as a function of clinical duration after an estimated preclinical duration of eleven years prior to PD symptom onset [3]. Several different diagnostic tools have been evaluated for their ability to detect nigrostriatal cell loss. The most widely used tests are dopamine transporter single-photon emission computed tomography (DAT SPECT), [18 F]DOPA positron emission tomography (PET), and transcranial sonography (TCS) [4]. A recent systematic review indicated that sensitivity and specificity of DAT SPECT imaging to detect nigrostriatal cell loss were 98 %, and it seems to be accurate in detecting nigrostriatal cell loss in patients with Parkinsonism [4]. SPECT-based brain scans have become increasingly common in routine PD diagnosis [2, 5, 6]. However, these scans are expensive and there are still technical issues which can lead to difficulties with interpretation in borderline cases. In this study, using DAT SPECT results as the clinical gold standard, we assessed the diagnostic accuracy of SS-16 on 52 patients diagnosed with PD based on clinical features in their early stage. Furthermore, this enabled us to also assess the ability of hyposmia defined by a SS-16 score to predict a DAT deficit.

Methods

Participants

A total of 52 PD patients were recruited in this study by consecutive referral at the movement disorders clinic in the Department of Neurology, Ruijin Hospital affiliated to Shanghai Jiao Tong University School of Medicine. Two senior movement disorders specialists clinically identified all patients in this study according to the United Kingdom Parkinson's Disease Society Brain Bank criteria. Patients with possible olfactory dysfunction secondary to other causes, such as nose surgery, chronic sinusitis, acute upper respiratory tract infection and other central nervous system diseases were excluded. Moreover, illiterate individuals were excluded from this study. All patients underwent the Chinese equivalent of the Mini Mental State Examination. We excluded participants with scores less than 20 for individuals that received 6 years or less of primary school education and participants with scores less than 24 for individuals that received more than 6 years of schooling. All subjects read and signed an informed consent prior to participation in the study. This study was approved by the Ethics Committee of Ruijin Hospital affiliated to Shanghai Jiao Tong University School of Medicine.

Experimental procedure

^{99m}Tc-TRODAT-1 SPECT

^{99m}Tc-TRODAT-1 SPECT was performed as described in our previous study [7]. Briefly,two hours after intravenous injection of ^{99m}Tc-TRODAT-1, prepared from a pre-formulated kit provided by Jiangsu Nuclear Medicine Institute (WuXi city, China), ^{99m}Tc-TRODAT-1 uptake was assessed by SPECT imaging. Images were acquired via a double-headed gamma camera (Simens, Symbia T16), with a 140 ± 14 keV energy window. Acquisition time for the projection was 30s, with a 1.45 zoom and 3 mm slice thickness at the level of the basal ganglia. Regions of interest (ROIs) for ^{99m}Tc-TRODAT-1 uptake were established by MRI (1.5 T, Siemens, Germany). Of note, if the average ^{99m}Tc-TRODAT-1 uptake was less than 1.21 for the right side or 1.31 for the left side, striatal uptake (a combination of putamen and caudate uptake) of the alternative side was considered pathological [8].

Odor identification test

Bilingual university graduate students translated the original SS-16 to Chinese (simplified) [9]. The content and wording of the questionnaires were discussed with the patients' representatives and caregivers, as well as public health experts. and the 16 odors in the original "Sniffin' Stick" odor identification test were kept the same but alternative descriptions were developed to accommodate the Chinese population. For example, the descriptions "pine tree" and "grapefruit" were replaced with the Mandarin equivalent of "wood," and "pomelo", which are common in mainland China and are similar odors. The test was continuously revised until it was considered unambiguous by the research committee. The odor sticks were placed approximately 2 cm in front of the nose of the subjects to smell for 3 s, and the subject was required to choose between four alternatives in a forced-choice paradigm. The interval between tests of various odors was about 30s. Each correct answer for each odor received a score of 1; thus, the total score expressed as the sum of correct responses ranged from 0 to 16. Subjects with scores lower than 9.5 were defined as olfactory impaired [2].

Statistical analysis

Statistical analysis was carried out using SPSS version 21. The diagnostic accuracy of SS-16 was determined by comparing their results to the surrogate gold standard: ^{99m}Tc-TRODAT-1 scans. Diagnostic accuracy is defined as the sensitivity, specificity, positive predictive value (PPV) and negative predictive value (NPV). Finally, we used Kappa test to compare the consistency of the two examinations. P values of less than 0.05 were considered statistically significant.

Results

Descriptives

The mean age of the 52 patients was 60.65 ± 7.82 years, and the majority (32/52) were male. The mean course of disease was 4.04 ± 3.54 years, and the mean Hoehn and Yahr score was 1.63 ± 0.83. The average UPDRS III score was 14.18 ± 11.23. The R/L-Striatal 99mTc-TRODAT-1 uptake was 0.81 ± 0.68. All recruited PD patients had the 16-item odor identification test from Sniffin' Sticks (SS-16), the score was 8.60 ± 3.16.

Accuracy of SS-16 in clinically diagnosed PD patients

For the complete overview of the results of the SS-16, ^{99m}Tc-TRODAT-1 SPECT in each subgroup of patients, see Fig. 1.

In the 52 subjects (20 women, 32 men) who underwent the 16-item odor identification test from Sniffin' Sticks (SS-16), 30 subjects (57.69 %) had distinct hyposmia (SS-16 scores <9.5). Of the 30 patients, 25 (83.33 %) had an abnormal 99mTc-TROD AT-1 uptake scan. 22 of the 52 patients had normal olfactory dysfunction, while only 3 had a normal ^{99m}Tc-TRODAT-1 uptake scan. Taking ^{99m}Tc-TROD AT-1 uptake results as the gold standard, the sensitivity of SS-16 was 56.8 % (25/(25 + 19)), and the specificity was 37.5 % (3/(5 + 3)).

Predictive value of SS-16 for the results of the DAT SPECT scans

To estimate the predictive values of SS-16 for the early-diagnosis of PD, all 52 patients were included in the analysis. In 28 patients (53.85 %), the result of the SS-16 was in accordance with the result of the ^{99m}Tc-TROD AT-1 scan. The PPV of a positive SS-16 test result for an abnormal scan was 83.3 % (25/30). However, the NPV of a negative SS-16 test result for a normal scan was only 13.6 %(3/22). The false negative rate of SS-16 test result for the DAT imaging result was 43.2 % (19/44). SS-16 and DAT-SPECT were both positive in 25 patients (48.1 %), while 3 patients (5.8 %) had double negative results. In summary, in 28 patients, the results of the SS-16 test were in accordance with the results of the DAT SPECT scan (Kappa test, Kappa = 0.269, P =0.004). Therefore, the consistency was poor (see Table 1).

Discussions

Olfactory dysfunction is a prodromal symptom in PD and can be found several years before the appearance of motor signs. In addition, it develops independent of treatment or age at onset. Olfactory tests, including ethnically specific odors, were recommended by the European Federation of Neurological Societies and the Movement Disorder Society as screening tests for pre-motor PD [10]. Moreover, the fact that α-synuclein deposits are present in the olfactory bulb and anterior olfactory nucleus at Braak stage I explains its high sensitivity in early PD [11]. A study that correlated diffusion tensor imaging (DTI) with olfactory deficit in early PD patients demonstrated that the Fractional anisotropy (FA) values of White Matter (WM) were significantly reduced in the early PD group versus healthy controls [12].

Prior studies have demonstrated SS-16 reliability in differentiating PD patients and healthy subjects in Asia and Latin America [1, 2]. Furthermore, a previous study suggested that the performance of Sniffin' Sticks was better than that of UPSIT, even among Children to whom discriminating different smells is more perplexing [7]. Thus, SS-16 showed capability in differentiating olfactory impairment in spite of the poor life experience of different smells. In the present study we try to investigate whether Sniffin' Sticks hold the qualification to detect early PD clinically with DAT SPECT as a gold standard.

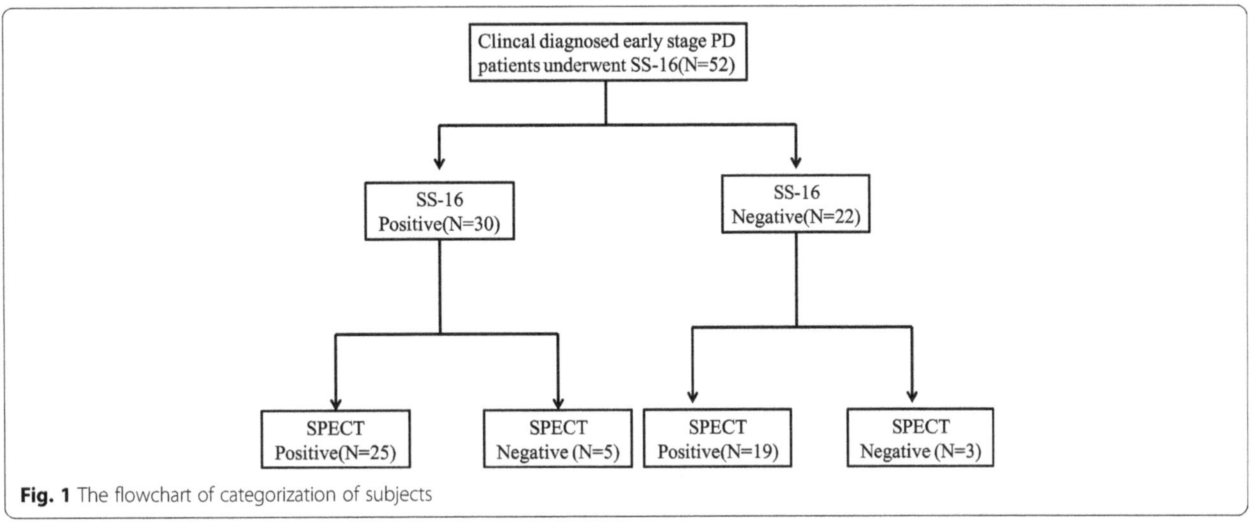

Fig. 1 The flowchart of categorization of subjects

Table 1 Predictive values of SS-16 for the results of the DAT-SPECT scan

	Sensitivity (%)	Specificity (%)	Positive predictive value (%)	Negative predictive value (%)	Kappa	*P* value
SS-16	56.8 %	37.5 %	83.3 %	13.6 %	0.269	0.004

Previous studies focus on identifying the diagnostic value of prodromal or early PD by combining smell tests with imaging examinations [13, 14]. Nevertheless, the investigation of consistency between olfactory impairment results and imaging diagnosis standards is lacking. In the present study, we found that the correlation between these two items is negative (Kappa = 0.269, $p = 0.004$). Taking ^{99m}Tc-TROD AT-1 uptake results as the gold standard, the sensitivity of SS-16 for DAT SPECT was 56.82 % with a false negative predictive value of 43.2 %. The negative predictive value was 13.6 %, and the specificity was only 37.5 %, while the positive predictive value was 83.3 %. The over misdiagnosis was reasonable to some degree and a number of factors might contribute to this outcome.

First, although olfactory impairment acts as a symptom of PD originating from extranigral neuropathological change according to Braak staging of Parkinson's disease, hyposmia is prevalent in Parkinson's disease with the deficiency of smell test ranging from 73 to 90 %, indicating a minority of PD patients not suffering from olfactory deficiency [15]. In a recent study, the utilization of SS-16 was compared among different countries with China included. The results suggested that the scores of several items called "component1" were significantly different across PD patients from different country groups because of culture, smell familiarity and environmental variations [11, 16]. Our previous study used the adapted SS-16 translational version evaluation (mentioned in the methods) in Chinese patients, resulting in a sensitivity of 86 % and the specificity of 81 % in discriminating PD patients from healthy controls. Among the 110 patients, 66.4 % were identified as having hyposmia. In addition, the cohort of 52 patients was in the early stage (Hoehn and Yahr score was 1.63 ± 0.83), thus, 57.7 % could be explained in the study and may not affect the results [2]. Thus, a certain rate of false negative and positive value exists in the particular SS-16 test and among a certain number of Chinese population. To that end, a larger sample size to evaluate the SS-16 test is in urgently needed to demonstrate stable scale characteristics.

Second, in the present study, the clinical PD diagnosis fulfilled the established UK Parkinson's Disease Society Brain Bank clinical diagnostic criteria. The clinical symptoms of PD were assessed by movement disorder specialists. Nevertheless, some atypical parkinsonism related disorders, such as MSA, essential tremor progressive supranuclear palsy and cortico-basal degeneration, might not be clearly discriminated from PD in the early disease course. However, olfactory function among the above diseases is impaired mildly and for monogenic PD, especially in recessive forms, the dysfunction is less serious than in PD. Consequently, there is a tendency for false negative predictive value elevation and with reduced specificity.

Third, with regard to DAT-SPECT diagnosistic capability, M. Menendez-Gonzalez [17] concluded that false negative values would become higher due to the quantitative analysis of SPECT scans and the existence of SWEDDs (scans without evidence of dopaminergic deficits). In addition, in early PD, 15 % patients might show normal brain scan results. The misdiagnosis could not be excluded in the assessment.

The present study is the first to take DAT SPECT as the gold standard to assess the correlation between SS-16 scores and ^{99m}Tc-TROD AT-1 uptake results from SPECT imaging in a Chinese population. The positive predictive value against SPECT was 83.3 %. Our previous study compared TCS with SPECT, finding the positive predictive value to be 91.7 % which was not much higher than SS-16 [8]. However, negative results of the SS-16 test could not exclude the diagnosis of PD. And there are some limitations in our study. For one thing, healthy subjects were not enrolled in the study. In addition, this study is limited by the small sample size of 52 patients, and larger samples are necessary in the future to produce results more representative of the population.

Conclusions

In conclusion, SS-16 is a non-invasive, low cost, rapid and convenient procedure recommended to be used as a clinical test in spite of the negative correlation with dopamine uptake results reflected via DAT SPECT. SS-16 would not be used as a diagnostic tool for early stage PD patients as a negative SS-16 test result could not exclude the diagnosis of PD.

Acknowledgements
We thank all the patients subjects for their generous donations. We also thank Linyuan Zhang, Qiong Yang, Xiaoying Wang, Wei Chen,Yu Zhang, for study coordination.

Funding
This work was supported by grants from the National Natural Science Foundation of China (81471287, 81071024, 81171202, 81371407, 30872729, 30870879,81501097), the Shanghai Shuguang Program (11SG20), the Shanghai Municipal Education Commission-Gaofeng Clinical Medicine Grant (20152201), and the Fifth National Undergraduate Student Innovating

Program (2011015). The Scientific Research Program of Shanghai Health and Family Planning Commission (20144Y0220).

Authors' contributions

JL and SC conceived and supervised the project. SC and JL were responsible for subject recruitment. WK, JL, TJQ and FD drafted the manuscript. WK, FD and DL were responsible for sample collection. WK and FD worked on Odor identification test and 99mTc-TRODAT-1 SPECT. WK worked on data management and statistical analyses. All authors critically reviewed the manuscript. All authors read and approved the final manuscript.

Competing interests

The authors declare that they have no competing interests.

Disclosure

This study was sponsored by Neurology & Institute of Neurology, Ruijin Hospital affiliated to Shanghai Jiaotong University School of Medicine.
Dr. Wenyan Kang reports no disclosures.
Dr. Fangyi Dong reports no disclosures.
Mr. Dunhui Li reports no disclosures.
Dr. Thomas J. Quinn reports no disclosures.
Dr. Shengdi Chen reports no disclosures.
Dr. Jun Liu reports no disclosures.

Author details

[1]Department of Neurology & Institute of Neurology, Ruijin Hospital affiliated to Shanghai Jiaotong University School of Medicine, Shanghai, China. [2]Department of Neurology, Ruijin Hospital North affiliated to Shanghai Jiaotong University School of Medicine, Shanghai, China. [3]Department of Radiation Oncology, Beaumont Health System, Royal Oak, MI 48073, USA.

References

1. Silveira-Moriyama L, Carvalho Mde J, Katzenschlager R, Petrie A, Ranvaud R, Barbosa ER, Lees AJ. The use of smell identification tests in the diagnosis of Parkinson's disease in Brazil. Mov Disord. 2008;23(16):2328–34. doi:10.1002/mds.22241.
2. Chen W, Chen S, Kang WY, Li B, Xu ZM, Xiao Q, Liu J, Wang Y, Wang G, Chen SD. Application of odoridentifycation test in Parkinson's disease in China: a matched case-control study. J Neurol Sci. 2012;316(1–2):47–50. doi:10.1016/j.jns.2012.01.033.
3. Fang YH, Chiu SC, Lu CS, Yen TC, Weng YH. Fully automated quantification of the Striatal uptake ratio of [(99m)Tc]-TRODAT with SPECTImaging: Evaluation of the diagnostic performance in Parkinson's disease and the temporal regression of Striatal tracer uptake. Biomed Res Int. 2015;2015: 461625. doi:10.1155/2015/461625.
4. Suwijn SR, van Boheemen CJ, de Haan RJ, Tissingh G, Booij J, de Bie RM. The diagnostic accuracy of dopamine transporter SPECT imaging to detect nigrostriatal cell loss in patients with Parkinson's disease or clinically uncertain parkinsonism: a systematic review. EJNM MI Res. 2015;5:12. doi:10.1186/s13550-015-0087-1.
5. Bajaj N, Hauser RA, Seibyl J, Kupsch A, Plotkin M, Chen C, Grachev ID. Association between Hoehn and Yahr, Mini-Mental State Examination, age, and clinical syndrome predominance and diagnostic effectiveness of ioflupane I 123 injection (DaTSCANTM) in subjects with clinically uncertain parkinsonian syndromes. Alzheimers Res Ther. 2014;6(5–8):67. doi:10.1186/s13195-014-0067–0.
6. Scherfler C, Schwarz J, Antonini A, Grosset D, Valldeoriola F, Marek K, Oertel W, Tolosa E, Lees AJ, Poewe W. Role of DAT-SPECT in the diagnostic work up of Parkinsonism. Mov Disord. 2007;22(9):1229–38. Review.
7. Hugh SC, Siu J, Hummel T, Forte V, Campisi P, Papsin BC, Propst EJ. Olfactory testing in children using objective tools: comparison of Sniffin' Sticks and University of Pennsylvania Smell Identific ation Test (UPSIT). Otolaryngol Head Neck Surg. 2015;44:10. doi:10.1186/s40463-015-0061-y.
8. Li DH, Zhang LY, Hu YY, Jiang XF, Zhou HY, Yang Q, Kang WY, Liu J, Chen SD. Transcranial sonography of the substantia nigra and its correlation with DAT-SPECT in the diagnosis of Parkinson's disease. Parkinsonism Relat Disord. 2015;21(8):923–8. doi:10.1016/j.parkreldis.
9. Tolosa E, Borght TV, Moreno E. DaTSCAN Clinically Uncertain Parkinsonian Syndromes Study Group. Accuracy of DaTSCAN (123I-Ioflupane) SPECT in diagnosis of patients with clinically uncertain parkinsonism: 2-year follow-up of an openlabel study. Mov Disord. 2007;22(16):2346–51.
10. Berardelli A, Wenning GK, Antonini A, Berg D, Bloem BR, Bonifati V, Brooks D, Burn DJ, Colosimo C, Fanciulli A, Ferreira J, Gasser T, Grandas F, Kanovsky P, Kostic V, Kulisevsky J, Oertel W, Poewe W, Reese JP, Relja M, Ruzicka E, Schrag A, Seppi K, Taba P, Vidailhet M. EFNS/MDS-ES/ENS [corrected] recommendations for the diagnosis of Parkinson's disease. Eur J Neurol. 2013;20:16–34. doi:10.1111/ene.12022.
11. Ubeda-Bañon I, Saiz-Sanchez D, de la Rosa-Prieto C, Martinez-Marcos A. α-Synuclein in the olfactory system in Parkinson's disease: role of neural connections on spreading pathology. Brain Struct Funct. 2014;219(5): 1513–26. doi:10.1007/s00429-013-0651-2.
12. Wang J, Eslinger PJ, Smith MB, Yang QX. Functional magnetic resonance imaging study of human olfaction and normal aging. J Gerontol A Biol Sci Med Sci. 2005;60:510–4.
13. Jennings D, Siderowf A, Stern M, Seibyl J, Eberly S, Oakes D, Marek K. PARS Investigators. Imaging prodromal Parkinson disease: the Parkinson Associated Risk Syndrome Study. Neurology. 2014;83(19):1739–46. doi:10.1212/WNL.0000000000000960.
14. Burke WJ. Association of anosmia with autonomic failure in Parkinson disease.Comment on. Neurology. 2010;74(3):245–51. doi:10.1212/WNL.0b013e3181e793fa.
15. Müller A, Reichmann H, Livermore A, Hummel T. Olfactory function in idiopathic Parkinson's disease: results from cross-sectional studies in IPD patients and long-term follow-up of de-novo IPD patients. J Neural Transm. 2002;109:805–11.
16. Rodríguez-Violante M, Gonzalez-Latapi P, Camacho-Ordoñez A, Martínez-Ramírez D, Morales-Briceño H, Cervantes-Arriaga A. Comparing the accuracy of different smell identification tests in Parkinson's disease: relevance of cultural aspects. Clin Neurol Neurosurg. 2014;123:9–14. doi:10.1016/j.clineuro.2014.04.030.
17. Menéndez-González M, Tavares F, Zeidan N, Salas-Pacheco JM, Arias-Carrión O. Diagnoses behind patients with hard-to-classify tremor and normal DaT-SPECT: a clinical follow up study. Front Aging Neurosci. 2014;6:56. doi:10.3389/fnagi.2014.00056.

11

Ubiquitin phosphorylation in Parkinson's disease: Implications for pathogenesis and treatment

Lih-Shen Chin and Lian Li*

Abstract

Parkinson's disease (PD) is the most common neurodegenerative movement disorder, characterized primarily by the loss of dopaminergic neurons in substantia nigra. The pathogenic mechanisms of PD remain unclear, and no effective therapy currently exists to stop neurodegeneration in this debilitating disease. The identification of mutations in mitochondrial serine/threonine kinase PINK1 or E3 ubiquitin-protein ligase parkin as the cause of autosomal recessive PD opens up new avenues for uncovering neuroprotective pathways and PD pathogenic mechanisms. Recent studies reveal that PINK1 translocates to the outer mitochondrial membrane in response to mitochondrial depolarization and phosphorylates ubiquitin at the residue Ser65. The phosphorylated ubiquitin serves as a signal for activating parkin and recruiting autophagy receptors to promote clearance of damaged mitochondria via mitophagy. Emerging evidence has begun to indicate a link between impaired ubiquitin phosphorylation-dependent mitophagy and PD pathogenesis and supports the potential of Ser65-phosphorylated ubiquitin as a biomarker for PD. The new mechanistic insights and phenotypic screens have identified multiple potential therapeutic targets for PD drug discovery. This review highlights recent advances in understanding ubiquitin phosphorylation in mitochondrial quality control and PD pathogenesis and discusses how these findings can be translated into novel approaches for PD diagnostic and therapeutic development.

Keywords: Mitophagy, Parkinson's disease, PINK1, Parkin, Ubiquitin-protein ligase, Ubiquitin phosphorylation, Mitochondrial quality control, Mitophagy

Background

Parkinson's disease (PD) is the most common neurodegenerative movement disorder with a prevalence of about 1 % at the age of 65 and of 4 %–5 % by the age of 85 [1, 2]. The disease occurs either in relatively rare, familial forms or in common, sporadic forms [3]. The different forms of PD share similar motor symptoms of rigidity, bradykinesia, postural instability, and resting tremor, which appear when there is a loss of 50 %–60 % of dopaminergic neurons in the substantia nigra pars compacta. Increasing evidence indicates that neurodegeneration is more widespread and occurs in multiple regions in the brain [4, 5]. The etiology of PD, particularly sporadic PD cases, is unknown, and there is no reliable biomarker for PD diagnosis. Current medications for PD only provide temporary relief of motor symptoms with no disease-modifying activity to delay or stop disease progression [3, 6]. Thus, there is clearly a need to develop new diagnostic approaches and more effective therapeutics for PD.

Although familial forms of PD account for less than 10 % of PD cases, the discovery of genes responsible for familial PD cases has provided insights into pathogenic mechanisms leading to neurodegeneration in PD. For example, the identification of loss-of-function mutations in mitochondrial serine/threonine kinase PINK1 as a cause of familial PD [7–9] provides genetic evidence for an involvement of mitochondrial dysfunction in PD pathogenesis. The finding of loss-of-function mutations in E3 ubiquitin-protein ligase parkin as a cause of familial PD [9–11] indicates a role of ubiquitination dysregulation in PD pathogenesis. Ubiquitination is a dynamic post-translational modification in which ubiquitin, a 76-amino-acid polypeptide, is conjugated to a lysine residue in substrate proteins through coordinated

* Correspondence: LLI5@emory.edu
Department of Pharmacology and Center for Neurodegenerative Disease, Emory University School of Medicine, Atlanta, GA 30322, USA

sequential actions of E1 ubiquitin-activating enzyme, E2 ubiquitin-conjugating enzyme, and E3 ubiquitin-protein ligase [12]. Proteins can be either monoubiquitinated or polyubiquitinated via successive conjugation of additional ubiquitin molecules to one of the seven internal lysine residues in the preceding ubiquitin. The different types of ubiquitination play distinct signaling roles in regulation of diverse cellular processes by modulating protein activity, localization, trafficking, or degradation [13, 14]. Ubiquitin-dependent signalling is also modulated by deubiquitinating enzymes, which catalyze the removal of ubiquitin from proteins [15]. Recent phosphoproteomic studies revealed that ubiquitin itself can be phosphorylated [16–18], adding a new layer of control over the ubiquitin signalling system. Interestingly, PINK1 was identified as a ubiquitin kinase for phosphorylation of ubiquitin, and the phosphorylated ubiquitin was shown to play novel signaling roles in activating parkin and recruiting autophagy receptors to promote mitophagy. In this review, we will summarize recent findings on the roles of ubiquitin phosphorylation in mitochondrial quality control and PD pathogenesis. We will also discuss the potential of ubiquitin phosphorylation as a PD biomarker and the strategies to target ubiquitin phosphorylation-dependent mitophagy for PD therapeutic intervention.

PINK1 phosphorylates ubiquitin at Ser65 in response to mitochondrial depolarization

Mitochondria are double membrane-bound organelles with four distinct submitochondrial compartments: the outer mitochondrial membrane (OMM), the inner mitochondrial membrane (IMM), the intermembrane space (IMS), and the matrix. The compartmentalization is crucial to mitochondria-mediated processes, including energy production, metabolism, redox control, calcium homeostasis, and programmed cell death [19, 20]. Mitochondrial dysfunction is implicated as a key factor in PD pathogenesis [21–23]. Human genetic studies revealed that homozygous mutations in mitochondrial kinase PINK1 cause autosomal recessive, early-onset PD [7–9, 24], whereas heterozygous mutations in PINK1 increase the risk for developing late-onset PD [25–27], highlighting the importance of knowing the sites and mechanisms of PINK1 action.

PINK1 is an ubiquitously expressed, 581-amino-acid protein Ser/Thr kinase with an N-terminal mitochondrial targeting sequence [28]. Under normal physiological conditions, PINK1 is imported into healthy mitochondria through the translocase of outer membrane (TOM) and translocase of inner membrane (TIM) complexes [29], where the 64-kDa full-length PINK1 can undergo sequential proteolytic cleavages by the matrix-localized mitochondrial processing peptidase (MPP) and the IMM-localized protease PARL to generate a 52-kDa processed form of PINK1 [30–33]. According to one model, the 52-kDa processed form of PINK1 is retrotranslocated to the cytosol for rapid degradation by the proteasome through the N-end rule pathway [34] and consequently, PINK1 protein levels are virtually undetectable under normal conditions, thus arguing against a function of PINK1 in healthy mitochondria [30, 34, 35]. In contrast, other studies reported significant levels of PINK1 protein under normal conditions, but localized PINK1 to either the OMM with its kinase domain facing the cytoplasm [36–38] or to the IMM/IMS with its kinase domain facing the IMS [39–43]. Recently, super-resolution imaging analyses using three-dimensional structured illumination microscopy (3D-SIM) [44] or a combination of tracking and localization microscopy (TALM) and fluorescence photoactivation localization microscopy (F-PALM) [45] clearly showed that, under normal conditions, PINK1 is not present on the OMM of healthy mitochondria, but rather PINK1 resides in the IMM/IMS where it is mainly localized to the cristae membrane and intracristae space. Furthermore, PINK1 was found to colocalize with the mitochondrial chaperone TRAP1, a previously identified PINK1 substrate [40, 46], in these submitochondrial compartments [44]. Together, these results support a model (Fig. 1) that PINK1 plays an intramitochondrial signaling role by phosphorylating TRAP1 [40] and potentially also other IMM/IMS-localized proteins, such as the complex I subunit NdufA10 [47] and the mitochondrial serine protease HtrA2 [48], to regulate activities of polarized mitochondria.

Super-resolution imaging analyses showed that, in response to mitochondrial depolarization, PINK1 changes its submitochondrial localization from the IMM/IMS to the OMM of depolarized mitochondria [44, 45], whereas TRAP remains in the IMM/IMS [44]. The PINK1 localization on the OMM of depolarized mitochondria is likely due to the blockade of PINK1 mitochondrial import through the IMM by the loss of mitochondrial membrane potential [29]. As expected, the mitochondrial import blockade prevents the cleavage of PINK1 by PARL, leading to accumulation of full-length PINK1 on damage mitochondria [29, 30, 33]. Recently, accumulation of misfolded proteins in the mitochondrial matrix was reported to cause PINK1 localization on the OMM without mitochondrial depolarization [49], which might be explained by the possibility that misfolded proteins may somehow inhibit PINK1 mitochondrial import through the TIM complex. Increasing evidence supports that mitochondrial dysfunction-triggered PINK1 localization on the OMM serves as a damage-sensing, quality-control mechanism to mark damaged mitochondria for clearance by mitophagy [29, 35, 44, 49, 50].

Mitochondrial depolarization not only causes PINK1 localization on the OMM of damaged mitochondria but also induces PINK1 dimerization and autophosphorylation

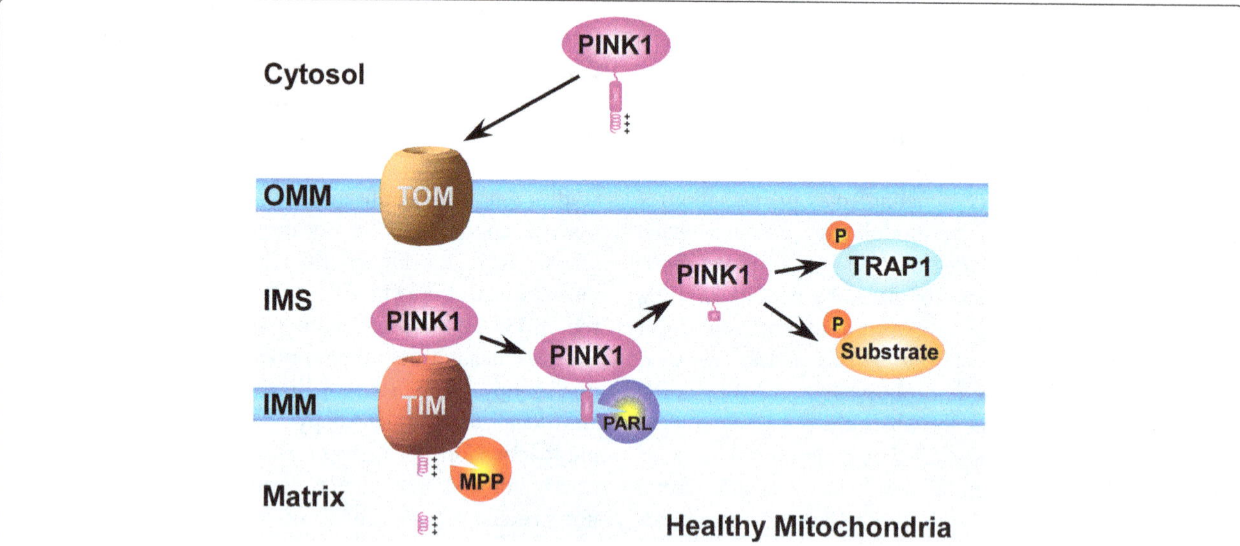

Fig. 1 PINK1-mediated intramitochondrial signaling in healthy mitochondria. PINK1 is imported into healthy mitochondria through the TOM and TIM complexes and is then cleaved sequentially by mitochondrial processing peptidase (MPP) and PARL to generate a processed form of PINK1 that resides in the intermembrane space. There, PINK1 can phosphorylate mitochondrial chaperone TRAP1 and perhaps also other substrates to regulate the activities of polarized mitochondria, such as respiration and redox control

at its Ser228 and Ser402 residues [51, 52], which could be an activation mechanism for enhancing PINK1 kinase activity [53]. Intriguingly, PINK1 was recently found to phosphorylate the residue Ser65 of either ubiquitin [54–57] or ubiquitin chains conjugated to mitochondrial proteins in response to mitochondrial depolarization [57, 58], indicating a function of PINK1 as a ubiquitin kinase. This finding is very exciting because previous phosphoproteomic analyses revealed that ubiquitin can be phosphorylated at multiple sites, including Ser65 [16, 17, 59], but the identity of the kinases for phosphorylating ubiquitin was unknown. Quantitative proteomic analysis showed that, under normal conditions, the Ser65-phosphorylated form of ubiquitin (phospho-Ser65-ubiquitin) is essentially undetectable on healthy mitochondria, but upon mitochondrial depolarization, the level of phospho-Ser65-ubiquitin increases to ~20 % of the total ubiquitin level on damaged mitochondria [57], indicating ubiquitin phosphorylation at Ser65 is a stress-responsive signal that can be induced by mitochondrial dysfunction. Interestingly, a study in yeast [18] demonstrated that ubiquitin phosphorylation at Ser65 can also be induced by oxidative stress, although another kinase must be involved because no PINK1 orthologue exists in yeast. Emerging data indicate that ubiquitin phosphorylation at Ser65 causes significant changes in the structures of ubiquitin and ubiquitin chains and affects ubiquitination and deubiquitination cascades catalyzed by a number of E2 ubiquitin-conjugating enzymes, E3 ligases, and deubiquitinating enzymes [18, 60]. Thus, ubiquitin phosphorylation can have a profound impact on the ubiquitin signalling system. Below, we will focus on the role of PINK1-mediated ubiquitin phosphorylation in activating parkin to promote mitophagy.

Ser65-phosphorylated ubiquitin activates parkin and recruits autophagy receptors on damaged mitochondria to promote mitophagy

There has been intense interest in understanding parkin-regulated neuroprotective processes because loss-of-function mutations in parkin are a major cause of familial PD [9–11] and oxidative/nitrosative stress-induced damage to parkin is associated with sporadic PD [61–63]. Parkin is a 465-amino-acid, cytosolic E3 ubiquitin-protein ligase with an N-terminal ubiquitin-like (Ubl) domain and four zinc-binding domains, RING0, RING1, IBR (in-between RING), and RING2 [64]. Parkin is expressed in many tissues and cell types, where it localizes in the cytosol under normal physiological conditions [10, 11]. *Drosophila* genetic studies provided first evidence that parkin functions downstream of PINK1 in a common pathway involved in the maintenances of mitochondrial homeostasis [65, 66]. Subsequent studies in mammalian cells showed that PINK1 is required for recruiting parkin from the cytosol to depolarized mitochondria to promote mitophagy [35, 37, 50, 67, 68]. Biochemical analyses revealed that parkin is a PINK1 substrate and identified the residue Ser65 within the Ubl domain of Parkin as the phosphorylation site by PINK1 [69–71].

Convergent data from recent studies support a model that PINK1-mediated ubiquitin phosphorylation and parkin phosphorylation work in concert to activate parkin and recruit autophagy receptors to promote mitophagy (Fig. 2).

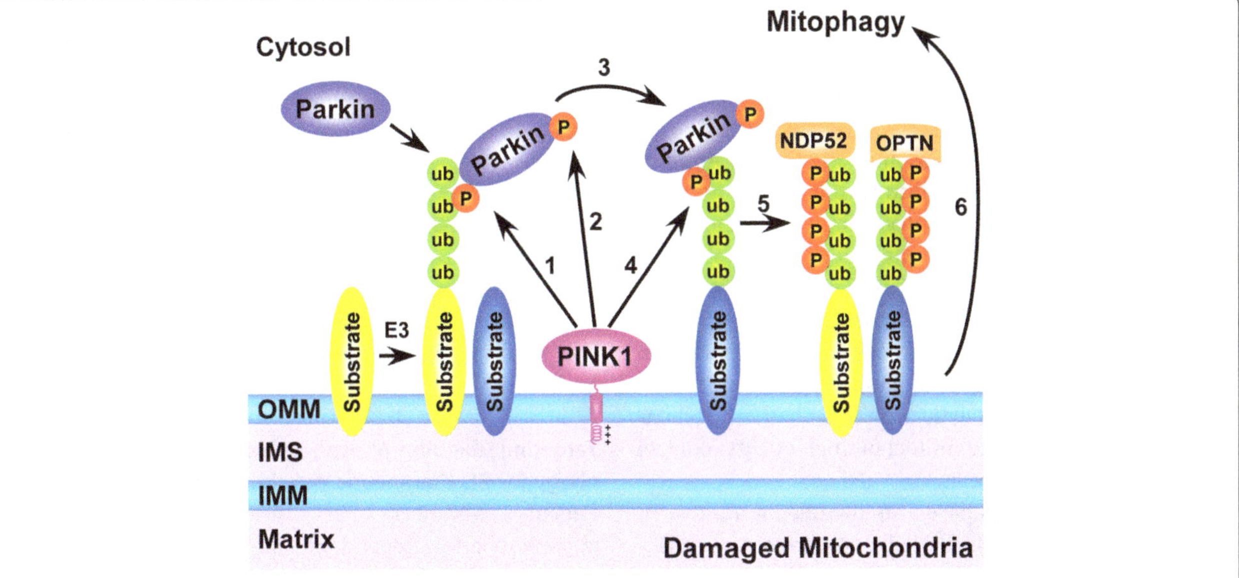

Fig. 2 PINK1-mediated phosphorylation of ubiquitin and parkin on damaged mitochondria in facilitation of mitophagy. Mitochondrial damage causes PINK1 localization and activation on the OMM, leading to Ser65-phosphorylation of pre-existing ubiquitin chains conjugated to OMM proteins (*1*). The phosphorylated ubiquitin recruits parkin, enables Ser65-phosphorylation of parkin by PINK1, and activates parkin (*2*). The activated parkin ubiquitinates additional OMM proteins (*3*) and thus provides more substrates for phosphorylation by PINK1 (*4*), leading to further recruitment and activation of parkin (*2*). This positive feed-forward cycle results in a rapid increase in the local concentration of Ser65-phosphorylated ubiquitin (*5*), which serves as a signal for recruiting autophagy receptors, such as OPTN and NDP52, to promote mitophagy (*6*)

Mitochondrial dysfunction triggers PINK1 localization and activation on the OMM of damaged mitochondria [29, 35, 44, 49, 50], resulting in Ser65-phosphorylation of ubiquitin chains that are already conjugated to OMM proteins by a yet unidentified E3 ligase(s) [51–53]. A function of Ser65-phosphorylated ubiquitin is to serve as a parkin receptor for binding and recruiting parkin from the cytosol to the OMM of damaged mitochondria [58]. Ser65-phosphorylated ubiquitin also functions as an allosteric activator of parkin E3 ligase activity [72–75]. Structural analyses showed that parkin normally exists in an inactive or autoinhibited conformation [64, 76] and that binding of Ser65-phosphorylated ubiquitin to parkin causes a substantial conformational change in parkin, which together with Ser65-phosphorylation parkin Ubl domain, converts parkin from the inactive conformation to an active conformation [72–75]. Once activated, parkin is able to ubiquitinate many OMM proteins [77, 78], which in turn provide additional substrates for phosphorylation by PINK1, leading to further recruitment and activation of parkin, thereby acting as a positive-feedback amplification mechanism to dramatically increase the local concentration of Ser65-phosphorylated ubiquitin on damaged mitochondria [57, 79]. In addition, Ser65-phosphorylated ubiquitin chains are resistant to deubiquitination by many deubiquitinating enzymes, including USP15 and USP30 [60], thereby further contributing to the accumulation of Ser65-phosphorylated ubiquitin on damaged mitochondria. Importantly, a recent study showed that the Ser65-phosphorylated ubiquitin on damaged mitochondria serves as a signal for recruiting autophagy receptors, such as optineurin (OPTN) and NDP52, which then recruit the components of the autophagy machinery to promote autophagic clearance of damaged mitochondria [80].

Dysregulation of ubiquitin phosphorylation in PD pathogenesis

Human genetic studies have identified numerous PD-causing, homozygous mutations in PINK1 and parkin, which are distributed throughout all domains of these two proteins [7–11]. Recent evidence from studying PD-linked PINK1 and parkin mutations indicates that impairment in ubiquitin phosphorylation-dependent mitochondrial quality control is critically involved in PD pathogenesis. A number of PD-linked mutations found in the PINK1 kinase domain, such as PINK1 G309D, L347P, C388R, and G409V mutations, have been shown to abolish the kinase activity of PINK1 for phosphorylating its substrates and the ability of PINK1 to promote parkin recruitment [40, 69, 81, 82], indicating that mutation-induced loss of PINK1 catalytic activity is a mechanism leading to impaired mitophagy and neurodegeneration. In addition, PD-linked C92F and W437X mutations which are located outside of the PINK1 kinase domain were recently shown to impair the ability of PINK1 to localize on the OMM of depolarized mitochondria [44], indicating that mutation-induced loss of mitochondrial damage-sensing function of PINK1 is another mechanism that triggers impaired mitochondrial quality control. In parkin, PD-linked L283P mutation found in the phospho-Ser65-ubiquitin-binding interface has been shown to impair parkin recruitment and activation on depolarized mitochondria [72–75], indicating that mutation-induced loss of phospho-Ser65-ubiquitin-binding ability of parkin can also lead to impaired mitochondrial quality control and neurodegeneration. Furthermore, a number of PD-linked mutations found in the parkin E3 ligase domain, such as parkin T240R and G430D mutations, are able to disrupt the E3 ligase activity of parkin for ubiquitinating its substrates and the ability of parkin to promote mitophagy [35, 50, 68], indicating that mutation-induced loss of parkin catalytic activity is another mechanism that causes impaired mitochondrial quality control and familial PD pathogenesis.

Human genetic studies have also identified a number of heterozygous mutations in PINK1 and parkin as risk factors for developing late-onset PD [9, 25–27]. In addition, oxidative damage to parkin has been detected in brains from patients with sporadic PD [61–63]. These findings suggest that dysregulation of PINK1/parkin-mediated, ubiquitin phosphorylation-dependent mitochondrial quality control may also contribute to the pathogenesis of sporadic PD.

Ubiquitin phosphorylation as a potential biomarker for PD diagnosis

A major challenge in the PD field is to identify biomarkers for PD diagnosis, particularly at the early stage of the disease. The recent finding of a link between ubiquitin phosphorylation and PD pathogenesis suggests the possibility of using phospho-Ser65-ubiquitin as a potential PD biomarker. One approach for detecting phospho-Ser65-ubiquitin is to use anti-phospho-Ser65-ubiquitin antibodies that specifically recognize the Ser65-phosphorylated form of ubiquitin but not the non-phosphorylated form of ubiquitin. Such antibodies have recently been generated and used for analyses of human postmortem brain samples to show the accumulation of phospho-Ser65-ubiquitin in cytoplasmic granules that were localized adjacent to, but not within the Lewy bodies and Lewy neurites - the pathological hallmarks of PD [83]. The phospho-Ser65-ubiquitin-positive granules were partially co-localized with mitochondrial and lysosomal markers [83], suggesting that phospho-Ser65-ubiquitin was accumulated in damaged mitochondria and/or in autolysosomes containing damaged mitochondria, perhaps as a result of increased mitochondrial damage and/or impaired mitophagy. The phospho-Ser65-ubiquitin-positive granules appear to increase with aging and sporadic PD [83], providing support for the potential of phospho-Ser65-ubiquitin as a biomarker for PD.

In addition to the anti-phospho-Ser65-ubiquitin antibody approach, a sensitive, quantitative proteomic approach was recently developed to measure the levels of phospho-Ser65-ubiquitin in cell and tissue lysates [57, 79, 84]. This approach has been used to show increased brain levels of phospho-Ser65-ubiquitin in a mouse model of mitochondria dysfunction caused by enhanced mitochondrial DNA mutagenic stress [84], indicating that accumulation of phospho-Ser65-ubiquitin could occur as a result of increased mitochondrial damage *in vivo*. The sensitivity and quantitative nature of the proteomic approach are particularly useful for its further development as a diagnostic tool for PD.

Targeting ubiquitin phosphorylation-dependent mitophagy for PD therapeutic development

Recent advances in understanding ubiquitin phosphorylation-dependent mitochondrial quality control have identified several potential targets for therapeutic intervention in PD. An attractive therapeutic target is the PINK1 kinase activity because PINK1-mediated phosphorylation of ubiquitin and other substrates is critically involved in neuroprotection against mitochondrial dysfunction [40, 54–56, 69, 85]. A novel PINK1-targeting approach was recently developed, which uses the ATP analogue kinetin triphosphate (KTP) or the KTP precursor kinetin to enhance the kinase activity of PINK1 [46]. Augmentation of PINK1 kinase activity by KTP or kinetin is able to promote parkin recruitment to damaged mitochondria and enhance cellular defense against oxidative stress-induced apoptosis [46], providing support for the therapeutic potential of PINK1 activation in PD treatment.

The E3 ubiquitin-protein ligase activity of parkin is another potential target for PD therapeutic development. The finding of phospho-Ser65-ubiquitin as an allosteric activator of parkin E3 ligase activity [72–75] that disrupts the autoinhibited conformation of parkin [64, 76] provides structural information for the development of small molecules that mimic the effect of phospho-Ser65-ubiquitin to activate parkin-dependent mitophagy. In addition, a recent study reported that parkin recruitment to damaged mitochondria is positively regulated by the deubiquitinating enzyme USP8 through its action to remove K6-linked ubiquitin chains from parkin [86], suggesting that USP8 activation could be another approach to promote clearance of damaged mitochondria. Furthermore, emerging data indicate that parkin-mediated mitochondrial protein ubiquitination and mitophagy are negatively regulated by deubiquitinating enzymes USP15 [87] and USP30 [88], which catalyze the removal of of ubiquitin from parkin substrates on damaged mitochondria. Knockdown of endogenous USP15 or USP30 is able to ameliorate mitochondrial and motor behavioral defects in parkin-deficient flies [87, 88] and enhance neuroprotection against paraquat toxicity [88], suggesting that USP15 and USP30 inhibition could provide potential therapeutic benefits for treating PD.

Phenotypic screening for chemical or genetic modifiers of PINK1 or parkin mutant phenotypes has emerged as a useful approach for PD drug discovery. Recent screens of a 2000-compound library using fibroblast cells from PD patients carrying parkin mutations have identified 15 compounds that can rescue mitochondrial dysfunction phenotypes of parkin-mutant patient cells [89]. Two of these compounds, ursocholanic acid and ursodeoxycholic acid, were further characterized and shown to ameliorate mitochondrial functional defects in parkin-mutant patient fibroblasts as well as in LRRK2-mutant patient fibroblasts, by acting through the glucocorticoid receptor and Akt signalling [89]. In addition, a *Drosophila* genetic screen using PINK1-deficient flies has identified UBIAD1/Heix, an enzyme involved in the synthesis of vitamin K_2, as a modifier of PINK1 mutant phenotype [90]. Further analyses showed that vitamin K_2 is able to improve the defective mitochondrial and behavioral phenotypes of PINK1 and parkin mutant flies, by acting as an electron carrier downstream of complex I [90]. These results support the therapeutic potential of vitamin K_2 supplementation in PD treatment.

Conclusions

An exciting, recent breakthrough from studying PD-linked proteins PINK1 and parkin is the discovery of a novel neuroprotective pathway in which PINK1 phosphorylates ubiquitin to activate parkin and promote mitophagy for maintaining mitochondrial and neuronal homeostasis. Emerging evidence has begun to indicate a link between the impairment of this neuroprotective pathway and the pathogenesis of familial PD as well as sporadic PD. These new mechanistic insights have revealed promising, novel avenues for PD diagnostic development and therapeutic intervention. Recent work supports the development of phospho-Ser65-ubiquitin as a potential biomarker for PD, and future studies using the quantitative proteomic approach [79, 84] to analyze phospho-Ser65-ubiquitin levels in PD patient samples, particularly in easily accessible body fluids such as blood or urine, should be pursued actively. In addition, newly gained insights into ubiquitin phosphorylation-dependent mitochondrial quality control have identified a number of potential therapeutic targets, which could be used in high-throughput screening for PD drug discovery. Furthermore, phenotypic screens for chemical or genetic modifiers of PINK1 and parkin mutant phenotypes have generated promising hits [89, 90], and future phenotypic screens using induced pluripotent stem cells (iPSCs) from PD patients will facilitate the development of new therapeutics to combat mitochondrial dysfunction and neurodegeneration in PD.

Competing interests

The authors declare that they have no competing interests.

Authors' contributions

LSC and LL wrote and approved the manuscript.

Acknowledgments

Work in the authors' laboratories is supported by grants from National Institutions of Health (NS093550, GM103613, and NS092343) and a pilot grant award from NIH-funded Emory Udall Parkinson's Disease Center (P50 NS071669).

References

1. Lang AE, Lozano AM. Parkinson's disease. First of two parts. N Engl J Med. 1998;339(15):1044–53.
2. Lang AE, Lozano AM. Parkinson's disease. Second of two parts. N Engl J Med. 1998;339(16):1130–43.
3. Savitt JM, Dawson VL, Dawson TM. Diagnosis and treatment of Parkinson disease: molecules to medicine. J Clin Invest. 2006;116(7):1744–54.
4. Braak H, Ghebremedhin E, Rub U, Bratzke H, Del Tredici K. Stages in the development of Parkinson's disease-related pathology. Cell Tissue Res. 2004;318(1):121–34.
5. Goedert M, Spillantini MG, Del Tredici K, Braak H. 100 years of Lewy pathology. Nat Rev Neurol. 2013;9(1):13–24.
6. Olanow CW, Schapira AH. Therapeutic prospects for Parkinson disease. Ann Neurol. 2013;74(3):337–47.
7. Valente EM, Abou-Sleiman PM, Caputo V, Muqit MM, Harvey K, Gispert S, et al. Hereditary early-onset Parkinson's disease caused by mutations in PINK1. Science. 2004;304(5674):1158–60.
8. Bonifati V, Rohe CF, Breedveld GJ, Fabrizio E, De Mari M, Tassorelli C, et al. Early-onset parkinsonism associated with PINK1 mutations: frequency, genotypes, and phenotypes. Neurology. 2005;65(1):87–95.
9. Tan EK, Skipper LM. Pathogenic mutations in Parkinson disease. Hum Mutat. 2007;28(7):641–53.
10. Kitada T, Asakawa S, Hattori N, Matsumine H, Yamamura Y, Minoshima S, et al. Mutations in the parkin gene cause autosomal recessive juvenile parkinsonism. Nature. 1998;392(6676):605–8.
11. Hattori N, Mizuno Y. Pathogenetic mechanisms of parkin in Parkinson's disease. Lancet. 2004;364(9435):722–4.
12. Weissman AM. Themes and variations on ubiquitylation. Nat Rev Mol Cell Biol. 2001;2(3):169–78.
13. Olzmann JA, Li L, Chin LS. Aggresome formation and neurodegenerative diseases: therapeutic implications. Curr Med Chem. 2008;15(1):47–60.
14. Komander D, Rape M. The ubiquitin code. Annu Rev Biochem. 2012;81:203–29.
15. Reyes-Turcu FE, Ventii KH, Wilkinson KD. Regulation and cellular roles of ubiquitin-specific deubiquitinating enzymes. Annu Rev Biochem. 2009;78:363–97.
16. Sharma K, D'Souza RC, Tyanova S, Schaab C, Wisniewski JR, Cox J, et al. Ultradeep human phosphoproteome reveals a distinct regulatory nature of Tyr and Ser/Thr-based signaling. Cell Rep. 2014;8(5):1583–94.
17. Lundby A, Secher A, Lage K, Nordsborg NB, Dmytriyev A, Lundby C, et al. Quantitative maps of protein phosphorylation sites across 14 different rat organs and tissues. Nat Commun. 2012;3:876.
18. Swaney DL, Rodriguez-Mias RA, Villen J. Phosphorylation of ubiquitin at Ser65 affects its polymerization, targets, and proteome-wide turnover. EMBO Rep. 2015;16(9):1131–44.
19. McBride HM, Neuspiel M, Wasiak S. Mitochondria: more than just a powerhouse. Curr Biol. 2006;16(14):R551–60.
20. Herrmann JM, Riemer J. The intermembrane space of mitochondria. Antioxid Redox Signal. 2010;13(9):1341–58.
21. Cookson MR, Bandmann O. Parkinson's disease: insights from pathways. Hum Mol Genet. 2010;19(R1):R21–7.
22. Schon EA, Przedborski S. Mitochondria: the next (neurode)generation. Neuron. 2011;70(6):1033–53.

23. Schapira AH. Mitochondrial dysfunction in Parkinson's disease. Cell Death Differ. 2007;14(7):1261–6.
24. Hatano Y, Li Y, Sato K, Asakawa S, Yamamura Y, Tomiyama H, et al. Novel PINK1 mutations in early-onset parkinsonism.[erratum appears in Ann Neurol. 2004 Oct;56(4):603]. Ann Neurol. 2004;56(3):424–7.
25. Zadikoff C, Rogaeva E, Djarmati A, Sato C, Salehi-Rad S, St George-Hyslop P, et al. Homozygous and heterozygous PINK1 mutations: considerations for diagnosis and care of Parkinson's disease patients. Mov Disord. 2006;21(6):875–9.
26. Hedrich K, Hagenah J, Djarmati A, Hiller A, Lohnau T, Lasek K, et al. Clinical spectrum of homozygous and heterozygous PINK1 mutations in a large German family with Parkinson disease: role of a single hit? Arch Neurol. 2006;63(6):833–8.
27. Toft M, Myhre R, Pielsticker L, White LR, Aasly JO, Farrer MJ. PINK1 mutation heterozygosity and the risk of Parkinson's disease. J Neurol Neurosurg Psychiatry. 2007;78(1):82–4.
28. Sim CH, Gabriel K, Mills RD, Culvenor JG, Cheng HC. Analysis of the regulatory and catalytic domains of PTEN-induced kinase-1 (PINK1). Hum Mutat. 2012; 33(10):1408–22.
29. Lazarou M, Jin SM, Kane LA, Youle RJ. Role of PINK1 binding to the TOM complex and alternate intracellular membranes in recruitment and activation of the E3 ligase Parkin. Dev Cell. 2012;22(2):320–33.
30. Jin SM, Lazarou M, Wang C, Kane LA, Narendra DP, Youle RJ. Mitochondrial membrane potential regulates PINK1 import and proteolytic destabilization by PARL. J Cell Biol. 2010;191(5):933–42.
31. Greene AW, Grenier K, Aguileta MA, Muise S, Farazifard R, Haque ME, et al. Mitochondrial processing peptidase regulates PINK1 processing, import and Parkin recruitment. EMBO Rep. 2012;13(4):378–85.
32. Deas E, Plun-Favreau H, Gandhi S, Desmond H, Kjaer S, Loh SH, et al. PINK1 cleavage at position A103 by the mitochondrial protease PARL. Hum Mol Genet. 2011;20(5):867–79.
33. Meissner C, Lorenz H, Weihofen A, Selkoe DJ, Lemberg MK. The mitochondrial intramembrane protease PARL cleaves human Pink1 to regulate Pink1 trafficking. J Neurochem. 2011;117(5):856–67.
34. Yamano K, Youle RJ. PINK1 is degraded through the N-end rule pathway. Autophagy. 2013;9(11):1758–69.
35. Narendra DP, Jin SM, Tanaka A, Suen DF, Gautier CA, Shen J, et al. PINK1 is selectively stabilized on impaired mitochondria to activate Parkin. PLoS Biol. 2010;8(1), e1000298.
36. Becker D, Richter J, Tocilescu MA, Przedborski S, Voos W. Pink1 kinase and its membrane potential (Deltapsi)-dependent cleavage product both localize to outer mitochondrial membrane by unique targeting mode. J Biol Chem. 2012;287(27):22969–87.
37. Vives-Bauza C, Zhou C, Huang Y, Cui M, de Vries RL, Kim J, et al. PINK1-dependent recruitment of Parkin to mitochondria in mitophagy. Proc Natl Acad Sci U S A. 2010;107(1):378–83.
38. Zhou C, Huang Y, Shao Y, May J, Prou D, Perier C, et al. The kinase domain of mitochondrial PINK1 faces the cytoplasm. Proc Natl Acad Sci U S A. 2008; 105(33):12022–7.
39. Gandhi S, Muqit MM, Stanyer L, Healy DG, Abou-Sleiman PM, Hargreaves I, et al. PINK1 protein in normal human brain and Parkinson's disease. Brain. 2006; 129(Pt 7):1720–31.
40. Pridgeon JW, Olzmann JA, Chin LS, Li L. PINK1 Protects against Oxidative Stress by Phosphorylating Mitochondrial Chaperone TRAP1. PLoS Biol. 2007;5:e172.
41. Mills RD, Sim CH, Mok SS, Mulhern TD, Culvenor JG, Cheng HC. Biochemical aspects of the neuroprotective mechanism of PTEN-induced kinase-1 (PINK1). J Neurochem. 2008;105(1):18–33.
42. Muqit MM, Abou-Sleiman PM, Saurin AT, Harvey K, Gandhi S, Deas E, et al. Altered cleavage and localization of PINK1 to aggresomes in the presence of proteasomal stress. J Neurochem. 2006;98(1):156–69.
43. Silvestri L, Caputo V, Bellacchio E, Atorino L, Dallapiccola B, Valente EM, et al. Mitochondrial import and enzymatic activity of PINK1 mutants associated to recessive parkinsonism. Hum Mol Genet. 2005;14(22):3477–92.
44. Fallaize D, Chin LS, Li L. Differential submitochondrial localization of PINK1 as a molecular switch for mediating distinct mitochondrial signaling pathways. Cell Signal. 2015;27(12):2543–54.
45. Beinlich FR, Drees C, Piehler J, Busch KB. Shuttling of PINK1 between Mitochondrial Microcompartments Resolved by Triple-Color Superresolution Microscopy. ACS Chem Biol. 2015;10(9):1970–6.
46. Hertz NT, Berthet A, Sos ML, Thorn KS, Burlingame AL, Nakamura K, et al. A neo-substrate that amplifies catalytic activity of parkinson's-disease-related kinase PINK1. Cell. 2013;154(4):737–47.
47. Morais VA, Haddad D, Craessaerts K, De Bock PJ, Swerts J, Vilain S, et al. PINK1 loss-of-function mutations affect mitochondrial complex I activity via NdufA10 ubiquinone uncoupling. Science. 2014;344(6180):203–7.
48. Plun-Favreau H, Klupsch K, Moisoi N, Gandhi S, Kjaer S, Frith D, et al. The mitochondrial protease HtrA2 is regulated by Parkinson's disease-associated kinase PINK1. Nat Cell Biol. 2007;Sep 30; [Epub ahead of print]
49. Jin SM, Youle RJ. The accumulation of misfolded proteins in the mitochondrial matrix is sensed by PINK1 to induce PARK2/Parkin-mediated mitophagy of polarized mitochondria. Autophagy. 2013;9(11):1750–7.
50. Matsuda N, Sato S, Shiba K, Okatsu K, Saisho K, Gautier CA, et al. PINK1 stabilized by mitochondrial depolarization recruits Parkin to damaged mitochondria and activates latent Parkin for mitophagy. J Cell Biol. 2010; 189(2):211–21.
51. Okatsu K, Uno M, Koyano F, Go E, Kimura M, Oka T, et al. A dimeric PINK1-containing complex on depolarized mitochondria stimulates Parkin recruitment. J Biol Chem. 2013;288(51):36372–84.
52. Okatsu K, Oka T, Iguchi M, Imamura K, Kosako H, Tani N, et al. PINK1 autophosphorylation upon membrane potential dissipation is essential for Parkin recruitment to damaged mitochondria. Nat Commun. 2012;3:1016.
53. Aerts L, Craessaerts K, De Strooper B, Morais VA. PINK1 kinase catalytic activity is regulated by phosphorylation on serines 228 and 402. J Biol Chem. 2015;290(5):2798–811.
54. Kane LA, Lazarou M, Fogel AI, Li Y, Yamano K, Sarraf SA, et al. PINK1 phosphorylates ubiquitin to activate Parkin E3 ubiquitin ligase activity. J Cell Biol. 2014;205(2):143–53.
55. Kazlauskaite A, Kondapalli C, Gourlay R, Campbell DG, Ritorto MS, Hofmann K, et al. Parkin is activated by PINK1-dependent phosphorylation of ubiquitin at Ser65. Biochem J. 2014;460(1):127–39.
56. Koyano F, Okatsu K, Kosako H, Tamura Y, Go E, Kimura M, et al. Ubiquitin is phosphorylated by PINK1 to activate parkin. Nature. 2014;510(7503):162–6.
57. Ordureau A, Sarraf SA, Duda DM, Heo JM, Jedrychowski MP, Sviderskiy VO, et al. Quantitative proteomics reveal a feedforward mechanism for mitochondrial PARKIN translocation and ubiquitin chain synthesis. Mol Cell. 2014;56(3):360–75.
58. Okatsu K, Koyano F, Kimura M, Kosako H, Saeki Y, Tanaka K, et al. Phosphorylated ubiquitin chain is the genuine Parkin receptor. J Cell Biol. 2015;209(1):111–28.
59. Peng J, Schwartz D, Elias JE, Thoreen CC, Cheng D, Marsischky G, et al. A proteomics approach to understanding protein ubiquitination. Nat Biotechnol. 2003;21(8):921–6.
60. Wauer T, Swatek KN, Wagstaff JL, Gladkova C, Pruneda JN, Michel MA, et al. Ubiquitin Ser65 phosphorylation affects ubiquitin structure, chain assembly and hydrolysis. EMBO J. 2015;34(3):307–25.
61. Chung KK, Thomas B, Li X, Pletnikova O, Troncoso JC, Marsh L, et al. S-nitrosylation of parkin regulates ubiquitination and compromises parkin's protective function. Science. 2004;304(5675):1328–31.
62. Yao D, Gu Z, Nakamura T, Shi ZQ, Ma Y, Gaston B, et al. Nitrosative stress linked to sporadic Parkinson's disease: S-nitrosylation of parkin regulates its E3 ubiquitin ligase activity. Proc Natl Acad Sci U S A. 2004;101(29):10810–4.
63. Lavoie MJ, Ostaszewski BL, Weihofen A, Schlossmacher MG, Selkoe DJ. Dopamine covalently modifies and functionally inactivates parkin. Nat Med. 2005;11(11):1214–21.
64. Trempe JF, Sauve V, Grenier K, Seirafi M, Tang MY, Menade M, et al. Structure of parkin reveals mechanisms for ubiquitin ligase activation. Science. 2013;340(6139):1451–5.
65. Clark IE, Dodson MW, Jiang C, Cao JH, Huh JR, Seol JH, et al. Drosophila pink1 is required for mitochondrial function and interacts genetically with parkin. Nature. 2006;441(7097):1162–6.
66. Park J, Lee SB, Lee S, Kim Y, Song S, Kim S, et al. Mitochondrial dysfunction in Drosophila PINK1 mutants is complemented by parkin. Nature. 2006; 441(7097):1157–61.
67. Narendra D, Tanaka A, Suen DF, Youle RJ. Parkin is recruited selectively to impaired mitochondria and promotes their autophagy. J Cell Biol. 2008; 183(5):795–803.
68. Geisler S, Holmstrom KM, Skujat D, Fiesel FC, Rothfuss OC, Kahle PJ, et al. PINK1/Parkin-mediated mitophagy is dependent on VDAC1 and p62/ SQSTM1. Nat Cell Biol. 2010;12(2):119–31.
69. Sha D, Chin LS, Li L. Phosphorylation of parkin by Parkinson disease-linked kinase PINK1 activates parkin E3 ligase function and NF-kappaB signaling. Hum Mol Genet. 2010;19(2):352–63.

70. Shiba-Fukushima K, Imai Y, Yoshida S, Ishihama Y, Kanao T, Sato S, et al. PINK1-mediated phosphorylation of the Parkin ubiquitin-like domain primes mitochondrial translocation of Parkin and regulates mitophagy. Sci Rep. 2012;2:1002.
71. Kondapalli C, Kazlauskaite A, Zhang N, Woodroof HI, Campbell DG, Gourlay R, et al. PINK1 is activated by mitochondrial membrane potential depolarization and stimulates Parkin E3 ligase activity by phosphorylating Serine 65. Open Biol. 2012;2(5):120080.
72. Wauer T, Simicek M, Schubert A, Komander D. Mechanism of phospho-ubiquitin-induced PARKIN activation. Nature. 2015;524(7565):370–4.
73. Kazlauskaite A, Martinez-Torres RJ, Wilkie S, Kumar A, Peltier J, Gonzalez A, et al. Binding to serine 65-phosphorylated ubiquitin primes Parkin for optimal PINK1-dependent phosphorylation and activation. EMBO Rep. 2015;16(8):939–54.
74. Sauve V, Lilov A, Seirafi M, Vranas M, Rasool S, Kozlov G, et al. A Ubl/ubiquitin switch in the activation of Parkin. EMBO J. 2015;34(20):2492–505.
75. Kumar A, Aguirre JD, Condos TE, Martinez-Torres RJ, Chaugule VK, Toth R, et al. Disruption of the autoinhibited state primes the E3 ligase parkin for activation and catalysis. EMBO J. 2015;34(20):2506–21.
76. Wauer T, Komander D. Structure of the human Parkin ligase domain in an autoinhibited state. EMBO J. 2013;32(15):2099–112.
77. Chan NC, Salazar AM, Pham AH, Sweredoski MJ, Kolawa NJ, Graham RL, et al. Broad activation of the ubiquitin-proteasome system by Parkin is critical for mitophagy. Hum Mol Genet. 2011;20(9):1726–37.
78. Sarraf SA, Raman M, Guarani-Pereira V, Sowa ME, Huttlin EL, Gygi SP, et al. Landscape of the PARKIN-dependent ubiquitylome in response to mitochondrial depolarization. Nature. 2013;496(7445):372–6.
79. Ordureau A, Heo JM, Duda DM, Paulo JA, Olszewski JL, Yanishevski D, et al. Defining roles of PARKIN and ubiquitin phosphorylation by PINK1 in mitochondrial quality control using a ubiquitin replacement strategy. Proc Natl Acad Sci U S A. 2015;112(21):6637–42.
80. Lazarou M, Sliter DA, Kane LA, Sarraf SA, Wang C, Burman JL, et al. The ubiquitin kinase PINK1 recruits autophagy receptors to induce mitophagy. Nature. 2015;524(7565):309–14.
81. Narendra DP, Wang C, Youle RJ, Walker JE. PINK1 rendered temperature sensitive by disease-associated and engineered mutations. Hum Mol Genet. 2013;22(13):2572–89.
82. Geisler S, Holmstrom KM, Treis A, Skujat D, Weber SS, Fiesel FC, et al. The PINK1/Parkin-mediated mitophagy is compromised by PD-associated mutations. Autophagy. 2010;6(7):871–8.
83. Fiesel FC, Ando M, Hudec R, Hill AR, Castanedes-Casey M, Caulfield TR, et al. (Patho-)physiological relevance of PINK1-dependent ubiquitin phosphorylation. EMBO Rep. 2015;16(9):1114–30.
84. Pickrell AM, Huang CH, Kennedy SR, Ordureau A, Sideris DP, Hoekstra JG, et al. Endogenous Parkin Preserves Dopaminergic Substantia Nigral Neurons following Mitochondrial DNA Mutagenic Stress. Neuron. 2015;87(2):371–81.
85. Kazlauskaite A, Kelly V, Johnson C, Baillie C, Hastie CJ, Peggie M, et al. Phosphorylation of Parkin at Serine65 is essential for activation: elaboration of a Miro1 substrate-based assay of Parkin E3 ligase activity. Open Bol. 2014; 4:130213.
86. Durcan TM, Tang MY, Perusse JR, Dashti EA, Aguileta MA, McLelland GL, et al. USP8 regulates mitophagy by removing K6-linked ubiquitin conjugates from parkin. EMBO J. 2014;33(21):2473–91.
87. Cornelissen T, Haddad D, Wauters F, Van Humbeeck C, Mandemakers W, Koentjoro B, et al. The deubiquitinase USP15 antagonizes Parkin-mediated mitochondrial ubiquitination and mitophagy. Hum Mol Genet. 2014;23(19):5227–42.
88. Bingol B, Tea JS, Phu L, Reichelt M, Bakalarski CE, Song Q, et al. The mitochondrial deubiquitinase USP30 opposes parkin-mediated mitophagy. Nature. 2014;510(7505):370–5.
89. Mortiboys H, Aasly J, Bandmann O. Ursocholanic acid rescues mitochondrial function in common forms of familial Parkinson's disease. Brain. 2013;136(Pt 10):3038–50.
90. Vos M, Esposito G, Edirisinghe JN, Vilain S, Haddad DM, Slabbaert JR, et al. Vitamin K2 is a mitochondrial electron carrier that rescues pink1 deficiency. Science. 2012;336(6086):1306–10.

12

The role of amyloid beta clearance in cerebral amyloid angiopathy: more potential therapeutic targets

Xue-mei Qi and Jian-fang Ma*

Abstract

Cerebral amyloid angiopathy (CAA) is characterized by the deposition of amyloid β-protein (Aβ) in the leptomeningeal and cortical blood vessels, which is an age-dependent risk factor for intracerebral hemorrhage (ICH), ischemic stroke and contributes to cerebrovascular dysfunction leading to cognitive impairment. However clinical prevention and treatment of the disease is very difficult because of its occult onset and severity of the symptoms. In recent years, many anti-amyloid β immunotherapies have not demonstrated clinical efficacy in subjects with Alzheimer's disease (AD), and the failure may be due to the deposition of Aβ in the cerebrovascular export pathway resulting in further damage to blood vessels and aggravating CAA. So decreased clearance of Aβ in blood vessels plays a crucial role in the development of CAA and AD, and identification of the molecular pathways involved will provide new targets for treatment. In this review, we mainly describe the mechanisms of Aβ clearance through vessels, especially in terms of some proteins and receptors involved in this process.

Keywords: Cerebral amyloid angiopathy, Alzheimer's disease, Amyloid β-protein, Clearance

Background

Cerebral amyloid angiopathy (CAA) is the second reason (after hypertension) causing cerebral hemorrhage in the elderly, accounting for 15–40% of non-traumatic cerebral hemorrhage in the elderly with a mortality of 30–50% [1]. Occasionally, CAA can be presented as cerebral ischemic attack, cognitive dysfunction and cerebral vasculitis [2, 3]. In addition, CAA is commonly found in Alzheimer's disease (AD) and nearly 80% of AD patients are accompanied by CAA [4].

The main pathological feature of CAA is the deposition of amyloid β-protein (Aβ) in the tunica media and adventitia of the arterioles and/or capillaries in the cerebral cortex and leptomeninges [5]. Aβ deposited in AD senile plaques is mainly $A\beta_{42}$, however it's usually $A\beta_{40}$ that deposited in the vascular wall of CAA. Sporadic CAA is commonly classified into two categories based on the presence or absence of Aβ on capillaries: CAA-type 1 is defined if the deposition of Aβ on cortical capillaries beside leptomeningeal, cortical arteries and arterioles, and CAA -type 2, not involving cortical capillaries.

In physiological conditions, human brain can produce Aβ without abnormal accumulation because Aβ can be moved out through several mechanisms quickly and effectively: (1) uptake and degradation by glial cells; (2) degradation by proteolytic enzymes; (3) clearance through blood brain barrier (BBB); (4) interstitial fluid bulk-flow clearance (perivascular drainage or clearance by glymphatic pathway); (5) complement-related clearance. One proposed pathogenesis of CAA is that inefficient Aβ clearance leads to abnormal Aβ accumulation in the brain and vessels, causing CAA in aged brain. Based on this assumption, several therapeutic interventions have been tried in CAA animal models by enhancing Aβ clearance and drainage systems. For example, experimental gene therapy to up-regulate neprilysin in the brains of aged Tg2576 mice has been reported to reduce Aβ levels [6]. Promoting perivascular drainage can facilitate $A\beta_{40}$ clearance and improve cognitive deficits in Tg-SwDI mice [7]. Administrating ponezumab, an anti- $A\beta_{40}$ selective antibody, to transgenic mice led to a reduction of Aβ deposition and an improvement of

* Correspondence: majifa@hotmail.com
Department of Neurology & Institute of Neurology, Ruijin Hospital Affiliated to Shanghai Jiaotong University School of Medicine, Shanghai 200025, China

vessel function [8]. How to make these basic neuroscience progresses into clinical effective therapies requires more comprehensive understanding of mechanisms involving Aβ clearance under pathological conditions. This review will focus on recent findings of Aβ clearance system and try to discuss the potential interventional targets for future CAA treatment.

Enzyme degradation

Aβ-degrading enzymes including neprilysin, insulin-degrading enzymes (IDE), angiotensin-converting enzyme (ACE), cathepsin, etc., play an important role in Aβ clearance and have a protective role in CAA by reducing the damage of Aβ to vascular smooth muscle cells. A previous review have summarized their crucial role in AD and CAA, and the up-regulation of cerebral Aβ degrading enzyme has potential therapeutic effect on AD [9]. Here we focus on their role in CAA pathology. For example the expression of vascular neprilysin reduced in CAA patients and the decrease was more obvious in Apoε4 carriers [10, 11]. Gene polymorphisms of neprilysin has also been reported to be related to sporadic CAA and disease severity [12]. Both vitro and vivo studies have demonstrated that up-regulation of neprilysin could reduce Aβ concentration and be beneficial to AD [13, 14]. A recent study suggests that neprilysin activity is suppressed directly or indirectly by dual-specificity tyrosine phosphorylation-regulated kinase 1A (DYRK1A), so DYRK1A inhibition may also be a promising therapeutic target for AD through up-regulating neprilysin [15]. Another Aβ degrading enzyme IDE isolated from human brain microvessels has been shown to be capable of degrading Aβ40, and the IDE protein levels was increasing in AD patients with CAA, however its degrading activity was reduced in CAA microvessels [16]. And for ACE, it's has been shown to cleave Aβ40 at the site Asp(7)-Ser(8). And the degradation products Aβ-(1-7) and Aβ-(8-40) peptides were less aggregated or cytotoxic [17]. The activity of ACE-1 was increased in AD patients and in moderate to severe CAA vessel-associated ACE-1 levels were higher [18]. Further study found that ACE variants are related to ICH recurrence in CAA, possibly by regulating ACE expression [19]. Up-regulation of Aβ degrading enzyme has potential therapeutic effect on AD and further studies are needed to assess their role in treatment for CAA pathology.

The transcytosis of Aβ across BBB

Blood brain barrier (BBB) refers to plasma and brain barrier composed of cerebral capillary wall and glial cells, as well as a barrier between plasma and cerebral spinal fluid (CSF) composed of choroid plexus named blood–cerebrospinal fluid barrier (BCSFB). BBB can limit the transport of polar molecules into the brain, but the necessary nutrients such as glucose, amino acids, and vitamins can permeate through BBB mediated by receptors on the vascular endothelium. BBB also allows the transport of larger molecules, such as neuroactive peptides and proteins, and plays an important role in the regulation of brain Aβ concentration.

Aβ can be transported bi-directionally through BBB by multiple receptors in the vascular endothelium (Fig. 1). Receptors involved transporting peripheral Aβ into the brain consist of advanced glycation end products (RAGE), organic anion transporting polypeptides (OATP) such as Oatp1a4. The receptors mediating Aβ clearance from the brain to the peripheral circulating system include low-density lipoprotein receptor family (LDLR family), ATP-binding cassette transporters (ABC transporters), insulin-sensitive transporter, natriuretic peptide receptor C (Npr-C). These receptors regulate the influx and efflux of brain Aβ and maintain the balance of Aβ under normal condition. So any dysfunction of this transportation system can disturb the balance of Aβ distribution and lead to Aβ aggregation in the vessels which contributes to CAA formation in the brain.

Receptors mediating Aβ influx

Advanced glycation end products (RAGE)

RAGE belongs to immunoglobulin receptor superfamilies and can interact with several ligands including soluble Aβ. The expression of RAGE was increased in capillary of CAA patients and APP transgenic mice, suggesting the association of RAGE with Aβ aggregation in the capillary [20]. Further study found that in 3xTg-AD transgenic mice, the exogenous pathogenic gene could up-regulate RAGE expression in endothelium cell [21]. RAGE can mediates the transport of $Aβ_{40}$ or $Aβ_{42}$ across BBB into brain, resulting in endothelial cell oxidative stress and expression of proinflammatory cytokines and NF-κB through redox-dependent activation of Ras-ERK1/2 pathway, p38 MAP (p38), Cdc42/Rac pathway and SAPK/JNK kinase pathways [22], which finally leads to cell apoptosis, inflammatory response and vascular dysfunction. And the inhibition of RAGE-ligand interaction reduces aggregation of Aβ in brain parenchyma in transgenic mouse [23]. Using an in vitro BBB model, Candela et al. [24] found that specific competitive inhibitor against RAGE could decrease the apical-to-basolateral transport of $Aβ_{40}$ and $Aβ_{42}$ significantly, which was a caveolae-dependent process through endothelial cells. And recently, a research observed that 1,25-dihydroxyvitamin D3 (1,25(OH)2D3) increased the efflux of Aβ40 from brain to blood through up-regulating LRP1 and down-regulating RAGE [25].

Several drugs targeting on RAGE have been tried for treating AD and CAA. Inhibition of RAGE-ligand

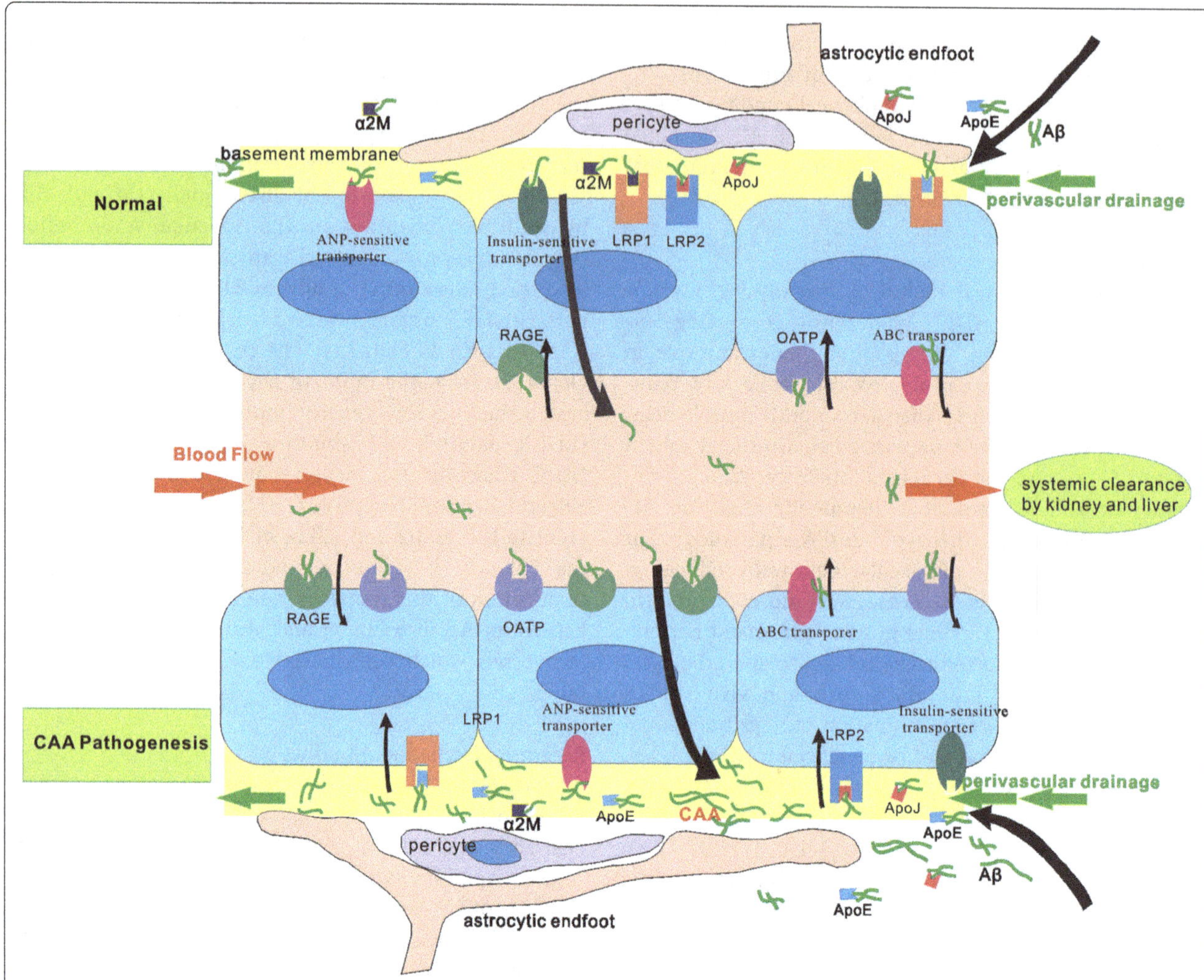

Fig. 1 Aβ can be transported bi-directionally through BBB by multiple receptors. In normal conditions the transportation of Aβ can be mediated by multiple receptors in endothelium. After binding to ApoE or α2M (α2-microglobulin) Aβ can be transported by LRP1 or it can be transported by LRP2 after binding to ApoJ (clusterin). Some other receptors also mediate Aβ efflux, such as ABC transporter, insulin-sensitive transporter and ANP-sensitive transporter. There's only little Aβ influx mediated by RAGE and OATP. In addition Aβ can be transported to perivascular spaces and eliminated through perivascular drainage. In CAA pathological condition, there's a change in the transporter profile of the BBB, with the efflux receptors decreasing and the influx receptors increasing, leading to the decrease of Aβ clearance and its deposition on the vessel wall. Consequently components changes of cerebrovascular basement membrane as well as the weakness of perivascular drainage results in the aggregation of Aβ in blood vessels aggregating CAA

interaction by using soluble RAGE (sRAGE) or anti-RAGE antibody can suppress the accumulation of Aβ in brain parenchyma in transgenic mouse models [23, 26]. Specific inhibitor against RAGE can alleviate amyloid deposition as well as improve cognitive function in APP transgenic mouse [27]. TransTech Pharma, Inc. discovered TTP488, which acts as an antagonist of RAGE-RAGE ligand interaction. Chronic oral dosing of this drug in AD transgenic mouse resulted in a reduction of amyloid deposition in the brain and an improvement of behavioral performance and in phase 2 clinical trial in mild to moderate AD, TTP488 has achieved positive results [28].

Organic anion transporting polypeptides (OATP)

Members of the OATP family, OATP1A2/SLCO1A2 (Oatpla4/Slcola4 in mice) and OATP14 (Oatp14/Slc21a14 in mice), are expressed on the luminal and abluminal sides of brain capillary endothelial cells. Statins are effective substrates for OATP and the uptake of statins in the liver is mainly dependent on OATP transport. As one kind of the cholesterol reducing drugs, statin has been shown helpful to prevent AD and the protective effect is probably not only related to their ability to reduce cholesterol levels, but also some other mechanisms may also be involved [29], such as competitively binding OATP with Aβ. Do et al. [30] found that rosuvastatin and taurocholate, two established Oatpla4 substrates, decreased Aβ influx, while its inhibitor L-thyroxine increased Aβ influx. So Oatpla4 might play an important role in the Aβ clearance from brain. More studies are needed to reveal the specific function between Oatpla4 and Aβ, as well as whether its inhibitor L-thyroxine contributes to the CAA and AD in pathological process.

Receptors mediate Aβ efflux

ATP-binding cassette transporters (ABC transporters)

ABC transporter is a member of the biggest protein superfamilies, existing in all living organism from micro-organism to human. The human ABC transporter is encoded by 49 genes and is divided into A to G 7 subfamilies based on sequence homology and functional similarity. ABC transporters utilize ATP to provide energy for transport of polar and non-polar molecules across cell membrane, which plays an important role in physiological conditions, and its function defects can lead to serious genetic diseases. The transporters are highly expressed in barrier structure (blood-brain barrier, blood-testis barrier, blood-placental barrier), excretory organs (liver, kidney) and absorption organs (small intestine, colon). Some members of the transporters in ABC transporter subfamilies B, C, G can discharge metabolic wastes, exogenous substances and many drugs from the central nervous system to the blood. Among them the most studied substances include multidrug resistance proteins (MDR1), ATP-binding cassette B1 (ABCB1) or P-glycoprotein (P-gp), multidrug resistance-associated protein (MRPs), ATP-binding cassette G2 (ABCG2), ATP-binding cassette G1 (ABCG1) or breast cancer resistance protein (BCRP) and ATP-binding cassette G4 (ABCG4). Recent studies have found that ABC transporters are involved in Aβ clearance.

ABCG2 is highly expressed in CAA and AD transgenic mouse brain and can inhibit the influx of $A\beta_{40}$ across BBB. In vitro study, inflammatory mediators released by Aβ-activated microglia enhance the expression of ABCG2 in vascular endothelial cell [31]. However Carrano et al. [32] observed that the expression of ABCG2 and ABCB1 decreased in capillary of CAA patients, but was not changed in AD and normal controls. And using a vitro BBB model, they further found that $A\beta_{42}$ oligomers or co-incubating $A\beta_{42}$ with clusterin (apolipoprotein J) down-regulated the expression of ABCB1 in the vascular endothelium without any change of ABCG2, suggesting the special function of ABCB1 in capillary CAA, and a recent study observed that Aβ40 could mediate the ubiquitination, internalization and proteasome-dependent degradation of ABCB1 in isolated rat brain capillaries, which indicates that the ubiquitin-proteasome pathway is associated with the lower ABCB1 protein levels in vascular endothelium exposing to Aβ40 [33]. 3xTg-AD transgenic mouse studies demonstrated that the expression of Aβ transporter protein differs in different disease stages. Although the exogenous APP gene can up-regulate the expression of influx transporter RAGE and down-regulate the expression of efflux transporter LRP1, mice can counteract this increased net influx by up-regulating ABCG4、ABCG2、ABCB1, and maintain the balance of Aβ influx and efflux in BBB [21]. Molecules in CSF including Aβ can also be removed via Aβ transporters at the BCSFB, such as ABCB1, LRP1, LRP2 [34]. During aging, there's a significant alterations in Aβ transporter profile expressed at BCSFB with Aβ efflux transporters increased and Aβ influx transporters decreased [35, 36]. So BBB and BCSFB is a dynamic barrier, which can adapt to different pathological conditions by changing its transporter profile. More researches are required to elucidate the role of ABCG2 in the pathogenesis of CAA and AD.

Low-density lipoprotein receptor family (LDLR family)

LDLR family includes at least 10 kinds of receptors, including LDLR, VLDLR, LRP1, LRP1B, LRP2, LRP3, LRP4, LRP5, LRP6 and LRP8. Previous studies revealed that LDLR family was of crucial importance for the development of the nervous system, aging and pathogenesis of AD [37]. The most well-known function of this receptor family is receptor-mediated endocytosis.

LRP1 expression decreases with aging especially for AD patients [38]. Along the progression of AD, hypoxia occurs and stimulates the overexpression of the serum response factor (SRF) and myocardin in cerebral vascular smooth muscle cells. SRF and myocardin can further activate sterol regulatory element binding protein-2, which could down-regulate LRP1 [39]. Many LRP1 ligands co-deposite with Aβ in senile plaques and are involved in Aβ clearance (Fig. 1), such as apoE, α2-microglobulin (α2M), lactoferrin, urokinase-type plasminogen activator, tissue-type plasminogen activator [40]. Studies have suggested that ApoE4 can block the clearance of soluble Aβ from brain by LRP1 [41], leading to the increasing Aβ deposition in the vascular wall and pathological changes of CAA in APP and ApoE4 double transgenic mice. ApoE4-expressing mice has an elevated ratio of Aβ40:42 in brain extracellular pools and a lower Aβ40:42 ratio in CSF, which suggests that ApoE4 leads to the altered transport and clearance of Aβ proteins by LDLR in different brain compartments [42], a possible explanation for the lower Aβ levels in CSF of AD patients with cortical microbleeds [43]. The lipidization level of different ApoE isoforms is not the same. The low lipidization level ApoE4 promotes Aβ deposition, while the higher lipidization level ApoE2 promotes Aβ clearance by LRP1 [44]. While ApoE2 genotype is protective for AD, it's related to intracerebral hemorrhage in CAA patients [45].

The cell surface LRP1 has been shown not only related to Aβ cell uptake and the lysosomal degradation of Aβ in vascular smooth muscle cells [46], but also mediating the Aβ efflux through BBB and further elimination by the liver, spleen and kidney [47]. And LRP1 may influence the phagocytosis or macropinocytosis of Aβ, because it has been respected to control cytoskeleton architectures through focal adhesion kinase (FAK)/paxillin and/or phosphoinositide 3-kinase (PI3K)/extracellular signal-regulated kinase (ERK) pathways [48, 49]. Recently Steffen E. Storck and colleges developed transgenic mouse models that allow for specific deletion of LRP1 within brain endothelial cells. The selective deletion of brain LRP1 in 5xFAD transgenic mouse can reduce plasma Aβ levels and elevate soluble brain Aβ, resulting in aggravated spatial learning and memory deficits [50]. So LRP1 plays an important role in Aβ clearance in BBB via various ligands. Apart from this LRP1 is a multifunctional receptor that can regulate several signaling pathways by binding to other receptors to play a role in the inflammation of atherosclerosis, cancer, and nervous system injury [51]. It can also regulate gene expression through the intracellular domain [49].

LRP2, also named as megalin, is the biggest receptor of the LDLR family, expressed in a variety of absorption epithelial cells such as small intestinal brush border cells and mainly expressed in endothelial cells and choroid plexus in the brain. LRP2 can recognize variety of ligands with different structure and functions including lipoprotein (apoE, clusterin), vitamin-binding proteins, hormones, neurotrophic factors and so on. Many studies have found that LRP2 could faciliate the endocytosis of Aβ as well as its clearance through blood cerebrospinal fluid barrier and blood-brain barrier [46, 52].

After binding of LRP2 to clusterin, the clearance of Aβ by LRP2 in BBB increases, indicating that the interaction between LRP2 and clusterin promotes Aβ efflux (Fig. 1) [53]. Further researchers observed that the efflux of clusterin increased when complexed to Aβ40 in vitro BBB model [54], so clusterin is important for the modulation of Aβ40 transcytosis across the BBB. Carro [55] found that selective deletion of LRP2 in the brain capillary endothelial cells of mice could originate behavioral impairments and neurodegeneration, which were the common clinical manifestations and pathological changes seen in AD brains. However there was no increase in the Aβ laden in the LRP2 deletion model and further studies are required to clarify the role of LRP2 in Aβ clearance. Serum insulin-like growth factor I (IGF-I) is neuroprotective, and in choroid plexus LRP2 can mediate the IGF-I-induced clearance of Aβ and promote the transport of IGF-I into the brain. So LRP2 is able to facilitate Aβ clearance and inhibit tau phosphorylation or amyloid neurotoxicity through mediating transport of IGF-1 [46].

Other receptors mediated Aβ efflux

As mentioned above many studies have proved that LRP and P-gp participate in the clearance of Aβ, however some researchers found that these two receptors do not play a major role in $A\beta_{40}$ clearance by BBB. [56] So there must be other molecules involved in $A\beta_{40}$ transport through BBB. It has been found that insulin can significantly inhibit [125I] $A\beta_{40}$ through BBB in rats, whereas insulin receptor-specific inhibitors cannot block the elimination of [125I] $A\beta_{40}$ across BBB into blood, [57] which suggests that there are unknown insulin-sensitive receptors involved in the elimination of [125I] $A\beta_{40}$.

Natriuretic peptide receptor C (Npr-C), expressed in the brain capillary endothelium, can mediate the elimination of atrial natriuretic peptide (ANP) across BBB. Ito [58] found that ANP elimination can be inhibited by $A\beta_{40}$, however, there was no direct interaction between Npr-C and $A\beta_{40}$, indicating that the clearance of $A\beta_{40}$ may be facilitated by other ANP-sensitive receptor expressed in cerebrovascular endothelium. Meanwhile in vitro study they found that insulin-degrading enzyme was involved in $A\beta_{40}$ clearance through insulin-sensitive transporter and ANP-sensitive receptor in addition to the direct degradation of the protein. As a result, high ANP level caused by cardio-cerebrovascular disease in the brain may suppress the transport of Aβ across BBB to some extent, which could aggravate Aβ-induced pathological changes. However the structure and the function of these receptors are not clear and more studies are required to elucidate their role in blood brain barrier and Aβ clearance.

Interstitial fluid bulk-flow clearance

Perivascular drainage

After released from the neuron, $A\beta_{42}$ tends to aggregate and form parenchyma senile plaques, but $A\beta_{40}$ is resistant to aggregation in parenchyma and can be removed through the drainage of interstitial fluid along the cerebral capillaries and arteries (Fig. 2), where part of the protein can be eliminated through BBB (Figure 1). Any dysfunction in this process can trigger or promote the accumulation of $A\beta_{40}$ in the vascular basement membrane leading to CAA pathological changes [59].

Vascular basement membrane

Vascular basement membrane is a special extracellular matrix of the endothelial basal surface, mainly secreted by endothelial cells. The main components include type IV collagen, laminin, nestin, heparan sulfate proteoglycan and other molecules. Cerebrovascular basement membrane plays a key role in vascular development,

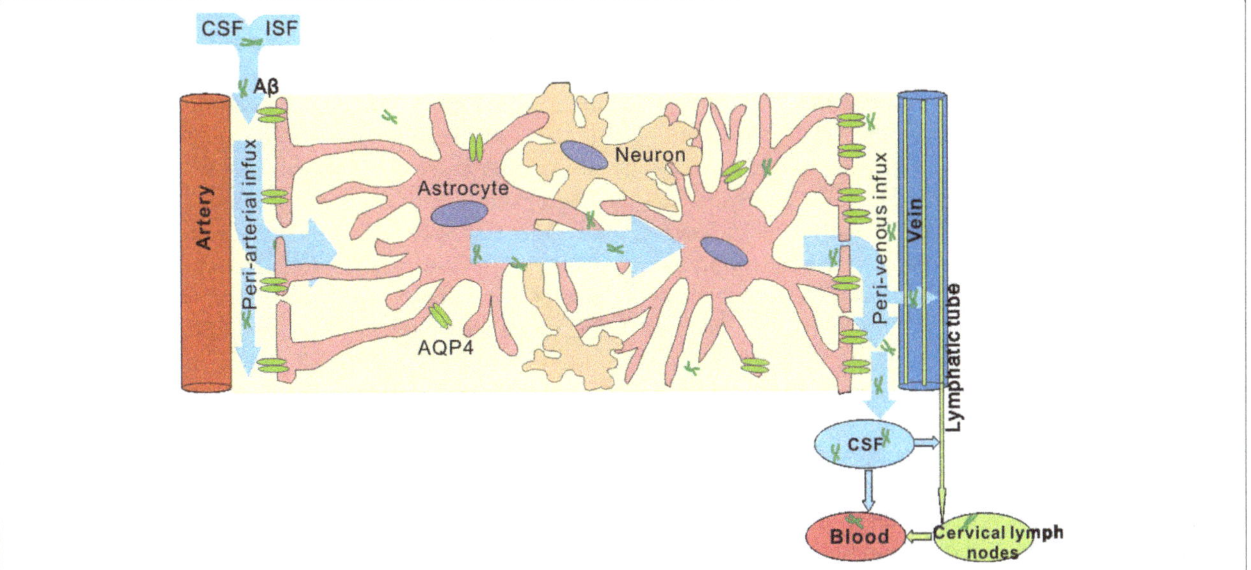

Fig. 2 Brain glymphatic pathway facilitates the drainage of excess Aβ in CSF and ISF. CSF can flows into perivascular space through Virchow-Robin space, and then enters into brain parenchyma mixing with extracellular ISF. The CSF and ISF can travel along the arterial and capillary membrane then flow into leptomeningeal blood vessels or subarachnoid space, or move to cervical lymphnodes by lymphatic drainage and finally flow into blood. The higher expression of AQP4 surrounding veins provides an arteriovenous hydrostatic gradient to drive glymphatic drainage

formation, BBB maintenance, and migration of peripheral cells including leukocytes [60]. There is continuity between brain extracellular matrix and cerebral capillary basement membrane (Fig. 1). So it is possible that interstitial fluid may be drained through the perivascular pathway to the peripheral which includes Aβ.

Increased age-related risk factors for cerebrovascular, such as arteriosclerosis, are also the risk factors for CAA and AD. Further study found that cerebrovascular basement membrane thickening, vacuolization, reduplication appeared in the elderly and the old mouse, were more predominant in the AD brain [61]. As to the workforce of the drainage system, it has been found that the drainage is only present in the live animals and it would stop when there is a cardiac arrest. So it is the blood flow that provides the main impetus for perivascular drainage [62]. After each heart beat the blood vessel will produce a reverse wave with the opposite direction of the blood flow, which appears to facilitate fluid and solute transport in perivascular drainage [63]. As a result, age-related cerebrovascular sclerosis, fibrosis, and loss of smooth muscle cells may reduce the artery contractile force, which leads to the weakness of the perivascular drainage and then induces the impairment of Aβ clearance and increases CAA risk.

Components' changes of cerebrovascular basement membrane

CAA transgenic mouse show a significant reduction in type IV collagen, laminin, nidogen and an obvious increase in heparan sulfate proteoglycan compared to wild type mouse. More importantly the morphological and functional effects of aging on cerebral basement membranes and perivascular drainage differ between brain regions, with a more obvious influence on hippocampus [61]. As a risk factor for sporadic AD and CAA, ApoE4 has been shown to interfere with perivascular drainage of soluble Aβ, which may be achieved by the alteration of protein expression in the vascular basement membrane [64].

The role of apolipoprotein in perivascular drainage

ApoE protein in the cerebral vascular wall increased after anti-amyloid β immunotherapy [65], and study has suggested the co-localization of ApoE and Aβ in the perivascular drainage route (Fig. 1) [66]. After intraventricular injection of $Aβ_{40}$ in ApoE transgenic mice, researchers found the co-deposition of ApoE4 and $Aβ_{40}$ in the vessel wall rather than ApoE3 [64], indicating that the drainage rate of Aβ40 mediated by ApoE4 is much slower. Probably because the binding force between ApoE4-Aβ complex and basement membrane laminin is much weaker than that of ApoE3-Aβ complex, which suggests the impaired clearance of ApoE4-Aβ complex through perivascular drain compared to other ApoE-Aβ complexes [67]. ApoE4 has lower antioxidant activity than other ApoE isoforms [68] thus accelerate the loss of vascular integrity, breakdown of BBB which contributes to CAA. Another apolipoprotein clusterin was found to have high immunoreactivity in the arterioles and capillaries of AD and CAA patients, indicating clusterin is more likely to co-locate with Aβ40 rather than

Aβ42 [69], so that clusterin might mediate the elimination of Aβ40 through perivascular drainage pathway.

Association between brain parenchymal and cerebrovascular Aβ deposition

Passive immunotherapy against Aβ in AD mice model and human has been confirmed to reduce amyloid deposition but it aggravates CAA pathological lesions [70]. Aβ deposition on the cerebral vessels flowing passive immunotherapy contains more $A\beta_{42}$, which suggests that the parenchymal insoluble Aβ can be transformed into soluble form by specific antibody and then transported into the vascular basement membrane, and the failure of periarterial drainage aggregates CAA in AD patients.

Diem et al. established a computational model to investigate the Aβ periarterial drainage in the context of diffusion in the brain, and their studies showed that periarterial drainage of Aβ along basal membranes was more rapid compared with diffusion [71]. These results demonstrate that periarterial drainage is involved in the pathogenesis of CAA and AD as well as immunotherapy related complications. Meanwhile this indicates, to some extent, that normal cerebrovascular function is critical to the success of AD immunotherapy. For example, vasoactive drug cilostazol, a selective inhibitor of phosphodiesterase (PDE) III, has recently shown to significantly improve cognitive decline in patients with mild cognitive impairment [72]. Further animal study revealed that cilostazol reduced $A\beta_{40}$ deposits and rescued cognitive decline in Tg-SwDI mice by promoting perivascular drainage of soluble $A\beta_{40}$ [7].

Therefore, the composition, protein expression and morphology changes of the cerebrovascular basement membrane can impair the perivascular drainage of Aβ, and the deposition of Aβ on the vessel wall can further aggravating Aβ drainage obstacles. This vicious cycle may be an important precipating factor for CAA pathology. Understanding the dynamics of perivascular drainage of the brain will help to find new therapeutic intervention for CAA and AD.

Glymphatic pathways

The glymphatic system is named based on its functional similarity to the peripheral lymphatic system, acting as a convective flux of CSF and ISF in the brain and strictly dependent on water channel aquaporin-4 (AQP4) expressed on the perivascular astrocytic endfeet [73]. Using in vivo two-photon microscopy in mice the dynamics of the glymphatic pathway was described for the first time. ISF solutes diffuse and finally enter the capillary and arterial basement membrane [74], then flow to the leptomeningeal blood vessels at the surface of the brain and finally move to cervical lymph nodes. CSF can flow into perivascular drainage route through Virchow-Robin space, and then enter into brain parenchyma mixing with extracellular ISF (Fig. 2) [75]. The perivascular drainage pathway was considered to be the lymphatic drainage in the brain, and it's still unclear whether these two pathways are distinct pathways or perhaps they just reflect the same transport pathway under different physiological or experimental conditions [36].

Recent animal studies found that AQP4-dependent glymphatic pathway played an important role in promoting clearance of soluble Aβ from CSF and extracellular fluid. In mouse lacking AQP4 in astrocytes, the Aβ clearance was reduced by 55–65% compared with wild mouse. And the expression of AQP4 surrounding veins is higher than arterial, perhaps providing an arteriovenous hydrostatic gradient in order to drive perivascular CSF and ISF bulk flow [76]. In aging mouse brain loss of perivascular AQP4 results in impairment of perivascular CSF recirculation and Aβ clearance [77]. And deletion of AQP4 in AD transgenic mice aggregates brain Aβ accumulation and memory impairment [78]. In postmortem human tissue studies AQP4 was shown to be abnormally expressed in AD and CAA brains [79], and loss of perivascular AQP4 localization was associated with AD status [80]. This is intriguing, for reason that AD is associated with reactive gliosis. We speculate that altered AQP4 expression and depolarization in perivascular astrocytic endfeet under neuropathological conditions may be a triggering factor that contribute to impaired interstitial bulk flow and renders the aging brain more vulnerable to Aβ accumulation in vessel walls. That needs more studies to clarify the internal mechanism.

Following the clearance of free Aβ from the brain ISF into CSF sink via bulk flow, the proteins must be removed into the circulation or possibly through the meningeal lymphatics into the lymphatic system (Fig. 2) [81]. In peripheral organs ISF drains from tissues to lymph nodes. Previously it was thought that the central nervous system (CNS) lacked lymphatic vessels. A recent study has discovered the meningeal lymphatic vessels which expressed the specific molecular markers of lymphatic endothelial cells and are able to drain CSF and ISF into the deep cervical lymph nodes [81]. So after the clearance of Aβ through ISF-to-CSF bulk flow these meningeal lymphatic vessels may provide a conventional path for its further elimination to the peripheral. As discussed above, cilostazol can improve cognitive function of MCI patients [82] and the protective effect is probably not only related to its antiplatelet and vasodilator ability, we suspect that its ability to improve lymphatic function [83] may also be involved, although this hypothesis needs further studies to improve.

Complement-related clearance system

Brain inflammation commonly occurs in CAA and AD, in which the accumulation of Aβ in the arterioles and capillaries of CAA patients might activate the complement system. The activated complement components, as a consequence, can produce a chronic, cumulating and low-level inflammatory response during disease course [84]. Aβ binding to C1q can activate complement system by classical pathway or by alternative pathway without C1q [85] (Fig. 3). These complement components are mainly expressed by neuron, microglial, astrocyte and cerebral microvascular endothelial cells (CMEC). Further study showed that complement proteins can also be produced by cerebrovascular smooth muscle cells and their activation aggravates vascular damage [86]. A recent study revealed that C3 secreted by astrocyte can interact with C3aR in microglial, mediating the inflammatory response induced by Aβ in central nervous system. Aβ can up-regulate the expression of NF-κB in astrocyte and promote the complement activation. Moreover, Aβ attenuated phagocytosis opsonized by complement and resulted in cognitive decline and Aβ deposition. C3aR antagonist can improve glial cell hyperplasia and Aβ deposition, exerting a therapeutic effect on the chronic inflammation of the nervous system [87]. However brain Aβ deposition increased when the activation of C3 was inhibited by expressing soluble complement receptor- related protein y (sCrry) in human amyloid precursor (hAPP) transgenic mice [88]. Complement activation components bind to Aβ-induced apoptotic cell surface, and the microglia complement receptors are implicated in their clearance [89]. So certain inflammatory response in the brain appears to be favorable to neurodegenerative disease.

CR1, also known as CD35 or C3b/C, is an impotent protein in the complement regulatory system, which can enhance the endocytosis of C3b, C4b, C1q coated particles by phagocytic cells and regulate complement activation by inhibiting C3 and C5 invertase activity. Immune complexes, aberrant antibodies or Aβ can be transported by erythrocyte CR1 receptors to the liver for removal. Rogers found that Aβ can be cleared from the bloodstream by CR1 receptors on erythrocyte after binding to C3b (Fig. 3) [90]. In addition, AD and MCI patients show lower levels of C3-opsonized erythrocyte Aβ compared to cognitive normal subjects. So CR1 may be involved in Aβ metabolism and the dysfunction of C3b-dependent Aβ adherence to CR1 can increase the risk of AD. However, it remained unclear how this additional C3b binding site of CR1 exerts its risk for CAA and AD.

In recent years, genome-wide association mapping studies (GWAS) have provided strong evidence for CR1 single nucleotide polymorphism (SNP) being a risk factor for sporadic AD, in which SNP rs6656401 was positively correlated with Aβ deposition in brain [91, 92, 93]. Given the overlap of CAA and AD pathological features, Biffi investigated whether this variant is also correlated with CAA risk and its pathological changes [94]. They found that rs6656401 aggravated CAA-related intracerebral hemorrhage (ICH), risk of recurrent CAA-ICH, as

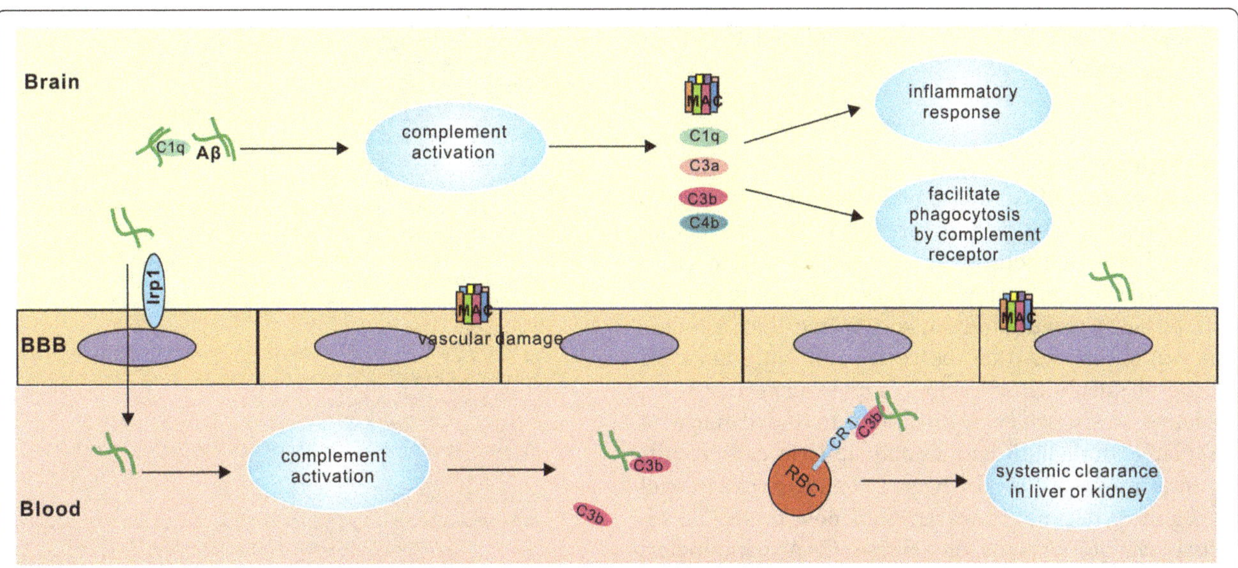

Fig. 3 Complement activation plays both protective and detrimental roles in CAA and AD. Complement activation caused by Aβ can trigger inflammatory response in CNS, and the released inflammatory mediators together with the formation of MAC complex further leads to neuronal and vascular damage. However in CNS complement activation components can bind to Aβ-induced apoptotic cell surface and assist their phagocytosis by microglia which expresses many complement receptors. And in peripheral bloodstream Aβ can be transported by CR1 on erythrocyte after binding to C3b and further cleared in liver or kidney

well as cerebrovascular Aβ deposition. So complement system may be an evoking factor for the pathogenesis of AD and CAA, not just being activated as a result of Aβ deposition. Rs6656401 is located on the non-coding region of CR1 gene and CR1 gene containing this SNP encodes CR1 protein with additional C3b binding sites [95]. It is possible that these additional C3b binding sites of CR1 increase the ability of CR1 to carry more Aβ for liver to degradation.

The only SNP found in the coding region of CR1 gene so far is rs4844609 which encodes a domain that binds to mannan-binding lectin (MBL) and fibronectin [96]. MBL are found to bind to Aβ [97], however the relationship between MBL and AD as well as CAA is unknown. Since C1q, C4b, and C3b are associated with Aβ plaques, it is speculated that rs4844609 and rs665401 may influence the affinity of CR1 with C1q, C4b, and C3b by altering the molecular structure of the receptor and further affect the clearance of Aβ. Rs4844609 can also regulate the cleavage site of the CR1 protein to produce soluble CR1 (sCR1) [98]. sCR1 could regulate complement activation on cell surface and may affect the removal of immune complex and Aβ. A recent study revealed that there is a slight difference in sCR1 levels among populations with different CR1 genotype, and CR1 has a better affinity for C1q and C3b in people with rs4844609, but these differences are not associated with changes in cognitive function [99]. Additionally, it's unknown whether different CR1 isoforms can influence the clearance of peripheral Aβ. So more precise methods are needed to determine the affinity of different CR1 isoforms with C1q, C3b and to identity the molecular pathways of these polymorphisms as related to AD or CAA susceptibility.

Conclusions

The aggregation of Aβ in the brain increases with aging, so age-related risk factors are also associated with impaired Aβ metabolism. As a result the incidence of CAA and AD significantly increases in the aging population, bringing great burden to society and their families. The deposition of Aβ on the vessel wall can induce the release of inflammatory factors, complement activation, oxidative stress, which further lead to the damage of vascular endothelium and smooth muscle cells resulting in intracerebral hemorrhage, ischemic stroke as well as cognitive decline. However, until now there's no effective way to prevent or reverse CAA pathological changes and the clearance of Aβ is regulated by variable factors and many of them are still unclear. So identification of molecular pathways involved in Aβ clearance will provide new targets for AD and CAA therapeutic intervention.

Abbreviations

ABC: ATP-binding cassette; AD: Alzheimer's disease; ANP: Atrial natriuretic peptide; APP: Amyloid precursor; Aβ: Amyloid β-protein; BBB: Blood brain barrier; BCRP: Breast cancer resistance protein; BCSFB: Blood–cerebrospinal fluid barrier; CAA: Cerebral amyloid angiopathy; CEMC: Cerebral microvascular endothelial cell; Crry: Complement receptor- related protein y; CSF: cerebral spinal fluid; ET-1: Endothelin-1; GWAS: Genome-wide association mapping studies; ICH: Intracerebral hemorrhage; IDE: Insulin-degrading enzyme; ISF: Interstitial fluid; LDLR: Low-density lipoprotein receptor; MBL: Mannan-binding lectin; MDR1: Multidrug resistance proteins; MRPs: Multidrug resistance-associated protein; Npr-C: Natriuretic peptide receptor; OATP: Organic anion transporting polypeptides; PDE: Phosphodiesterase; P-gp: P-glycoprotein; RAGE: Advanced glycation end products; SRF: Serum response factor; α2M: α2-microglobulin

Acknowledgements

Not applicable.

Funding

This work was supported by national natural science grant (81570035).

Authors' contributions

XMQ drafted the manuscript. JFM revised the manuscript. Both authors read and approved the final manuscript.

Competing interests

The authors declare that they have no competing interests.

References

1. Biffi A, Halpin A, Towfighi A, Gilson A, Busl K, Rost N, et al. Aspirin and recurrent intracerebral hemorrhage in cerebral amyloid angiopathy. Neurology. 2010;75:693–8.
2. Boyle PA, Yu L, Nag S, Leurgans S, Wilson RS, Bennett DA, et al. Cerebral amyloid angiopathy and cognitive outcomes in community-based older persons. Neurology. 2015;85:1930–6.
3. Scolding NJ, Joseph F, Kirby PA, Mazanti I, Gray F, Mikol J, et al. Abeta-related angiitis: primary angiitis of the central nervous system associated with cerebral amyloid angiopathy. Brain. 2005;128:500–15.
4. Jellinger KA. Alzheimer disease and cerebrovascular pathology: an update. J Neural Transm. 2002;109:813–36.
5. Yamada M. Cerebral amyloid angiopathy: emerging concepts. J Stroke. 2015;17:17–30.
6. Iwata N, Mizukami H, Shirotani K, Takaki Y, Muramatsu S, Lu B, et al. Presynaptic localization of neprilysin contributes to efficient clearance of amyloid-beta peptide in mouse brain. J Neurosci. 2004;24:991–8.
7. Maki T, Okamoto Y, Carare RO, Hase Y, Hattori Y, Hawkes CA, et al. Phosphodiesterase iii inhibitor promotes drainage of cerebrovascular beta-amyloid. Ann Clin Transpl Neurol. 2014;1:519–33.
8. Bales KR, O'Neill SM, Pozdnyakov N, Pan F, Caouette D, Pi Y, et al. Passive immunotherapy targeting amyloid-beta reduces cerebral amyloid angiopathy and improves vascular reactivity. Brain. 2016;139:563–77.
9. Saito S, Ihara M. New therapeutic approaches for alzheimer's disease and cerebral amyloid angiopathy. Frontiers Aging Neuroscience. 2014;6:290.
10. Carpentier M, Robitaille Y, DesGroseillers L, Boileau G, Marcinkiewicz M. Declining expression of neprilysin in alzheimer disease vasculature: possible involvement in cerebral amyloid angiopathy. J Neuropathol Exp Neurol. 2002;61:849–56.

11. Miners JS, Van Helmond Z, Chalmers K, Wilcock G, Love S, Kehoe PG. Decreased expression and activity of neprilysin in alzheimer disease are associated with cerebral amyloid angiopathy. J Neuropathol Exp Neurol. 2006;65:1012–21.
12. Yamada M. Cerebral amyloid angiopathy and gene polymorphisms. J Neurol Sci. 2004;226:41–4.
13. Lim CS, Alkon DL. Pkcepsilon promotes hud-mediated neprilysin mrna stability and enhances neprilysin-induced abeta degradation in brain neurons. PLoS One. 2014;9:e97756.
14. Iwata N, Sekiguchi M, Hattori Y, Takahashi A, Asai M, Ji B, et al. Global brain delivery of neprilysin gene by intravascular administration of aav vector in mice. Sci Rep. 2013;3:1472.
15. Kawakubo T, Mori R, Shirotani K, Iwata N, Asai M. Neprilysin is suppressed by dual-specificity tyrosine-phosphorylation regulated kinase 1a (dyrk1a) in down-syndrome-derived fibroblasts. Biol Pharm Bull. 2017;40:327–33.
16. Morelli L, Llovera RE, Mathov I, Lue LF, Frangione B, Ghiso J, et al. Insulin-degrading enzyme in brain microvessels: proteolysis of amyloid {beta} vasculotropic variants and reduced activity in cerebral amyloid angiopathy. J Biol Chem. 2004;279:56004–13.
17. Hu J, Igarashi A, Kamata M, Nakagawa H. Angiotensin-converting enzyme degrades alzheimer amyloid beta-peptide (a beta); retards a beta aggregation, deposition, fibril formation; and inhibits cytotoxicity. J Biol Chem. 2001;276:47863–8.
18. Miners JS, Ashby E, Van Helmond Z, Chalmers KA, Palmer LE, Love S, et al. Angiotensin-converting enzyme (ace) levels and activity in alzheimer's disease, and relationship of perivascular ace-1 to cerebral amyloid angiopathy. Neuropathol Appl Neurobiol. 2008;34:181–93.
19. Domingues-Montanari S, Hernandez-Guillamon M, Fernandez-Cadenas I, Mendioroz M, Boada M, Munuera J, et al. Ace variants and risk of intracerebral hemorrhage recurrence in amyloid angiopathy. Neurobiol Aging. 2011;32(551):e513–22.
20. Carrano A, Hoozemans JJ, van der Vies SM, Rozemuller AJ, van Horssen J, de Vries HE. Amyloid beta induces oxidative stress-mediated blood-brain barrier changes in capillary amyloid angiopathy. Antioxid Redox Signal. 2011;15:1167–78.
21. Do TM, Dodacki A, Alata W, Calon F, Nicolic S, Scherrmann JM, et al. Age-dependent regulation of the blood-brain barrier influx/efflux equilibrium of amyloid-beta peptide in a mouse model of alzheimer's disease (3xtg-ad). J Alzheimers Dis. 2015;49:287–300.
22. Origlia N, Arancio O, Domenici L, Yan SS. Mapk, beta-amyloid and synaptic dysfunction: the role of rage. Expert Rev. Neurother. 2009;9:1635–45.
23. Deane R, Du Yan S, Submamaryan RK, LaRue B, Jovanovic S, Hogg E, et al. Rage mediates amyloid-beta peptide transport across the blood-brain barrier and accumulation in brain. Nature Med. 2003;9:907–13.
24. Candela P, Gosselet F, Saint-Pol J, Sevin E, Boucau MC, Boulanger E, et al. Apical-to-basolateral transport of amyloid-beta peptides through blood-brain barrier cells is mediated by the receptor for advanced glycation end-products and is restricted by p-glycoprotein. J Alzheimers Dis. 2010; 22:849–59.
25. Guo YX, He LY, Zhang M, Wang F, Liu F, Peng WX. 1,25-dihydroxyvitamin d3 regulates expression of lrp1 and rage in vitro and in vivo, enhancing abeta1-40 brain-to-blood efflux and peripheral uptake transport. Neuroscience. 2016;322:28–38.
26. Rocken C, Kientsch-Engel R, Mansfeld S, Stix B, Stubenrauch K, Weigle B, et al. Advanced glycation end products and receptor for advanced glycation end products in aa amyloidosis. Am J Pathol. 2003;162:1213–20.
27. Deane R, Singh I, Sagare AP, Bell RD, Ross NT, LaRue B, et al. A multimodal rage-specific inhibitor reduces amyloid beta-mediated brain disorder in a mouse model of alzheimer disease. J Clin Invest. 2012;122:1377–92.
28. Burstein AH, Grimes I, Galasko DR, Aisen PS, Sabbagh M, Mjalli AM. Effect of ttp488 in patients with mild to moderate alzheimer's disease. BMC Neurol. 2014;14:12.
29. Shinohara M, Sato N, Kurinami H, Takeuchi D, Takeda S, Shimamura M, et al. Reduction of brain beta-amyloid (abeta) by fluvastatin, a hydroxymethylglutaryl-coa reductase inhibitor, through increase in degradation of amyloid precursor protein c-terminal fragments (app-ctfs) and abeta clearance. J Biol Chem. 2010;285:22091–102.
30. Do TM, Bedussi B, Chasseigneaux S, Dodacki A, Yapo C, Chacun H, et al. Oatp1a4 and an l-thyroxine-sensitive transporter mediate the mouse blood-brain barrier transport of amyloid-beta peptide. J Alzheimers Dis. 2013;36:555–61.
31. Xiong H, Callaghan D, Jones A, Bai J, Rasquinha I, Smith C, et al. Abcg2 is upregulated in alzheimer's brain with cerebral amyloid angiopathy and may act as a gatekeeper at the blood-brain barrier for abeta (1-40) peptides. J Neuroradiol. 2009;29:5463–75.
32. Carrano A, Snkhchyan H, Kooij G, van der Pol S, van Horssen J, Veerhuis R, et al. Atp-binding cassette transporters p-glycoprotein and breast cancer related protein are reduced in capillary cerebral amyloid angiopathy. Neurobiol Aging. 2014;35:565–75.
33. Hartz AM, Zhong Y. Abeta40 reduces p-glycoprotein at the blood-brain barrier through the ubiquitin-proteasome pathway. J Neurosci. 2016;36: 1930–41.
34. Erickson MA, Banks WA. Blood-brain barrier dysfunction as a cause and consequence of alzheimer's disease. J Cereb Blood Flow Metab. 2013;33: 1500–13.
35. Pascale CL, Miller MC, Chiu C, Boylan M, Caralopoulos IN, Gonzalez L, et al. Amyloid-beta transporter expression at the blood-csf barrier is age-dependent. Fluids Barriers CNS. 2011;8:21.
36. Tarasoff-Conway JM, Carare RO, Osorio RS, Glodzik L, Butler T, Fieremans E, et al. Clearance systems in the brain-implications for alzheimer disease. Nat Rev. Neurol. 2015;11:457–70.
37. Auderset L, Landowski LM, Foa L. Low density lipoprotein receptor related proteins as regulators of neural stem and progenitor cell function. Stem Cells Int. 2016;2016:2108495.
38. Kang DE, Pietrzik CU, Baum L, Chevallier N, Merriam DE, Kounnas MZ, et al. Modulation of amyloid beta-protein clearance and alzheimer's disease susceptibility by the ldl receptor-related protein pathway. J Clin Invest. 2000;106:1159–66.
39. Bell RD, Deane R, Chow N, Long X, Sagare A, Singh I, et al. Srf and myocardin regulate lrp-mediated amyloid-beta clearance in brain vascular cells. Nat Cell Biol. 2009;11:143–53.
40. Rebeck GW, Harr SD, Strickland DK, Hyman BT. Multiple, diverse senile plaque-associated proteins are ligands of an apolipoprotein e receptor, the alpha 2-macroglobulin receptor/low-density-lipoprotein receptor-related protein. Ann Neurol. 1995;37:211–7.
41. Deane R, Sagare A, Hamm K, Parisi M, Lane S, Finn MB, et al. Apoe isoform-specific disruption of amyloid beta peptide clearance from mouse brain. J Clin Investig. 2008;118:4002–13.
42. Fryer JD, Simmons K, Parsadanian M, Bales KR, Paul SM, Sullivan PM, et al. Human apolipoprotein e4 alters the amyloid-beta 40:42 ratio and promotes the formation of cerebral amyloid angiopathy in an amyloid precursor protein transgenic model. J Neurosci. 2005;25:2803–10.
43. Noguchi-Shinohara M, Komatsu J, Samuraki M, Matsunari I, Ikeda T, Sakai K, et al. Cerebral amyloid angiopathy-related microbleeds and cerebrospinal fluid biomarkers in alzheimer's disease. J Alzheimers Dis. 2017;55(3):905–13.
44. Hu J, Liu CC, Chen XF, Zhang YW, Xu H, Bu G. Opposing effects of viral mediated brain expression of apolipoprotein e2 (apoe2) and apoe4 on apoe lipidation and abeta metabolism in apoe4-targeted replacement mice. Mol Neurodegener. 2015;10:6.
45. Charidimou A, Martinez-Ramirez S, Shoamanesh A, Oliveira-Filho J, Frosch M, Vashkevich A, et al. Cerebral amyloid angiopathy with and without hemorrhage: evidence for different disease phenotypes. Neurology. 2015;84:1206–12.
46. Carro E, Spuch C, Trejo JL, Antequera D, Torres-Aleman I. Choroid plexus megalin is involved in neuroprotection by serum insulin-like growth factor i. J Neuroradiol. 2005;25:10884–93.
47. Shibata M, Yamada S, Kumar SR, Calero M, Bading J, Frangione B, et al. Clearance of alzheimer's amyloid-ss (1-40) peptide from brain by ldl receptor-related protein-1 at the blood-brain barrier. J Clin Investig. 2000;106:1489–99.
48. Dedieu S, Langlois B. Lrp-1: a new modulator of cytoskeleton dynamics and adhesive complex turnover in cancer cells. Cell Adhes Migr. 2008;2:77–80.
49. Kanekiyo T, Bu G. The low-density lipoprotein receptor-related protein 1 and amyloid-beta clearance in alzheimer's disease. Front Aging Neurosci. 2014;6:93.
50. Storck SE, Meister S, Nahrath J, Meissner JN, Schubert N, Di Spiezio A, et al. Endothelial lrp1 transports amyloid-beta1-42 across the blood-brain barrier. J Clin Invest. 2016;126:123–36.
51. Gonias SL, Campana WM. Ldl receptor-related protein-1: a regulator of inflammation in atherosclerosis, cancer, and injury to the nervous system. Am J Pathol. 2014;184:18–27.

52. Deane R, Wu Z, Sagare A, Davis J, Du Yan S, Hamm K, et al. Lrp/amyloid beta-peptide interaction mediates differential brain efflux of abeta isoforms. Neuron. 2004;43:333–44.
53. Bell RD, Sagare AP, Friedman AE, Bedi GS, Holtzman DM, Deane R, et al. Transport pathways for clearance of human alzheimer's amyloid beta-peptide and apolipoproteins e and j in the mouse central nervous system. J Cereb Blood Flow Metab. 2007;27:909–18.
54. Merino-Zamorano C, Fernandez-de Retana S, Montanola A, Batlle A, Saint-Pol J, Mysiorek C, et al. Modulation of amyloid-beta1-40 transport by apoa1 and apoj across an in vitro model of the blood-brain barrier. J Alzheimers Dis. 2016;53:677–91.
55. Dietrich M, Antequera D, Pascual C, Castro N, Bolos M, Carro E. Alzheimer's disease-like impaired cognition in endothelial-specific megalin-null mice. J Alzheimers Dis. 2014;39:711–7.
56. Ito S, Ueno T, Ohtsuki S, Terasaki T. Lack of brain-to-blood efflux transport activity of low-density lipoprotein receptor-related protein-1 (lrp-1) for amyloid-beta peptide (1-40) in mouse: involvement of an lrp-1-independent pathway. J Neurochem. 2010;113:1356–63.
57. Shiiki T, Ohtsuki S, Kurihara A, Naganuma H, Nishimura K, Tachikawa M, et al. Brain insulin impairs amyloid-beta (1-40) clearance from the brain. J Neurosci. 2004;24:9632–7.
58. Ito S, Ohtsuki S, Murata S, Katsukura Y, Suzuki H, Funaki M, et al. Involvement of insulin-degrading enzyme in insulin- and atrial natriuretic peptide-sensitive internalization of amyloid-beta peptide in mouse brain capillary endothelial cells. J Alzheimers Dis. 2014;38:185–200.
59. Weller RO, Massey A, Newman TA, Hutchings M, Kuo YM, Roher AE. Cerebral amyloid angiopathy: Amyloid beta accumulates in putative interstitial fluid drainage pathways in alzheimer's disease. Am J Pathol. 1998;153:725–33.
60. Wu C, Ivars F, Anderson P, Hallmann R, Vestweber D, Nilsson P, et al. Endothelial basement membrane laminin alpha5 selectively inhibits t lymphocyte extravasation into the brain. Nature Med. 2009;15:519–27.
61. Hawkes CA, Gatherer M, Sharp MM, Dorr A, Yuen HM, Kalaria R, et al. Regional differences in the morphological and functional effects of aging on cerebral basement membranes and perivascular drainage of amyloid-beta from the mouse brain. Aging Cell. 2013;12:224–36.
62. Ball KK, Cruz NF, Mrak RE, Dienel GA. Trafficking of glucose, lactate, and amyloid-beta from the inferior colliculus through perivascular routes. J Cereb Blood Flow Metab. 2010;30:162–76.
63. Wang P, Olbricht WL. Fluid mechanics in the perivascular space. J Theor Biol. 2011;274:52–7.
64. Hawkes CA, Sullivan PM, Hands S, Weller RO, Nicoll JA, Carare RO. Disruption of arterial perivascular drainage of amyloid-beta from the brains of mice expressing the human apoe epsilon4 allele. PLoS One. 2012;7:e41636.
65. Sakai K, Boche D, Carare R, Johnston D, Holmes C, Love S, et al. Abeta immunotherapy for alzheimer's disease: effects on apoe and cerebral vasculopathy. Acta Neuropathol. 2014;128:777–89.
66. Rolyan H, Feike AC, Upadhaya AR, Waha A, Van Dooren T, Haass C, et al. Amyloid-beta protein modulates the perivascular clearance of neuronal apolipoprotein e in mouse models of alzheimer's disease. J Neural Transm. 2011;118:699–712.
67. Zekonyte J, Sakai K, Nicoll JA, Weller RO, Carare RO. Quantification of molecular interactions between apoe, amyloid-beta (abeta) and laminin: relevance to accumulation of abeta in alzheimer's disease. Biochim Biophys Acta. 1862;2016:1047–53.
68. Miyata M, Smith JD. Apolipoprotein e allele-specific antioxidant activity and effects on cytotoxicity by oxidative insults and beta-amyloid peptides. Nature Genet. 1996;14:55–61.
69. Craggs L, Taylor J, Slade JY, Chen A, Hagel C, Kuhlenbaeumer G, et al. Clusterin/apolipoprotein j immunoreactivity is associated with white matter damage in cerebral small vessel diseases. Neuropathol Appl Neurobiol. 2016;42:194–209.
70. Boncoraglio GB, Piazza F, Savoiardo M, Farina L, DiFrancesco JC, Prioni S, et al. Prodromal alzheimer's disease presenting as cerebral amyloid angiopathy-related inflammation with spontaneous amyloid-related imaging abnormalities and high cerebrospinal fluid anti-abeta autoantibodies. J Alzheimers Dis. 2015;45:363–7.
71. Diem AK, Tan M, Bressloff NW, Hawkes C, Morris AW, Weller RO, et al. A simulation model of periarterial clearance of amyloid-beta from the brain. Frontiers Aging Neuroscience. 2016;8:18.
72. Taguchi A, Takata Y, Ihara M, Kasahara Y, Tsuji M, Nishino M, et al. Cilostazol improves cognitive function in patients with mild cognitive impairment: a retrospective analysis. Psychogeriatrics. 2013;13:164–9.
73. Hitscherich K, Smith K, Cuoco JA, Ruvolo KE, Mancini JD, Leheste JR, et al. The glymphatic-lymphatic continuum: opportunities for osteopathic manipulative medicine. J Am Optom Assoc. 2016;116:170–7.
74. Pullen RG, DePasquale M, Cserr HF. Bulk flow of cerebrospinal fluid into brain in response to acute hyperosmolality. Am J Phys. 1987;253:F538–45.
75. Rennels ML, Gregory TF, Blaumanis OR, Fujimoto K, Grady PA. Evidence for a 'paravascular' fluid circulation in the mammalian central nervous system, provided by the rapid distribution of tracer protein throughout the brain from the subarachnoid space. Brain Res. 1985;326:47–63.
76. Iliff JJ, Wang M, Liao Y, Plogg BA, Peng W, Gundersen GA, et al. A paravascular pathway facilitates csf flow through the brain parenchyma and the clearance of interstitial solutes, including amyloid beta. Sci Transl Med. 2012;4:147ra111.
77. Kress BT, Iliff JJ, Xia M, Wang M, Wei HS, Zeppenfeld D, et al. Impairment of paravascular clearance pathways in the aging brain. Ann Neurol. 2014;76: 845–61.
78. Xu Z, Xiao N, Chen Y, Huang H, Marshall C, Gao J, et al. Deletion of aquaporin-4 in app/ps1 mice exacerbates brain abeta accumulation and memory deficits. Mol Neurodegener. 2015;10:58.
79. Hoshi A, Yamamoto T, Shimizu K, Ugawa Y, Nishizawa M, Takahashi H, et al. Characteristics of aquaporin expression surrounding senile plaques and cerebral amyloid angiopathy in alzheimer disease. J Neuropathol Exp Neurol. 2012;71:750–9.
80. Zeppenfeld DM, Simon M, Haswell JD, D'Abreo D, Murchison C, Quinn JF, et al. Association of perivascular localization of aquaporin-4 with cognition and alzheimer disease in aging brains. JAMA Neurol. 2017;74:91–9.
81. Louveau A, Smirnov I, Keyes TJ, Eccles JD, Rouhani SJ, Peske JD, et al. Structural and functional features of central nervous system lymphatic vessels. Nature. 2015;523:337–41.
82. Saito S, Kojima S, Oishi N, Kakuta R, Maki T, Yasuno F, et al. A multicenter, randomized, placebo-controlled trial for cilostazol in patients with mild cognitive impairment: the comcid study protocol. Alzheimer's & Dementia: Trans Res Clin Interven. 2016;2:250–7.
83. Kimura T, Hamazaki TS, Sugaya M, Fukuda S, Chan T, Tamura-Nakano M, et al. Cilostazol improves lymphatic function by inducing proliferation and stabilization of lymphatic endothelial cells. J Dermatol Sci. 2014;74:150–8.
84. Shen Y, Lue L, Yang L, Roher A, Kuo Y, Strohmeyer R, et al. Complement activation by neurofibrillary tangles in alzheimer's disease. Neurosci Lett. 2001;305:165–8.
85. Bradt BM, Kolb WP, Cooper NR. Complement-dependent proinflammatory properties of the alzheimer's disease beta-peptide. J Exp Med. 1998;188: 431–8.
86. Walker DG, Dalsing-Hernandez JE, Lue LF. Human postmortem brain-derived cerebrovascular smooth muscle cells express all genes of the classical complement pathway: a potential mechanism for vascular damage in cerebral amyloid angiopathy and alzheimer's disease. Micro Res. 2008;75:411–9.
87. Lian H, Litvinchuk A, Chiang AC, Aithmitti N, Jankowsky JL, Zheng H. Astrocyte-microglia cross talk through complement activation modulates amyloid pathology in mouse models of alzheimer's disease. J Neurosci. 2016;36:577–89.
88. Wyss-Coray T, Yan F, Lin AH, Lambris JD, Alexander JJ, Quigg RJ, et al. Prominent neurodegeneration and increased plaque formation in complement-inhibited alzheimer's mice. Proc Natl Acad Sci U S A. 2002;99: 10837–42.
89. Crehan H, Hardy J, Pocock J. Microglia, alzheimer's disease, and complement. Int J Alzheimers Dis. 2012;2012:983640.
90. Rogers J, Li R, Mastroeni D, Grover A, Leonard B, Ahern G, et al. Peripheral clearance of amyloid beta peptide by complement c3-dependent adherence to erythrocytes. Neurobiol Aging. 2006;27:1733–9.
91. Lambert JC. Genome-wide association study identifies variants at clu and cr1 associated with alzheimer's disease. Nat Genet. 2009;41:1094–9.
92. Chibnik LB, Shulman JM, Leurgans SE, Schneider JA, Wilson RS, Tran D, et al. Cr1 is associated with amyloid plaque burden and age-related cognitive decline. Ann Neurol. 2011;69:560–9.
93. Farfel JM, Yu L, Buchman AS, Schneider JA, De Jager PL, Bennett DA. Relation of genomic variants for alzheimer disease dementia to common neuropathologies. Neurology. 2016;87:489–96.

94. Biffi A, Shulman JM, Jagiella JM, Cortellini L, Ayres AM, Schwab K, et al. Genetic variation at cr1 increases risk of cerebral amyloid angiopathy. Neurology. 2012;78:334–41.
95. Brouwers N, Van Cauwenberghe C, Engelborghs S, Lambert JC, Bettens K, Le Bastard N, et al. Alzheimer risk associated with a copy number variation in the complement receptor 1 increasing c3b/c4b binding sites. Mol Psychiatry. 2012;17:223–33.
96. Jacquet M, Lacroix M, Ancelet S, Gout E, Gaboriaud C, Thielens NM, et al. Deciphering complement receptor type 1 interactions with recognition proteins of the lectin complement pathway. J Immunol. 2013;190:3721–31.
97. Larvie M, Shoup T, Chang WC, Chigweshe L, Hartshorn K, White MR, et al. Mannose-binding lectin binds to amyloid beta protein and modulates inflammation. J Biomed Biotechnol. 2012;2012:929803.
98. Chen CH, Ghiran I, Beurskens FJ, Weaver G, Vincent JA, Nicholson-Weller A, et al. Antibody cr1-2b11 recognizes a non-polymorphic epitope of human cr1 (cd35). Clin Exp Immunol. 2007;148:546–54.
99. Fonseca MI, Chu S, Pierce AL, Brubaker WD, Hauhart RE, Mastroeni D, et al. Analysis of the putative role of cr1 in alzheimer's disease: genetic association, expression and function. PLoS One. 2016;11:e0149792.

13

The study of brain functional connectivity in Parkinson's disease

Lin-lin Gao[1,2] and Tao Wu[1,2*]

Abstract

Parkinson's disease (PD) is a neurodegenerative disorder primarily affecting the aging population. The neurophysiological mechanisms underlying parkinsonian symptoms remain unclear. PD affects extensive neural networks and a more thorough understanding of network disruption will help bridge the gap between known pathological changes and observed clinical presentations in PD. Development of neuroimaging techniques, especially functional magnetic resonance imaging, allows for detection of the functional connectivity of neural networks in patients with PD. This review aims to provide an overview of current research involving functional network disruption in PD relating to motor and non-motor symptoms. Investigations into functional network connectivity will further our understanding of the mechanisms underlying the effectiveness of clinical interventions, such as levodopa and deep brain stimulation treatment. In addition, identification of PD-specific neural network patterns has the potential to aid in the development of a definitive diagnosis of PD.

Keywords: Parkinson's disease, Functional connectivity, fMRI

Background

Parkinson's disease (PD) is the second most common neurodegenerative disorder in the aging population. PD is characterized by progressive deterioration of motor function, such as bradykinesia, rigidity, resting tremor, gait disturbance, and postural instability. Patients with PD also experience non-motor symptoms such as cognitive deficits, anxiety, apathy, hallucination, and depression. The pathological hallmark of PD is progressive decrease in dopamine concentrations and neuronal cell loss within the substantia nigra and other brain structures combined with the appearance of intracytoplasmic inclusions composed of α-synuclein aggregates known as Lewy bodies [1]. However, the precise mechanism by which the pathological changes in the brain result in the described clinical symptoms is unknown. It is well known that PD affects a large scale of neural networks. For example, dysfunction of cortico-basal ganglia-thalamo-cortical pathway is well known to be critical for the development of parkinsonian symptoms [2]. Therefore, further examination of neuronal network integrity may provide more valuable information for understanding the pathophysiological changes of PD than investigations of local brain activity, and may be helpful to bridge the gap between pathological changes and clinical presentations in PD.

The development of techniques such as functional magnetic resonance imaging (fMRI), electroencephalography (EEG), magnetoencephalography MEG), and transcranial magnetic stimulation (TMS) has greatly enhanced the ability to evaluate functional network integrity in vivo [3, 4]. In recent years, extensive studies have investigated PD-related disruption of functional networks, and have provided useful information regarding neurophysiological mechanisms underlying parkinsonian symptoms. In addition, these studies have served to identify mechanisms of anti-parkinsonian interventions, and suggest that brain networks have the potential to be developed as a biomarker for the diagnosis of PD. The aim of this review is to provide a comprehensive overview of the application of functional network connectivity in investigating neural mechanisms underlying parkinsonian symptoms and interventions, and as a potential biomarker in patients with PD. The reviewed publications were selected by the authors on the basis of relevance to the

* Correspondence: wutao69@gmail.com
[1]Department of Neurobiology, Key Laboratory on Neurodegenerative Disorders of Ministry of Education, Beijing Institute of Geriatrics, Xuanwu Hospital, Capital Medical University, Beijing 100053, China
[2]Beijing Key Laboratory on Parkinson's Disease, Parkinson Disease Center of Beijing Institute for Brain Disorders, Beijing, China

topic. The functional connectivity studies included in the current study is summarized in Table 1.

Techniques to assess network integrity

EEG, fMRI, and MEG are the most widely used techniques that enable researchers to assess large-scale neural networks at different spatial and temporal resolutions. With the advantages of being noninvasive and having high spatial resolution, fMRI is now the most used method to investigate functional integrity of networks in PD. In broad definition, fMRI includes all magnetic resonance imaging (MRI) methods that detect neural functional changes, such as blood oxygen level-dependent (BOLD) contrast imaging, perfusion, or diffusion. However, fMRI typically refers to BOLD fMRI, which detects changes in oxygen saturation levels of the blood [5]. In this review, the applications of BOLD fMRI on network integrity in PD will be discussed. The methods used to explore network integration involve the analysis of functional or effective connectivity [6–10]. Functional connectivity is defined as a temporal correlation between spatially remote neurophysiological events, whereas effective connectivity is defined as the influence that one neuronal system exerts over another [11]. Findings from both methods will be presented in this review.

Motor symptoms-related network changes

Bradykinesia

Bradykinesia is an important feature contributing to motor difficulties in PD. In this review, we use bradykinesia to describe bradykinesia (slowness of movement), hypokinesia (smallness of movement), and akinesia (lack of movement). Although extensive research has been conducted in this area, the pathophysiological mechanisms underlying bradykinesia remain unclear. Several neuroimaging studies have investigated network connectivity during performance of various motor tasks in patients with PD. During the performance of self-initiated movement, the functional connectivity between the striatum and cortical motor areas, i.e., primary motor cortex (M1), premotor cortex (PMC), and supplementary motor area (SMA), is weakened in PD [12]. In addition, the connectivity between the prefrontal cortex, PMC and SMA is disrupted [12–15]. The SMA is critical in planning and decision of movements and plays a primary role in the preparation of self-initiated movements [16–18]. The SMA is one of the main receiving regions of the basal ganglia motor circuit [19]. The dysfunction of the SMA has been correlated with motor difficulty, and the administration of levodopa has been shown to relatively normalize the function of the SMA in patients with PD resulting in improved motor performance [20, 21]. Thus, the disconnection of the striato-SMA pathway due to the deficit of the nigrostriatal dopamine system is likely to be an important factor contributing to bradykinesia in PD.

Motor automaticity has been proposed as a possible mechanism underlying bradykinesia [22]. Automaticity is the ability to perform movements without attention directed toward the details of the movement [23]. In healthy people, the processing of motor automaticity is accompanied by the more efficiency of neural network and less significant of attentional network. The automated motor program is likely stored in the sensorimotor striatum (posterior putamen), and is resistant to interference [22, 24–26]. Most bradykinesia-related motor problems are associated with deterioration of motor automaticity, as PD patients tend to perform all daily behaviors slower or with smaller amplitude, e.g., akinesia, reduced arm swing, freezing of gait (FOG), and micrographia [27]. Motor automaticity dysfunction is already apparent in the early stages of PD [28, 29]. During automatic processing, the connectivity of striato-cortical motor pathways is decreased, the activity in the sensorimotor striatum is not enhanced, and the attentional networks remain active in PD compared to controls [22, 29, 30].

Based on these studies of neural networks, neural mechanisms for impaired motor automaticity in PD includes less efficient neural coding of movement, failure to shift automated motor skills to the sensorimotor striatum, instability of the automatic mode within the striatum, and use of attentional control efforts to execute movements usually performed automatically in healthy people [22]. As a consequence, PD patients lose previously acquired automatic skills and have difficulty in acquiring new automatic skills or restoring lost motor skills, which results in bradykinesia.

Tremor

As tremor may disturb fMRI signals, tremor-related network connectivity has been much less investigated compared to bradykineisa. In an elegant study, Helmich and colleagues described the use of electromyography to monitor tremor during fMRI scanning, and measured functional connectivity between basal ganglia nuclei and the cerebellothalamic circuit [31]. The authors reported that the basal ganglia nuclei were transiently activated at the onset of tremor, while activity in the cerebellothalamic circuit correlated with tremor amplitude. The internal globus pallidus and putamen had increased functional connectivity with the cerebellothalamic circuit. These findings suggest that parkinsonian tremor may result from a pathological interaction between the basal ganglia and the cerebellothalamic circuit, which is supported by the following studies [30].

Functional connectivity experiments have also been used to explore the underlying mechanisms for several

Table 1 Summary of the characteristics of the reviewed studies

Paper	Number of patients	Task	Type of connectivity	Main findings
Wu T et al., 2011 [12]	18 PD patients 18 controls	A self-initiated right hand tapping task	Effective connectivity psychophysiological interaction (PPI)	The striatum-cortical connections were weakened, while the cortico-cerebellar connections were strengthened in PD
Rowe J et al., 2002 [13]	12 PD patients 12 controls	An overlearned motor sequence task, with and without attention	Effective connectivity • Structural equation modeling (SEM)	Attention to action did not increase the connectivity between the prefrontal cortex, lateral premotor cortex and SMA in PD
Wu T et al., 2010 [14]	12 patients 12 age-and sex-matched healthy subjects	two sequences of right hand finger tapping	Effective connectivity psychophysiological interaction (PPI)	The pre-SMA, cerebellum, and cingulate motor area had increased effective connectivity with brain networks in PD
Rowe JB et al., 2010 [15]	16 PD patients 42 controls	A visually paced finger-tapping task	Effective connectivity Dynamic causal modelling (DCM)	The coupling between the prefrontal cortex and the pre-SMA was enhanced in PD
Wu T et al., 2016 [27]	36 PD patients 18 controls	Handwriting	Functional connectivity	Dysfunction of basal ganglia motor circuit in both consistent and progressive. Progressive micrographia was also associated with disconnections between the pre-SMA, rostral cingulated motor area and cerebellum
Wu T et al., 2015 [22, 29]	22 PD patients 22 controls	Visuomotor association task	Effective connectivity Granger causality analysis (GCA)	The connectivity from the putamen to the motor cortex was decreased in PD
Ma H et al., 2015 [30]	50 PD patients 29 age-matched health controls	Resting state	Functional connectivity	The bilateral dentate nucleus had higher connectivity with the bilateral cerebellar anterior lobe, and lower connectivity with the bilateral prefrontal cortex in tremor-dominant PD
Tessitore A et al., 2012 [32]	29 PD patients 15 controls	Resting state	Functional connectivity	Reduced connectivity within both executive-attention and visual networks
Liu H et al., 2013 [34]	9 PD patients 9 controls	Resting state	Functional connectivity	Decreased connectivity of the dentate nucleus with the bilateral cerebellar posterior lobe in tremor-dominant PD
Hu X et al., 2015 [35, 43]	21 tremor-dominant (TD)-PD 29 akinetic-rigid (AR)-PD patients 26 controls	Resting state	Voxel-mirrored homotopic connectivity (VMHC)	TD-PD exhibited significantly lower VMHC values in the posterior lobe of the cerebellum. AR-PD exhibited lower VMHC values in the precentral gyrus.
Seibert TM et al., 2012 [36]	19 cognitively unimpaired controls, 19 cognitively unimpaired PD patients, 18 patients with dementia	Resting state	Functional connectivity	Decreased striato-prefrontal connectivity in patients with dementia
Gorges M et al., 2015 [37]	14 cognitively unimpaired PD patients, 17 cognitively impaired PD patients 22 controls	Resting state	Functional connectivity	Decreased default mode network connectivity in cognitively impaired PD patients.
Disbrow EA et al., 2014 [38]	14 non-demented PD patients, 20 controls.	Resting state	Functional connectivity	Decreased default mode network connectivity in PD
Manza P et al., 2016 [41]	62 early-stage PD patients	Resting state	Functional connectivity	Motor deficit was associated with weaker coupling between anterior putamen and midbrain, cognitive impairment was associated with stronger coupling between the dorsal caudate and the rostral anterior cingulate cortex
Luo C et al., 2014 [42]	29 PD patients with depression, 30 PD patients without depression, 30 controls	Resting state	Functional connectivity	Reduced connectivity in the prefrontal-limbic network in the depression group

Table 1 Summary of the characteristics of the reviewed studies *(Continued)*

Hu X et al., 2015 [35, 43]	20 depressed PD patients, 40 non-depressed PD patients, 43 controls	Resting state	Functional connectivity	Stronger connectivity between the left median cingulate cortex and default mode network in the depressed PD
Sunwoo MK et al., 2015 [46]	110 PD patients subdivided into three groups based on olfactory performance	Resting state	Functional connectivity	Enhancement of striatocortical connectivity in the bilateral occipital areas and right frontal areas in patients with olfactory impairment
Baggio HC et al., 2015 [47]	62 PD patients, 31 controls	Resting state	Functional connectivity	Reduced connectivity in left-sided circuits, predominantly involving limbic, striatal and frontal territories in apathetic PD patients
Yao N et al., 2015 [48]	12 PD patients without hallucinations, 12 PD patients with visual hallucinations, 14 controls	Resting state	Functional connectivity	Increased occipital-corticostriatal connectivity in PD patients with visual hallucinations
Kwak Y et al., 2010 [50]	24 mild to moderate stage PD patients, 24 controls	Resting state	Functional connectivity	Increased cortico-striatal connectivity in PD patients
Agosta F et al., 2014 [51]	69 PD patients, 25 drug-naïve, 44 dopamine treated, 27 controls	Resting state	Functional connectivity	Decreased striato-thalamic connectivity, increased striato-temporal, and thalamo-cortical connections in dopaminergic treated PD
Bell PT et al., 2015 [52]	39 PD patients, controls	Resting state	Functional connectivity	Decoupling between the striatum and thalamic and sensorimotor networks in PD
Szewczyk-Krolikowski K et al., 2014 [53]	19 PD patients, 19 controls	Resting state	Functional connectivity	Reduced basal ganglia network connectivity in PD
Herz DM et al., 2015 [54]	26 PD patients	Visually cued movement	Effective connectivity Dynamic causal modelling (DCM)	Increase in the putamen and primary motor cortex connectivity after levodopa intake during movement suppression in patients who later developed levodopa-induced dyskinesias
Herz DM et al., 2016 [55]	12 PD patients with dyskinesias, 12 patients without dyskinesias	Resting state	Functional connectivity	Increased connectivity between the primary sensorimotor cortex and putamen after levodopa intake in patients with dyskinesias
Kahan J et al., 2014 [57]	12 PD patients	Resting state	Effective connectivity Dynamic causal modelling (DCM)	The strength of effective subthalamic nucleus afferents and efferents were reducedm cortico-striatal, thalamo-cortical and direct pathways were strengthened by DBS
Schweder PM et al., 2010 [58]	1 PD patient	Resting state	Functional connectivity	Normalization of pathological pedunculopontine nucleus (PPN) connectivity after PPN-DBS
Long D et al., 2012 [59]	19 early PD patients, 27 controls	Resting state	RFCS (regional functional connectivity strength)	The PD patients showed significant RFCS increases in the left parahippocampal gyrus, left angular gyrus and right middle temporal gyrus

other parkinsonian motor symptoms. For example, Tessitore and colleagues reported that PD patients with FoG had impaired functional connectivity within the frontoparietal networks sub-serving attentional functions [32]. Functional neuroimaging studies suggest that the disturbances in frontal cortical regions, the basal ganglia, and the midbrain locomotor region are possibly the origins of FoG [33]. Network connectivity also can be used to identify the neural characters in different subtypes of PD [2, 34, 35].

Non-motor symptoms

In addition to symptoms related to motor function, most PD patients present with some non-motor symptoms such as cognitive, emotional, or olfactory impairments. In recent years, more focus has been applied to characterizing the neural network of these non-motor symptoms. Cognitive deficits are common in PD patients. PD with dementia is associated with selective disruption of corticostriatal connectivity [36]. Moreover, it has been shown that the connectivity of the so called "default mode network" (DMN) is disrupted in PD patients with cognitive deficits [37, 38]. The DMN is a network showing consistent task-related deactivations, and includes the medial prefrontal cortex, anterior cingulate cortex, posterior cingulate cortex, precuneus, and inferior parietal lobe [39, 40]. The DMN is thought to facilitate cognitive performance by allocating neural resources to critical brain regions. The disruption of the DMN was associated with the progress of cognitive decline [37], while the decline in cognitive function, particularly in the memory and visuospatial domains, was associated with stronger coupling between the dorsal caudate and the rostral anterior cingulate cortex [41]. These findings suggest that malfunctioning of the DMN may contribute to the executive function deficits in PD.

Depression is the most frequent psychiatric disorder reported in patients with PD. Abnormal prefrontal-limbic network connectivity has been demonstrated in depressed PD patients [31, 42]. PD patients with depression are associated with disrupted functional connectivity between the median cingulate cortex and precuneus, prefrontal cortex, and cerebellum [43]. The cingulate cortex plays key roles in integrating multimodal information that is important for emotional, sensorimotor, and cognitive functions [44]. The median cingulate cortex also appears to be involved in many emotion-related cognitive processes such as meditation, self-related rumination, aversive conditioning, and the anticipation and perception of pain [45]. The impaired median cingulate cortex-related networks may play a role in depression experienced by patients with PD.

Network connectivity in some other non-motor symptoms, such as olfactory impairment, apathy, and hallucination has also been investigated. PD patients with olfactory impairment had decreased connectivity between the posterior cingulate cortex and bilateral primary sensory areas, right frontal areas, and right parietal areas, and had an enhancement of striatocortical connectivity compared to PD patients with normal olfaction [46]. Apathetic PD patients showed reduced functional connectivity mainly involving limbic striatal and frontal territories. In addition, the limbic division of the left striatum showed reduced connectivity with the ipsilateral frontal cortex and with the rest of the left striatum [47]. In PD patients with visual hallucinations, occipital-cortico-striatal connectivity was significantly higher than in patients without hallucinations [48]. Hallucinations have been associated with functional abnormalities in primary visual cortex and visual associative cortices [49].

Intervention-related network changes

Functional connectivity can be also used to investigate neural mechanisms underlying anti-parkinsonian interventions. Levodopa treatment has been reported to normalize the function of the basal ganglia motor pathways (e.g., by enhancing neural activity in the SMA and striatum) and restore striato-cortical motor pathway connectivity [4, 50–53] in a manner associated with improvements in motor function.

Although levodopa remains the most effective medication for the management of PD symptoms, many PD patients develop daily fluctuations in mobility and involuntary movements known as levodopa-induced dyskinesias (LID). The neural correlates in the genesis of LID remain poorly understood. A recent study found an increase in connectivity between the putamen and M1 after levodopa intake in patients developed LID [54]. This excessive striato-cortical connectivity in response to levodopa may play a role in the pathophysiology of LID [54, 55]. Another study showed that the connectivity of inferior frontal cortex was decreased with M1 and increased with the putamen in patients with LID [56]. This finding suggests that the neural network centered on the inferior frontal cortex may also involve in the pathophysiological mechanisms underlying LID.

Deep brain stimulation (DBS) is another effective therapy for PD, but the neural mechanism underlying therapeutic effects of DBS remain unclear. It has been shown that DBS on the subthalamic nucleus (STN) can modulate the connectivity of striato-thalamo-cortical and STN-cortical pathways in association with symptom improvements [57]. The pedunculopontine nucleus (PPN) is a target in treating primarily gait and posture symptoms. PPN-DBS has been reported to normalize pathological PPN connectivity [58].

Diagnosis

The diagnosis of PD is based mainly on clinical assessments. Some studies have combined fMRI and various pattern analysis methods to try to establish an imaging methodology for PD diagnosis [53, 59–61]. In a recent study, the authors of this review have identified a PD-related spatial covariance pattern that was characterized by decreased activity in the striatum, supplementary motor area, middle frontal gyrus, and occipital cortex, and also by increased activity in the thalamus, cerebellum, precuneus, superior parietal lobule, and temporal cortex. This pattern had a high accuracy (90 %) to discriminate PD patients from healthy controls [59]. These studies have proven that network connectivity approach can identify characteristic PD-specific neural changes, and has the potential of network pattern as a biomarker for PD diagnosis. However, functional connectivity cannot directly reveal pathological changes in PD, therefore, whether this method can be applied in clinical practice needs further investigation.

Conclusions

Future directions

Studies on functional connectivity have provided important information on PD-related functional and pathophysiological changes. At present, functional connectivity is primarily used to further understand how pathological changes lead to parkinsonian symptoms, and is far from being a method in routine clinical investigations. As shown in the Table 1, the analytic methods of "functional connectivity" studies vary a lot from study to study. Few studies have used the same "functional connectivity" procedure. Therefore, it is hard to perform meta-analysis on these studies. In contrast, voxel-level analysis, like most PET studies and some resting-state fMRI studies focusing the local activity support coordinate-based meta-analysis and, hence, are more helpful to clinical studies. Additional research should focus on increased efforts to develop neural network pattern as a neuroimaging biomarker for early diagnosis of PD; this might well require further technical and methodological improvements. These developments will improve early diagnosis, better evaluate disease progression, differentiate PD from other parkinsonisms on an individual basis, and may guide novel targets for future therapies.

Acknowledgements
Not applicable.

Funding
This research did not receive any specific grant from funding agencies in the public, commercial, or not-for-profit sectors.

Authors' contributions
L-lG: execution of the research, analysis of the data, writing of the manuscript; TW: conception, organization of the research, and critique of the manuscript. Both authors read and approved the final manuscript.

Competing interests
Not applicable.

References

1. Jankovic J. Parkinson's disease: clinical features and diagnosis. J Neurol Neurosurg Psychiatry. 2008;79:368–76.
2. DeLong MR, Wichmann T. Circuits and circuit disorders of the basal ganglia. Arch Neurol. 2007;64:20–4.
3. Fox MD, Raichle ME. Spontaneous fluctuations in brain activity observed with functional magnetic resonance imaging. Nat Rev Neurosci. 2007;8:700–11.
4. Wu T, Long X, Zang Y, Wang L, Hallett M, Li K, Chan P. Regional homogeneity changes in patients with Parkinson's disease. Hum Brain Mapp. 2009;30:1502–10.
5. Ogawa S, Lee TM, Kay AR, Tank DW. Brain magnetic resonance imaging with contrast dependent on blood oxygenation. Proc Natl Acad Sci U S A. 1990;87:9868–72.
6. Sporns O, Chialvo DR, Kaiser M, Hilgetag CC. Organization, development and function of complex brain networks. Trends Cogn Sci. 2004;8:418–25.
7. Horwitz B. The elusive concept of brain connectivity. Neuroimage. 2003;19: 466–70.
8. Stam CJ. Characterization of anatomical and functional connectivity in the brain: a complex networks perspective. Int J Psychophysiol. 2010;77:186–94.
9. Bullmore E, Sporns O. Complex brain networks: graph theoretical analysis of structural and functional systems. Nat Rev Neurosci. 2009;10:186–98.
10. Stam CJ, Reijneveld JC. Graph theoretical analysis of complex networks in the brain. Nonlinear Biomed Phys. 2007;1:3.
11. Friston K. Functional and effective connectivity in neuroimaging: A synthesis [J]. Hum Brain Mapp. 1994;2:56–78.
12. Wu T, Wang L, Hallett M, Chen Y, Li K, Chan P. Effective connectivity of brain networks during self-initiated movement in Parkinson's disease. Neuroimage. 2011;55:204–15.
13. Rowe J, Stephan KE, Friston K, Frackowiak R, Lees A, Passingham R. Attention to action in Parkinson's disease: impaired effective connectivity among frontal cortical regions. Brain. 2002;125:276–89.
14. Wu T, Chan P, Hallett M. Effective connectivity of neural networks in automatic movements in Parkinson's disease. Neuroimage. 2010;49: 2581–7.
15. Rowe JB, Hughes LE, Barker RA, Owen AM. Dynamic causal modelling of effective connectivity from fMRI: are results reproducible and sensitive to Parkinson's disease and its treatment? Neuroimage. 2010;52:1015–26.
16. Deiber MP, Passingham RE, Colebatch JG, Friston KJ, Nixon PD, Frackowiak RS. Cortical areas and the selection of movement: a study with positron emission tomography. Exp Brain Res. 1991;84:393–402.
17. Cunnington R, Windischberger C, Deecke L, Moser E. The preparation and execution of self-initiated and externally-triggered movement: a study of event-related fMRI. Neuroimage. 2002;15:373–85.
18. Jenkins IH, Jahanshahi M, Jueptner M, Passingham RE, Brooks DJ. Self-initiated versus externally triggered movements. II. The effect of movement predictability on regional cerebral blood flow. Brain. 2000;123(Pt 6):1216–28.
19. Schell GR, Strick PL. The origin of thalamic inputs to the arcuate premotor and supplementary motor areas. J Neurosci. 1984;4:539–60.
20. Haslinger B, Erhard P, Kampfe N, Boecker H, Rummeny E, Schwaiger M, Conrad B, Ceballos-Baumann AO. Event-related functional magnetic resonance imaging in Parkinson's disease before and after levodopa. Brain. 2001;124:558–70.
21. Buhmann C, Glauche V, Sturenburg HJ, Oechsner M, Weiller C, Buchel C. Pharmacologically modulated fMRI–cortical responsiveness to levodopa in drug-naive hemiparkinsonian patients. Brain. 2003;126:451–61.
22. Wu T, Hallett M, Chan P. Motor automaticity in Parkinson's disease. Neurobiol Dis. 2015;82:226–34.
23. Bernstein ME, Hughes FW, Forney RB. The influence of a new chlordiazepoxide analogue on human mental and motor performance. J Clin Pharmacol J New Drugs. 1967;7:330–5.
24. Redgrave P, Rodriguez M, Smith Y, Rodriguez-Oroz MC, Lehericy S, Bergman H, Agid Y, DeLong MR, Obeso JA. Goal-directed and habitual control in the basal ganglia: implications for Parkinson's disease. Nat Rev Neurosci. 2010;11:760–72.
25. Wu T, Kansaku K, Hallett M. How self-initiated memorized movements become automatic: a functional MRI study. J Neurophysiol. 2004;91:1690–8.
26. Wu T, Hallett M. Neural correlates of dual task performance in patients with Parkinson's disease. J Neurol Neurosurg Psychiatry. 2008;79:760–6.
27. Wu T, Zhang J, Hallett M, Feng T, Hou Y, Chan P. Neural correlates underlying micrographia in Parkinson's disease. Brain. 2016;139:144–60.
28. Wu T, Hallett M. A functional MRI study of automatic movements in patients with Parkinson's disease. Brain. 2005;128:2250–9.
29. Wu T, Liu J, Zhang H, Hallett M, Zheng Z, Chan P. Attention to Automatic Movements in Parkinson's Disease: Modified Automatic Mode in the Striatum. Cereb Cortex. 2015;25:3330–42.
30. Ma H, Chen H, Fang J, Gao L, Ma L, Wu T, Hou Y, Zhang J, Feng T. Resting-state functional connectivity of dentate nucleus is associated with tremor in Parkinson's disease. J Neurol. 2015;262:2247–56.
31. Surdhar I, Gee M, Bouchard T, Coupland N, Malykhin N, Camicioli R. Intact limbic-prefrontal connections and reduced amygdala volumes in Parkinson's disease with mild depressive symptoms. Parkinsonism Relat Disord. 2012;18:809–13.

32. Tessitore A, Amboni M, Esposito F, Russo A, Picillo M, Marcuccio L, Pellecchia MT, Vitale C, Cirillo M, Tedeschi G, Barone P. Resting-state brain connectivity in patients with Parkinson's disease and freezing of gait. Parkinsonism Relat Disord. 2012;18:781–7.
33. Nutt JG, Bloem BR, Giladi N, Hallett M, Horak FB, Nieuwboer A. Freezing of gait: moving forward on a mysterious clinical phenomenon. Lancet Neurol. 2011;10:734–44.
34. Liu H, Edmiston EK, Fan G, Xu K, Zhao B, Shang X, Wang F. Altered resting-state functional connectivity of the dentate nucleus in Parkinson's disease. Psychiatry Res. 2013;211:64–71.
35. Hu X, Zhang J, Jiang X, Zhou C, Wei L, Yin X, Wu Y, Li J, Zhang Y, Wang J. Decreased interhemispheric functional connectivity in subtypes of Parkinson's disease. J Neurol. 2015;262:760–7.
36. Seibert TM, Murphy EA, Kaestner EJ, Brewer JB. Interregional correlations in Parkinson disease and Parkinson-related dementia with resting functional MR imaging. Radiology. 2012;263:226–34.
37. Gorges M, Muller HP, Lule D, Pinkhardt EH, Ludolph AC, Kassubek J. To rise and to fall: functional connectivity in cognitively normal and cognitively impaired patients with Parkinson's disease. Neurobiol Aging. 2015;36:1727–35.
38. Disbrow EA, Carmichael O, He J, Lanni KE, Dressler EM, Zhang L, Malhado-Chang N, Sigvardt KA. Resting state functional connectivity is associated with cognitive dysfunction in non-demented people with Parkinson's disease. J Parkinsons Dis. 2014;4:453–65.
39. Salvador R, Suckling J, Coleman MR, Pickard JD, Menon D, Bullmore E. Neurophysiological architecture of functional magnetic resonance images of human brain. Cereb Cortex. 2005;15:1332–42.
40. Greicius MD, Krasnow B, Reiss AL, Menon V. Functional connectivity in the resting brain: a network analysis of the default mode hypothesis. Proc Natl Acad Sci U S A. 2003;100:253–8.
41. Manza P, Zhang S, Li CS, Leung HC. Resting-state functional connectivity of the striatum in early-stage Parkinson's disease: Cognitive decline and motor symptomatology. Hum Brain Mapp. 2016;37:648–62.
42. Luo C, Chen Q, Song W, Chen K, Guo X, Yang J, Huang X, Gong Q, Shang HF. Resting-state fMRI study on drug-naive patients with Parkinson's disease and with depression. J Neurol Neurosurg Psychiatry. 2014;85:675–83.
43. Hu X, Song X, Li E, Liu J, Yuan Y, Liu W, Liu Y. Altered Resting-State Brain Activity and Connectivity in Depressed Parkinson's Disease. PLoS One. 2015; 10:e131133.
44. Taylor KS, Seminowicz DA, Davis KD. Two systems of resting state connectivity between the insula and cingulate cortex. Hum Brain Mapp. 2009;30:2731–45.
45. Vogt BA, Berger GR, Derbyshire SW. Structural and functional dichotomy of human midcingulate cortex. Eur J Neurosci. 2003;18:3134–44.
46. Sunwoo MK, Cha J, Ham JH, Song SK, Hong JY, Lee JM, Sohn YH, Lee PH. Olfactory performance and resting state functional connectivity in non-demented drug naive patients with Parkinson's disease. Hum Brain Mapp. 2015;36:1716–27.
47. Baggio HC, Segura B, Garrido-Millan JL, Marti MJ, Compta Y, Valldeoriola F, Tolosa E, Junque C. Resting-state frontostriatal functional connectivity in Parkinson's disease-related apathy. Mov Disord. 2015;30:671–9.
48. Yao N, Pang S, Cheung C, Chang RS, Lau KK, Suckling J, Yu K, Mak HK, McAlonan G, Ho SL, Chua SE. Resting activity in visual and corticostriatal pathways in Parkinson's disease with hallucinations. Parkinsonism Relat Disord. 2015;21:131–7.
49. Meppelink AM, de Jong BM, Renken R, Leenders KL, Cornelissen FW, van Laar T. Impaired visual processing preceding image recognition in Parkinson's disease patients with visual hallucinations. Brain. 2009;132:2980–93.
50. Kwak Y, Peltier S, Bohnen NI, Muller ML, Dayalu P, Seidler RD. Altered resting state cortico-striatal connectivity in mild to moderate stage Parkinson's disease. Front Syst Neurosci. 2010;4:143.
51. Agosta F, Caso F, Stankovic I, Inuggi A, Petrovic I, Svetel M, Kostic VS, Filippi M. Cortico-striatal-thalamic network functional connectivity in hemiparkinsonism. Neurobiol Aging. 2014;35:2592–602.
52. Bell PT, Gilat M, O'Callaghan C, Copland DA, Frank MJ, Lewis SJ, Shine JM. Dopaminergic basis for impairments in functional connectivity across subdivisions of the striatum in Parkinson's disease. Hum Brain Mapp. 2015; 36:1278–91.
53. Szewczyk-Krolikowski K, Menke RA, Rolinski M, Duff E, Salimi-Khorshidi G, Filippini N, Zamboni G, Hu MT, Mackay CE. Functional connectivity in the basal ganglia network differentiates PD patients from controls. Neurology. 2014;83:208–14.
54. Herz DM, Haagensen BN, Christensen MS, Madsen KH, Rowe JB, Lokkegaard A, Siebner HR. Abnormal dopaminergic modulation of striato-cortical networks underlies levodopa-induced dyskinesias in humans. Brain. 2015; 138:1658–66.
55. Herz DM, Haagensen BN, Nielsen SH, Madsen KH, Lokkegaard A, Siebner HR. Resting-state connectivity predicts levodopa-induced dyskinesias in Parkinson's disease. Mov Disord. 2016;31:521–9.
56. Cerasa A, Donzuso G, Morelli M, Mangone G, Salsone M, Passamonti L, Augimeri A, Arabia G, Quattrone A. The motor inhibition system in Parkinson's disease with levodopa-induced dyskinesias. Mov Disord. 2015;30: 1912–20.
57. Kahan J, Urner M, Moran R, Flandin G, Marreiros A, Mancini L, White M, Thornton J, Yousry T, Zrinzo L, et al. Resting state functional MRI in Parkinson's disease: the impact of deep brain stimulation on 'effective' connectivity. Brain. 2014;137:1130–44.
58. Schweder PM, Joint C, Hansen PC, Green AL, Quaghebeur G, Aziz TZ. Chronic pedunculopontine nucleus stimulation restores functional connectivity. Neuroreport. 2010;21:1065–8.
59. Long D, Wang J, Xuan M, Gu Q, Xu X, Kong D, Zhang M. Automatic classification of early Parkinson's disease with multi-modal MR imaging. PLoS One. 2012;7:e47714.
60. Skidmore FM, Yang M, Baxter L, von Deneen KM, Collingwood J, He G, White K, Korenkevych D, Savenkov A, Heilman KM, et al. Reliability analysis of the resting state can sensitively and specifically identify the presence of Parkinson disease. Neuroimage. 2013;75:249–61.
61. Wu T, Ma Y, Zheng Z, Peng S, Wu X, Eidelberg D, Chan P. Parkinson's disease-related spatial covariance pattern identified with resting-state functional MRI. J Cereb Blood Flow Metab. 2015;35:1764–70.

14

A survey of impulse control disorders in Parkinson's disease patients in Shanghai area

Xue-Ping Wang, Ming Wei and Qin Xiao*

Abstract

Background: Levodopa and dopamine agonists are the main treatments for Parkinson's disease (PD) in recent years. Increased drug dosages are linked to some severe side effects, one of which is impulse control disorders (ICD). Many studies have reported the related risk factors of ICDs, such as dopamine agonist, male sex, younger age, earlier age of onset and so on. This study aims to investigate the incidence of ICD in Chinese PD patients from Shanghai area, explore the association of ICD with dopamine replacement therapy (DRT).

Methods: Two hundred seventeen PD patients were consecutively recruited from the Movement Disorder Clinic of Ruijin Hospital from March to October 2013. Minnesota Impulsive Disorders Interview was used to assess the PD patients. PD patients with possible ICD would undergo a further interview by a movement disorder specialist to confirm the diagnosis. Clinical information was also collected.

Results: Nine PD patients (4.15 %) showed ICD behaviors as follows: hypersexuality (4, 1.84 %), pathological gambling (3, 1.38 %), binge eating (1, 0.46 %), compulsive shopping (1, 0.46 %). Compared with the non-ICD PD group, ICD PD group took more dopamine agonists (LED 119.4 ± 86.4 mg/d vs 60.5 ± 80.5 mg/d, $P = 0.019$), had higher total levodopa equivalent dosage (TLED 912.81 ± 878.73 mg/d vs 503.78 ± 359.14 mg/d, $P = 0.031$), and had higher H&Y stage (2.33 ± 0.87 vs 1.41 ± 0.52, $p = 0.013$). However, logistic regression analysis didn't reveal the above factors as independent risk factors of ICD behaviors in our study.

Conclusion: The incidence of ICDs behaviors in PD patients in our study is much lower than in western countries. ICD-PD group took higher dopamine agonists and higher total levodopa equivalent dosage, even though logistic regression analysis didn't reveal them as independent risk factors.

Keyword: Parkinson's disease, ICD, Dopamine replacement therapy

Background

Parkinson's disease is associated with progressive degeneration of the nigrostriatal pathway that often impairs motor skills (resting tremor, rigidity, bradykinesia and postural instability). Dopaminergic replacement therapy (DRT), including levodopa and dopamine agonists (DA agonists), relieves the motor symptoms and improves quality of life. However, a series of motor complications, such as dyskinesia and wearing off, appear with the increased dosage of levodopa and DA agonists [1, 2]. In recent years, PD patients have been evidenced having increased risk of developing impulse control disorders (ICDs) mainly because of DRT medication. ICDs have four major symptoms, pathological gambling (PG), hypersexuality (HS), compulsive shopping (CS) and binge-eating (BE) disorder. Excessive dopaminergic medication usage, punding and aimless walkabout are also considered as impusive/compulsive behaviors (ICB) [3, 4].

Lots of studies were conducted to explore the prevalence and associated risk factors of ICDs. The most well-known was DOMINION cross-sectional study ($N = 3090$ patients) conducted by multi-centers in North America. In this study, ICD prevalence was 13.6 % (PG 5.0 %, HS 3.5 %, CS 5.7 %, and BE 4.3 %). A wide spectrum of prevalence, ranging from 3.53 % to 34.8 %, has been reported from different studies [4–12], with higher prevalence in Western

* Correspondence: xiaoqin67@medmail.com.cn
Department of Neurology and Institute of Neurology, Ruijin Hospital affiliated to Shanghai Jiao Tong University School of Medicine, Shanghai, China

populations than in Asian generally. Different variables associated with ICDs have been revealed, including DA agonist [4–6, 8, 10, 11], male sex (mainly in HS and PG) [4, 6–8, 12], younger age [6–9], earlier age of onset [9], prior personal or family history of alcohol addiction or gambling problems etc. [6, 10, 13]. But, DA agonist was the most consistent risk factor in those studies. In DOMINION study, DA agonist treatment increased about 2- to 3.5-fold odds of having an ICD, suggesting that there existed a close relationship between DA agonists and ICDs [6]. Therefore we tried to investigate the prevalence of ICDs among Chinese PD patients from Shanghai area and explore the associated risk factors, especially DA agonist medication. The underlying reasons for different prevalence between Western population and Asians were also discussed by reviewing literature.

Methods

Two hundred seventeen idiopathic PD patients, based on UK Brain Bank clinical diagnostic criteria [14], were recruited from the Movement Disorder Clinic at the Department of Neurology of Ruijin Hospital from March to October in 2013. Exclusion criteria included atypical parkinsonism, secondary parkinsonism, and cognitive abnormality that might have problem in understanding and giving feedback of questionnaire. The study was approved by ethics committee of Ruijin Hospital.

The modified version of Minnesota Impulsive Disorders Interview (Chinese version) was used to assess gambling, compulsive shopping, hypersexuality, binge eating, and punding. The questionnaire was performed by two graduates who had been well trained and the screened positive patients were interviewed by a movement disorder specialist, and a final diagnosis was made according to the diagnostic criteria listed in Voon et al's paper [13].

Statistics

Statistical analysis was performed using SPSS 18.0, and $P < 0.05$ was considered to be significant. Independent-sample t-tests, non-parametric test and Fisher's exact test were used to compare age, disease duration, Hohn-Yahr stage, gender, and dosage of anti-parkinsonian drugs between PD patients with and without ICD behaviors. Logistic regression was used to investigate the correlation among the potential risk factors for ICD behaviors.

Results

Demographic characteristics

The clinical characteristics are listed in Table 1. There were 120 male (55.3 %), and 97 female (44.7 %). The mean age was 67.15 ± 0.61 years old (range: 40–85) and mean disease duration was 5.78 ± 4.32 years (range:1–23). All PD patients were taking anti-parkinsonian drugs. Totally, 193(88.9 %) patients were taking levodopa with an average daily dose 494.94 ± 348.03 mg/d (100-2825 mg/d), 101(46.5 %) patients were taking DA agonists, with a dopamine agonists levodopa equivalent dosage (DA-LED) 135.15 ± 66.8 mg in average per day (ranging from 50 to 300 mg) and total levodopa equivalent dosage (TLED) 548.53 ± 382.12 mg/d (ranging from 50 to 3000 mg) (Table 1).

Table 1 The demographic and clinical characteristics of PD patients

Item	mean ± SD	Range
Number of cases	217	
Male, n(%)	120 (55.3 %)	
Age, year	67.15 ± 0.61	40-85
Disease duration, year	5.78 ± 4.32	1-23
H&Y stage	1.43 ± 0.55	1-4
Use of levodopa, n(%)	193 (88.9 %)	
Use of DA agonists, n(%)	101 (46.5 %)	
Levodopa, (mg/d)	494.94 ± 348.03	100-2825
DA agonist LED, (mg/d)	135.15 ± 66.8	50-300
TLED, (mg/d)	548.53 ± 382.12	50-3000

Note:DA agonist-LED (DA-LED, mg/d) = piribedil (mg/d) × 1 + pramipexole (mg/d) × 100. Total LED (TLED, mg/d) = regular levodopa dose (mg/d) × 1 + levodopa CR dose (mg/d) × 0.75 + DA-LED, and plus [regular levodopa dose (mg/d) + CR levodopa dose(mg/d) × 0.75] × 0.33 if taking COMT-I [24]

Point prevalence and clinical features of ICD

Among 217 PD patients interviewed, 9 (4.15 %) patients fulfilled criteria for ICDs and their behaviors and medications were listed in Table 2. Seven patients among ICD group took both DA agonists and levodopa, two patients took levodopa only. Overall, there was 1(0.46 %) patient had CS, 1(0.46 %) patient had BE, 3(1.38 %) patients had PG, 4(1.84 %) PD patients were diagnosed with HS. All those patients showed ICD symptoms after DRT therapy.

Clinical characteristics of PD with ICD group and non-ICD PD group were listed in Table 3. There was no significant difference of age, gender, and disease duration between these two groups. But, for H-Y stage, ICD-PD group had more severe disease condition than non-ICD PD group (2.33 ± 0.87 vs1.41 ± 0.52, $p = 0.013$). In ICD group, 7 (77.8 %) out of 9 patients took DA agonists, the DA-LED was 119.4 ± 86.4 mg/d, 94 (45.2 %) of non-ICD patients took DA agonists (DA-LED 60.5 ± 80.5 mg/d). The dosage of DA agonists in ICD group was much higher than non-ICD patients ($P = 0.019$). Patients in ICD group also took more levodopa (791.67 ± 802.73 mg/d) than those in non-ICD group (425.0 ± 327.26 mg/d), although this difference didn't reach the significant level ($P = 0.066$). TLED was also calculated, ICD group took 912.81 ± 878.73 mg/d TLED, which was much higher than that of non-ICD group (503.78 ± 359.13 mg/d) ($P = 0.031$). Variables entered into the multiple logistic regression

Table 2 ICD behaviors in patients with Parkinson's disease

case	gender	age	PD duration	H&Y stage	concurrent medication	DA-LED	TLED	ICD behaviors
1	M	75	6	3	L-DA+ pra	200	1100	PG
2	M	67	4	2	L-DA	0	300	PG
3	M	69	3	2	L-DA+ pra	150	450	HS
4	F	62	5	1	L-DA+ pra	150	825	CS
5	M	49	8	3	L-DA+ pra	225	3000	HS
6	M	50	5	3	L-DA+ pra	200	500	HS
7	F	73	10	3	L-DA	0	600	BE
8	F	51	4	2	L-DA + pir	100	300	PG
9	M	68	10	3	L-DA + pir + ent	50	1014.25	HS

Note: *pra* = pramipexole; *pir* = piribedil; *ent* = entacapone
PG = pathological gambling; *HS* = hypersexuality; *CS* = compulsive buying; *BE* = binge-eating disorder

analysis were: gender, age, disease duration, use of agonists, dosage of levodopa, DA-LED, TLED and H-Y stage. Our results didn't reveal any independent risk factors for ICD behaviors (data was not shown).

Comparison with Previous studies

A wide range of ICDs prevalence and variable risk factors of ICDs from different studies have been reported (Table 4). Generally, prevalence of ICDs in Asian countries (3.53 %-5.9 %) [4, 10, 11] was lower than Western countries (8.1 %-34.8 %) [5–8], except studies from Japan with 12.9 % of ICD [9] and Malaysia with 15.4 % of screen positive ICD [12]. Lower DA agonist medication, ethnic differences, social factors, and culture differences have been considered as potential factors influencing different prevalence [4, 10, 11]. But we found that screening instruments might be another influencing factor. As listed in Table 4, a variety of screen questionaires, such as Questionnaire for Impulsive Compulsive Disorders in Parkinson's Disease (QUIP), Minnesota Impulsive Disorders Interview (MIDI) and a list of screen/diagnostic tests for PG, HS and CS, were used in these studies. Studies using QUIP as screen instrument reported high rate of screen positive ICD patients, 28 % in Japan [9], 15.4 % in Malaysia [12], 34.8 % in Finland [7] and 18.4 % in Brazil [5]. In this Japan study, the actual prevalence of ICDs assessed by various diagnostic criteria for each ICD turned out to be 12.9 %. Thus, QUIP might be an optimal instrument for screening ICDs because of its high sensitivity, but further diagnostic criteria is needed for confirmative diagnosis.

Table 3 Comparison between patients with and without ICD behaviors (mean ± SD, n, %, p)

	Non-ICD	ICD	*P* value
Number of case	208	9	
Age, year	67.25 ± 8.82	63.67 ± 10.55	0. 469
Male, n(%)	114 (54.8 %)	6 (66.7 %)	0.521
Disease duration, year	5.76 ± 4.38	6.44 ± 3.17	0.33
Dose of levodopa, (mg/d)	425.0 ± 327.26	791.67 ± 802.73	0.066
DA - LED, (mg/d)	60.5 ± 80.5	119.4 ± 86.4	0.019*
TLED, (mg/d)	503.78 ± 359.13	912.81 ± 878.73	0.031*
H&Y stage	1.41 ± 0.52	2.33 ± 0.87	0.013*
Use of agonists, n(%)	94(45.2 %)	7 (77.8 %)	0.055

*$p < 0.05$ ICD vs Non-ICD group

Discussion

Previous reports estimated the frequency of ICDs in PD patients ranged from 3.53 % to 34.8 % [4–12]. Two reports from Xuanwu Hospital Beijing China and ChangGung Memorial Hospital Taiwan reported the rates of ICDs in PD patients are 3.53 % and 4.48 % respectively [4, 10]. ICD frequency in our study was estimated at 4.15 %. These studies carried out among Chinese PD patients got similar results.

By comparison with Western countries reports, results from Asian studies showed a relatively low incidence of ICD except studies from Japan with 12.9 % of ICD [9] and Malaysia with 15.4 % of ICD [12]. Point prevalence of ICDs from China, Taiwan, South Korea and present study showed a range from 3.53 % to 5.9 % [4, 10, 11], while data from North America, Brazil, Italy, Finland showed higher prevalence 8.1 % ~ 34.8 % [5–8]. Note that studies from Malaysia, Brazil and Finland reported high frequency of ICDs only by QUIP screen without further confirmative diagnosis. Besides that, a variety of reasons have been considered for different prevalence. Lower dosage of DA agonists because of medication practice, cost burden, limited availability and health insurance [10] has been suggested as a potential factor affecting different prevalence. Other factors, such as ethnic differences, social factors, study design, culture difference, were also considered [4–12]. Genetic factors

Table 4 Comparison between previous studies and present study

Study population	Sample Size	Screen instruments	Frequency of compulsive behaviors	Risk factors	Dosage of drugs(ICD vs non ICD mg/d, mean)	Reference
Taiwan	268	DSM-IV-TR criteria forPG and BE,McElroy's criteria for CSVoon's criteria (2006) for HS	ICD 4.48 % PG 1.49 %, HS 2.99 % CS 0 %, BE 0.37 %	Dopamine agonistTLEDMale gender	TLED (ICD group): 741.94 DA-LED (ICD group): 105	4
Brazil	152	QUIP	QUIP results:ICD 18.4 % PG 1.3 %, HS 11.8 % CS 10.5 %, BE 7.9 %	SmokingUse of pramipexole	TLED: 732.8 vs 644.4Pramipexole: 2.9 vs 0.85(equivalent to 290 vs 85)	5
North America	3090	Massachusetts Gambling ScreenMIDIDSM-IV-TR	ICD 13.6 % PG 5 %, HS 3.5 % CS 5.7 %, BE 4.3 %	DAcombination of DA & Levodopayounger age, male sexcurrent smokingbeing unmarriedliving in the United Statesfamily history of gambling	DA-LED: 200 ~ 450 vs 150 ~ 400(listed as interquartile in patients taking DA)Levodopa: 621 vs 461 (in patients taking levodopa only)	6
Finland	575	SOGSQUIP	QUIP results:ICD 34.8 % PG 8.8 %, HS 22.8 % CS 10.1 %, BE 11.8 %	Depression, Male sexYounger ageAge of disease onsetCurrent alcohol use	NA	7
Italy	805	QUIP for screenOther criteria for confirmation	ICD 8.1 % PG 3.2 %, HS 3.0 % CS 1.0 %, BE 2.4 %	dopamine agonistMale sex, levodopayounger age, Amantadine	NA	8
Japan	118	QUIP for screenOther criteria for confirmation	QUIP results vs Actual prevalenceICD 28 % vs 12.9 % PG 14 % vs 6.5 % HS 14 % vs 3.2 % CS 10.8 % vs 3.2 % BE 10.8 % vs 3.2 %	younger agelonger disease durationTLEDD, LevodopaEarlier age of onset	ICB vs non-ICBLevodopa: 676 vs 520DA-LED: 139 vs 71.6	9
China	312	SOGS, DSM-IVLejoyeux's Compulsive Shopping questionnaire;specially designed hypersexuality questionnaire;	ICD 3.53 % PG 0.32 %, HS 1.92 % CS 0.32 %, BE 0.32 %	Dopamine agonistAlcohol use	Levodopa: 345.5 vs 357.01DA-LED: 142.37 vs 35.45	10
South Korea	1167	MIDI	ICD 5.9 % PG 1.3 %, HS 2.8 % CS 2.5 %, BE 3.4 %	Dopamine agonistLevodopa	Levodopa: 656 vs 544DA-LED: 145 vs 99	11
Malaysian	200	QUIP	QUIP results based on patient reportICD 15.4 % PG 2.6 %, HS 8.2 % CS 3.6 %, BE 8.7 %	Male genderLonger PD duration	PD patients:TLED: 527.7DA-LED: 73.7	12
Present study	217	MIDIVoon's criteria (2007) for each ICD	ICD 4.15 % PG 1.38 %, HS 1.84 % CS 0.46 %, BE 0.46 %	None	Levodopa: 791.67 vs 425.0DA-LED: 119.4 vs 60.5	–

SOGS: modified South Oaks Gambling Screen. *QUIP*: Questionnaire for Impulsive Compulsive Disorders in Parkinson's Disease
MIDI: Minnesota Impulsive Disorders Interview. *ICB*: impulsive compulsive behavior
DA-LED: Dopamine agonist levodopa equivalent dosage. *TLED*: Total levodopa equivalent dosage

have also been revealed. Polymorphism of dopamine receptor D3 and D2, serotonin 2A receptor gene (HTR2A) have been linked with ICDs [15–17].

However, here we want to emphasize screen instruments as a potential reason for different prevalence. Study from Japan reported 28 % ICDs by QUIP screen and 12.9 % actual prevalence by other diagnostic criteria [9], indicating QUIP is a screening test with high sensitivity but relatively low specificity. QUIP is a comprehensive screening test and can evaluate a wide range of impulsive compulsive behaviors [18]. In our study, we used MIDI for screen test. MIDI and QUIP are different in design. MIDI has 5 modules with 1 module for each ICD. Each module has one Yes/No question for preliminary screen, and the Yes/No answer largely depends on the patients or informants' rough judgement. In QUIP test with session 1 as an example, for each ICD there are 5 specific questions from different perspectives collecting patients' feelings and experiences, and patients or informants can make a fine judgement based on those 5 questions. Thus, MIDI is a quick and convenient battery for clinical work, while QUIP is more comprehensive and sensitive for both research and clinical work. But, to get a final diagnosis, other diagnostic criteria were needed. In our study, diagnostic criteria listed by Voon et.al [13] were adopted.

With regard to potential risk factors for ICDs identified in previous analyses, such as younger age, male sex, earlier age of disease onset, were not revealed as independent risk factors for development of ICDs in our study. Many researchers have confirmed that DA agonist was a main risk factor for ICDs [4–6, 8–11, 19]. However, logistic regression analysis didn't reveal it as an independent risk factor for ICD in our study. Failing to identify DA agonist as a risk factor might due to several reasons. First, the main reason might be lower average daily dosage of DA agonists (ICD vs non-ICD: 119.4 ± 86.4 vs 60.5 ± 80.5 mg/d) taken by our patients compared with other studies listed in Table 4. Study from Malaysia didn't find correlation between DA agonist and ICD either. There were less than 50 % PD patients taking DA agonist and the average daily dosage of DA agonist was 73.7 ± 84.3 mg in that study [12]. Therefore, high dosage of DA agonist places patients in a higher risk condition. Lower dosage might cover the potential relationship between drugs and development of ICD in this study. Second, it might be due to sample and area limitation in our study. PD patients enrolled in our study were mainly from Shanghai. Larger sample and a multi-center based study would be a better option to explore risk factors in Chinese population.

Although failing to identify DA agonist as a risk factor, we found a higher percentage of ICDs patients took DA agonists and a higher average daily DA agonist dosage than that of non-ICD patients, which also indicates DA agonist might be a potential risk factor for those PD-ICD patients. One patient with HS behavior in our study got recovered by discontinuation of pramipexole. Previous study showed successful management of the PD patient with ICD by reduction or discontinuation of DA agonist therapy [19–23]. Seven of 18 PD patients with an ICD had resolution of the behavior by discontinuation or dosage reduction of a DA agonist [22]. A 43 months follow–up study showed that nearly 73 % of PD patients with ICD behaviors were completely recovered after reducing dosage of DA drugs [23]. At present, there were very limited data to support an effective medicine for treatment of ICD behaviors in PD. Reduction or discontinuation of DA agonist is generally accepted as the first line management strategy of ICDs [23], especially for those PD patients had ICD behaviors after DRT therapy.

Conclusions

In conclusion, the incidence of ICDs behaviors in PD patients in our study is much lower than in western countries. Routine screening of ICDs in PD patients is necessary to discover PD-ICD patients and give early intervention.

Competing interests

The authors declare that they have no competing interests.

Authors' contributions

QX was responsible for study design and manuscript revision. XPW and MW were responsible for the patient recruitment and data integration, analysis and statistical analyses. XPW wrote the manuscript. All authors read and approved the final manuscript.

Acknowledgments

This work was supported by the National Natural Science Foundation of China (Grant No.81071023) and the Natural Science Foundation of Shanghai (Grant No.14ZR1425700).

References

1. Hoehn MM. The natural history of Parkinson's disease in the pre-levodopa and post-levodopa eras. Neurol Clin. 1992;10(2):331–9.
2. Fahn S. The spectrum of levodopa-induced dyskinesias. Ann Neurol. 2000; 47(4 Suppl 1):S2-9; discussion S9-11.
3. Lim SY, Evans AH, Miyasaki JM. Impulse control and related disorders in Parkinson's disease: review. Ann N Y Acad Sci. 2008;1142:85–107.
4. Chiang HL et al. Are there ethnic differences in impulsive/compulsive behaviors in Parkinson's disease? Eur J Neurol. 2012;19(3):494–500.
5. Valenca GT et al. Past smoking and current dopamine agonist use show an independent and dose-dependent association with impulse control disorders in Parkinson's disease. Parkinsonism Relat Disord. 2013;19(7):698–700.
6. Weintraub D et al. Impulse control disorders in Parkinson disease: a cross-sectional study of 3090 patients. Arch Neurol. 2010;67(5):589–95.
7. Joutsa J et al. Impulse control disorders and depression in Finnish patients with Parkinson's disease. Parkinsonism Relat Disord. 2012;18(2):155–60.
8. Poletti M et al. A single-center, cross-sectional prevalence study of impulse control disorders in Parkinson disease: association with dopaminergic drugs. J Clin Psychopharmacol. 2013;33(5):691–4.
9. Tanaka K et al. Impulsive compulsive behaviors in Japanese Parkinson's disease patients and utility of the Japanese version of the Questionnaire for Impulsive-Compulsive Disorders in Parkinson's disease. J Neurol Sci. 2013; 331(1–2):76–80.
10. Fan W et al. Impulse control disorders in Parkinson's disease in a Chinese population. Neurosci Lett. 2009;465(1):6–9.
11. Lee JY et al. Association between the dose of dopaminergic medication and the behavioral disturbances in Parkinson disease. Parkinsonism Relat Disord. 2010;16(3):202–7.
12. Lim SY et al. Impulsive-compulsive behaviors are common in Asian Parkinson's disease patients: assessment using the QUIP. Parkinsonism Relat Disord. 2011;17(10):761–4.
13. Voon V, Fox SH. Medication-related impulse control and repetitive behaviors in Parkinson disease. Arch Neurol. 2007;64(8):1089–96.
14. Gibb WR, Lees AJ. The relevance of the Lewy body to the pathogenesis of idiopathic Parkinson's disease. J Neurol Neurosurg Psychiatry. 1988;51(6):745–52.
15. Lee JY et al. Genetic variant of HTR2A associates with risk of impulse control and repetitive behaviors in Parkinson's disease. Parkinsonism Relat Disord. 2012;18(1):76–8.
16. Blum K et al. Dopamine D2 receptor gene variants: association and linkage studies in impulsive-addictive-compulsive behaviour. Pharmacogenetics. 1995;5(3):121–41.
17. Lee JY et al. Association of DRD3 and GRIN2B with impulse control and related behaviors in Parkinson's disease. Mov Disord. 2009;24(12):1803–10.
18. Weintraub D et al. Validation of the questionnaire for impulsive-compulsive disorders in Parkinson's disease. Mov Disord. 2009;24(10):1461–7.
19. Klos KJ et al. Pathological hypersexuality predominantly linked to adjuvant dopamine agonist therapy in Parkinson's disease and multiple system atrophy. Parkinsonism Relat Disord. 2005;11(6):381–6.
20. Galpern WR, Stacy M. Management of impulse control disorders in Parkinson's disease. Curr Treat Options Neurol. 2007;9(3):189–97.
21. Uitti RJ et al. Hypersexuality with antiparkinsonian therapy. Clin Neuropharmacol. 1989;12(5):375–83.
22. Weintraub D et al. Association of dopamine agonist use with impulse control disorders in Parkinson disease. Arch Neurol. 2006;63(7):969–73.
23. Sohtaoglu M et al. Long term follow-up of Parkinson's disease patients with impulse control disorders. Parkinsonism Relat Disord. 2010;16(5):334–7.
24. Tomlinson CL et al. Systematic review of levodopa dose equivalency reporting in Parkinson's disease. Mov Disord. 2010;25(15):2649–53.

15

Caregiver burden is increased in Parkinson's disease with mild cognitive impairment (PD-MCI)

Ann J. Jones[1,2*], Roeline G. Kuijer[2], Leslie Livingston[1,3], Daniel Myall[1,3], Kyla Horne[1,2,3], Michael MacAskill[1,3], Toni Pitcher[1,3], Paul T. Barrett[2,4], Tim J. Anderson[1,3,5,6] and John C. Dalrymple-Alford[1,2,3,6]

Abstract

Background: There is limited evidence on caregiver outcomes associated with mild cognitive impairment in patients with Parkinson's disease (PD-MCI) and the coping strategies used by these caregivers.

Methods: To investigate this relationship, we examined levels of burden, depression, anxiety, coping strategies and positive aspects of caregiving in the informal caregivers of 96 PD patients. The PD patients were classified using MDS-Task Force Level II criteria as showing either normal cognition (PD-N; n = 51), PD-MCI (n = 30) or with dementia (PDD; n = 15).

Results: Mean Zarit Burden Interview (ZBI) score increased significantly between carers of PD-N (M = 13.39, SD = 12.22) compared to those of PD-MCI patients (M = 22.00, SD = 10.8), and between carers of PD-MCI and PDD patients (M = 29.33, SD = 9.59). Moreover, the proportion of carers showing clinically significant levels of burden (ZBI score ≥ 21) also increased as the patients' cognitive status declined (18% for PD-N; 60% for PD-MCI; and 80% for PDD) and was mirrored by an increasing amount of time spent providing care by the caregivers. Caregiver ZBI score was independent of patient neuropsychiatric symptoms, motor function, disease duration and time that caregivers spent caregiving. Caregiver use of different coping strategies increased with worsening cognition. However, we found only equivocal evidence that the use of problem-focused, emotion-focused and dysfunctional coping mediated the association between patient cognitive status and caregiver burden, because the inverse models that used caregiver burden as the mediator were also significant.

Conclusions: The study highlights the impact of Parkinson's disease on those providing care when the patient's cognition is poor, including those with MCI. Caregiver well-being has important implications for caregiver support, nursing home placement and disease course.

Keywords: Parkinson's disease, Mild cognitive impairment, Zarit caregiver burden interview, Coping, Depression, Anxiety, Positive aspects of caregiving

Background

Cognitive problems are an integral part of Parkinson's disease because dementia (PDD) eventuates in 75%–90% of patients and is associated with substantial health and economic burden [1]. Patients who present with mild cognitive impairment (PD-MCI) are at high risk of progression to PDD and are a growing research focus to assess the impact of increasing cognitive impairment and to facilitate early intervention [2–5]. The impact of cognitive status on the informal caregiver is a relatively neglected dimension of PD-MCI and there is limited research on the specific effects of cognitive decline on the well-being of caregivers of these PD patients. Understanding these relationships is important because improving caregiver support and well-being may have a bearing on disease management and delay formal care and nursing home placement.

* Correspondence: anniejones@xtra.co.nz

[1]New Zealand Brain Research Institute, 66 Stewart Street, Christchurch 8011, New Zealand

[2]Department of Psychology, University of Canterbury, Christchurch, New Zealand

Full list of author information is available at the end of the article

It is well-established that there is higher caregiver burden and reduced quality of life in caregivers once dementia onset has commenced in PD [6, 7]. Recent assessments of well-being in PD-MCI caregivers has revealed mixed results, in that reduced quality of life measures were found in these caregivers [8] but explicit measures of burden using the Zarit Burden Interview (ZBI), did not show elevated levels of burden for PD-MCI caregivers as compared to PD-N caregivers [9, 10]. Such results contrast with reports of increased caregiver burden in carers of people with MCI who are at risk of Alzheimer's dementia [11], although additional factors may contribute to PD caregiver difficulties [12]. The failure to find increased Zarit burden scores in carers of PD-MCI patients is unexpected, but may reflect the over-riding impact of motor disabilities and other non-motor symptoms in PD even prior to dementia.

The Zarit Burden Interview provides a well-validated global measure of the physical, emotional and socioeconomic impact of caring for neurologically compromised individuals [13]. While motor and neuropsychiatric symptoms present one explanation of the response of the caregiver to the patient with PD, an alternative reason for the failure to identify increased burden with PD-MCI patients may be that caregiving strategies develop within the context of ostensibly a movement disorder that has a dominant influence on the interaction between patient and caregiver. For example, the response by caregivers to the presence of MCI in the context of an already established disease such as PD may evoke compensatory positive attitudes in carers or may influence their coping strategies before problems associated with dementia become overwhelming. In the wider literature in the context of dementia, the use of three coping strategies (problem-focused, emotion-focused and dysfunctional coping) has been found useful to explain variability in caregiver outcomes in that dementia caregivers who use more emotion-focused coping and less dysfunctional coping express lower anxiety and depression [14]. Dysfunctional strategies include substance use, distraction, and disengagement, while emotion-focused coping concerns attempts to reduce distress by regulating emotions which may prove adaptive in the context of PD caregiving. Problem-focused coping relates to managing distress through confronting and altering the situation, but findings for this strategy are less clear [14]. Identifying these strategies has the benefit of providing a focus for interventions to improve caregiver well-being [15, 16]. We therefore examined caregiver coping strategies and positive aspects of caregiving as potential mediators of the relationship between patients' cognitive status and caregiver burden.

In the current study we employed a cross-sectional design to examine burden expressed by caregivers of patients who met the current Movement Disorders Society – Task Force (MDS-TF) Level II criteria for PD-MCI and PDD [17, 18] and by caregivers of patients with normal levels of cognition (PD-N). Previous studies that assessed caregivers of PD-MCI patients employed Level I criteria, in which the range of tests employed are restricted either to global measures of cognition or a relatively restricted range of cognitive measures [8–10]. We have found that specific Level II criteria, in which two impairments are required within a single domain, capture PD-MCI patients who are at greatest risk of decline to PDD in the subsequent 4 years [4] and who may thus pose a greater challenge to caregiver well-being. The MDS-TF level II criteria also enabled an assessment of caregiver outcomes associated with PD-MCI subtypes [10] including attentional deficits, which have been shown to be associated with lower Quality of Life in PD carers [8].

We hypothesized that caregivers of patients meeting Level II PD-MCI criteria would express a level of burden (ZBI) that was intermediate to that experienced by PD-N and PDD caregivers. It was also anticipated that attentional deficits in PD patients would be associated with increased caregiver burden [10]. Further, it was hypothesized that, similar to Alzheimer's caregivers, [19] use of emotion-focused-coping strategies would reduce this level of distress (ZBI) but that use of problem-focused coping and dysfunctional coping would not.

Methods

A convenience sample of 96 PD patients (UK Parkinson's Society criteria), part of a longitudinal study, were recruited through the New Zealand Brain Research Institute. Caregivers were identified as any person who was directly involved in the patient's care and provided some form of support with respect to everyday activities. These caregivers either lived with the patients (n = 82), were spouses, partners or children and spent a minimum of 4 hours per week caring for the patient. At the time when caregivers were interviewed for this study, 15 patients met criteria for PDD, while the remaining PD patients were assessed as showing either PD-MCI (n = 30) or cognitive abilities within a normal range of scores (PD-N; n = 51). The PD patients met MDS-TF level II criteria by completing neuropsychological assessments over 2 sessions using 23 measures across the recommended five cognitive domains (attention, working memory and processing speed; executive function; visuoperceptual/visuospatial; learning and memory; language) within 6 months of the caregiver burden and coping assessments. A diagnosis of PD-MCI was confirmed when any two (or more) impaired neuropsychological test scores were present within any single domain but everyday independent function as reported by the caregiver [20] was generally preserved and indicated cognitive independence. A score 1.5SD or more below normative data was considered an impaired score [4]. Evidence of PDD was determined when the caregiver reported inability by the patient on everyday tasks in the context of impaired cognition in two or more cognitive domains [20], which was supplemented by assessment of the patient's performance during interview and caregiver responses on the neuropsychiatric inventory (NPI) [21]. Motor function was assessed with the Unified Parkinson's disease Rating Scale part III (UPDRS-III) [22]. All patients were in an 'on' state during neuropsychological assessment. Table 1 provides individual neuropsychological test and domain scores for the three patient groups. Caregiver demographical information and clinical characteristics of the caregivers and patients are provided in Tables 2 and 3.

Measures

The Zarit burden interview (ZBI)

This 22-item scale identifies the impact of the patient's disability in terms of caregiver health, finances, emotion, social life and interpersonal relations [13]. For each item, the caregiver rates how often they have felt the suggested feeling or perception, from never (score 0) to nearly always (score 4), generating a score ranging from 0 to 88. In dementia caregivers, the measure has good internal consistency with a Cronbach's alpha of .92. A score ≥ 21 signifies mild to moderate burden [13].

The brief coping orientations for problems experienced (COPE)

This 28-item version of the 60-item inventory assesses coping strategies [23]. Caregivers were asked to consider their current PD-caregiving situation. Responses were scored on a 4-point Likert scale ranging from 'I usually don't do this at all' through to 'I usually do this a lot'. Principal component factor analysis identified three dimension scores involving problem-focused, emotion-focused and dysfunctional coping (Additional file 1: Table A and Table B).

Positive aspects of caregiving (PAC)

This 9-item instrument provided a positive dimension score of the caregiving experience [24].

Depression/anxiety

The 15-item Geriatric Depression Scale (GDS) [25] was used to screen for depressive symptoms in caregivers and patients while anxiety symptoms in caregivers were assessed with the Geriatric Anxiety Inventory (GAI) [26].

Hours per week spent caregiving

Caregivers were asked to estimate the average amount of time they spent each day providing care to the PD patient, which was multiplied by 7 to give a total of hours per week. Caregivers were asked to consider the provision of care relating to PD symptoms.

Neuropsychiatric inventory

The Neuropsychiatric Inventory (NPI) [21] assesses 10 behavioural disturbances: delusions, hallucinations, dysphoria, anxiety, agitation/aggression, euphoria, disinhibition, irritability/lability, apathy, and aberrant motor activity. Information for the NPI is obtained from the caregiver about the patient's behaviour. Only those domains with positive responses to screening questions are used for scoring. The frequency of the symptoms is scored on a 4-point scale, severity on a 3-point scale, and distress caused by the patient's symptoms on a 5-point scale.

Activities of daily living – International scale

The Activities of Daily living – International scale (ADL-IS) [20] consists of 40 questions such as "Does [the patient] have difficulty putting household items in the right places?" to which the informant is asked to respond using a Likert scale of 0 = 'never has difficulty' to 3 = 'always has difficulty'. A response of 4 = 'activity no longer performed (ie. has given up initiating the activity)'; 8 = 'activity was never performed' and 9 = 'unknown'. A score between 0 and 4 is generated based on the number of items that the patient was known to perform prior to their illness.

Statistical analysis

All variables in the study were screened for outliers and deviations from normality. Single outliers were detected for disease duration, Hoehn & Yahr score, caregiver age and the ZBI. Since none of the results changed when outliers were excluded from analysis, it was decided to retain these data points. The distribution of the GDS (patient and caregiver), the NPI, hours of caregiving and the GAI violated assumptions of normality. A log transformation was used to ensure that skewness and kurtosis of these variables were within the acceptable range (means and standard deviations prior to transformation are presented in the tables to assist interpretability). Comparison of demographic and clinical variables across the three cognitive status groups, for both patients and caregivers, was assessed using Analysis of Variance (ANOVA) and Chi square. Newman-Keuls (N-K) tests for equal group variances and Tamhane's T2 (T2) tests for unequal group variances were used for post-hoc comparisons. Additional analyses of covariance examined whether any effects of cognitive status on caregiver burden remained after controlling for patient clinical variables and time spent caregiving. Pearson's correlations between PD patient cognitive status (defined as 1 = PD-N, 2 = PD-MCI, 3 = PD-D) [27],

Table 1 Neuropsychological assessments used for level II criteria (n = 96)

Patient groups	PD-N(n = 51)	PD-MCI(n = 30)	PD-D(n = 15)	Analysis ($F_{2,93}$)
MoCA[a]	26.64 ± 2.16	24.53 ± 3.08	21.33 ± 2.32	27.12, p < .0001
Attention, Working Memory and Processing Speed				
DigitsF/B	.54 ± 0.93	.14 ± 0.69	−.37 ± 0.64	7.69, p < .01
Digit Ordering	−.60 ± 1.06	−1.33 ± 1.10	−2.16 ± 0.89	13.52, p < .001
TEA (Map Search)	−.46 ± 0.84	−1.40 ± 0.85	−1.91 ± 0.72	23.6, p < .001
Stroop colour	.09 ± 0.80	−.60 ± 1.14	−1.13 ± 1.07	15.03, p < .001
Stroop word	.15 ± 0.73	−.34 ± 1.06	−.68 ± 1.07	6.17, p < .01
Trails A	.32 ± 0.69	−.41 ± 0.99	−1.7 ± 1.22	8.83, p < .001
Domain Score	.01 ± 0.50	−.65 ± 0.51	−1.40 ± 0.52	47.78, p < .001
Domain Pass/Fail	51/0	13/17	2/13	
Executive Function				
Letter Fluency	.61 ± 1.45	.28 ± 1.24	−.42 ± 1.40	3.32, p < .05
Action Fluency	−.78 ± 1.08	−1.45 ± 1.09	−1.76 ± 1.03	6.56, p < .01
Category Fluency	.68 ± 1.14	.07 ± 1.09	−.95 ± 1.17	12.55, p < .001
Category Switching	.27 ± 1.12	−.52 ± 1.27	−1.95 ± .89	22.80, p < .001
Trails B	.28 ± 0.83	−.30 ± 1.13	−2.31 ± 0.84	44.03, p < .0001
Stroop Interference	.31 ± 1.04	−.45 ± 0.78	−1.66 ± 0.70	35.01, p < .0001
Domain Score	.23 ± 0.74	−.40 ± 0.72	−1.05 ± 0.55	36.05, p < .0001
Domain Pass/Fail	51/0	15/15	2/13	
Learning & Memory				
CVLT Free recall	.59 ± 1.13	−.29 ± 0.96	−1.44 ± 0.90	23.26, p < .001
CVLT Short delay	.31 ± 1.32	−.33 ± 1.28	−1.43 ± 0.53	12.17, p < .001
CVLT Long delay	.38 ± 0.90	−.23 ± 0.98	−.76 ± 0.53	11.38, p < .001
Rey Immediate	.59 ± 1.71	−.56 ± 1.08	−1.34 ± 1.03	12.84, p < .001
Rey Delayed	.58 ± 1.77	−.85 ± 1.15	−1.82 ± 1.08	18.13, p < .001
Domain Score	.50 ± 1.06	−.45 ± 0.80	−1.41 ± 0.46	28.50, p < .0001
Domain Pass/Fail Visuospatial	51/0	24/6	4/11	
JOL	−.15 ± 0.81	−.99 ± 0.81	−.94 ± 0.84	10.55, p < .001
Fragmented letters	.62 ± 0.58	.10 ± 9.99	.20 ± .08	7.9, p < .05
Rey Copy	.02 ± 1.04	−.85 ± 1.27	−1.61 ± 1.11	14.11, p < .01
Domain Score	.44 ± 0.55	−.31 ± 0.63	−.76 ± 0.57	31.94, p < .0001
Domain Pass/Fail	51/0	26/4	11/4	
Language				
Boston Naming	.21 ± 0.86	.05 ± 1.07	−.11 ± 1.21	$F_{2,64}$ = .87, p = .42
ADAS-Cog	.01 ± 0.65	−.18 ± 0.78	−1.16 ± 0.59	14.89, p < .001
DRS-2	.01 ± 0.57	−.18 ± 0.66	−.62 ± 0.88	5.45, p < .01
Domain Score	.06 ± 0.47	−.10 ± 0.46	−.67 ± 0.57	13.64, p < .001
Domain Pass/Fail	51/0	29/1	14/1	
Global neuropsychological z score	.29 ± 0.57	−.45 ± 0.41	−1.29 ± 0.41	62.23, p < .001

Values reported as mean ± standard deviation

[a]MoCA Montreal Cognitive Assessment, with one missed test; Age and education z scores for all tests except MoCA; global performance was expressed by an aggregate z score by first averaging standardized scores within four cognitive domains and then taking the mean of these four values; the language domain scores were not included in this z score due to the distributions of the normative data

Table 2 Demographic and clinical characteristics of the Parkinson's disease patient groups $n = 96$

Patient groups	PD-N ($n = 51$)	PD-MCI ($n = 30$)	PDD ($n = 15$)	Analysis	Significant post-hoc differences (N-K or T2)
Age	68.23 ± 7.60	69.5 ± 6.86	72.73 ± 4.85	$F_{2,93} = 2.39, p = .09$	
Female: Male	16/35	9/21	3/12	$X^2 = .74, p = .69$	
Education (yrs)	13.14 ± 3.03	12.56 ± 1.99	12.26 ± 2.49	$F_{2,93} = .82, p = .44$	
GDS	1.45 ± 2.88	0.73 ± 1.79	2.13 ± 3.14	$F_{2,93} = 1.29, p = .28$	
H&Y	2.10 ± 0.52	2.30 ± 0.75	2.33 ± 0.59	$F_{2, 90} = 1.48, p = .23$	
NPI	3.14 ± 5.21	4.37 ± 4.62	8.13 ± 9.26	$F_{2, 89} = 4.83, p < .05$	PD-N v PDD, $p < .05$
ADL-IS	.51 ± 0.51	.78 ± 0.47	2.04 ± 0.54	$F_{2,91} = 55.35, p < .0001$	PD-N v PDD, $p < .001$ PD-MCI v PDD, $p < .001$
Disease Duration (yrs)	7.54 ± 4.00	9.10 ± 4.44	11.63 ± 6.92	$F_{2, 93} = 4.59, p < .05$	
UPDRS-III	25.64 ± 10.80	29.2 ± 13.07	34.83 ± 10.42	$F_{2,92} = 3.84, p < .05$	PD-N v PDD, $p < .05$

Values reported as mean ± standard deviation: GDS-Geriatric Depression Scale; H&Y- Hoehn & Yahr; NPI - Neuropsychiatric Inventory; ADL-IS Activities of Daily Living - International Scale (max = 4.0); UPDRS-III Unified Parkinson's Disease Rating Scale Part III

caregiver burden and the three coping strategies were assessed to see whether criteria for path analysis (mediation) were met. The PROCESS macro developed by Hayes [28] was used to test for mediation using linear regression. In this procedure the mediated effect (indirect effect) is calculated via bootstrapping using a 95% confidence interval (CI) [29]. A mediator is significant when the 95% CI does not include zero. Separate analyses for each of the three coping strategies as intended mediators were conducted. Reverse causation, with caregiver burden as the mediator, was also assessed. All analyses employed an alpha level of $p < 0.05$ and were two-tailed.

Results

Patients in the 3 cognitive status groups did not differ significantly in mean age, years of education, depression symptoms or disease stage (Table 2). There were, however, significant differences between the three groups in neuropsychiatric inventory (NPI) symptoms, abilities at everyday tasks (ADL-IS score), motor features (UPDRS III score) and disease duration. Scores for these patient measures increased linearly from PD-N to PD-MCI through to PDD, with significant differences between the PD-N versus the PDD groups on all measures apart from disease duration, and between PD-MCI and PDD on the ADL-IS.

Table 3 Demographic and clinical characteristics of the caregivers ($n = 96$)

Caregivers of patient groups	PD-N ($n = 51$)	PD-MCI ($n = 30$)	PDD ($n = 15$)	Analysis	Significant post-hoc differences (N-K or T2)
Age	65.53 ± 9.68	62.33 ± 13.61	66.87 ± 11.34	$F_{2,93} = 1.07, p = .35$	
Female/Male	33/18	21/9	12/3	$X^2 = 0.74, p = .36$	
Years Education	12.41 ± 2.36	12.33 ± 2.45	11.60 ± 1.88	$F_{2,93} = 0.73, p = .49$	
Spouse/Other[a]	47/4	24/6	12/3	$X^2 = 3.02, p = .22$	
Lives separately	3	6	5	$X^2 = 8.04, p = .98$	
Hours/week caregiving	5.40 ± 14.30	16.47 ± 27.06	25.01 ± 27.23	$F_{2,93} = 10.17, p < .001$	PD-MCI v PDD, $p < .05$ PD-N v PDD, $p < .001$
Zarit Burden Interview	13.39 ± 12.22	22.00 ± 10.86	29.33 ± 9.59	$F_{2,93} = 13.89, p < .001$	PD-N v PD-MCI, $p < .01$ PD-N v PDD, $p < .001$ PD-MCI v PDD, $p < .05$
Coping Strategies					
Problem-Focused	1.88 ± .67	2.20 ± .62	2.35 ± .65	$F_{2,93} = 4.09, p < .05$	PD-N v PDD, $p < .05$
Emotion-Focused	1.93 ± .55	2.24 ± .64	2.27 ± .47	$F_{2,93} = 3.61, p < .05$	
Dysfunctional	1.28 ± .40	1.43 ± .38	1.55 ± .37	$F_{2,93} = 3.32, p < .05$	PD-N v PDD, $p < .05$
GDS	1.21 ± 1.94	0.73 ± 1.41	0.40 ± .83	$F_{2,93} = 1.59, p = .21$	
GAI	2.47 ± 3.85	2.47 ± 3.81	0.80 ± 1.61	$F_{2,93} = 1.52, p = .22$	
Positive Aspects of Caregiving	27.12 ± 8.85	27.316 ± 9.20	24.87 ± 9.36	$F_{2,93} = 0.40, p = .67$	

Values reported as mean ± standard deviation

[a]Daughter, son, daughter-in-law, brother or friend

The caregivers were aged between 23 and 83 years old, and predominantly a slightly younger spouse (85.4%) and female (70.8%). Caregivers of the PD patients in the three cognitive status groups did not differ in mean age, years of education, positive aspects of caregiving, depression or anxiety symptoms (Table 3). Caregiver burden (ZBI), however, increased significantly across the 3 cognitive status groups ($F_{2,\ 93}$ = 13.89, p < .00001) with post-hoc tests (N-K) showing significant differences between all 3 groups. Moderate to large effect sizes were found for the differences between PD-N versus PD-MCI (Cohen's d = .73; [CI = .27, 1.20]) and between PD-MCI versus PDD (Cohen's d = .70; [CI = .064, 1.33]). A large effect size was found for the difference between PD-N versus PDD (Cohen's d = 1.36; [CI = .74, 1.98]). The proportion of carers showing mild to moderate burden (ZBI ≥ 21) [13] was 18% for PD-N, 60% for PD-MCI and 80% for PDD; these proportions were significantly different to chance (χ^2 = 32.45, p < .0001). There were no significant correlations between caregiver ZBI or coping strategies and any of the five individual cognitive domain scores used to assess the PD-MCI group. Mean caregiver ZBI scores did not differ significantly when PD-MCI patients were subdivided according to possible cognitive subtypes: PD-MCI with attention deficit only, n = 10, M = 20.9 (SD = 12.88); executive only, n = 8, M = 24.15 (SD = 6.22); memory only, n = 4, M = 25.25 (SD = 20.13); visuoperception only, n = 1; and any multidomain impairments, n = 7, M = 19 (SD = 8.18). Lack of clear effects of multidomain were also evident when the multidomain classification focused on either attention plus any other domain, n = 7, M = 19 (SD = 8.18) or executive plus any other domain, n = 7, M = 19 (SD = 8.18), although there was some suggestion of less burden than the multidomain impairment derived from memory plus any other domain, n = 2, M = 8.5 (SD = .71) and visuoperceptual plus any other domain, n = 3, M = 15.33 (SD = 5.5).

The number of hours that caregivers spent per week caring for PD patients also increased significantly for caregivers across the 3 cognitive status groups (Table 3). Post-hoc tests (T2) confirmed significant differences in time spent caregiving between PD-MCI versus PDD: medium to large effect size, Cohen's d = .74 [CI = .09, 1.37]) and PD-N versus PDD: large effect size, Cohen's d = 1.49 [CI = .86, 2.11), but the difference between PD-N versus PD-MCI did not reach significance: Cohen's d = .43 [CI = −.04, .88].

Additional covariance analyses showed that the significant effect of patient cognitive status on the ZBI scores remained after controlling for disease duration (F(2,92) = 9.16, p < .001), patient neuropsychiatric symptoms [NPI] (F(2, 88) = 16.04, p < .001), ability to perform everyday tasks [ADL-IS] (F(2, 88) = 6.70 p < .05), motor difficulties (UPDRS-III) (F(2, 91) = 12.74, p < .001) and even time spent caregiving (F(2, 92) = 9.09, p < .001). There was no difference in ZBI scores between the caregivers of PD-MCI patients who converted to PDD within 2 years of the caregiver interview compared to those who did not convert t(5) = 1.8, p = .13. There was also no difference in ZBI scores between female (M = 19.26, SE = 1.58) and male (M = 16.17, SE =2.15) caregivers (t = 1.15, p = 2.00) and no significant interaction between the effects of patient cognitive status and gender of caregiver (F(2, 92) = .60, p = .43).

One aim of this study was to examine whether coping strategies may provide a mechanism to explain variability in caregiver outcomes. There were significant differences across the groups in the use of problem-focused, emotion-focused and dysfunctional coping (Table 3). Post-hoc tests (N-K) identified significant differences between PD-N and PDD caregivers only for problem-focused coping (Cohen's d = .71[CI = .12, 1.29]) and dysfunctional coping (Cohen's d = .69 [CI = .10, 1.27]). There were no differences between the three caregiver groups in terms of positive aspects of caregiving.

Correlational analyses identified that all 3 coping strategies correlated with both cognitive status and with caregiver ZBI score and thus met criteria for path analysis (Table 4). Support for (partial) mediation requires that the relationship between cognitive status and caregiver burden decreases significantly once the mediator is added to the regression model. A mediator is significant when the 95% CI of the mediated effect does not include zero. The bootstrapping procedure provided support for mediation when problem-focused coping was used as the intended mediator, (b = 2.02, SE = 0.97, [CI = 0.58, 4.47]). The same was true for the analyses with emotion-focused coping as the intended mediator (bootstrapping procedure: b = 0.82, SE = .59, [CI = .06, 2.47]) and dysfunctional coping (b = 2.70 SE = 1.04 [CI = .85–4.94]). Thus, problem-focused coping, emotion-focused coping and dysfunctional coping all partially mediated the relationship between patients' cognitive status and caregiver burden (Fig. 1). However, given the cross-sectional nature of our design, it was also necessary to examine the reverse models in which caregiver burden (ZBI) may instead mediate the relationship between cognitive status and problem-focused coping, emotion-focused coping

Table 4 Pearson's correlations between caregiver burden, cognitive status, and coping strategies (n = 96)

	ZBI	CogSt	P-F Coping	E-F Coping
CogSt	0.48***			
P-F Coping	0.53***	0.28**		
E-F Coping	0.30***	0.25*	0.41***	
Dysf Coping	0.70***	0.26**	0.41***	0.26**

ZBI Zarit burden interview, *CogSt* Cognitive status, *P-F* Problem-focused, *E-F* Emotion-focused, Dysf = dysfunctional. *p < .05, **p < .01, ***p < .001

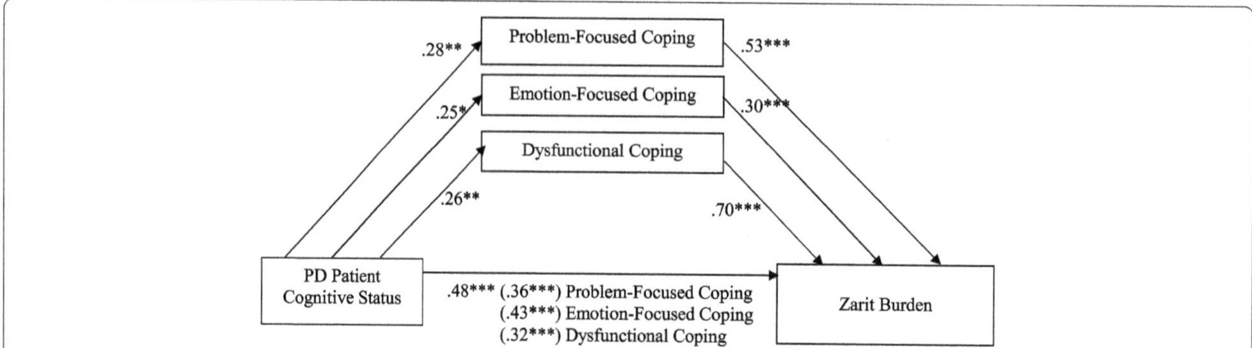

Fig. 1 Standardized regression coefficients for the relationship between PD patient cognitive status and caregiver burden as mediated by use of problem-focused, emotion-focused and dysfunctional coping strategies (n = 96). The standardized regression coefficients between cognitive status and burden controlling for coping strategies are in parentheses $^{*}p$ < .05, $^{**}p$ < .01, $^{***}p$ < .001

and dysfunctional coping. This reverse analysis was significant for all three coping measures: problem-focused: b = .22 SE = .06 [CI = .12, .37], emotion-focused: b = .09, SE = .06 [CI = .01, .24], and dysfunctional: b = .19, SE = .03 [CI = .13, .27]. Given these bidirectional mediating relationships, we cannot be certain that coping strategies mediated the association between patient's cognitive status and caregiver ZBI score.

Discussion

Assessing the impact of PD-MCI on patients and caregivers is seen as a 'crucial unmet need' [18] but has been scarcely studied. PD patients in the present study were classified as PD-N, PD-MCI or PDD according to level II criteria. Unlike previous work using Level I criteria, we identified increased burden among carers of PD-MCI patients compared with those of PD-N. Further, PDD caregivers had significantly higher ZBI scores compared to both PD-N and PD-MCI caregivers. The use of all three coping strategies increased as the patient's cognitive status worsened. There were no differences in terms of positive caregiving aspects, depression or anxiety across the carers of the different PD patient groups. The current study's ZBI findings on burden in caregivers of PD-MCI patients are in contrast to previous research by Leroi et al. [9] and Szeto et al. [10].

Leroi and colleagues identified moderate burden in PD-MCI caregivers which was significantly lower than that of PDD caregivers but not significantly higher than PD-N carers. Levels of ZBI in the PD-MCI and PDD caregivers reported by Leroi (23.61 and 35.48) respectively, were similar to the differences found in the current study (22.00 and 29.33). One disparity compared to the current study was higher levels of burden reported by PD-N caregivers (20.00) in the Leroi study. Perhaps Leroi's predominantly male caregivers found the caregiving role demanding in the early stages of PD, although previous research suggests female caregivers experience higher perceived burden [30] and we found no significant gender differences in the extent to which the current study's PD-N male and female caregivers reported ZBI [$t(49)$ = .88, p = .38]. Another possible explanation for the contrasting finding is that continuous involvement in the New Zealand Brain Research's longitudinal study has provided a sense of support to the caregivers of PD-N patients involved in this research and has thereby lowered their feelings of burden. Also relevant is that the PD-MCI criteria used in the current study is associated with high levels of conversion to PDD over a four-year period [4].

The study by Szeto et al. [10] compared caregivers for PD-N and PD-MCI patients only. While the authors reported significantly lower quality of life scores with regard to physical health and interruptions to usual activities among PD-MCI caregivers, they mention that there was no difference in caregiver burden. They did not, however, report the actual levels of burden, but stated that the results were similar to those of Leroi et al. [9] These two studies used level I criteria to establish PD-MCI status, whereas the current study employed the more comprehensive level II criteria, which has been shown to be suitable in terms of stability and increased risk of progression to PDD [4]. Also, level I criteria may underestimate the proportion of PD-MCI patients and thus misclassify some PD-MCI patients as PD-N [31]. In another study of PD carers Lawson et al. [8] used a range of cognitive tests, though using modified Level II criteria, to identify PD-MCI patients. Lawson et al. reported that quality of life scores for PD-MCI carers were intermediate to that of caregivers for patients classified as PD-N (higher) and PDD (lower). Their results support the findings of the current study, which identified intermediate levels of distress among PD-MCI caregivers relative to caregivers of patients meeting PDD and PD-N classification. Unlike the Lawson study we were unable to find support that attentional deficits were related to caregiver distress.

Elevated burden among PDD caregivers in the current study compared with PD-N caregivers is consistent with previous research. Indeed 80% of PDD caregivers scored above the 21-point threshold on the ZBI, indicating mild to severe burden [13]. This threshold of burden was also frequent in PD-MCI caregivers (60%), and even apparent in a substantial number of caregivers of PD-N patients (30%) [11]. Given the high rates of burden irrespective of cognitive status, it is possible that neuropsychiatric and motor symptoms associated with PD and disease progression play a significant part towards negative caregiver outcomes. The significant effects of PD patient cognitive status nonetheless remained significant after controlling for neuropsychiatric symptoms and motor severity even though these features increased progressively with worsening cognition. Notably caregiver burden was also independent of disease duration. The difference in the number of hours spent caregiving between the three patient cognitive status groups suggests that even in the early stages of the disease the presence of impaired cognition places an additional load on caregivers. These observations lend support for the notion of PD-MCI as a clinical identity that has a significant impact not just on the person with PD but also the primary carer.

This is the first study to examine caregiver coping strategies as potential mediators of the relationship between patients' cognitive status and caregiver burden in PD. The use of all three coping strategies increased as the patient's cognitive status worsened. However, no evidence was found to suggest that the use of any of these coping strategies reduced caregiver burden in the current study. In fact, increased use of all three coping strategies was related to higher burden scores across the whole PD sample. For dysfunctional coping (disengaging from the situation or emotions) these findings are in line with other studies on dementia [14], and for problem-focused coping these findings add to a growing literature suggesting that responding with problem-focused strategies to situations that are beyond one's control, such as when caring for an individual with a deteriorating illness, may not be effective [19]. For emotion-focused coping, however, these findings are not in line with studies of dementia caregivers showing that emotion-focused coping (managing one's emotional response to stress) was associated with better caregiver outcomes (lower levels of anxiety and depression) [14]. Because of its correlational design the current study was unable to draw conclusions about causality. Although the three coping strategies mediated the relationship between cognitive status and caregiver burden, the reverse causation models (with burden mediating the relationship between cognitive status and coping) were also significant. The complex and possibly bidirectional relationship between caregiver outcomes and coping strategies was also illustrated in a longitudinal study of dementia caregivers by Cooper et al. [19]. They found that cross-sectionally caregiver burden was related to increased emotion-focused, problem-focused and dysfunctional coping (in line with findings from the current study), but that longitudinally an increased use of emotion-focused coping was related to lower anxiety.

Limitations

Further evidence on burden and coping strategies in PD-MCI patients is needed because the current study had a relatively low number of participants and group sizes differed. Another limitation is the cross-sectional design. Longitudinal data could better assess the temporal course of caregiver outcomes and disentangle the directional causality between ZBI, cognitive impairment and coping strategies.

Conclusions

The current study showed that caregivers of PD-MCI patients, known to have a high risk of dementia, often experience high levels of burden. PD without cognitive impairment is less often associated with caregiver burden, but this is also apparent even in a subset of these carers. The association between cognitive impairment and caregiver burden is relatively independent of neuropsychiatric and motor symptoms, disease duration and patient ability to engage in tasks of daily living. The findings add weight to the need for greater awareness of cognitive decline in PD patients and in particular to provide better support frameworks for caregivers before the onset of dementia. Increased support for caregivers may benefit patients and help delay the need for nursing home placement.

Acknowledgements
Not applicable.

Funding
The authors are grateful for the support of the University of Canterbury Department of Psychology, New Zealand Neurological Foundation, Canterbury Medical Research Foundation, Christchurch Neurology Trust and Brain Research New Zealand.

Authors' contributions
AJ: Study design, data collection, statistical analysis. RK: Study design, statistical analysis. LL: Data collection. DM: Data management and statistical analysis. KH: Data collection, data management, statistical analysis. MM: Data management, statistical analysis. TP: Data collection, data management. PB: Statistical analysis. TA: Study design. JD-A: Study design. All authors contributed to the preparation and review for the final manuscript.

Competing interests

The authors declare that they have no competing interests.

Author details

[1]New Zealand Brain Research Institute, 66 Stewart Street, Christchurch 8011, New Zealand. [2]Department of Psychology, University of Canterbury, Christchurch, New Zealand. [3]Department of Medicine, University of Otago, Christchurch, New Zealand. [4]Cognadev, UK Ltd., Sandton, South Africa. [5]Department of Neurology, Christchurch Hospital, Christchurch, New Zealand. [6]Brain Research New Zealand Centre of Research Excellence, Christchurch, New Zealand.

References

1. Hely MA, et al. The Sydney multicenter study of Parkinson's disease: the inevitability of dementia at 20 years. Mov Disord. 2008;23(6):837–44.
2. Broeders M, et al. Evolution of mild cognitive impairment in Parkinson disease. Neurology. 2013;81(4):346–52.
3. Pedersen KF, et al. Prognosis of mild cognitive impairment in early Parkinson disease: the Norwegian ParkWest study. JAMA Neurol. 2013;70(5):580–6.
4. Wood K-L, et al. Different PD-MCI criteria and risk of dementia in Parkinson's disease: 4-year longitudinal study. Npj Parkinson's Disease. 2016;2:15027.
5. Hobson P, Meara J. Mild cognitive impairment in Parkinson's disease and its progression onto dementia: a 16-year outcome evaluation of the Denbighshire cohort. Int J Geriatr Psychiatry. 2015;30(10):1048–55.
6. Cifu DX, et al. Caregiver distress in parkinsonism. J Rehabil Res Dev. 2006;43(4):499–508.
7. Martinez-Martin P, et al. Burden, perceived health status, and mood among caregivers of Parkinson's disease patients. Mov Disord. 2008;23(12):1673–80.
8. Lawson RA, et al. Cognitive impairment in Parkinson's disease: impact on quality of life of carers. Int J Geriatr Psychiatry. 2016;27:47–53.
9. Leroi I, et al. Cognitive impairment in Parkinson disease: impact on quality of life, disability, and caregiver burden. J Geriatr Psychiatry Neurol. 2012;25(4):208–14.
10. Szeto JY, et al. Mild cognitive impairment in Parkinson's disease: impact on caregiver outcomes. J Parkinsons Dis. 2016;6(3):589–96.
11. Bruce JM, et al. Burden among spousal and child caregivers of patients with mild cognitive impairment. Dement Geriatr Cogn Disord. 2008;25(4):385–90.
12. Shin H, et al. Caregiver burden in Parkinson disease with dementia compared to Alzheimer disease in Korea. J Geriatr Psychiatry Neurol. 2012;25(4):222–6.
13. Zarit SH, Reever KE, Bach-Peterson J. Relatives of the impaired elderly: correlates of feelings of burden. Gerontologist. 1980;20(6):649–55.
14. Li R, et al. Coping strategies and psychological morbidity in family carers of people with dementia: a systematic review and meta-analysis. J Affect Disord. 2012;139(1):1–11.
15. Cooper C, et al. Systematic review of the effectiveness of non-pharmacological interventions to improve quality of life of people with dementia. Int Psychogeriatr. 2012;24(6):856–70.
16. Schulz R, et al. Resources for enhancing Alzheimer's caregiver health (REACH): overview, site-specific outcomes, and future directions. Gerontologist. 2003;43(4):514–20.
17. Emre M, et al. Clinical diagnostic criteria for dementia associated with Parkinson's disease. Mov Disord. 2007;22(12):1689–707. quiz 1837
18. Litvan I, et al. Diagnostic criteria for mild cognitive impairment in Parkinson's disease: Movement Disorder Society Task Force guidelines. Mov Disord. 2012;27(3):349–56.
19. Cooper C, et al. Coping strategies, anxiety and depression in caregivers of people with Alzheimer's disease. Int J Geriatr Psychiatry. 2008;23(9):929–36.
20. Reisberg B, et al. The Alzheimer's disease activities of daily living international scale (ADL-IS). Int Psychogeriatr. 2001;13(2):163–81.
21. Cummings JL. The neuropsychiatric inventory: assessing psychopathology in dementia patients. Neurology. 1997;48(5 Suppl 6):S10–6.
22. The Unified Parkinson's Disease Rating Scale (UPDRS). Status and recommendations. Mov Disord. 2003;18(7):738–50.
23. Carver CS, Scheier MF, Weintraub JK. Assessing coping strategies: a theoretically based approach. J Pers Soc Psychol. 1989;56(2):267–83.
24. Tarlow B, et al. Positive aspects of caregiving: contributions of the REACH project to the development of new measures for Alzheimer's caregiving. Research on Aging. 2004;26:429.
25. Weintraub D, et al. Test characteristics of the 15-item geriatric depression scale and Hamilton depression rating scale in Parkinson disease. Am J Geriatr Psychiatry. 2006;14(2):169–75.
26. Pachana NA, et al. Development and validation of the geriatric anxiety inventory. Int Psychogeriatr. 2007;19(1):103–14.
27. Field A. Discovering statistics using SPSS. 4th ed. London: EC1Y 1SP: Sage Publications; 2009.
28. Hayes AF. Introduction to mediation, moderation, and conditional process analysis: a regression-based approach. New York: Guilford Press; 2013.
29. Preacher KJ, Hayes AF. SPSS and SAS procedures for estimating indirect effects in simple mediation models. Behav Res Methods Instrum Comput. 2004;36(4):717–31.
30. Yee JL, Schulz R. Gender differences in psychiatric morbidity among family caregivers: a review and analysis. Gerontologist. 2000;40(2):147–64.
31. Galtier I, et al. Mild cognitive impairment in Parkinson's disease: diagnosis and progression to dementia. J Clin Exp Neuropsychol. 2016;38(1):40–50.

Methylation status of DJ-1 in leukocyte DNA of Parkinson's disease patients

Yuyan Tan[1†], Li Wu[2†], Dunhui Li[1], Xiaoli Liu[1], Jianqing Ding[1] and Shengdi Chen[1,3*]

Abstract

Background: DJ-1 has been thought as a candidate biomarker for Parkinson's disease (PD). It was found reduced in PD brains, CSF and saliva, although there were conflicting results. How DJ-1 expression may be regulated is not clear. Recently, blood-based DNA methylation represents a highly promising biomarker for PD by regulating the causative gene expression. Thus, in this study, we try to explore whether blood-based DNA methylation of DJ-1 could be used as a biomarker to differentiate PD patients from normal control (NC), and whether DNA methylation could regulate DJ-1 expression in a SH-SY5Y cell model.

Methods: Forty PD patients and 40 NC were recruited in this study. DNA was extracted from peripheral blood leukocytes (PBLs). Methylation status of two CpG islands (CpG1 and CpG2) in promoter region of DJ-1 was explored by bisulfite specific PCR-based sequencing method. Methylation inhibitor 5-Aza-dC was used to treat SH-SY5Y cell line, DJ-1 level was detected in both mRNA and protein level.

Results: CpG sites in these two CpG islands (CpG1 and CpG2) of DJ-1 were unmethylated in both PD and NC group. In SH-SY5Y cell model treated by methylation inhibitor, there was no significant change of DJ-1 expression in either mRNA level or protein level.

Conclusions: Our results indicated that DNA methylation inhibitor didn't alter DJ-1 gene expression in SH-SY5Y cell model, and DNA methylation of DJ-1 promoter region in PBLs level might not be an efficient biomarker for PD patients.

Keywords: Parkinson's disease, DJ-1, DNA methylation, Peripheral blood leukocytes

Background

Parkinson's disease (PD) is the second most common neurodegenerative disorders, pathologically characterized by a progressive degeneration of dopaminergic neurons and the presence of intracytoplasmic Lewy bodies (LBs). The mechanisms responsible for neuronal degeneration in PD are complex and remain to be fully elucidated.

Mutations of DJ-1 are linked to autosomal recessive early-onset PD [1]. Extensive studies showed that DJ-1 has neuroprotective functions in anti-oxidative stress, anti-inflammation, mitochondrial regulation [2]. Loss of DJ-1 function was shown to cause autosomal recessive PD [1]. In sporadic PD patients, the level of total DJ-1 protein was significantly reduced in the substantia nigra (SN) and CSF [3–5], although there were conflicting results [6]. These results suggested that lower DJ-1 level in PD patients may contribute to the pathogenesis of PD. However, the molecular mechanisms underlying the decreased DJ-1 level are not yet clear.

In recent years, epigenetic mechanisms such as DNA methylation, histone modification, chromatin remodeling and non-coding RNA regulation have been evidenced to play a role in regulating gene expression in neurodegenerative diseases [7–9]. DNA methylation at the 5-carbon position of cytosine residues located in dinucleotide CpG sites has the specific effect of reducing gene expression and unmethylated CpG sites are mostly linked to gene activation [10]. Reduced CpG island methylation in intron 1 of SNCA has been evidenced in

* Correspondence: chen_sd@medmail.com.cn
†Equal contributors
[1]Department of Neurology, and Institute of Neurology, Ruijin Hospital Affiliated to Shanghai Jiao Tong University School of Medicine, Shanghai 200025, China
[3]Parkinson's Disease Center, Beijing Institute for Brain Disorders, Beijing 100069, China
Full list of author information is available at the end of the article

PD brain tissue [11, 12], and hypomethylation of CpG was associated with increased a-synuclein expression [12]. Our previous results showed that the hypomethylation of SNCA in PD can also be detected in the blood-based DNA methylation [13]. Eliezer Masliah et al. identified concordant methylation alterations in brain and blood by investigating genome-wide DNA methylation in brain and blood samples from PD patients and NC [14]. These reports from both of Eliezer Masliah et al. and us indicated that DNA extracted from leukocytes in peripheral blood might be a potential effective noninvasive source for screening epigenetic biomarker for PD diagnosis. Until now, no data on the methylation status of DJ-1 has been reported. In our study, we aimed to detect whether there was differential DNA methylation of DJ-1 in the peripheral blood between PD and NC groups and determine whether DNA methylation of DJ-1 in peripheral blood could represent the reduced expression of DJ-1 in PD patients. In SH-SY5Y cell model we tested whether DNA methylation can regulate DJ-1 expression by using methylation inhibitor.

Methods

Subjects

Forty PD patients, diagnosed by the UK PD brain bank criteria, were enrolled from the Department of Neurology, Ruijin Hospital affiliated to Shanghai Jiao Tong University School of Medicine, Shanghai, China; 40 NC were recruited from our previous epidemiological studies. For each subject, 5 ml of blood samples and clinical data, such as name, gender, age, age of onset, duration, disease stage (H-Y stage) were collected. The PD and NC groups were well matched for age (PD: 63.7 ± 6.16 years; NC: 61.28 ± 9.21 years, $p = 0.228$) and gender (PD: 24/16; NC: 24/16). All the subjects have signed the informed consent form, and the study was approved by the Ruijin Hospital Ethics Committee, Shanghai Jiao Tong University School of Medicine.

DNA extraction and bisulfite specific PCR-based sequencing method

Genomic DNA was extracted from peripheral blood according to the standard procedures. CPGPLOT (http://emboss.bioinformatics.nl/cgi-bin/emboss/cpgplot) was used to identify and plot CpG islands in DJ-1 promoter region. Primer3 (http://frodo.wi.mit.edu/) was used to design PCR bisulfite conversion-specific primers (Table 1).

Bisulfite Specific PCR-based sequencing method was described in our previous report [13]. 1 μg DNA was treated with EZ DNA Methylation-GoldKit (ZYMO RESEARCH) following the manufacture's protocol. After bisulfite conversion, unmethylated cytosines were converted to uracils, the converted product was purified followed by PCR amplification and sequencing. A 20 μl mixture was prepared for each reaction and included 1× HotStarTaq buffer, 2.0 mM Mg^{2+}, 0.2 mM dNTP, 0.2 μM of each primer, 1 U HotStarTaq polymerase (Qiagen Inc.) and 1 μl template DNA. The cycling program was 95 °C for 15 mins; 11 cycles of 94 °C for 20s, 60–0.5 °C per cycle for 40 s, 72 °C for 1 min; 24 cycles of 94 °C for 20 s, 54 °C for 30 s, 72 °C for 1 min; 72 °C for 2 mins. 1U SAP and 6U Exo I were added into 8 μl PCR products for PCR purification. The mixtures were incubated at 37 °C for 60mins, followed by incubation at 70 °C for 10mins. In PCR amplification, the uracils were amplified as thymines, whereas 5-MeC residues were amplified as cytosines. The PCR products were purified to remove any primer dimers and sequenced on an ABI 3730 XL analyzer (Applied Biosystems and Life Technologies, USA). DNA methylation in the PCR target region was then read by scoring the remaining cytosine residues in the sequence. The degree of methylation at each CpG site from the direct sequencing profile was estimated by measuring the relative peak height of the cytosine (C) versus cytosine plus thymine (T) profile (C/(C + T)%). As this can only be regarded as semi-quantitative, the degree

Table 1 Primers for PCR assays

Primer	Sequence (5′ > 3′)	Tm (°C)	Amplicon (bp)
DJ-1- CpG1-methylation-PCR-F	GTTYGGGAGGTTTGGATTAGAGTT	56	170
DJ-1- CpG1-methylation-PCR-R	ACRACTCRATCCCACATAATACCC		
DJ-1- CpG2-methylation-PCR-F	TTGYGTAGTGTGGGGTTGAGG	58	141
DJ-1- CpG2-methylation-PCR-R	ACCRTCCAACACAAAAACACC		
DJ-1- CpG1-methylation-Seq-R	ACRACTCRATCCCACATAATACCC		
DJ-1- CpG2-methylation-Seq-R	ACCRTCCAACACAAAAACACC		
DJ-1- Realtime-F	CGGGGTGCAGGCTTGTAAA	58	150
DJ-1- Realtime-R	TCCGGTTTTCCTGCTCCTTC		

Table 2 Clinical characteristics of subjects

	NC ($n = 40$)	PD ($n = 40$)	*P*-Value
Age, years mean ± sd(lowest,highest)	61.28 ± 9.21(59,80)	63.7 ± 6.16(45,83)	0.228
Gender (male/female)	24/16	24/16	1.0
H&Y stage			
1–2	–	28	–
3	–	8	–
4-5	–	4	–
Duration, years mean ± sd(lowest,highest)	–	5 ± 2.7(2,14)	–

of methylation was expressed as 0, 25, 50, 75 or 100 %.

Cell culture and treatment with 5-Aza-dC

SH-SY5Y cells (ATCC) were cultured in DMEM with 10 % FBS, 100 U/ml penicillin/streptomycin (Invitrogen) and maintained at 37 °C with 5 % CO2. SH-SY5Y cells were chemically treated with 5-Aza-dC (2.5 or 5 mM; Sigma). Real time PCR and Western blot were used to detect the mRNA and protein level of DJ-1. Total RNA was extracted from SH-SY5Y cells after 24 h 5-Aza-dC treatment by a standard method with TRIZOL Reagent (Invitrogen), and reverse-transcribed by using the Prime-Script® RT reagent Kit (Takara) according to the manufacture's instruction. The mRNA levels were detected through real-time PCR by a standard method with Real-time PCR Master Mix (SYBR Green) kit (Takara). The primers for real-time PCR have been summarized in Table 1. We extracted the total protein of SH-SY5Y cells after 5-Aza-dC 48 h treatment. Rabbit anti-DJ-1 antibody (1:1000, sigma) were used for immunoblotting. The results were analyzed in three independent experiments.

Statistical analysis

Statistical analysis was performed using SPSS13.0 and $P < 0.05$ was considered as significant. Statistical analysis included t tests for age. One-way ANOVA was used to evaluate the differences in mRNA and protein levels among SH-SY5Y cells treated by AZA, DMSO and mock groups.

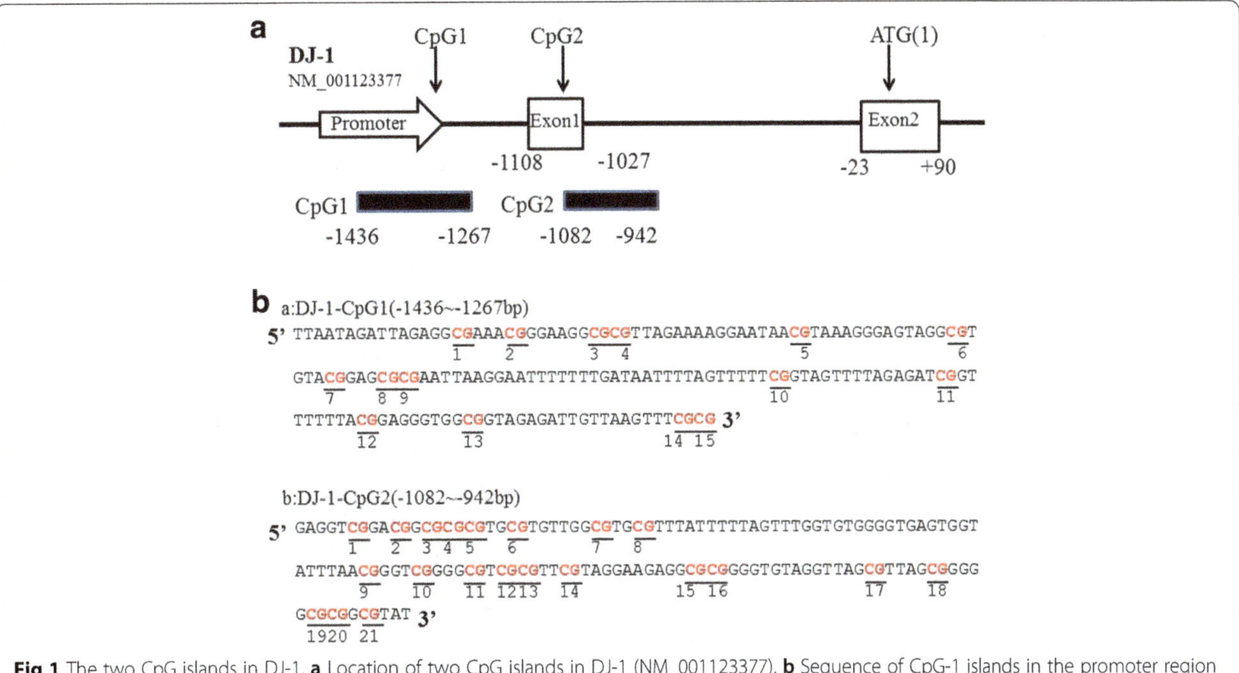

Fig 1 The two CpG islands in DJ-1. **a** Location of two CpG islands in DJ-1 (NM_001123377). **b** Sequence of CpG-1 islands in the promoter region of DJ-1(a), sequence of CpG-2 islands in exon 1 of DJ-1(b)

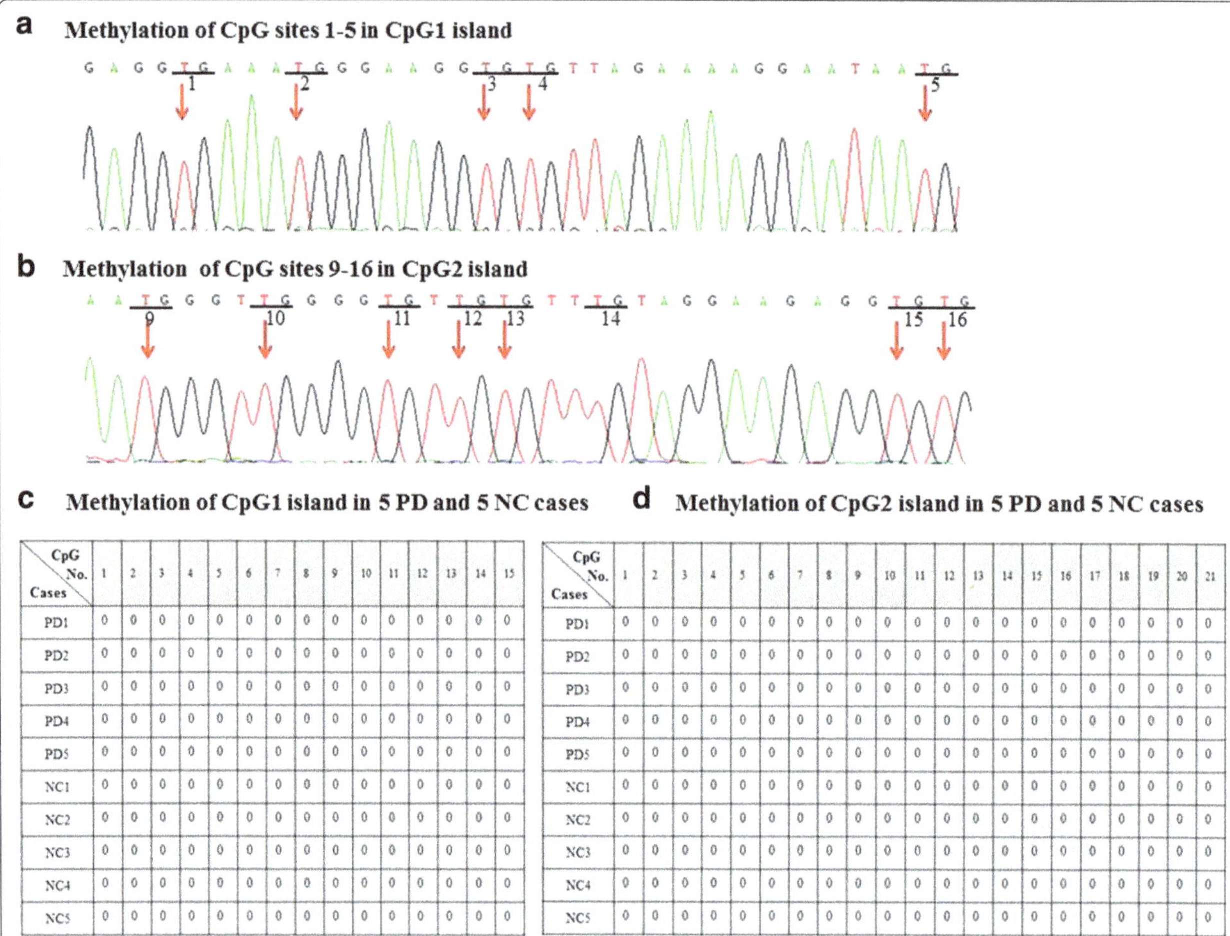

Cases \ CpG No.	1	2	3	4	5	6	7	8	9	10	11	12	13	14	15
PD1	0	0	0	0	0	0	0	0	0	0	0	0	0	0	0
PD2	0	0	0	0	0	0	0	0	0	0	0	0	0	0	0
PD3	0	0	0	0	0	0	0	0	0	0	0	0	0	0	0
PD4	0	0	0	0	0	0	0	0	0	0	0	0	0	0	0
PD5	0	0	0	0	0	0	0	0	0	0	0	0	0	0	0
NC1	0	0	0	0	0	0	0	0	0	0	0	0	0	0	0
NC2	0	0	0	0	0	0	0	0	0	0	0	0	0	0	0
NC3	0	0	0	0	0	0	0	0	0	0	0	0	0	0	0
NC4	0	0	0	0	0	0	0	0	0	0	0	0	0	0	0
NC5	0	0	0	0	0	0	0	0	0	0	0	0	0	0	0

Cases \ CpG No.	1	2	3	4	5	6	7	8	9	10	11	12	13	14	15	16	17	18	19	20	21
PD1	0	0	0	0	0	0	0	0	0	0	0	0	0	0	0	0	0	0	0	0	0
PD2	0	0	0	0	0	0	0	0	0	0	0	0	0	0	0	0	0	0	0	0	0
PD3	0	0	0	0	0	0	0	0	0	0	0	0	0	0	0	0	0	0	0	0	0
PD4	0	0	0	0	0	0	0	0	0	0	0	0	0	0	0	0	0	0	0	0	0
PD5	0	0	0	0	0	0	0	0	0	0	0	0	0	0	0	0	0	0	0	0	0
NC1	0	0	0	0	0	0	0	0	0	0	0	0	0	0	0	0	0	0	0	0	0
NC2	0	0	0	0	0	0	0	0	0	0	0	0	0	0	0	0	0	0	0	0	0
NC3	0	0	0	0	0	0	0	0	0	0	0	0	0	0	0	0	0	0	0	0	0
NC4	0	0	0	0	0	0	0	0	0	0	0	0	0	0	0	0	0	0	0	0	0
NC5	0	0	0	0	0	0	0	0	0	0	0	0	0	0	0	0	0	0	0	0	0

Fig 2 Bisulfite specific PCR-based sequencing analysis of two CpG islands methylation in 40 PD patients and 40 normal controls. **a** and **b** Unmethylated cytosines (**c**) were converted to uracil (U) after bisulfite treatment and amplified as thymines (T) in PCR amplication. Unmethylated CpG sites 1–5 in CpG1 island and CpG sites 9–16 in CpG2 island were shown here as an example. **c** and **d** All the CpG sites of these two CpG islands were unmethylated. Here are the methylation of CpG1 island and CpG2 island from 5 PD and 5 NC cases, and the rest cases showed the exact same methylation pattern

Results

1. Demographic characteristics

   The clinical characteristics are listed in Table 2. Each group comprised 24 men and 16 women, and there was no significant difference in age ($P = 0.228$) between the PD patients (63.7 ± 6.16 years) and NC (61.28 ± 9.21 years). Among the PD patients, 28 had mild degree of the disease (H &Y stage 1–2), 8 moderate (H& Y stage 3), and 4 severe (H&Y stage 4–5). Disease duration of 40 PD patients was 5 ± 2.7 years.
2. DNA Methylation of DJ-1 promoter region detected by Bisulfite specific PCR-based sequencing method

   Based on the NCBI database, the promoter region of human DJ-1 gene (NM_001123377) has two CpG islands (CGIs), locating at−1545 ~ −1244 bp(CpG1),−1178 ~−732 bp(CpG2) upstream of the translation initiation site (Fig. 1a). CpG1 has 15 CpG sequences (Fig. 1b, a). CpG2 contains 21 CpG sequences (Fig. 1b, b). Bisulfite specific PCR-based sequencing method was used to examine the average methylation level at each CpG site (See methods). Our results showed that all the CpG sites probed in the two CGIs were unmethylated in both PD and NC (Fig. 2). The stable unmethylated status of CpG sites in both PD and NC group indicated that CpG methylation in the promoter region of DJ-1 in PBLs might have very limited or no regulatory effects on DJ-1 expression.
3. No effects of methylation inhibitor on the DJ-1 expression in SH-SY5Y cell model

   Previous whole genome bisulfite sequencing (WGBS) study showed that DNA methylation can be detected in various regions, including CGIs, gene

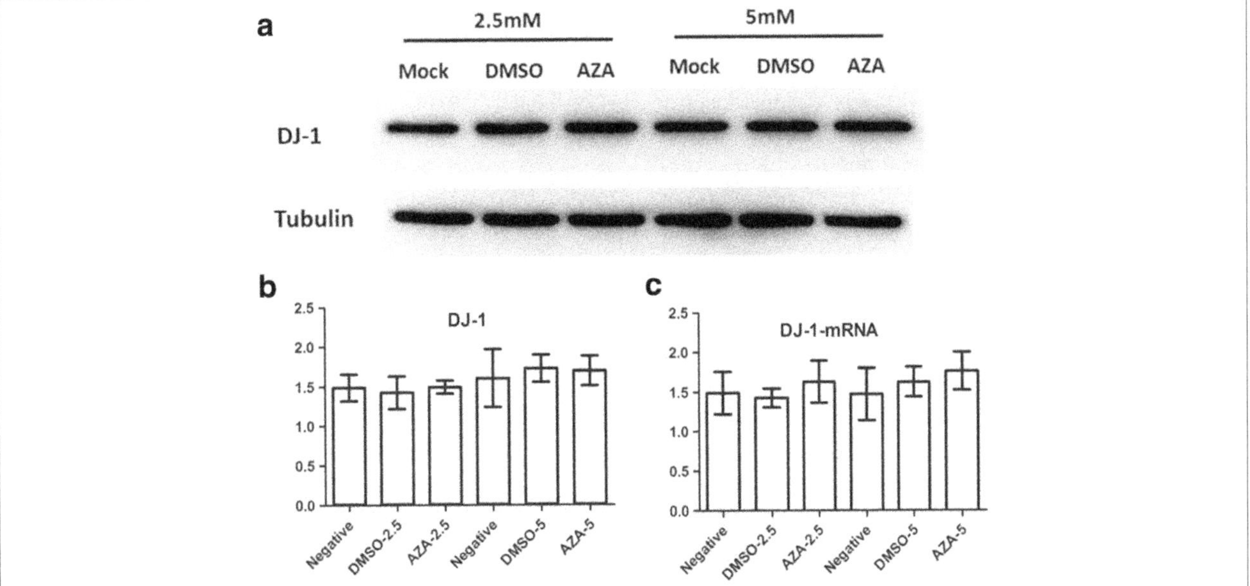

Fig 3 The mRNA and protein levels of DJ-1 did not change in 5-Aza-dC treated SH-SY5Y cells. Western blot and RT-PCR showed no significant change of DJ-1 protein level (**a** & **b**) and mRNA level (**c**) among 5-Aza-dC treated, DMSO treated and mock cells. Bar plot indicated the statistical analysis of DJ-1 protein level (**b**) and mRNA level (**c**) (Mean ± SD, *$p < 0.05$)

bodies and tandem repeating-containing regions [15]. Moreover, methylation levels in these regions can regulate the transcription levels [15, 16]. Although the CpG sites probed in this study were unmethylated in both PD and NC group, the other CpG sites out of the promoter region haven't been determined. In order to test whether CpG methylation level can regulate the DJ-1 expression, methylation inhibitor 5-Aza-dC was used to demethylate the CpG sites in a SH-SY5Y cell model, then DJ-1 expression was detected in the mRNA and protein level. Our results showed DJ-1 expression didn't have significant change in both the mRNA and protein level in SH-SY5Y cells treated with 2.5 mM or 5 mM 5-Aza-dC compared with the untreated cells (Fig. 3). Thus, the results indicated that DNA methylation had no regulatory effects on DJ-1 expression in SH-SY5Y cell model.

Discussion

PD can begin years before the appearance of clinical motor symptoms when a significant number of nigrostriatal dopaminergic neurons have already been degenerated. The detection of PD prior to the emergence of motor symptoms is important for early diagnosis, neuroprotective treatment, monitoring disease progression and response to therapy. Thus, reliable biomarkers, which can represent a pathological process and can be easily detected, are needed. DJ-1 detected from brain [3], CSF [4, 5] and saliva [17] has been thought as a candidate biomarker of PD [18]. Recently, blood-based DNA methylation represents a highly promising biomarker for PD [13, 14] by regulating the causative gene expression. Thus, in the present study, we explored whether there was different DNA methylation level of DJ-1 in the PBLs between PD patients and NC.

Our results showed that in the two CGIs that we probed, all the CpG sites were unmethylated in both PD group and NC group, indicating that CpG methylation in the promoter region of DJ-1 in PBLs might have very limited or no regulatory effects on DJ-1 expression and could not be used as a biomarker to reflect DJ-1 expression changes in brains of PD patients and NC. However, previous WGBS study showed that DNA methylation can be detected in various regions, including CGIs, gene bodies and tandem repeating-containing regions [15]. Methylation levels in these regions can also regulate the transcription levels [15, 16]. Bisulfite specific PCR-based sequencing method used in our study only favored those CpG sites contained within CGIs and promoter regions [16]. Thus all other CpG sites out of the CGIs and promoter region can't be probed by this method. In order to confirm whether CpG methylation can regulate the DJ-1 expression, we used methylation inhibitor to treat SH-SY5Y cells, then DJ-1 expression was detected in the mRNA and protein level. Our results revealed that there was no significant expression change of DJ-1 between the cells treated with methylation inhibitor and non-treated cells. Thus, our results indicated that DNA methylation might not be the key factor in regulating DJ-1 expression.

Generally, gene expression can be regulated in three different levels, transcriptional, mature mRNA processing and translational level. In the transcriptional level, both Sp1 and X-box-binding protein-1S (XBP-1S) were identified as transcription regulatory factor interacting with the DJ-1 promoter, thereby enhancing its promoter trans-activation, mRNA levels and protein expression [19, 20]. In mRNA processing level, miR-494 was found to decrease DJ-1 expression by binding to the 3'UTR of DJ-1 [21]. Till now, the epigenetic mechanism in modulating DJ-1 expression has not been fully explored. Zhou W et al. reported that phenylbutyrate, a HDAC inhibitor, can up-regulate the DJ-1 protein, indicating that DJ-1 expression can be regulated by histone modification [22]. In our study, we explored the possibility that whether DJ-1 expression can be regulated by the DNA methylation. We did not find differential CpG sites methylation in the CGIs of DJ-1 promoter region between PD and NC group, and there was no significant change of DJ-1 expression in a SH-SY5Y cell model treated by methylation inhibitor.

However, there were some limitations in our study. First, the sample size is small, and brain tissue as a standard control is not available in our country. Second, bisulfite specific PCR-based sequencing method used in our study is a convenient and economic method for DNA methylation screening, but it is a semi-quantitative method and only favored those CpG sites in the CGIs and promoter region [16]. Usually, we use PCR-based sequencing method for screening, if it provides any clue of different methylation, we would use bisulfite specific cloning-based sequencing, which is a more accurate and sensitive method to test the cytosine methylation at each CpG site in individual molecules [23], for further study. In this study, no methylated CpG sites were found in both PD and NC. Thus, the results would be the same even bisulfite specific cloning-based sequencing was used. As bisulfite specific PCR-based method only favors those CpG sites in CGIs and promoter region, in order to detect any regulatory effect of CpG sites methylation out of CGIs and promotor region on DJ-1 expression, we treated SH-SY5Y cells with methylation inhibitor and tested the DJ-1 expression level from both the mRNA and protein level, and our results confirmed no regulatory effects of DNA methylation on DJ-1 expression. In this study, we tried our best to get the truth, but the objective limits still exist. For further study, WGBS would be a good way to obtain an unbiased and more complete representation of the methylome by testing in both human brain tissue and PBLs.

Conclusions

CpG sites are unmethylated in DJ-1 promoter region of PBLs from both PD patients and NC. DNA methylation inhibitor didn't alter DJ-1 gene expression in SH-SY5Y cell model. Our results indicated that methylation status of DJ-1 had no obvious regulatory effects on DJ-1 expression, and might not be an efficient biomarker for PD patients.

Competing interests
We declare we have no competing interests.

Authors' contributions
Chen SD, Ding JQ, Tan YY participated in the design of the study; Wu L, Li DH, Liu XL performed the research; Wu L performed the statistical analysis. Tan YY prepared the manuscript. Chen SD revised the manuscript. All authors read and approved the final manuscript.

Acknowledgments
This work was supported by the National Program of Basic Research (2011CB504104) of China, Natural Science Fund (81430022, 81371407, 30872729, 30971031), The Twelfth Five-year National Science and Technology Support Program (2012BAI10B03), Shanghai Key Project of Basic Science Research (10411954500). We acknowledge all the patients and healthy subjects for their generous donations of blood samples without which this study could not be carried out.

Author details
[1]Department of Neurology, and Institute of Neurology, Ruijin Hospital Affiliated to Shanghai Jiao Tong University School of Medicine, Shanghai 200025, China. [2]Department of Neurology, Shanghai Ninth People's Hospital Affiliated to Shanghai Jiao Tong University School of Medicine, Shanghai 200011, China. [3]Parkinson's Disease Center, Beijing Institute for Brain Disorders, Beijing 100069, China.

References

1. Bonifati V, Rizzu P, van Baren MJ, Schaap O, Breedveld GJ, Krieger E, Dekker MC, Squitieri F, Ibanez P, Joosse M, van Dongen JW, Vanacore N, van Swieten JC, Brice A, Meco G, van Duijn CM, Oostra BA, Heutink P. Mutations in the DJ-1 gene associated with autosomal recessive early-onset parkinsonism. Science. 2003;299(5604):256–9.
2. Ariga H, Takahashi-Niki K, Kato I, Maita H, Niki T, Iguchi-Ariga SM. Neuroprotective function of DJ-1 in Parkinson's disease. Oxid Med Cell Longev. 2013;2013:683920.
3. Nural H, He P, Beach T, Sue L, Xia W, Shen Y. Dissembled DJ-1 high molecular weight complex in cortex mitochondria from Parkinson's disease patients. Mol Neurodegener. 2009;4:23.
4. Hong Z, Shi M, Chung KA, Quinn JF, Peskind ER, Galasko D, Jankovic J, Zabetian CP, Leverenz JB, Baird G, Montine TJ, Hancock AM, Hwang H, Pan C,Bradner J, Kang UJ, Jensen PH, Zhang J. DJ-1 and alpha-synuclein in human cerebrospinal fluid as biomarkers of Parkinson's disease. Brain. 2010; 133(Pt 3):713–26.
5. Shi M, Bradner J, Hancock AM, Chung KA, Quinn JF, Peskind ER, Galasko D, Jankovic J, Zabetian CP, Kim HM, Leverenz JB, Montine TJ, Ginghina C, Kang UJ, Cain KC, Wang Y, Aasly J, Goldstein D, Zhang J. Cerebrospinal fluid biomarkers for Parkinson disease diagnosis and progression. Ann Neurol. 2011;69(3):570–80.
6. Waragai M, Wei J, Fujita M, Nakai M, Ho GJ, Masliah E, Akatsu H, Yamada T, Hashimoto M. Increased level of DJ-1 in the cerebrospinal fluids of sporadic Parkinson's disease. Biochem Biophys Res Commun. 2006;345(3):967–72.
7. Qureshi IA, Mehler MF. Advances in epigenetics and epigenomics for neurodegenerative diseases. Curr Neurol Neurosci Rep. 2011;11(5):464–73.
8. Marques SC, Oliveira CR, Pereira CM, Outeiro TF. Epigenetics in neurodegeneration: a new layer of complexity. Prog Neuropsychopharmacol Biol Psychiatry. 2011;35(2):348–55.
9. Migliore L, Coppedè F. Genetics environmental factors and the emerging role of epigenetics in neurodegenerative diseases. Mutat Res. 2009;667(1–2): 82–97.
10. Jiricny J, Menigatti M. DNA cytosine demethylation: are we getting close? Cell. 2008;135:1167e9.
11. Jowaed A, Schmitt I, Kaut O, Wullner U. Methylation regulates alpha-synuclein expression and is decreased in Parkinson's disease patients' brains. J Neurosci. 2010;30:6355e9.
12. Matsumoto L, Takuma H, Tamaoka A, Kurisaki H, Date H, Tsuji S, Iwata A. CpG demethylation enhances alpha-synuclein expression and affects the pathogenesis of Parkinson's disease. PLoS One. 2010;5(11), e15522.

13. Tan YY, Wu L, Zhao ZB, Wang Y, Xiao Q, Liu J, Wang G, Ma JF, Chen SD. Methylation of α-synuclein and leucine-rich repeat kinase 2 in leukocyte DNA of Parkinson's disease patients. Parkinsonism Relat Disord. 2014;20(3): 308–13.
14. Masliah E, Dumaop W, Galasko D. Desplats. PD distinctive patterns of DNA methylation associated with Parkinson disease: identification of concordant epigenetic changes in brain and peripheral blood leukocytes. Epigenetics. 2013;8(10):1030–8.
15. Okae H, Chiba H, Hiura H, Hamada H, Sato A, Utsunomiya T, Kikuchi H, Yoshida H, Tanaka A, Suyama M, Arima T. Genome-wide analysis of DNA methylation dynamics during early human development. PLoS Genet. 2014; 10(12), e1004868.
16. Kobayashi H, Sakurai T, Imai M, Takahashi N, Fukuda A, Yayoi O, Sato S, Nakabayashi K, Hata K, Sotomaru Y, Suzuki Y, Kono T. Contribution of intragenic DNA methylation in mouse gametic DNA methylomes to establish oocyte-specific heritable marks. PLoS Genet. 2012;8(1), e1002440.
17. Kang WY, Yang Q, Jiang XF, Chen W, Zhang LY, Wang XY, Zhang LN, Quinn TJ, Liu J, Chen SD. Salivary DJ-1 could be an indicator of Parkinson's disease progression. Front Aging Neurosci. 2014;6:102.
18. Haas BR, Stewart TH, Zhang J. Premotor biomarkers for Parkinson's disease - a promising direction of research. Transl Neurodegener. 2012;1(1):11.
19. Taira T, Takahashi K, Kitagawa R, Iguchi-Ariga SM, Ariga H. Molecular cloning of human and mouse DJ-1 genes and identification of Sp1-dependent activation of the human DJ-1 promoter. Gene. 2001;263(1–2):285–92.
20. Duplan E, Giaime E, Viotti J, Sévalle J, Corti O, Brice A, Ariga H, Qi L, Checler F, Alves da Costa C. ER-stress-associated functional link between Parkin and DJ-1 via a transcriptional cascade involving the tumor suppressor p53 and the spliced X-box binding protein XBP-1. J Cell Sci. 2013;126(9):2124–33.
21. Xiong R, Wang Z, Zhao Z, Li H, Chen W, Zhang B, Wang L, Wu L, Li W, Ding J, Chen S. MicroRNA-494 reduces DJ-1 expression and exacerbates neurodegeneration. Neurobiol Aging. 2014;35(3):705–14.
22. Zhou W, Bercury K, Cummiskey J, Luong N, Lebin J, Freed CR. Phenylbutyrate up-regulates the DJ-1 protein and protects neurons in cell culture and in animal models of Parkinson disease. J Biol Chem. 2011; 286(17):14941–51.
23. Clark SJ, Statham A, Stirzaker C, Molloy PL, Frommer M. DNA methylation: bisulphite modification and analysis. Nat Protoc. 2006;1(5):2353e64.

17

Endoplasmic reticulum-mitochondria tethering in neurodegenerative diseases

Yi Liu and Xiongwei Zhu*

Abstract

Endoplasmic reticulum (ER) and mitochondria are tubular organelles with a characteristic "network structure" that facilitates the formation of inter-organellar connections. As a result, mitochondria-associated ER membranes (MAMs), a subdomain of the ER that is tightly linked to and communicates with mitochondria, serve multiple physiological functions including lipid synthesis and exchange, calcium signaling, bioenergetics, and apoptosis. Importantly, emerging evidence suggests that the abnormality and dysfunction of MAMs have been involved in various neurodegenerative disorders including Alzheimer's disease, amyotrophic lateral sclerosis, and Parkinson's disease. This review will focus on the architecture and function of MAMs and its involvement in the neurodegenerative diseases.

Keywords: Mitochondria-associated ER membrane, Mitochondria-ER tethering, Alzheimer's disease, Parkinson's disease, Amyotrophic lateral sclerosis

Background

In 1990, Vance [1] found that crude rat liver mitochondrial fraction was capable of rapid and linked synthesis of phospholipids and also contained phosphatidylserine synthase (PSS) and phosphatidylethanolamine methyltransferase activities which were absent from highly purified mitochondria. This could be attributed to the presence of a membrane fraction 'X' in the crude but not highly purified mitochondria. It turns out that this fraction 'X', now commonly regarded as the mitochondrial associated membrane (MAMs), is a specialized subdomain of the endoplasmic reticulum (ER) with specific lipid and protein composition that is involved in the crosstalk with mitochondria. Phospholipid synthesis and exchange was the first identified function of MAMs. Later, it was demonstrated by electron tomography that ER and mitochondria are linked by high electron-dense tethers (10 nm at the smooth ER and 25 nm at the rough ER) termed as mitochondria-ER tethers (a.k.a., *M*itochondria-*ER* contact/crosslink/crosstalk/communication or MERC) [2, 3]. In fact, approximately 5 ~ 20% of the mitochondrial surface is juxtaposed (10–30 nm distances) to specialized regions of the ER tubules [4–7]. Such a short distance suggests that the two organelles are tethered together by proteins on the juxtaposed membranes [7]. MERC appear to be stable structures. Although the ER and mitochondrial membranes form multiple and specific crosslink sites, it must be emphasized that they do not fuse but instead still maintain the organelles' distinct structures and characteristics which is crucial for them to serve as a major platform to carry out important physiological roles in the regulation of intracellular calcium homeostasis [6, 8–12], lipid metabolism [1, 13], mitochondrial fission [14], autophagosome formation [15] and apoptosis progression [16, 17]. In this review, we will focus on recent data addressing the structural composition and function of the MAMs in mammalian system and its potential involvement in various neurodegenerative diseases.

ER–mitochondria tethering protein complexes

The molecular details of ER–mitochondria tethers are largely unknown. Electron microscopic studies showed that the cleft of a MERC is typically dotted by electron-dense areas that are widely accepted to be formed by protein complexes. The MAM fraction can be detached from mitochondria through the limited digestion with trypsin or Proteinase K which is suggestive of proteinaceous characteristics [7]. Indeed, several pairs of integral membrane proteins located on mitochondria and ER important for MERC formation and physical

* Correspondence: xiongwei.zhu@case.edu
Department of Pathology, Case Western Reserve University, Cleveland, OH, USA

tethering of the organelles were identified (Fig. 1) [5]. Additional proteins that localize in the cleft of the MERC and participate in its biochemical activity or functional regulation might also, directly or indirectly, participate in MERC formation or maintenance such as by spacing apart the opposing membranes of the ER and the mitochondrion at a distance that allows the formation of MERC tethers.

1. **Mfn2 Tether**
   Mitofusin 2 (Mfn2) is a large GTPase involved in the fusion of mitochondrial outer membrane. After the initial report from Luca Scorrano's group suggesting the potential involvement of Mfn2 in ER-mitochondrial tethering, Mfn2 is among the most widely studied ER-mitochondria tethering protein factors but its exact role in MERC regulation is still in hot debate. In 2008, Luca Scoranno and colleagues found that Mfn2 ablation caused dramatic defects in ER morphology in vitro in mouse embryonic fibroblasts(MEFs) and HeLa cells [18]. It turned out that Mfn2 is enriched at MERC and is required for the juxtaposition of ER to mitochondria [18]. ER-located Mfn2 interacts *in trans* with mitochondrial mitofusins (i.e., Mfn1 or Mfn2) to form trans-organelle hetero- or homo- dimer tethers to bridge the mitochondria onto ER which allows efficient calcium transfer between ER and mitochondria [18, 19]. The confocal microscopy analysis revealed that the distance between ER and mitochondria increases in cells lacking Mfn2 which impairs mitochondrial calcium uptake [18, 19]. Indeed, the presence and enrichment of Mfn2 in the interface between ER and mitochondria is directly demonstrated by immunoelectron microscopy in Melanocytes [20]. Moreover, Mfn2-mediated ER-mitochondria tethering is regulated by MitoL-dependent activation of mitochondrial Mfn2 through ubiquitination and MitoL ablation inhibited Mfn2 complex formation and caused Mfn2 mislocalization from MAM to non-MAM ER [21]. Owing to its well-known role in the tethering of adjacent membranes, Mfn2 is widely accepted as a major regulator of MERC in different tissues [18, 19, 22]. However, such a view was challenged by a quantitative electron microscopic study followed by a series morphological and functional studies from multiple groups: In 2012, Pierre C et al. reported that the percentage of mitochondria in close contact with ER tubules was increased in Mfn2 defective MEFs when compared to wildtype MEFs (4.91% vs 2.25%,

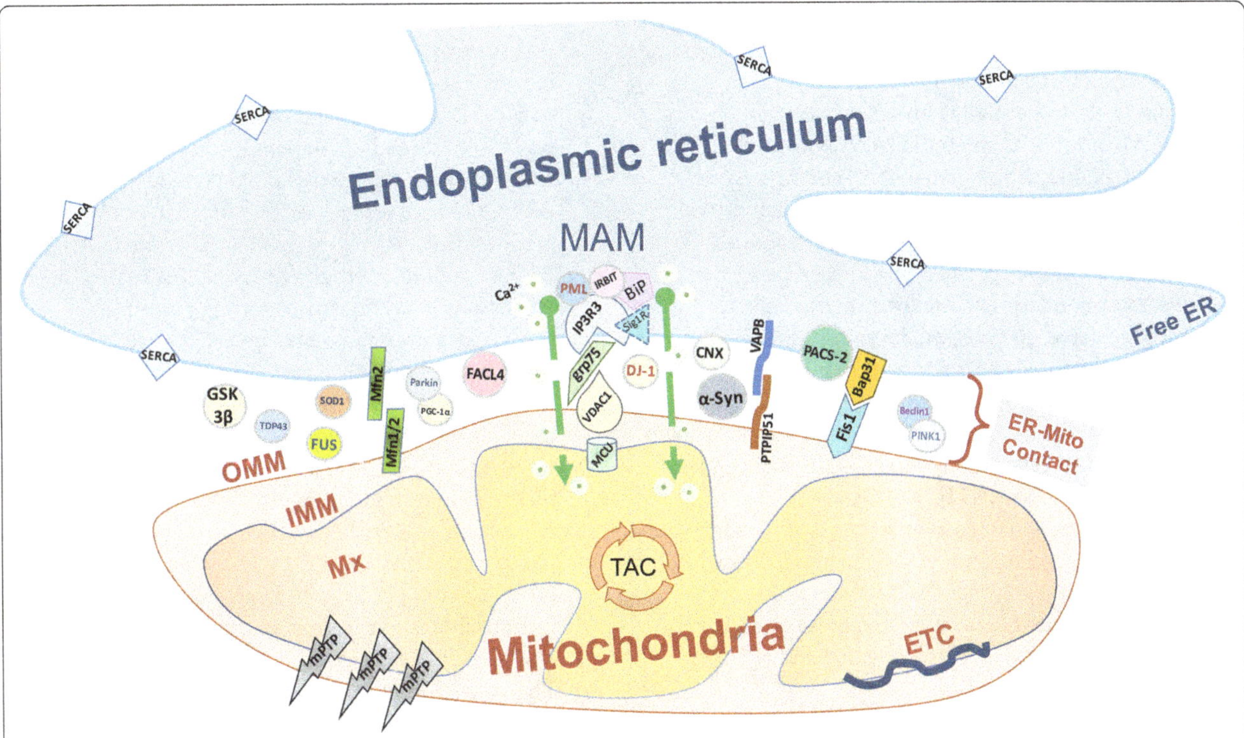

Fig. 1 Global view of the architecture/choreography of ER–mitochondria contacts. As depicted, a part of ER tubule and mitochondria form quasi-synaptic structure. Several pairs of integral membrane proteins located on mitochondria and ER important for MERC formation and physical tethering of the organelles were identified, including Mfn1/2 tether, Fis1-Bap31 tether, VAPB-PTPIP51 tether and IP3R-grp75-VDAC1 tripartite complex. The latter is essential for the efficient Ca^{2+} transfer from the ER to mitochondria. MAM: mitochondria associated ER membrane, OMM = outer mitochondrial membrane, IMM: inner mitochondrial membrane, Mx = matrix, ETC: electron transport chain, TAC: tricarboxylic acid cycle

the distance between ER and mitochondria was restricted to <20 nm in the study). In 2015, Riccardo Filadia et al. confirmed this EM findings that the ER-mitochondria crosslink was increased in Mfn2 defective MEFs and SH-SY5Y cells and provided functional evidence of an elevated calcium flow from ER to mitochondria in Mfn2 defective MEFs [23]. While they also confirmed the confocal microscopy results from Scoranno's group that Mfn2 deficiency caused a net decrease in the overlapping area between ER and mitochondria, they noted that the dramatic changes in mitochondrial morphology caused by Mfn2 ablation resulted in changes in mitochondrial area which could make classical colocalization analysis unsuitable. Excluding the confounding effects of area change, they found that mitochondrial perimeter colocalizing with the ER actually increased in Mfn2 deficient cells [23]. Other groups also reported that Mfn2 knockdown increased ER-mitochondria tethering and calcium transfer from ER to mitochondria [24]. Along this line, deficiency in Gp78 (a.k.a. autocrine motility factor receptor, AMFR), an endoplasmic-reticulum (ER)-associated protein degradation E3 ubiquitin ligase involved in the degradation of Mfn2, caused significantly decreased rough ER-mitochondria crosstalk as evaluated by EM which could be blocked by Mfn2 knockdown, suggesting that Gp78 might promote ER-mitochondria interaction through degradation of Mfn2 [25]. Collectively, these studies strongly challenges the role of Mfn2 as an essential component of ER-mitochondrial tethering but argues for a role of Mfn2 as a negative regulator of organelle apposition. Most recently, Luca Scorrano's group responded to these challenges by providing further ultramorphometric and confocal microscopic evidence based on unbiased fluorescent probes of ER-mitochondrial proximity to demonstrate that Mfn2 ablation increases ER-mitochondria distance which resulted in impaired mitochondrial calcium uptake in an mitochondrial calcium uniporter (MCU)-independent manner in MEF cells [22], yet the number of ER-mitochondria contacts were not directly addressed in this study and it is not clear whether and how larger ER-mitochondrial distance may affect ER-mitochondrial tethering. Further research is needed to fully elucidate the role of Mfn2 at MERC.

2. **VAPB-PTPIP51 Tether**
   Vesicle-associated membrane protein-associated protein B (VAPB) is an integral protein in the ER membrane involved in ER unfolded protein response and the regulation of cellular calcium homeostasis [26]. Most recently, it was demonstrated that VAPB interacts with mitochondrial outer membrane protein tyrosine phosphatase-interacting protein-51 (PTPIP51) [27]. Overexpression of either proteins increase, while knockdown of either protein decreases, ER-mitochondria tethering along with functional changes such as calcium exchange between the two organelles, suggesting that this pair of proteins forms another molecular scaffold to tether the two organelles [28].
3. **Fis1-Bap31 Tether**
   As an ER protein-sorting factor, B-cell receptor-associated protein 31 (Bap31), an abundant 28-kDa integral membrane chaperone protein of the ER, forms several large protein complexes and controls the fate of newly synthesized integral membrane proteins. An earlier study demonstrated that outer membrane associated active caspase 8 could cleave ER-associated Bap31 and the cleavage product p20Bap31 mediated mitochondrion-ER cross talk through a calcium-dependent mechanism [29]. The overexpression of P20Bap31 could lead to early release of calcium from ER and concomitant uptake of calcium into mitochondria [30], implicating the functional involvement of Bap31 in ER-mitochondrial tethering. More recently, it was demonstrated that mitochondrial fission protein Fission 1 homologue (Fis1) interacts with Bap31 and forms an ER-mitochondrial platform which is essential in the recruitment and activation of procaspase 8 and the conveyance of the apoptotic signal from mitochondria to ER [31]. Given that Fis1-Bap31 interaction is also present in normal, non-apoptotic cells [31], it likely constitutes a preformed scaffold complex to tether ER-mitochondria together that may have roles broader than apoptotic signaling. The role of Bap31 in ER-mitochondria tethering may be modulated by phosphofurin acidic cluster sorting protein 2 (PACS-2), a multifunctional cytosolic sorting protein: depletion of PACS-2 caused Bap-31-dependent mitochondrial fragmentation and uncoupling from the ER along with inhibition of calcium signal transmission [32]. More recently, it was demonstrated that mammalian target of rapamycin complex 2 regulates the integrity of MAM by Akt-dependent phosphorylation of PACS-2 [33] although how PACS-2 promotes MAM integrity and regulates its composition is not entirely clear.
4. **IP3R3-Grp75-VDAC1**
   The voltage-dependent anion channel (VDAC) of the outer mitochondrial membrane interacts with the ER calcium-release channel inositol 1,4,5-trisphosphate receptor (IP3R) through the molecular chaperone glucose-regulated protein 75 (grp75), which is essential for the efficient calcium transfer from the ER to mitochondria [34, 35].

Despite such an important functional role, this tripartite complex may not have a tethering role, but rather a MERC spacing/filling function that derives from functionally coupling ER and mitochondria in calcium exchanges. Nevertheless, the ER-resident protein Sigma1R (Sig-1R) stabilizes MAM by interacting with VDAC and IP3R and prolongs the calcium signaling in MAMs [36].

Functions of MAM

Mitochondria and ER have crucial but distinctive roles in mammalian cells. ER-mitochondria tethering provides a platform facilitating the crosstalk between these two organelles which appears essential for the function of these organelles. Indeed, it becomes increasingly clear that MAM plays an important role in various cellular processes critical for cell survival and death, which is briefly discussed below.

1. **Phospholipid Synthesis and Exchange**
   While lipid synthesis largely occurs in the ER, it needs the assistance of other organelles since several of the key enzymes are located on the membrane of other organelles such as mitochondria [13, 37]. MAMs were initially described as an ER subdomain enriched in proteins involved in lipid metabolism such as PSS1 and PSS2 with an ascribed function as a platform for lipid biosynthesis and exchange [1, 38]. Indeed, phosphatidylserine is first synthesized in the MAM by PSS1 and PSS2 [39]; then transferred to the closely apposed mitochondrion, where a decarboxylase in the inner mitochondrial membrane converts it to phosphatidylethanolamine; to make phosphotidylcholine, phosphatidylethanolamine is transferred back to the ER, where a methyltransferase converts it into phosphatidylcholine, a major component of the cell membrane. Phosphotidylcholine must be transferred back to mitochondria again since it is present in mitochondrial membrane [13]. Later studies revealed that MAMs are also the site of triacylglycerol synthesis and steroidogenesis [40]. Another lipid metabolism associated enzyme enriched in MAMs is Long-chain-fatty-acid-CoA ligase 4 (FACL4), also known as acyl-CoA synthetase long-chain family member 4, which mediates the ligation of fatty acids to coenzyme A (CoA) and other cholesterol metabolites. Acyl-coenzyme A:cholesterol acyltransferase-1 that catalyzes the formation of cholesterol esters and diacylglycerol acyltransferase are also enriched in MAMs [41, 42].
2. **Calcium Transfer**
   The calcium homeostasis of mitochondria is of vital significance to mitochondria and cell as a whole. On one hand, moderate loading of mitochondrial calcium has an important physiological function to stimulate ATP production through calcium-dependent activation of the key metabolic enzymes in the Krebs cycle such as pyruvate dehydrogenase and α-ketoglutarate dehydrogenase [43]. On the other hand, calcium overloading of mitochondria causes the opening of mitochondrial permeability transition pore (mPTP) and leads to cell apoptosis [44]. ER is the intracellular calcium store and MAMs facilitate the calcium transfer between ER and mitochondria [9, 11]. While outer mitochondrial membrane is permeable to calcium through VDAC1, the inner mitochondrial membrane is not and calcium needs to go through MCU in the inner mitochondrial membrane [45–47]. As a low affinity calcium channel, MCU requires high calcium levels which can be efficiently achieved by the MAM through IP3R3-grp75-VDAC1 complex: the calcium released from ER through IP3R to the VDAC1 on the OMM leads to localized sites of calcium influx in the intermembrane space and creates the microdomain of high [Ca^{2+}] (calcium puff) close to MCU and thus facilitate the calcium uptake by MCU [48, 49]. The IP3R3-grp75-VDAC1 complex also serves as a molecular scaffold for other calcium handling players (Sig-1R [36], BiP, Bcl-2 [50], IRBIT [51], etc.), which may be essential for the fine-tuning of the calcium signaling of IP3R3-grp75-VDAC1 axis at the MAM.
3. **Regulation of Mitochondrial Fission**
   Mitochondria are highly dynamic organelles that undergo continuous fusion and division which is critical for the homeostasis of mitochondria [52]. Mitochondrial fission involves the translocation of cytosolic dynamin-like protein (DLP1) to the outer membrane of mitochondria where it oligomerizes into ring-like structures that wrap around the mitochondrial constriction sites [14, 53, 54]. Interestingly, during fission, mitochondria appeared to be constricted at the point of contact with the ER. In both yeast and mammalian cells, Dnm1 (DLP1 yeast ortholog)/DLP1 localizes to the mitochondrial membrane constriction site wrapped by ER tubules [14]. Three-dimensional electron microscopic study of the structure of MERC in *Saccharomyces cerevisiae* revealed that mitochondria-associated ER tubules might mediate the formation of mitochondrial constriction sites [14]. The presence of ER tubules at mitochondrial constriction and fission sites has been further evidenced using a two-color STORM super-resolution study [55]. In fact, the perimeter of mitochondria tubules circumscribed by ER decreased by ~30% when compared with the uncircumscribed which better fit for the action of narrower DLP1 ring [14]. A later

study revealed that the ER-localized protein inverted formin 2 is activated during fission to polymerize actin, which in turn might generate the driving force for initial mitochondrial constriction at the ER-mitochondria contact site [56].

4. **Apoptosis**
Both mitochondria and ER play a role in apoptosis and MERC provides a platform for the two organelles to exchange signals to regulate and coordinate a rapid and orderly cell demise [57]. The Fis1-Bap31 tethering complex (as discussed in "Fis1-Bap31 tether" earlier) allows for apoptotic signals being transferred from mitochondria to the ER by recruiting and activating caspase 8 which cleaves Bap31 into the pro-apoptotic p20Bap31 [31]. P20Bap31 propagates the apoptotic signal from ER back to mitochondria by stimulating the ER calcium release which activates and opens the mPTP and thus amplifies the death signal [58]. IP3R-Grp75-VDAC1 complex at the MAM is crucial for mitochondrial calcium uptake which could thus participate in the apoptotic signal through mitochondrial calcium overload. SUMOylation of DLP1 was also reported to stabilize the MERC and promote calcium crosstalk and cytochrome c release [59].

Disturbed ER-mitochondria tethering in neurodegenerative disorders

Alzheimer's disease (AD), Parkinson's disease (PD), and amyotrophic lateral sclerosis with associated frontotemporal dementia (ALS/FTD) are major neurodegenerative diseases. These neurodegenerative diseases are characterized by damage to various cellular processes, many of which are regulated by ER-mitochondria tethering. Indeed, abnormal MAM signaling is reported in all these neurodegenerative diseases as reviewed below.

1. **Alzheimer's Disease**
Presenilins are the catalytic subunits of the gamma secretase responsible for the generation of amyloid-β (Aβ) [60]. Mutations in presenilin 1 (PS1) and 2 (PS2) cause human familial AD. Presenilins were present in many compartments in the cell including ER and mitochondria [61]. Eric Schon's group first demonstrated the enrichment of presenilins in the MAM and suggested that MAM is the predominant subcellular location for PS1/PS2 and gamma secretase activity and later further demonstrated significantly increased MAM function and ER-mitochondrial communication in presenilin-deficient cells and in fibroblasts from patients with both the familial and sporadic forms of AD, suggesting that upregulated MAM function and increased ER-mitochondria crosstalk may be involved in the pathogenesis of AD [60, 62, 63]. Indeed, expression of MAM-associated proteins were significantly increased in postmortem brain of human AD patients and in the APP transgenic mice although direct evidence of specific alterations in the ER-mitochondria interaction was lacking [64]. Consistent with this notion, Aβ treatment leads to increased MAM protein expression and increased MERC in cultured neurons and ApoE4 allele also upregulated MAM function [65]. However, another group, although agreeing upon the notion that presenilin modulates MAM function, disagreed on the specific effects of PS2 on MAM: Pizzo's group reported that the expression of the PS2, but not of PS1, facilitates the physical interaction and functional coupling between ER and mitochondria in Mfn2-dependent manner [66]. The reason for the discrepancy is not clear.

2. **Amyotrophic Lateral Sclerosis with associated Frontotemporal Dementia**
Mutations in genes encoding several different MAM proteins, including a tethering protein, were associated with familial ALS which provides strong evidence to support the involvement of disturbed MAM function in the pathogenesis of ALS although it is hard to reconcile whether upregulated or disrupted MAM function plays the pathogenic role. VAPB interacts with the OMM protein PTPIP51 to form a MAM tether complex [27]. P56S mutation of VAPB causes autosomal-dominant ALS and VAPB-P56S mutant demonstrated higher affinity for PTPIP51 and consequently, increased Ca^{2+} transfer into mitochondria [27]. On the other hand, Sig-1R is another MAM protein that participates in the IP3R function to facilitate calcium signaling at MAM [36]. Mutations in Sig-1R caused juvenile ALS although in an autosomal recessive pattern [67]. Loss of Sig-1R function by gene mutation or downregulation has been shown to break ER–mitochondria associations [68]. ALS-causing superoxide dismutase 1 (SOD1) mutants aggregated and accumulated at MAM which compromised the integrity and activity of MAM [69]. ALS/FTD-associated TAR DNA-binding protein 43 (TDP-43), and fused in sarcoma (FUS) could also disrupt the MERC and perturb mitochondrial calcium uptake from ER through activation of glycogen synthase kinase 3β (GSK3β) which in turn perturbs VAPB-PTPIP51 interaction [28].

3. **Parkinson's Disease**
Mutations in α-synuclein gene cause autosomal dominant PD and α-synuclein aggregates were major components of Lewy bodies. α-synuclein is present

in MAM [70, 71], but pathogenic point mutations of α-synuclein result in its reduced association with MAM, coincident with a lower degree of apposition of ER with mitochondria, a decrease in MAM function, and an increase in mitochondrial fragmentation. Mutations in PARK2 gene (encoding Parkin protein) is associated with juvenile onset autosomal recessive forms of PD. Parkin is ATF4-dependently upregulated during mitochondrial and ER stress, which regulates the functional interplay between ER and mitochondria to help promote cell survival under stress [72]. Interestingly, Parkin is translocated to endoplasmic reticulum (ER) and mitochondrial/ER junctions following excitotoxicity, implicating a potential role for Parkin in MAM [73]. Indeed, a confocal microscopic study showed that Parkin overexpression resulted in enhanced physical coupling between ER and mitochondria and favored calcium transfer from the ER to the mitochondria following 1,4,5 inositol trisphosphate (InsP3) generating agonist and increased the agonist-induced ATP production in vitro [74]. Such a positive effect of Parkin on the ER-mitochondria interaction has been confirmed in nigral neurons by EM analysis [75]. However, a recent study demonstrated enhanced ER-mitochondria tethering in primary fibroblasts from Parkin knockout mice and PD patients with PARK2 gene mutations as well as in neurons derived from induced pluripotent stem cells of a patient with PARK2 gene mutations along with ER-to-mitochondria calcium transfers likely due to increased Mfn2 in MAMs [76]. PINK1, another familial PD and mitochondria quality control associated protein, and the pro-autophagic protein BECN1/Beclin1 were both found at MAM, the PINK1 and Beclin1 interaction enhanced ER-mitochondria contact and promoted the formation of autophagosome following mitophagy induction [77]. Mutations or deletion of DJ-1 are associated with autosomal recessive early onset familial PD. It was reported that DJ-1 is also present in the MAMs. DJ-1 overexpression caused increased Mitochondria-ER colocalization as demonstrated by confocal microscopy [78]. Whether this represents true increase in the MERC needs to be confirmed by other methods since confocal microscopy does not permit accurate quantification of the <30 nm distance.

Conclusions

Although it remains to be fully characterized how ER-mitochondria contacts are maintained and regulated, it is becoming increasingly clear that MERC provide an important platform to intertwine various signaling pathways to carry out many cellular processes of importance to neuronal function including the regulation of calcium homeostasis, phospholipid synthesis and exchange, mitochondrial biogenesis and dynamics and apoptosis. It is interesting that disturbance in MERC are involved in most of the neurodegenerative diseases studied such as AD, PD and ALS as discussed above. Indeed, disturbance in MERC provides a connection for the various seemingly disparate features of these neurodegenerative diseases which may suggest that the disturbance in MERC may serve as a common convergent mechanism underlying neurodegeneration. Admittedly appealing, this hypothesis faces several challenges. First, the many conflicting observations, likely due to the different methods used, need to be reconciled. For example, the fundamental involvement of Mfn2 in the ER-mitochondria tethering is under hot debate and the effects of PS2 on MAM need clarification. Secondly, it appears that both upregulated and disrupted MAM functions are implicated in neurodegenerative diseases, even in the same disease. For example, VAPB-P56S mutant caused enhanced ER-mitochondria crosstalk while TDP43 and FUS disrupted ER-mitochondria contacts. While both upregulated and disrupted MAM function could lead to cellular dysfunction and neurodegeneration, this highlights the need to characterize the effects of specific neurodegenerative disease insults on the ER–mitochondria axis. Thirdly, the detailed mechanism of MAM disturbance in these conditions needs to be worked out. Is there a common mechanism? TDP43 and FUS disrupt the VAPB-PTPIP51 tethering through GSK3β activation. While GSK3β is activated in many of these neurodegenerative diseases, it may not elicit the same outcome since PS1 mutation caused GSK3β activation [79] but led to increased ER-mitochondria tethering [80]. Fundamentally, therefore, the pathophysiological relevance of these observations also need to be firmly established.

Abbreviations

AD: Alzheimer's disease; ALS: Amyotrophic lateral sclerosis; Aβ: Amyloid-β; Bap31: B-cell receptor-associated protein 31; CoA: Coenzyme A; DLP1: Dynamin-like protein; ER: Endoplasmic reticulum; FACL4: Long-chain-fatty-acid-CoA ligase 4; Fis1: Mitochondrial fission 1 protein; FTD: Frontotemporal dementia; FUS: Fused in sarcoma; grp75: Glucose-regulated protein 75; GSK3β: Glycogen synthase kinase 3β; IP3R: Inositol 1,4,5-trisphosphate receptor; MAMs: Mitochondrial associated membrane; MCU: Mitochondrial calcium uniporter; MERC: Mitochondria-ER contact/crosslink/crosstalk/communication; Mfn: Mitofusin; mPTP: Mitochondrial permeability transition pore; PACS-2: Phosphofurin acidic cluster sorting protein 2; PARK2: Parkin; PD: Parkinson's disease; PS: Presenilin; PSS: Phosphatidylserine synthase; PTPIP51: Protein tyrosine phosphatase-interacting protein-51; SERCA: Sarco–endoplasmic reticulum Ca^{2+} ATPase; Sig-1R: Sigma1R; SOD1: Superoxide dismutase 1; TCA: Tricarboxylic acid cycle; TDP-43: TAR DNA-binding protein 43; VAPB: Vesicle-associated membrane protein-associated protein B; VDAC: Voltage-dependent anion channel

Acknowledgements

Not applicable.

Funding

This work is partly supported by National Institute of Health (grant numbers NS083385 and AG049479 to XZ) and Alzheimer's Association (AARG-16-443584 to XZ).

Authors' contributions

YL and XZ conceived and wrote the manuscript. Both authors read and approved the final manuscript.

Competing interests

X.Z. is a paid consultant of Sierra Research Group LLC.

References

1. Vance JE. Phospholipid synthesis in a membrane fraction associated with mitochondria. J Biol Chem. 1990;265(13):7248–56.
2. Montisano DF, et al. Association between mitochondria and rough endoplasmic reticulum in rat liver. Anat Rec. 1982;203(4):441–50.
3. Pickett CB, et al. The physical association between rat liver mitochondria and rough endoplasmic reticulum. I. Isolation, electron microscopic examination and sedimentation equilibrium centrifugation analyses of rough endoplasmic reticulum-mitochondrial complexes. Exp Cell Res. 1980;128(2):343–52.
4. Rowland AA, Voeltz GK. Endoplasmic reticulum-mitochondria contacts: function of the junction. Nat Rev Mol Cell Biol. 2012;13(10):607–25.
5. Kornmann B. The molecular hug between the ER and the mitochondria. Curr Opin Cell Biol. 2013;25(4):443–8.
6. Rizzuto R, et al. Close contacts with the endoplasmic reticulum as determinants of mitochondrial Ca2+ responses. Science. 1998;280(5379):1763–6.
7. Csordas G, et al. Structural and functional features and significance of the physical linkage between ER and mitochondria. J Cell Biol. 2006;174(7):915–21.
8. Boehning D, et al. Cytochrome c binds to inositol (1,4,5) trisphosphate receptors, amplifying calcium-dependent apoptosis. Nat Cell Biol. 2003;5(12):1051–61.
9. Patergnani S, et al. Calcium signaling around mitochondria associated membranes (MAMs). Cell Commun Signal. 2011;9(1):19.
10. Hajnoczky G, Csordas G, Yi M. Old players in a new role: mitochondria-associated membranes, VDAC, and ryanodine receptors as contributors to calcium signal propagation from endoplasmic reticulum to the mitochondria. Cell Calcium. 2002;23(5):363–77.
11. Pinton P, et al. Calcium and apoptosis: ER-mitochondria Ca2+ transfer in the control of apoptosis. Oncogene. 2008;27(50):6407–18.
12. Wang HJ, et al. Calcium regulates the association between mitochondria and a smooth subdomain of the endoplasmic reticulum. J Cell Biol. 2000;150(6):1489–98.
13. Vance JE. MAM (mitochondria-associated membranes) in mammalian cells: lipids and beyond. Biochim Biophys Acta. 2014;1841(4):595–609.
14. Friedman JR, et al. ER tubules mark sites of mitochondrial division. Science. 2011;334(6954):358–62.
15. Hamasaki M, et al. Autophagosomes form at ER-mitochondria contact sites. Nature. 2013;495(7441):389–93.
16. van Vliet AR, Verfaillie T, Agostinis P. New functions of mitochondria associated membranes in cellular signaling. Biochim Biophys Acta. 2014;1843(10):2253–62.
17. Cardenas C, et al. Essential regulation of cell bioenergetics by constitutive InsP3 receptor Ca2+ transfer to mitochondria. Cell. 2010;142(2):270–83.
18. de Brito OM, Scorrano L. Mitofusin 2 tethers endoplasmic reticulum to mitochondria. Nature. 2008;456(7222):605–10.
19. Merkwirth C, Langer T. Mitofusin 2 builds a bridge between ER and mitochondria. Cell. 2008;135(7):1165–7.
20. Daniele T, Hurbain I, Vago R, Casari G, Raposo G, Tacchetti C, Schiaffino MV. Mitochondria and melanosomes establish physical contacts modulated by Mfn2 and involved in organelle biogenesis. Curr Biol. 2014;24(4):393–403.
21. Sugiura A, et al. MITOL regulates endoplasmic reticulum-mitochondria contacts via Mitofusin2. Mol Cell. 2013;51(1):20–34.
22. Naon, D., Zaninello, M., Giacomello, M., Varanita, T., Grespi, F., Lakshminaranayan, S., ... & Zorzano, A., Critical reappraisal confirms that Mitofusin 2 is an endoplasmic reticulum–mitochondria tether. Proc Natl Acad Sci 2016. 113(40): p. 11249-11254.
23. Filadi R, et al. Mitofusin 2 ablation increases endoplasmic reticulum-mitochondria coupling. Proc Natl Acad Sci U S A. 2015;112(17):E2174–81.
24. Leal NS, et al. Mitofusin-2 knockdown increases ER-mitochondria contact and decreases amyloid beta-peptide production. J Cell Mol Med. 2016;20(9):1686–95.
25. Wang PT, et al. Distinct mechanisms controlling rough and smooth endoplasmic reticulum contacts with mitochondria. J Cell Sci. 2015;128(15):2759–65.
26. Kanekura K, et al. Characterization of amyotrophic lateral sclerosis-linked P56S mutation of vesicle-associated membrane protein-associated protein B (VAPB/ALS8). J Biol Chem. 2006;281(40):30223–33.
27. De Vos KJ, et al. VAPB interacts with the mitochondrial protein PTPIP51 to regulate calcium homeostasis. Hum Mol Genet. 2012;21(6):1299–311.
28. Stoica R, et al. ER-mitochondria associations are regulated by the VAPB-PTPIP51 interaction and are disrupted by ALS/FTD-associated TDP-43. Nat Commun. 2014;5:3996.
29. Chandra D, et al. Association of active caspase 8 with the mitochondrial membrane during apoptosis: potential roles in cleaving BAP31 and caspase 3 and mediating mitochondrion-endoplasmic reticulum cross talk in etoposide-induced cell death. Mol Cell Biol. 2004;24(15):6592–607.
30. Breckenridge DG, et al. Caspase cleavage product of BAP31 induces mitochondrial fission through endoplasmic reticulum calcium signals, enhancing cytochrome c release to the cytosol. J Cell Biol. 2003;160(7):1115–27.
31. Iwasawa R, et al. Fis1 and Bap31 bridge the mitochondria-ER interface to establish a platform for apoptosis induction. EMBO J. 2011;30(3):556–68.
32. Simmen T, et al. PACS-2 controls endoplasmic reticulum–mitochondria communication and bid-mediated apoptosis. EMBO J. 2005;24(4):717–29.
33. Betz C, et al. mTOR complex 2-Akt signaling at mitochondria-associated endoplasmic reticulum membranes (MAM) regulates mitochondrial physiology. Proc Natl Acad Sci U S A. 2013;110(31):12526–34.
34. Szabadkai G, et al. Chaperone-mediated coupling of endoplasmic reticulum and mitochondrial Ca2+ channels. J Cell Biol. 2006;175(6):901–11.
35. De Stefani D, et al. VDAC1 selectively transfers apoptotic Ca2+ signals to mitochondria. Cell Death Differ. 2012;19(2):267–73.
36. Hayashi T, Su TP. Sigma-1 receptor chaperones at the ER-mitochondrion interface regulate ca(2+) signaling and cell survival. Cell. 2007;131(3):596–610.
37. Voelker DR. Bridging gaps in phospholipid transport. Trends Biochem Sci. 2005;30(7):396–404.
38. Stone SJ, Vance JE. Phosphatidylserine synthase-1 and -2 are localized to mitochondria-associated membranes. J Biol Chem. 2000;275(44):34534–40.
39. Achleitner G, et al. Synthesis and intracellular transport of aminoglycerophospholipids in permeabilized cells of the yeast, Saccharomyces Cerevisiae. J Biol Chem. 1995;270(50):29836–42.
40. Prasad M, et al. Mitochondria-associated endoplasmic reticulum membrane (MAM) regulates steroidogenic activity via steroidogenic acute regulatory protein (StAR)-voltage-dependent anion channel 2 (VDAC2) interaction. J Biol Chem. 2015;290(5):2604–16.
41. Lewin TM, et al. Acyl-CoA synthetase isoforms 1, 4, and 5 are present in different subcellular membranes in rat liver and can be inhibited independently. J Biol Chem. 2001;276(27):24674–9.
42. Lewin TM, et al. Rat liver acyl-CoA synthetase 4 is a peripheral-membrane protein located in two distinct subcellular organelles, peroxisomes, and mitochondrial-associated membrane. Arch Biochem Biophys. 2002;404(2):263–70.
43. Gellerich FN, et al. The regulation of OXPHOS by extramitochondrial calcium. Biochim Biophys Acta. 2010;1797(6-7):1018–27.
44. Baumgartner HK, et al. Calcium elevation in mitochondria is the main Ca2+ requirement for mitochondrial permeability transition pore (mPTP) opening. J Biol Chem. 2009;284(31):20796–803.
45. Baughman JM, et al. Integrative genomics identifies MCU as an essential component of the mitochondrial calcium uniporter. Nature. 2011;476(7360):341–5.
46. Qi H, Li L, Shuai J. Optimal microdomain crosstalk between endoplasmic reticulum and mitochondria for Ca2+ oscillations. Sci Rep. 2015;5:7984.
47. Patron M, et al. The mitochondrial calcium uniporter (MCU): molecular identity and physiological roles. J Biol Chem. 2013;288(15):10750–8.

48. Bononi A, et al. Mitochondria-associated membranes (MAMs) as hotspot ca(2+) signaling units. Adv Exp Med Biol. 2012;740:411–37.
49. Horne JH, Meyer T. Elementary calcium-release units induced by inositol trisphosphate. Science. 1997;276(5319):1690–3.
50. White C, et al. The endoplasmic reticulum gateway to apoptosis by Bcl-X(L) modulation of the InsP3R. Nat Cell Biol. 2005;7(10):1021–8.
51. Bonneau B, et al. IRBIT controls apoptosis by interacting with the Bcl-2 homolog, Bcl2l10, and by promoting ER-mitochondria contact. Elife. 2016;5:e19896.
52. Smirnova E, et al. Mitochondria: dynamic organelles in disease, aging, and development. Cell. 2006;125(7):1241–52.
53. Smirnova E, et al. Dynamin-related protein Drp1 is required for mitochondrial division in mammalian cells. Mol Biol Cell. 2011;12(8):2245–56.
54. Yoon Y, Pitts KR, McNiven MA. Mammalian dynamin-like protein DLP1 tubulates membranes. Mol Biol Cell. 2001;12(9):2894–905.
55. Shim SH, et al. Super-resolution fluorescence imaging of organelles in live cells with photoswitchable membrane probes. Proc Natl Acad Sci U S A. 2012;109(35):13978–83.
56. Korobova F, Ramabhadran V, Higgs HN. An actin-dependent step in mitochondrial fission mediated by the ER-associated formin INF2. Science. 2013;339(6118):464–7.
57. Grimm S. The ER–mitochondria interface: the social network of cell death. Mol Cell Res. 2012;1823(2):327–34.
58. Wang B, et al. Fis1, Bap31 and the kiss of death between mitochondria and endoplasmic reticulum. EMBO J. 2011;30(3):451–2.
59. Prudent J, et al. MAPL SUMOylation of Drp1 stabilizes an ER/mitochondrial platform required for cell death. Mol Cell. 2015;59(6):941–55.
60. Area-Gomez E, et al. Presenilins are enriched in endoplasmic reticulum membranes associated with mitochondria. Am J Pathol. 2009;175(5):1810–6.
61. Zampese E, et al. Presenilin 2 modulates endoplasmic reticulum (ER)–mitochondria interactions and Ca2+ cross-talk. Proc Natl Acad Sci U S A. 2011;108(7):2777–82.
62. Schon EA, Area-Gomez E. Is Alzheimer's disease a disorder of mitochondria-associated membranes? J Alzheimers Dis. 2010;20(Suppl 2):S281–92.
63. Schreiner B, et al. Amyloid-β peptides are generated in mitochondria-associated endoplasmic reticulum membranes. J Alzheimers Dis. 2015;43(2):369–74.
64. Hedskog L, et al. Modulation of the endoplasmic reticulum–mitochondria interface in Alzheimer's disease and related models. Proc Natl Acad Sci U S A. 2013;110(19):7916–21.
65. Tambini MD, et al. ApoE4 upregulates the activity of mitochondria-associated ER membranes. EMBO Rep. 2016;17(1):27–36.
66. Filadi R, et al. Presenilin 2 modulates endoplasmic reticulum-mitochondria coupling by tuning the antagonistic effect of Mitofusin 2. Cell Rep. 2016;15(10):2226–38.
67. Al-Saif A, Al-Mohanna F, Bohlega S. A mutation in sigma-1 receptor causes juvenile amyotrophic lateral sclerosis. Ann Neurol. 2011;70(6):913–9.
68. Su TP, et al. The sigma-1 receptor chaperone as an inter-organelle signaling modulator. Trends Pharmacol Sci. 2010;31(12):557–66.
69. Watanabe S, et al. Mitochondria-associated membrane collapse is a common pathomechanism in SIGMAR1- and SOD1-linked ALS. EMBO Mol Med. 2016;8(12):1421–37.
70. Guardia-Laguarta C, et al. Alpha-Synuclein is localized to mitochondria-associated ER membranes. J Neurosci. 2014;34(1):249–59.
71. Cali T, et al. Alpha-Synuclein controls mitochondrial calcium homeostasis by enhancing endoplasmic reticulum-mitochondria interactions. J Biol Chem. 2012;287(22):17914–29.
72. Bouman L, et al. Parkin is transcriptionally regulated by ATF4: evidence for an interconnection between mitochondrial stress and ER stress. Cell Death Differ. 2011;18(5):769–82.
73. Van Laar VS, et al. Glutamate excitotoxicity in neurons triggers mitochondrial and endoplasmic reticulum accumulation of Parkin, and, in the presence of N-acetyl cysteine, mitophagy. Neurobiol Dis. 2015;74:180–93.
74. Cali T, et al. Enhanced parkin levels favor ER-mitochondria crosstalk and guarantee ca(2+) transfer to sustain cell bioenergetics. Biochim Biophys Acta. 2013;1832(4):495–508.
75. Zheng L, et al. Parkin functionally interacts with PGC-1alpha to preserve mitochondria and protect dopaminergic neurons. Hum Mol Genet. 2017;26(3):582–98.
76. Gautier CA, et al. The endoplasmic reticulum-mitochondria interface is perturbed in PARK2 knockout mice and patients with PARK2 mutations. Hum Mol Genet. 2016;25(14):2972–84.
77. Gelmetti V, et al. PINK1 and BECN1 relocalize at mitochondria-associated membranes during mitophagy and promote ER-mitochondria tethering and autophagosome formation. Autophagy. 2017;13(4):654–69.
78. Ottolini D, et al. The Parkinson disease-related protein DJ-1 counteracts mitochondrial impairment induced by the tumour suppressor protein p53 by enhancing endoplasmic reticulum-mitochondria tethering. Hum Mol Genet. 2013;22(11):2152–68.
79. Pigino G, et al. Alzheimer's presenilin 1 mutations impair kinesin-based axonal transport. J Neurosci. 2003;23(11):4499–508.
80. Area-Gomez E, et al. Upregulated function of mitochondria-associated ER membranes in Alzheimer disease. EMBO J. 2012;31(21):4106–23.

18

Aberrant functional connectivity network in subjective memory complaint individuals relates to pathological biomarkers

Kaicheng Li[1†], Xiao Luo[1†], Qingze Zeng[1], Yeerfan Jiaerken[1], Xiaojun Xu[1], Peiyu Huang[1], Zhujing Shen[1], Jingjing Xu[1], Chao Wang[1], Jiong Zhou[2], Min-Ming Zhang[1*] and for the Alzheimer's Disease Neuroimaging Initiative

Abstract

Background: Individuals with subjective memory complaints (SMC) feature a higher risk of cognitive decline and clinical progression of Alzheimer's disease (AD). However, the pathological mechanism underlying SMC remains unclear. We aimed to assess the intrinsic connectivity network and its relationship with AD-related pathologies in SMC individuals.

Methods: We included 44 SMC individuals and 40 normal controls who underwent both resting-state functional MRI and positron emission tomography (PET). Based on graph theory approaches, we detected local and global functional connectivity across the whole brain by using degree centrality (DC) and eigenvector centrality (EC) respectively. Additionally, we analyzed amyloid deposition and tauopathy via florbetapir-PET imaging and cerebrospinal fluid (CSF) data. The voxel-wise two-sample T-test analysis was used to examine between-group differences in the intrinsic functional network and cerebral amyloid deposition. Then, we correlated these network metrics with pathological results.

Results: The SMC individuals showed higher DC in the bilateral hippocampus (HP) and left fusiform gyrus and lower DC in the inferior parietal region than controls. Across all subjects, the DC of the bilateral HP and left fusiform gyrus was positively associated with total tau and phosphorylated tau_{181}. However, no significant between-group difference existed in EC and cerebral amyloid deposition.

Conclusion: We found impaired local, but not global, intrinsic connectivity networks in SMC individuals. Given the relationships between DC value and tau level, we hypothesized that functional changes in SMC individuals might relate to pathological biomarkers.

Keywords: Subjective memory complaint, Functional connectivity, Graph theoretical analysis, Neuropathology, Eigenvector centrality, Degree centrality

Background

Subjective memory complaint (SMC) refers to self-perceived cognitive decline with normal objective cognitive performance [1]. Prior studies showed that SMC individuals might precede amnestic mild cognitive impairments (aMCI) and exhibit a high conversion risk of Alzheimer's disease (AD) [2]. Moreover, longitudinal studies noted that the risk for SMC individuals to convert to MCI or AD is 4.5-6.5 times higher than healthy aging individuals [3–7]. Therefore, SMC might serve as the typical presymptomatic stage along the AD continuum [1].

Recent neuroimaging studies found that SMC individuals is accompanied by cortical atrophy [8, 9] and white matter (WM) abnormalities [10] in AD-related regions, such as the medial temporal lobe. Functionally, SMC individuals feature both functional connectivity and metabolic alterations in the medial temporal and occipitoparietal regions [11–15]. These results jointly suggested SMC as the middle stage between MCI and normal controls (NC) and

* Correspondence: zhangminming@zju.edu.cn
†Kaicheng Li and Xiao Luo contributed equally to this work.
1Department of Radiology, 2nd Affiliated Hospital of Zhejiang University School of Medicine, No.88 Jie-fang Road, Shang-cheng District, Hangzhou 310009, China
Full list of author information is available at the end of the article

demonstrated that SMC might be among the earliest AD clinical symptoms. Pathological changes may explain these neuroimaging abnormalities. For example, autopsy studies have found higher levels of amyloid-β deposits and tau tangles in SMC individuals than healthy aging [16]. Further, PET study found increased entorhinal cortical tauopathy in SMC individuals and noted that tauopathy might be the most suggestive sign of SMC [17]. Despite these findings, the link between AD-related biomarkers and functional changes in SMC individuals is unclear.

To cover this gap, we combined graph theoretical approaches based on resting-state functional MRI (rsfMRI) and pathological biomarkers. By definition, graph theoretical centrality considers the brain as one vast network and measures the overall importance of individual brain regions. In the present study, we assessed two representative centrality metrics, degree centrality (DC) and eigenvector centrality (EC), across the entire brain. These metrics could capture the functional relationships of a given voxel (node) within the entire connectivity matrix of the brain (connectome). Specifically, DC is a local metric, calculating the number of direct connections for a given node [18]. In other words, a higher DC represents more direct connections with the node. In contrast, EC is a global metric calculating both the number and the weight of the connections [19, 20]. A brain region with a higher EC value means strong connection with more nodes and with higher weighting (i.e., there is a central role for the region in the whole-brain connectome). Furthermore, we assessed amyloid deposition in a voxel-wise manner and explored pathological changes in SMC individuals. Additionally, we examined the possible amyloid burden, neuronal death, and accumulation of tangles based on cerebrospinal fluid (CSF) data [21] .

We aimed to explore the intrinsic functional network and its corresponding pathologies in SMC individuals. Based on previous studies, we hypothesized that SMC individuals had more severe topological network impairment and a higher pathological burden than controls, especially in regions susceptible to AD pathologies such as the temporal and parietal lobes [22]. Moreover, aberrant functional connectivity metrics might relate to pathological change.

Methods

Alzheimer's disease neuroimaging and initiative

Data used in the preparation of this article were obtained from the Alzheimer's Disease Neuroimaging Initiative (ADNI) database (http://adni.loni.usc.edu). The ADNI was initially launched in 2004 (ADNI-1), and additional recruitment was made through ADNI-GO in 2009, ADNI-2 in 2010 and ADNI-3 in 2016. The primary goal of the ADNI has been to identify serial MRI, PET, biomarkers and genetic characteristics that would support the early detection and tracking of AD, and improve clinical trial design. For up-to-date information, see http://www.adni-info.org.

Study participants

This study was approved by the Institutional Review Boards of all participating institutions, and informed written consent was obtained from all participants at each site. We included 44 SMC individuals and 40 well-matched normal controls (NC) from the ADNI database (Additional file 1). All participants underwent structural scans, rsfMRI scans, florbetapir PET amyloid scans, and comprehensive neuropsychological assessments at the same time point. The inclusion criteria for NC included the following: (a) having an Mini-Mental State Examination (MMSE) score between 24 and 30; (b) having a clinical dementia rating (CDR) score of 0; (c) having a normal Wechsler Memory Scale Logical Memory, WMS-LM, delay recall performance (in detail: ≥ 9 for subjects with 16 or more years of education; ≥ 5 for subjects with 8–15 years of education; and ≥ 3 for 0–7 years of education); (d) non-clinical depression (geriatric depression scale-15, GDS-15 score < 6) [23]; and (e) non-demented.

The inclusion criteria for SMC individuals included the following: (a) having a self-reported persistent memory decline assessed by using the Cognitive Change Index (CCI; the total score from the first 12 items ≥ 16, Additional file 1) [9]; (b) having a normal cognitive performance (as for memory: having a normal WMS-LM delay recall performance; as for general mental status: having a normal MMSE (between 24 and 30) and a CDR score of 0) [1].

We excluded subjects with the following manifestations: (a) significant medical, neurological, and psychiatric illness; (b) obvious head trauma history; (c) use of non-AD-related medications known to influence cerebral function; (d) clinical depression; (e) alcohol or drug abuse; (f) left-handedness. After careful screening, we excluded 14 SMC individuals (three subjects with abnormal cognitive abilities, three subjects scanned with different rsfMRI acquisition parameters, six subjects with amyloid-PET data missing, two subjects with excessive head motion, Additional file 1) Table 1 shows the demographics of the included 44 SMC subjects and 40 well-matched NC subjects.

Neuropsychological and CSF data acquisition

All subjects underwent comprehensive neuropsychological tests, including assessment of general mental status (Mini-Mental State Examination, MMSE) and other cognitive domains, involving memory function (Auditory Verbal Learning Test, AVLT; WMS-LM, immediate and delayed memory), attention (Trail-Making Test part A,

Table 1 The demographic, cognitive and neuropathological information

Variables	NC	SMC	T/χ^2- value	*P* value
Number	40	44		
Demographic characteristics				
Age, y, mean (SD)	75.10±5.39	73.78±5.81	1.08	0.28
Female, *n* (%)	22/18	24/20	0.002	0.57
Education (y), mean (SD)	16.70±2.39	16.66±2.60	0.08	0.94
Family, yes/no	23/17	14/30	7.28	0.03*
APOE	27/13	35/9	1.57	0.16
CSF				
$A\beta_{1-42}$ (pg/ml)	1389.89±755.77	1552.79±683.30	-0.75	0.46
T-Tau (pg/ml)	235.32±83.46	259.52±68.76	-1.05	0.30
P-Tau_{181} (pg/ml)	21.80±8.80	23.50±6.10	-0.73	0.47
Neuropsychiatric Scores				
CCI		31.37±8.30		
GDS	0.68±0.89	1.14±0.90	-2.36	0.02*
General mental status				
MMSE	29.05±1.18	29.36±0.75	-1.44	0.15
Memory function				
WMS-LM immediate	15.00±2.67	15.25±3.01	-0.39	0.70
WMS-LM delay	14.38±2.83	14.23±3.40	0.22	0.83
AVLT sum of trials 1–5	44.95±9.43	48.84±9.59	-1.86	0.07
AVLT30	7.18±4.14	8.88±4.18	-1.85	0.07
Attention				
Log-transformed TMT-A	1.50±0.12	1.48±0.14	0.59	0.55
Decision-making function				
Log-transformed TMT-B	1.79±0.16	1.84±0.17	-1.36	0.18
Language				
BNT total	28.94±1.05	28.52±1.50	1.14	0.26
Category fluency	21.75±4.06	22.20±5.02	-0.45	0.65
Visuospatial processing				
CDT	4.85±0.36	4.86±0.35	-0.18	0.86
Ecog PT: memory	1.53±0.41	1.94±0.60	-3.73	<0.001*
Ecog PT: global	1.35±0.26	1.55±0.38	-2.85	0.006*
Ecog Inf: memory	1.24±0.40	1.59±0.59	-3.18	0.002*
Ecog Inf: global	1.22±0.34	1.43±0.52	-2.15	0.03*

Data are presented as means ± standard deviations.
Abbreviation: *SMC* Significant Memory Complaint, *NC* Normal Controls, *GDS* Geriatric Depression Scale, *MMSE* Mini-Mental State Examination, *WMS-LM* Wechsler Memory Scale Logical Memory, *AVLT* Auditory Verbal Learning Test, *TMT* Trail-Making Test, *BNT* Boston Naming Test, *CDT* Clock Drawing Test, *E-Cog* Measurement of Everyday Cognition, *PT* patient-based, *Inf* Informant-based;
*$p<0.05$, significant difference between NC and SMC
Notably: The CSF data in Table 1 only represents the subjects who had CSF sample.

TMT-A), visuospatial function (Clock-Drawing Test, CDT), executive function (Trail-Making Test part B, TMT-B), and language ability (Boston Naming Test, BNT). Moreover, we also used Everyday Cognition (Ecog, Participant version and Informant version) to assess the subjective and partner-based cognitive complaints.

CSF biomarkers included amyloid-beta 1–42 ($A\beta_{1-42}$), total tau (t-tau), and phosphorylated tau at position 181 (p-tau_{181}), measured by the fully automated Roche Elecsys and Cobas e immunoassay analyzer system as previously described [24]. Notably, not all subjects had CSF sample since lumbar puncture is an invasive procedure. To ensure that pathology biomarkers accurately reflected the functional profile, we only included CSF samples at the same time as the rsfMRI acquisition (Additional file 1). Thus, 19 out of 44 SMC individuals and 28 out of 40 NC had CSF samples available.

MRI acquisition and pre-processing

We acquired the T1-weighted images using the following parameters: repetition time (TR)=2300 ms; echo time (TE)=2.98 ms; inversion time (TI)=900 ms; 170 sagittal slices; within plane FOV=256 × 240 mm^2; voxel size=1.1 × 1.1×1.2 mm^3; flip angle=9°; bandwidth=240 Hz/pix. The rsfMRI images were obtained using an echo-planar imaging sequence with the following parameters: TR=3000 ms; TE=30 ms; the number of slices=48; slice thickness=3.3 mm; spatial resolution=3.31×3.31×3.31 mm^3. According to the scan protocol, all subjects were instructed to open their eyes and keep at rest calmly during the scan.

We pre-processed all neuroimaging data using the Data Processing Assistant and Resting-State FMRI (DPARSF; www.rfmri.org/DPASFA) [25] based on the platform of Statistical Parametric Mapping 8 (SPM8; www.fil.ion.ucl.ac.uk/spm) [26]. First, we discarded the first ten image volumes of rsfMRI scans for the signal equilibrium and subject's adaptation to the scanning noise. Then, we corrected the remaining 130 images for timing differences and head motion [27]. Here, we discarded the image data with more than 2.5 mm maximum displacement in any of the x, y, or z directions or 2.5° of any angular motion. Subsequently, based on rigid-body transformation, we co-registered T1-weighted images to the mean rsfMRI image and spatially normalized these images to the Montreal Neurological Institute (MNI) standard space. The standardized image was subsequently re-sampled into 3 mm × 3 mm × 3 mm cubic voxel. Then, we performed a detrend and filter procedure (0.01 Hz < f < 0.08 Hz) to remove the bias from the high-frequency physiological noise and the low-frequency drift. Finally, we scrubbed the data to reduce motion-related artifacts by using a framewise displacement (FD) threshold of 0.5, deleting one time point before and two time points after "bad" time points [28]. To remove residual effects of motion and other non-neuronal factors, we corrected covariates including 24 head motion parameters and signals of white matter and CSF signal. Moreover, considering the possible effect of autocorrelation in fMRI time series, we additionally performed pre-whitening [29, 30] in the pre-processing by using FSL (Additional file 1).

Centrality metrics

For each subject, we computed Pearson's correlations between the time series of all pairs within the whole brain to produce the functional connectivity matrix. The procedure constrained by the gray matter mask generated by setting a threshold of 0.3 on the mean gray matter probability map. Then, we calculated the DC and EC metrics in a voxel-wise manner to quantify the local and global brain network integrity (Additional file 1) [18]. In detail, we calculated DC by counting, for each voxel, the number of voxels it was connected to at a threshold of r ≥ 0.25. More details regarding DC processing are available in the literature [18, 31–34]. On the other hand, we calculated EC by counting the weighted number of correlations based on fast ECM (fECM) toolbox [31, 35, 36]. Then, all DC and EC maps underwent smoothing with full width at half maximum with a Gaussian kernel of 6 mm × 6 mm × 6 mm and Fisher's Z transformation.

PET acquisition and pre-processing

We downloaded amyloid PET data from LONI in the most fully pre-processed format (series description in LONI Advanced Search: "AV45 Coreg, Avg, Std Img and Vox Siz, Uniform Resolution"). Subsequently, we coregistered the T1-weighted image to the mean amyloid PET image and spatially normalized these images to the Montreal Neurological Institute (MNI) space. A standardized image was subsequently re-sampled into 3 mm × 3 mm × 3 mm cubic voxel. Finally, each amyloid PET image was normalized to the whole cerebellum to create standardized uptake value ratio (SUVR) images.

Statistical analyses

We analyzed the demographic data using the chi-squared test for categorical data and t-test for continuous data (SPSS version 19.0). Then, we examined the neuroimaging metric differences (including DC, EC, and SUVR images) between the SMC and NC groups in a voxel-wise manner based on REST software (www.restfmri.net). In detail, we performed a two-sample t-test with age, gender, education, and GDS as the covariates, by setting the statistical threshold at $P<0.001$ and cluster size > ten voxels (uncorrected).

We defined regions showing significant differences between groups as the region of interest (ROIs) and extracted the mean features (DC, EC, and SUVR values) from them. Then, based on Spearman's correlation, we correlated these neuroimaging metrics with neuropathological and neuropsychological results. To reduce the selection bias, we extended the CSF data and repeated the correlation analyses (Additional file 1).

Moreover, to examine the stability of our results across time, we selected a subgroup of SMC individuals with both baseline and follow-up data from our original SMC subjects and repeated our analysis (Additional file 1).

Results

Demographic and neuropsychological data

Descriptive data are presented as the mean ± standard deviation for continuous variables and percentage for dichotomous variables. The SMC individuals matched well with NC for age, gender, education, and APOE status. However, the SMC individuals showed higher GDS than the NC individuals. Regarding the cognitive performance and mean FD value (micromotion index), no significant difference existed between groups (Table 1, Additional file 1). Moreover, SMC individuals had greater self-based/informant-based complaints than NC individuals in memory and global state.

Centrality metrics

The SMC individuals showed higher DC in the bilateral hippocampus (HP) and left fusiform gyrus and lower DC in the right inferior parietal region than NC individuals. However, no significant differences in EC existed between groups (Fig. 1 and Table 2). Moreover, we adopted different statistical thresholds to explore the stability of our results (Additional file 1).

PET and CSF data

The voxel-wise comparison of SUVR images showed no significant difference between the SMC and NC groups. No significant differences in CSF biomarkers existed between groups (Table 1).

Correlation analyses

Across groups, the DC value of bilateral HP and left fusiform gyrus was positively related with T-tau and P-tau$_{181}$. Specifically, the DC value of the left HP was related to T-tau and P-tau$_{181}$ (r=0.32, P<0.05; r=0.37, P<0.05, respectively); the DC value of the right HP was related to T-tau and P-tau$_{181}$ (r=0.47, P<0.05; r=0.45, P<0.05, respectively); the DC value of the left fusiform gyrus was related to T-tau and P-tau$_{181}$ (r=0.39, P<0.05; r=0.40, P<0.05, respectively) (Fig. 2). More information is provided in Additional file 1.

Discussion

Our study initially combined rsfMRI and pathological data to explore the intrinsic functional network and its possible pathological mechanism in SMC individuals. Based on centrality analyses, we found that the SMC individuals showed both impairment and compensation in the default mode network (DMN) at the local level

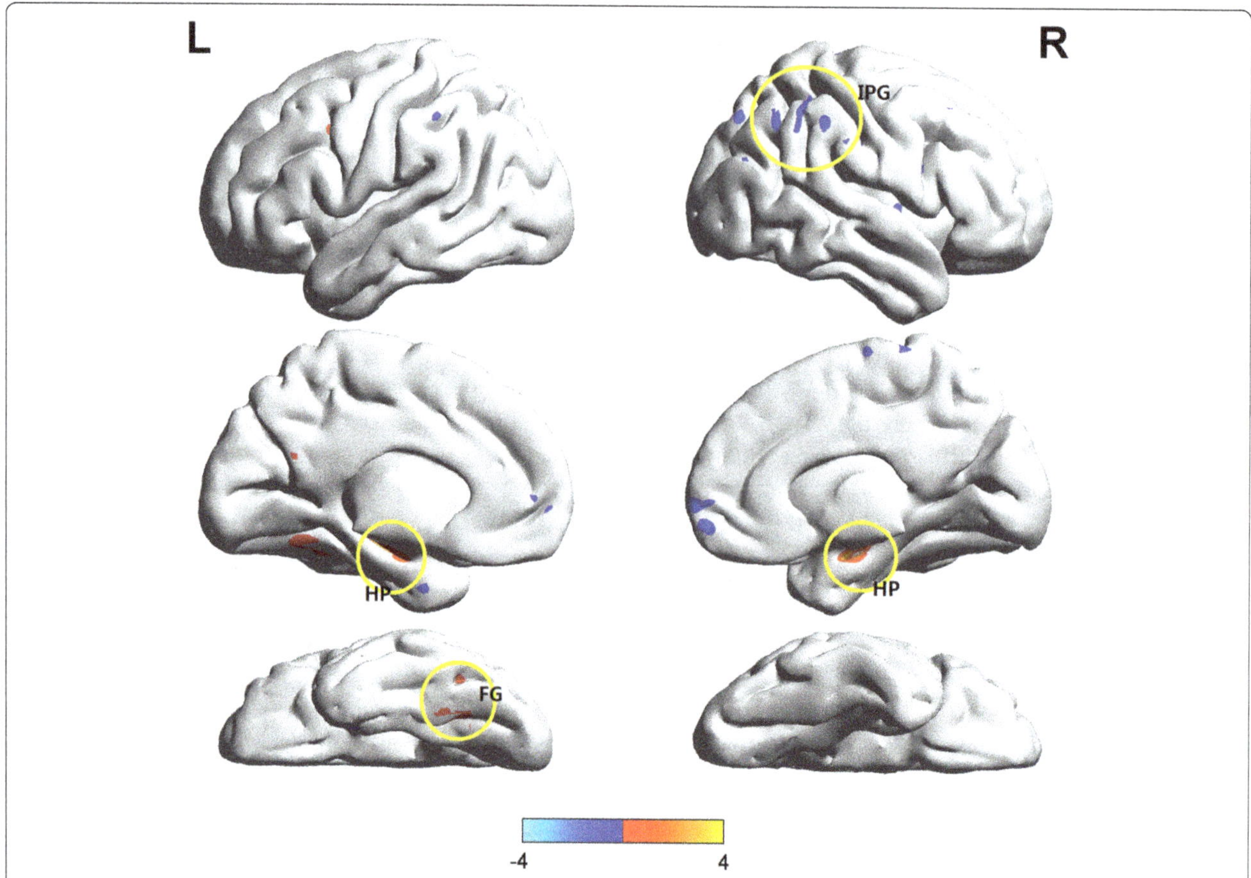

Fig. 1 Shows the DC differences between SMC individuals and controls. SMC individuals showed higher DC (hot color) in the bilateral HP, left fusiform gyrus and lower DC (cold color) in the right inferior parietal region than controls (P<0.001, cluster size > 10 voxels, uncorrected, covariates including age, gender, education and geriatric depression scale). *Abbreviations: DC* degree centrality, *SMC* subjective memory complaint, *HP* hippocampus, *IPG* inferior parietal region

Table 2 Results of degree centrality differences between SMC individuals and NC

Brain regions	Cluter-size	Coordinates (MNI)			Peak intensity
		X	Y	Z	
R Hippocampus	23	27	-3	-24	3.89
L Hippocampus	11	-30	-18	-21	4.12
L Fusiform	16	-27	-45	-18	4.02
R Inferior parietal region	13	54	-21	27	-4.21

(reflected by DC) but not at the global level (reflected by EC). Moreover, the links between the DC value and CSF tau level in the temporal regions suggested that the functional alternation in SMC individuals may result from tau-related pathologies.

SMC is at a stage of mild neuronal damage but still with sufficient functional compensation [37]. This stage may reflect the first effects of AD pathology on cognitive functioning between full compensation and the very first decline. Here, we found no difference in EC between groups, which suggested that SMC individuals have relatively intact global connectivity. This result was in line with the work of Wang et al. which reported similar global efficiency in SMC individuals and NC by examining the white matter connectivity network [38]. On the other hand, we found that the SMC individuals displayed increased DC in the medial temporal region (MTL, including the HP and fusiform gyrus) and decreased DC in the inferior parietal gyrus (IPG), suggesting aberrant local connectivity in the DMN. Another functional study came to similar conclusions, reporting that DMN function was alternated in SMC individuals and proposed it as the early AD-related connectivity failure [39]. Moreover, one study also reported reduced parietal activation while increased HP activation [40] in normal aging, demonstrating that successful memory encoding requires the coordination of neural activity in hippocampal and parietal regions. Accordingly, we hypothesized that reduced functional activity in the inferior parietal gyrus might indicate network deficiency, but increased activity in MTL might compensate for decreased memory in SMC individuals.

Supporting evidence for our hypothesis also comes from studies using different modalities. The inferior

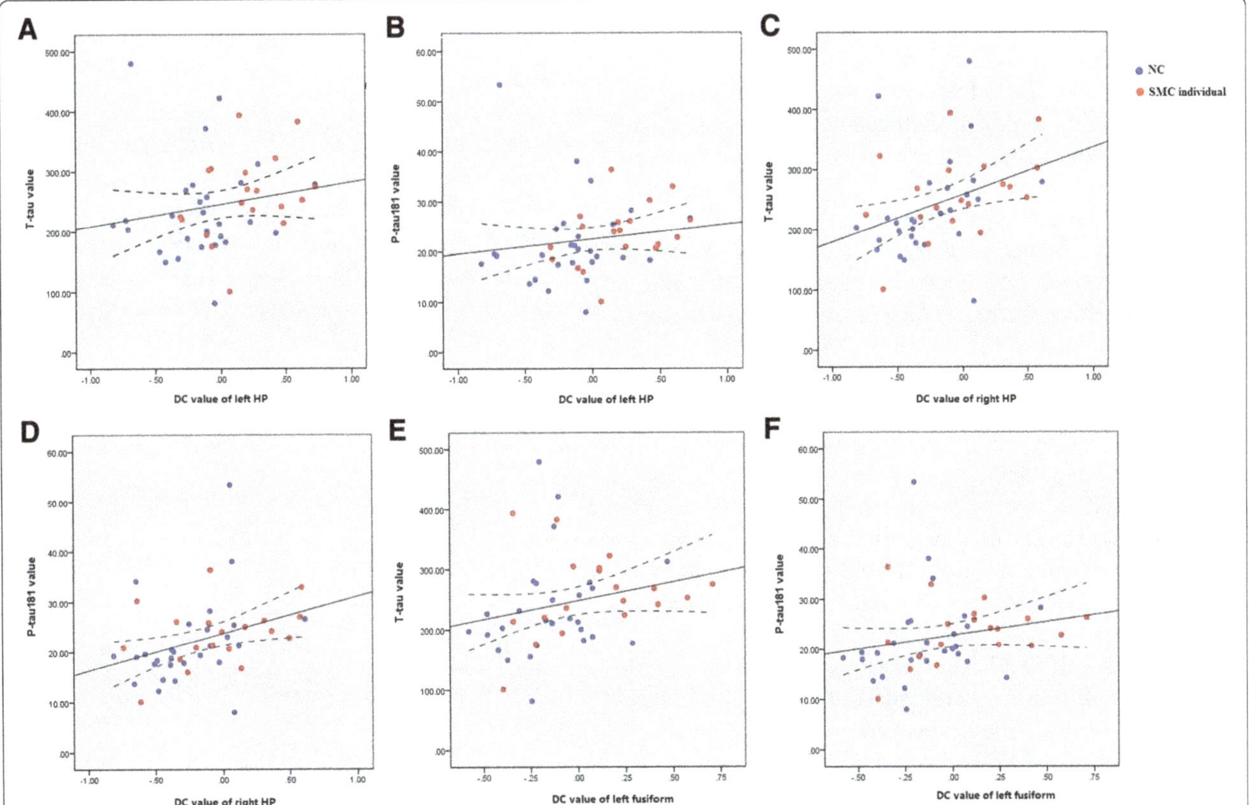

Fig. 2 Shows the association between tau and DC value. Across groups, the DC value of the bilateral HP and left fusiform gyrus was positively associated with the T-tau and P-tau$_{181}$ levels. **a** DC value of left HP related to T-tau (r=0.32, P<0.05); **b** DC value of left HP related to P-tau$_{181}$ (r=0.37, P<0.05); **c** DC value of right HP related to T-tau (r=0.47, P<0.05); **d** DC value of right HP related to P-tau$_{181}$ (r=0.45, P<0.05); **e** DC value of left fusiform gyrus related to T-tau (r=0.39, P<0.05); **f** the DC value of left fusiform gyrus related to P-tau$_{181}$ (r=0.40, P<0.05). The scatter plot diagram displays the 95% confidence band of the best-fit line. *Abbreviations*: *DC* degree centrality, *HP* hippocampus, *T-tau* total tau, *P-tau$_{181}$* phosphorylated tau; the unit of CSF: (pg/ml)

parietal region, as a functional core of the DMN, is vulnerable to functional connectivity breakdown in AD patients [32, 41]. Similar results can also be found in white matter network studies, demonstrating decreased nodal strength in the parietal region in SMC individuals [38, 42]. Moreover, early suffering from decreased glucose metabolic rates in the inferior parietal lobe in SMC individuals may help explain these connectivity abnormalities. [11]. Therefore, we proposed that the inferior parietal region is the primary target of functional decrease in SMC individuals which may further lead to cognition decline. Meanwhile, we observed that MTL exhibited increased function at the local level, which may help maintain cognitive performance in SMC individuals. Similarly, several memory encoding-related fMRI studies found increased activation in the MTL in SMC individuals [13, 14, 43], suggesting that this region may be involved in memory compensation [14]. Additionally, one white matter connectivity study reported impaired WM microstructure and integrity in MTL in SMC individuals [44]. Previous literature has hypothesized that before a global connectivity failure, brain regions with high activity could reflect an attempted compensation of early pathophysiological processes [45, 46]. Combined with the correlation between tau level and functional connectivity in the MTL, we proposed that the hyperconnectivity in SMC individuals is a result of brain plasticity after damage to the neural system. Conclusively, we hypothesized that both functional impairment and compensation simultaneously existed in SMC individuals, and such a functional pattern works jointly to maintain normal cognition in SMC individuals.

Regarding the pathological results, we did not observe significant amyloid differences between the SMC and NC groups. However, correlation analyses showed the links between MTL DC value and CSF tau level in all subjects. One possible explanation is that tau-mediated neuronal dysfunction [47, 48], but not amyloid burden is the initial pathology in SMC individuals. Some PET studies supported this interpretation to some extent [49–52]. Specifically, the SMC individuals tend to suffer tau pathology accumulation early in the MTL, in regions involved in memory function [17, 53–56]. In addition, Risacher et al. [57] reported that olfactory identification was more related to tauopathy than amyloid deposition in individuals with SMC. Another explanation is that the SMC group consists of a heterogeneous population [58]. Here, we included SMC individuals according to the framework and tried to meet the plus criteria [1]. Evidence such as informant-based complaints provides additional predictive ability for the progression to dementia in SMC individuals [59]. Notably, apart from AD-related pathologies, other neuropsychiatric factors such as depression or anxiety may also contribute to SMC [60–64]. These symptoms may also be manifestations of preclinical AD and can further lead to increases in amyloid formation and tau accumulation [65, 66] at the early stage of AD and could constitute a risk factor for subsequent dementia [67]. In our study, SMC individuals had a higher depression score (but within the clinically normal range), which was controlled to eliminate its possible effect according to the framework [1]. Considering the mixed function of subthreshold symptoms and pathologies, we still inferred that these possible mixed factors might affect the results to some extent.

There exist several limitations in our study. First, the sample size was relatively small, which reduced the statistical power. Future studies with larger sample sizes are required. Second, the SMC group is a heterogeneous group, easily resulted from other neuropsychological factors apart from AD-related pathologies. Future studies should consider these neuropsychiatric factors associated with SMC [58]. Moreover, the pathological ATN classification can help to define the SMC due to AD and should be used in the further analysis [68, 69]. Third, some CSF data are missing, which may lead to a selection bias. We performed a complementary correlation analysis based on extended CSF, which may support the stability of our findings to some extent. However, further studies with larger CSF sample sizes are urgent.

Conclusion

We found an impaired local, but not global, intrinsic functional network in SMC individuals, mainly involving the DMN. We hypothesized that the co-existence of functional impairment and compensation helped keep the normal cognitive in SMC individuals. Moreover, our results suggested that functional changes in SMC individuals may result from tau-related pathologies.

Additional file

Additional file 1: Flow chart of subjects inclusion. Details regarding CCI. Analysis based on extended CSF data. Analysis based on data after pre-whitening. Details regarding DC and EC calculation. Analysis based on the follow-up data. Head motion parameters of SMC individuals and NC. Results under different thresholds. (DOCX 1176 kb)

Abbreviations

AD: Alzheimer's disease; ADNI: Alzheimer's disease Neuroimaging Initiative; AVLT: Auditory Verbal Learning Test; Aβ1-42: amyloid-beta 1-42; BNT: Boston Naming Test; CCI: Cognitive Change Index; CDR: Clinical dementia rating; CDT: Clock-Drawing Test; CSF: Cerebrospinal fluid; DC: Degree centrality; DMN: Default mode network; EC: Eigenvector centrality; FD: Frame-wise displacement; fECM: Fast ECM; GDS: Geriatric depression scale; HP: Hippocampus; MCI: Mild cognitive impairments; MNI: Montreal Neurological Institute; MTL: Medial temporal lobe; NC: Normal control; PET: Positron emission tomography; P-tau_{181}: Hosphorylated tau at position 181; rsfMRI: Resting-state functional MRI; SMC: Subjective memory complaints; SUVR: Standardized uptake value ratio; TE: Echo time; TI: Inversion time; TMT-A: Trail-Making Test, Part A; TMT-B: Trail-Making Test, Part B; TR: Epetition time; T-tau: Total tau; WM: White matter; WMS-LM: Wechsler Memory Scale Logical Memory

Acknowledgements

Data collection and sharing for this project was funded by the Alzheimer's Disease Neuroimaging Initiative (ADNI) (National Institutes of Health Grant U01 AG024904) and DOD ADNI (Department of Defense award number W81XWH-12-2-0012). ADNI is funded by the National Institute on Aging, the National Institute of Biomedical Imaging and Bioengineering, and through generous contributions from the following: AbbVie, Alzheimer's Association; Alzheimer's Drug Discovery Foundation; Araclon Biotech; Bio Clinica, Inc.;Biogen; Bristol-Myers Squibb Company; CereSpir, Inc.; Eisai Inc.; ElanPharmaceuticals, Inc.; Eli Lilly and Company; EuroImmun; F. Hoffmann-La Roche Ltd. and its affiliated company Genentech, Inc.; Fujirebio; GE Healthcare; IXICO Ltd.; Janssen Alzheimer Immunotherapy Research & D development t , LLC.; J Johnson & Johnson Pharmaceutical Research & Development LLC.; Lumosity; Lundbeck; Merck & Co., Inc.; Meso Scale Diagnostics, LLC.; NeuroRx Research; Neurotrack Technologies; Novartis Pharmaceuticals Corporation; Pfizer Inc.; Piramal Imaging; Servier; Takeda Pharmaceutical Company; and Transition Therapeutics. The Canadian Institutes of Health Research is providing funds to support ADNI clinical sites in Canada. Private sector contributions are facilitated by the foundation for the National Institutes of Health (www.fnih.org). The grantee organization is the Northern California Institute for Research and Education, and the study is coordinated by the Alzheimer's Disease Cooperative Study at the University of California, San Diego.ADNI data are disseminated by the Laboratory for NeuroImaging at the University ofSouthern California. Data used in the preparation of this article were obtained from the Alzheimer's disease Neuroimaging Initiative (ADNI) database (http://www.adni.loni.usc.edu). As such, the investigators within the ADNI contributed to the design and implementation of ADNI and provided data but did not participate in analysis or writing of this report. A complete listing of ADNI investigators can be found at http://adni.loni.usc.edu/wp-content/uploads/how_to_apply/ADNI_Acknowledgement_List.pdf.

Funding

This study was funded by National Key Research and Development Program of China (Grant No. 2016YFC1306600), Zhejiang Provincial Natural Science Foundation of China (Grant Nos. LZ14H180001 and Y16H090026), Young ResearchTalents Fund, Chinese Medicine Science, and Technology Project of Zhejiang Province (Grant No. 2018ZQ035), the Fundamental Research Funds for the Central Universities (No.2017XZZX001-01), Zhejiang Medicine and Health Science and Technology Program (2018KY418).

Authors' contributions

KL and XL contributed equally to this work. KL designed the study and wrote the first draft of the manuscript. XL analysed the MRI data and wrote the protocol. JY modified the manuscript. QZ and JX collected the clinical and MRI data. JZ, CW, XX, PH, ZS and MZ assisted with study design and interpretation of findings. All authors have contributed to and approved the final manuscript. All authors read and approved the final manuscript.

Competing interests

The authors declare that they have no competing interests.

Author details

[1]Department of Radiology, 2nd Affiliated Hospital of Zhejiang University School of Medicine, No.88 Jie-fang Road, Shang-cheng District, Hangzhou 310009, China. [2]Department of Neurology, 2nd Affiliated Hospital of Zhejiang University School of Medicine, Zhejiang, China.

References

1. Jessen F, Amariglio RE, van Boxtel M, Breteler M, Ceccaldi M, Chételat G, Dubois B, Dufouil C, Ellis KA, van der Flier WM, Glodzik L, van Harten AC, de Leon MJ, McHugh P, et al. A conceptual framework for research on subjective cognitive decline in preclinical Alzheimer's disease. Alzheimers Dement. 2014;10:844–52.
2. Reisberg B, Prichep L, Mosconi L, John ER, Glodzik-Sobanska L, Boksay I, Monteiro I, Torossian C, Vedvyas A, Ashraf N, Jamil IA, de Leon MJ. The pre-mild cognitive impairment, subjective cognitive impairment stage of Alzheimer's disease. Alzheimers Dement. 2008;4:S98–S108.
3. Reisberg B, Shulman MB, Torossian C, Leng L, Zhu W. Outcome over seven years of healthy adults with and without subjective cognitive impairment. Alzheimers Dement. 2010;6:11–24.
4. Jessen F, Wiese B, Bachmann C, Eifflaender-Gorfer S, Haller F, Kolsch H, Luck T, Mosch E, van den Bussche H, Wagner M, Wollny A, Zimmermann T, Pentzek M, Riedel-Heller SG, Romberg HP, Weyerer S, Kaduszkiewicz H, Maier W, Bickel H, German Study on Aging Cognition, Dementia in Primary Care Patients Study Group. Prediction of dementia by subjective memory impairment: effects of severity and temporal association with cognitive impairment. Arch Gen Psychiatry. 2010;67:414–22.
5. Jessen F, Wolfsgruber S, Wiese B, et al. AD dementia risk in late MCI, in early MCI, and in subjective memory impairment. Alzheimers Dement. 2014;10:76–83.
6. Kaup AR, Nettiksimmons J, LeBlanc ES, Yaffe K. Memory complaints and risk of cognitive impairment after nearly 2 decades among older women. Neurology. 2015;85:1852–8.
7. R€ o MS€ o A, Adolfsson R, Nilsson LG. Subjective memory impairment in older adults predicts future dementia independent of baseline memory performance: Evidence from the Betula prospective cohort study. Alzheimers Dement. 2015;11:1385–92.
8. Schultz SAOJM, Koscik RL, Dowling NM, Gallagher CL, Carlsson CM, Bendlin BB, LaRue A, Hermann BP, Rowley HA, Asthana S, Sager MA, Johnson SC, Okonkwo OC. Subjective memory complaints, cortical thinning, and cognitive dysfunction in middle-aged adults at risk for AD. Alzheimers Dement. 2015;1:33–40.
9. Saykin AJ, Wishart HA, Rabin LA, Santulli RB, Flashman LA, West JD, McHugh TL, Mamourian AC. Older adults with cognitive complaints show brain atrophy similar to that of amnestic MCI. Neurology. 2006;67:834–42.
10. Li XY, Tang ZC, Sun Y, Tian J, Liu ZY, Han Y. White matter degeneration in subjective cognitive decline: a diffusion tensor imaging study. Oncotarget. 2016;7:54405–14.
11. Mosconi L, De Santi S, Brys M, et al. Hypometabolism and altered cerebrospinal fluid markers in normal apolipoprotein E E4 carriers with subjective memory complaints. Biol Psychiatry. 2008;63:609–18.
12. Scheef L, Spottke A, Daerr M, Joe A, Striepens N, K€ o H, et al. Glucose metabolism, gray matter structure, and memory decline in subjective memory impairment. Neurology. 2012;79:1332–9.
13. Rodda J, Dannhauser T, Cutinha DJ, Shergill SS, Walker Z. Subjective cognitive impairment: Functional MRI during a divided attention task. Eur Psychiatry. 2011;26:457–62.
14. Rodda JE, Dannhauser TM, Cutinha DJ, Shergill SS, Walker Z. Subjective cognitive impairment: increased prefrontal cortex activation compared to controls during an encoding task. Int J Geriatr Psychiatry. 2009;24:865–74.
15. Sun Y, Dai Z, Li Y, Sheng C, Li H, Wang X, Chen X, He Y, Han Y. Subjective Cognitive Decline: Mapping Functional and Structural Brain Changes-A Combined Resting-State Functional and Structural MR Imaging Study. Radiology. 2016;281:185–92.
16. Barnes LL, Schneider JA, Boyle PA, Bienias JL, Bennett DA. Memory complaints are related to Alzheimer disease pathology in older persons. Neurology. 2006;67:1581–5.
17. Buckley RF, Hanseeuw B, Schultz AP, Vannini P, Aghjayan SL, Properzi MJ, Jackson JD, Mormino EC, Rentz DM, Sperling RA, Johnson KA, Amariglio RE. Region-Specific Association of Subjective Cognitive Decline With Tauopathy Independent of Global beta-Amyloid Burden. JAMA Neurol. 2017;74:1455–63.
18. Zuo XN, Ehmke R, Mennes M, Imperati D, Castellanos FX, Sporns O, Milham MP. Network centrality in the human functional connectome. Cereb Cortex. 2012;22:1862–75.

19. Wink AM, de Munck JC, van der Werf YD, van den Heuvel OA, Barkhof F. Fast eigenvector centrality mapping of voxel-wise connectivity in functional magnetic resonance imaging: implementation, validation, and interpretation. Brain Connect. 2012;2:265–74.
20. Binnewijzend MA, Adriaanse SM, Van der Flier WM, Teunissen CE, de Munck JC, Stam CJ, Scheltens P, van Berckel BN, Barkhof F, Wink AM. Brain network alterations in Alzheimer's disease measured by eigenvector centrality in fMRI are related to cognition and CSF biomarkers. Hum Brain Mapp. 2014;35:2383–93.
21. Blennow K, Hampel H. CSF markers for incipient Alzheimer's disease. Lancet Neurol. 2003;2:605–13.
22. Frisoni GB, Pievani M, Testa C, Sabattoli F, Bresciani L, Bonetti M, et al. The topography of grey matter involvement in early and late onset Alzheimer's disease. Brain. 2007;130:720–30.
23. Sheikh JI, Yesavage JA. Geriatric Depression Scale (GDS): recent evidence and development of a shorter version. In: Brink TL, editor. Clinical Gerontology: A Guide to Assessment and Intervention. New York, NY: The Haworth Press; 1986. p. 165–73.
24. Schindler SE, Gray JD, Gordon BA, Xiong C, Batrla-Utermann R, Quan M, Wahl S, Benzinger TLS, Holtzman DM, Morris JC, Fagan AM. Cerebrospinal fluid biomarkers measured by Elecsys assays compared to amyloid imaging. Alzheimers Dement. 2018.
25. Chao-Gan Y, Yu-Feng Z. DPARSF: A MATLAB Toolbox for "Pipeline" Data Analysis of Resting-State fMRI. Front Syst Neurosci. 2010;4:13.
26. Song XW, Dong ZY, Long XY, Li SF, Zuo XN, Zhu CZ, He Y, Yan CG, Zang YF. REST: a toolkit for resting-state functional magnetic resonance imaging data processing. PLoS One. 2011;6:e25031.
27. Friston KJ, Williams S, Howard R, Frackowiak RS, Turner R. Movement-related effects in fMRI time-series. Magn Reson Med. 1996;35:346–55.
28. Yan CG, Cheung B, Kelly C, Colcombe S, Craddock RC, Di Martino A, Li Q, Zuo XN, Castellanos FX, Milham MP. A comprehensive assessment of regional variation in the impact of head micromovements on functional connectomics. Neuroimage. 2013;76:183–201.
29. Fiecas M, Cribben I, Bahktiari R, Cummine J. A variance components model for statistical inference on functional connectivity networks. Neuroimage. 2017;149:256–66.
30. Arbabshirani MR, Damaraju E, Phlypo R, Plis S, Allen E, Ma S, Mathalon D, Preda A, Vaidya JG, Adali T, Calhoun VD. Impact of autocorrelation on functional connectivity. Neuroimage. 2014;102(Pt 2):294–308.
31. García-García I, Jurado MÁ, Garolera M, Marqués-Iturria I, Horstmann A, Segura B, Pueyo R, Sender-Palacios MJ, Vernet-Vernet M, Villringer A, Junqué C, Margulies DS, Neumann J. Functional network centrality in obesity: A resting-state and task fMRI study. Psychiatry Research. 2015;233:331–8.
32. Buckner RL, Sepulcre J, Talukdar T, Krienen FM, Liu H, Hedden T, Andrews-Hanna JR, Sperling RA, Johnson KA. Cortical hubs revealed by intrinsic functional connectivity: mapping, assessment of stability, and relation to Alzheimer's disease. J Neurosci. 2009;29:1860–73.
33. Li S Ma X, Huang R, Li M, Tian J, Wen H, Lin C, Wang T, Zhan W, Fang J, Jiang G. Abnormal degree centrality in neurologically asymptomatic patients with end-stage renal disease: A resting-state fMRI study. Clin Neurophysiol. 2016;127:602–9.
34. Takeuchi H, Taki Y, Nouchi R, Sekiguchi A, Hashizume H, Sassa Y, Kotozaki Y, Miyauchi CM, Yokoyama R, Iizuka K, Nakagawa S, Nagase T, Kunitoki K, Kawashima R. Degree centrality and fractional amplitude of low-frequency oscillations associated with Stroop interference. Neuroimage. 2015;119:197–209.
35. Wink AM, de Munck JC, van der Werf YD, van den Heuvel OA, Barkhof F. Fast eigenvector centrality mapping of voxel-wise connectivity in functionalmagnetic resonance imaging: Implementation, validation, and interpretation. Brain Connect. 2012;2:265–74.
36. Lohmann G, Margulies DS, Horstmann A, Pleger B, Lepsien J, Goldhahn D, Schloegl H, Stumvoll M, Villringer A, Turner R. Eigenvector centrality mapping for analyzing connectivity patterns in fMRI data of the human brain. PLoS One. 2010;5:e10232.
37. Sperling RA, Jack CR Jr, Aisen PS. Testing the right target and right drug at the right stage. Sci Trans Med. 2011;3:111cm133.
38. Wang XN, Zeng Y, Chen GQ, Zhang YH, Li XY, Hao XY, Yu Y, Zhang M, Sheng C, Li YX, Sun Y, Li HY, Song Y, Li KC, Yan TY, Tang XY, Han Y. Abnormal organization of white matter networks in patients with subjective cognitive decline and mild cognitive impairment. Oncotarget. 2016;7:48953–62.
39. Verfaillie SCJ, Pichet Binette A, Vachon-Presseau E, Tabrizi S, Savard M, Bellec P, Ossenkoppele R, Scheltens P, van der Flier WM, Breitner JCS, Villeneuve S, Group Prevent-Ad Research. Subjective Cognitive Decline Is Associated With Altered Default Mode Network Connectivity in Individuals With a Family History of Alzheimer's Disease. Biol Psychiatry Cogn Neurosci Neuroimaging. 2018;3:463–72.
40. Miller SL, Celone K, DePeau K, Diamond E, Dickerson BC, Rentz D, Pihlajamaki M, Sperling RA. Age-related memory impairment associated with loss of parietal deactivation but preserved hippocampal activation. Proc Natl Acad Sci U S A. 2008;105:2181–6.
41. Buckner RL, Andrews-Hanna JR, Schacter DL. The brain's default network: anatomy, function, and relevance to disease. Ann N Y Acad Sci. 2008;1124:1–38.
42. Zhuang L, Sachdev PS, Trollor JN, Kochan NA, Reppermund S, Brodaty H, Wen W. Microstructural white matter changes in cognitively normal individuals at risk of amnestic MCI. Neurology. 2012;79:748–54.
43. Hafkemeijer A, Altmann-Schneider I, Oleksik AM, van de Wiel L, Middelkoop HA, van Buchem MA, van der Grond J, Rombouts SA. Increased Functional Connectivity and Brain Atrophy in Elderly with Subjective Memory Complaints. Brain Connect. 2013;3:353–62.
44. Wang Y, West JD, Flashman LA, Wishart HA, Santulli RB, Rabin LA, Pare N, Arfanakis K, Saykin AJ. Selective changes in white matter integrity in MCI and older adults with cognitive complaints. Biochim Biophys Acta. 2012; 1822:423–30.
45. Elman JA, Oh H, Madison CM, Baker SL, Vogel JW, Marks SM, Crowley S, O'Neil JP, Jagust WJ. Neural compensation in older people with brain amyloid-beta deposition. Nat Neurosci. 2014;17:1316–8.
46. Hillary FG, Grafman JH. Injured Brains and Adaptive Networks: The Benefits and Costs of Hyperconnectivity. Trends Cogn Sci. 2017;21:385–401.
47. Myeku N, Clelland CL, Emrani S, Kukushkin NV, Yu WH, Goldberg AL, Duff KE. Tau-driven 26S proteasome impairment and cognitive dysfunction can be prevented early in disease by activating cAMP-PKA signaling. Nat Med. 2016;22:46–53.
48. Ballatore C, Lee VM, Trojanowski JQ. Tau-mediated neurodegeneration in Alzheimer,s disease and related disorders. Nat Rev Neurosci. 2007;8:663–72.
49. Beckett LA, Donohue MC, Wang C, Aisen P, Harvey DJ, Saito N, Initiative A's DN. The Alzheimer's Disease Neuroimaging Initiative phase 2: Increasing the length, breadth, and depth of our understanding. Alzheimers Dement. 2015; 11:823–31.
50. Rodda J, Okello A, Edison P, Dannhauser T, Brooks DJ, Walker Z. (11)C-PIB PET in subjective cognitive impairment. Eur Psychiatry. 2010;25:123–5.
51. Chetelat G, Villemagne VL, Bourgeat P, Pike KE, Jones G, Ames D, Ellis KA, Szoeke C, Martins RN, O'Keefe GJ, Salvado O, Masters CL, Rowe CC, Australian Imaging Biomarkers, Lifestyle Research Group. Relationship between atrophy and beta-amyloid deposition in Alzheimer disease. Ann Neurol. 2010;67:317–24.
52. Ivanoiu A, Dricot L, Gilis N, Grandin C, Lhommel R, Quenon L, Hanseeuw B. Classification of non-demented patients attending a memory clinic using the new diagnostic criteria for Alzheimer's disease with disease-related biomarkers. J Alzheimers Dis. 2015;43:835–47.
53. Schwarz AJ, Yu P, Miller BB, Shcherbinin S, Dickson J, Navitsky M, Joshi AD, Devous MD Sr, Mintun MS. Regional profiles of the candidate tau PET ligand 18F-AV-1451 recapitulate key features of Braak histopathological stages. Brain. 2016;139:1539–50.
54. Braak H, Braak E. Neuropathological staging of Alzheimer-related changes. Acta Neuropathologica. 1991;82:239–59.
55. Andrews-Hanna JR, Reidler JS, Sepulcre J, Poulin R, Buckner RL. Functional-anatomic fractionation of the brain's default network. Neuron. 2010;65:550–62.
56. Mormino EC, Kluth JT, Madison CM, Rabinovici GD, Baker SL, Miller BL, Koeppe RA, Mathis CA, Weiner MW, Jagust WJ, Initiative A's DN. Episodic memory loss is related to hippocampal-mediated beta-amyloid deposition in elderly subjects. Brain. 2009;132:1310–23.
57. Risacher SL, Tallman EF, West JD, Yoder KK, Hutchins GD, Fletcher JW, Gao S, Kareken DA, Farlow MR, Apostolova LG, Saykin AJ. Olfactory identification in subjective cognitive decline and mild cognitive impairment: Association with tau but not amyloid positron emission tomography. Alzheimers Dement (Amst). 2017;9:57–66.
58. Blackburn DJ, Wakefield S, Shanks MF, Harkness K, Reuber M, Venneri A. Memory difficulties are not always a sign of incipient dementia: a review of the possible causes of loss of memory efficiency. Br Med Bull. 2014;112:71–81.
59. Caselli RJ, Chen K, Locke DE, Lee W, Roontiva A, Bandy D, Fleisher AS, Reiman EM. Subjective cognitive decline: self and informant comparisons. Alzheimers Dement. 2014;10:93–8.
60. Caracciolo B, Gatz M, Xu W, Marengoni A, Pedersen NL, Fratiglioni L. Relationship of subjective cognitive impairment and cognitive impairment

no dementia to chronic disease and multimorbidity in a nation-wide twin study. J Alzheimers Dis. 2013;36:275–84.
61. Comijs HC, Deeg DJ, Dik MG, Twisk JW, Jonker C. Memory complaints; the association with psycho-affective and health problems and the role of personality characteristics. A 6-year follow-up study. J Affect Disord. 2002;72:157–65.
62. Steffens DC, Potter GG. Geriatric depression and cognitive impairment. Psychol Med. 2008;38:163–75.
63. Derouesne C, Lacomplez L, Thibault S, LePoncin M. Memory complaints in young and elderly subjects. Int J Geriatr Psychiat. 1999;14:291–301.
64. Jorm AF, Butterworth P, Anstey KJ, et al. Memory complaints in a community sample aged 60–64 years: associations with cognitive functioning, psychiatric symptoms, APOE genotype, hippocampus and amygdale volumes, and white matter hyperintensities. Psychol Med. 2004; 34:1495–506.
65. Ramakers IH, Verhey FR, Scheltens P, et al. Anxiety is related to Alzheimer cerebrospinal fluid markers in subjects with mild cognitive impairment. Psychol Med. 2013;43:911–20.
66. Green KN, Billings LM, Roozendaal B, et al. Glucocorticoids increase amyloid-beta and tau pathology in a mouse model of Alzheimer's disease. J Neurosci. 2006;26:9047–56.
67. Kaup AR, Byers AL, Falvey C, Simonsick EM, Satterfield S, Ayonayon HN, et al. Trajectories of Depressive Symptoms in Older Adults and Risk of Dementia. JAMA Psychiatry. 2016;73:525–31.
68. Jack CR Jr, Bennett DA, Blennow K, Carrillo MC, Dunn B, Haeberlein SB, Holtzman DM, Jagust W, Jessen F, Karlawish J, Liu E, Molinuevo JL, Montine T, Phelps C, Rankin KP, Rowe CC, Scheltens P, Siemers E, Snyder HM, Sperling R, Contributors. NIA-AA Research Framework: Toward a biological definition of Alzheimer's disease. Alzheimers Dement. 2018;14:535–62.
69. Jack CR Jr, Knopman DS, Chetelat G, Dickson D, Fagan AM, Frisoni GB, Jagust W, Mormino EC, Petersen RC, Sperling RA, van der Flier WM, Villemagne VL, Visser PJ, Vos SJ. Suspected non-Alzheimer disease pathophysiology--concept and controversy. Nat Rev Neurol. 2016;12:117–24.

Identification of Ser465 as a novel PINK1 autophosphorylation site

Ji-feng Guo[1,2,3,4], Ling-yan Yao[1], Qi-ying Sun[1], Yi-ting Cui[1], Yang Yang[1], Qian Xu[1], Xin-xiang Yan[1,3,4] and Bei-sha Tang[1,2,3,4,5,6,7*]

Abstract

Background: PINK1 (PTEN-induced putative kinase 1) gene is the causal gene for recessive familial type 6 of Parkinson's disease (PARK6), which is an early-onset autosomal recessive inherited neurodegenerative disease. PINK1 has been reported to exert both autophosphorylation and phosphorylation activity, affecting cell damage under stress and other physiological responses. However, there has been no report on the identification of PINK1 autophosphorylation sites and their physiological functions.

Methods: (1) We adopted mass spectrometry assay to identify the autophosphorylation site of PINK1, and autoradiography assay was further conducted to confirm this result. (2) Kinase activity assay was used to compare the kinase activity of both Ser465 mutant PINK1 and disease-causing mutant PINK1. (3) We use Pulse-chase analysis to measure whether Ser465 may affect PINK1 degradation. (4) Immunocytochemistry staining was used to study the PINK1 subcellular localization and Parkin transition in subcellular level.

Result: In our study, we identified the 465th serine residue (Ser465) as one of the autophosphorylation sites in PINK1 protein. The inactivation of Ser465 can decrease the kinase activity of PINK1. Either dissipated or excessive Ser465 site phosphorylation of PINK1 can slow down its degradation. PINK1 autophosphorylation contributes to the transit of Parkin to mitochondria, and has no effect on its subcellular localization. PARK6 causal mutations, T313 M and R492X, display the same characteristics as Ser465A mutation PINK1 protein, such as decreasing PINK1 kinase activity and affecting its interaction with Parkin.

Conclusion: Ser465 was identified as one of the autophosphorylation sites of PINK1, which affected PINK1 kinase activity. In addition, Ser465 is involved in the degradation of PINK1 and the transit of Parkin to mitochondria. T313 M and R492X, two novel PARK6 mutations on Thr313 and Arg492, were similar to Ser465 mutation, including decreasing PINK1 phosphorylation activity and Parkin subcellular localization.

Keywords: Parkinson's disease, PINK1, Autophosphorylation sites, Kinase activity

Background

Parkinson's disease (PD) is one of the most pervasive neurodegenerative diseases. Currently, the etiology and mechanism of PD are not fully clear. But, aging, environmental and genetic factors appear to play the key role in PD [2, 7, 21].

PINK1 (*PTEN-induced putative kinase 1*) gene is the causative gene for PARK6, which was cloned in 2004 by Valente et al. [20]. Encoded by the *PINK1* gene, PINK1 protein contains 581 amino acids, including a mitochondrial localization domain (34 amino acids) and a serine/threonine kinase domain (354 amino acids). The kinase domain (KD) is highly conserved, capable of catalyzing by binding to the peptide substrate and transferring ATP phosphate group [20]. Recent studies showed that PINK1 may directly phosphorylate other proteins, exerting anti-oxidative stress and anti-apoptosis effects. TRAP1 protein is found to be the substrate of PINK1 [14], through which, PINK1 can reduce the release of mitochondrial cytochrome c and fill the gap caused by cell damage and even cell death under stress. In 2008,

* Correspondence: bstang7398@163.com
[1]Department of Neurology, Xiangya Hospital, Central South University, Changsha, Hunan 410008, People's Republic of China
[2]Laboratory of Medical Genetics, Central South University Changsha, Changsha, Hunan 410078, China
Full list of author information is available at the end of the article

Kim et al. [8] found that PINK1 can phosphorylate Parkin directly, regulating their transfer to the mitochondria. In addition, PINK1 kinase domain possesses both autophosphorylation [11] and phosphorylation activity in vitro, such as phosphorylating histone H1 or casein [17, 18]. In our previous work, we found two novel *PINK1* homozygous disease-causing mutations (T313 M, R492X) [6], both located in the kinase domain. Matenia et al. [9] found that microtubule affinity regulating kinase 2 (MARK2) can phosphorylate PINK1, and Thr313 was proved to be the phosphorylation site. When T313 M mutation occurs, PINK1 cannot be phosphorylated, leading to mitochondrial toxicity and abnormal distribution in nerve cells. Arg492 is located at the junction of PINK1 protein kinase domain and the carboxyl terminus. R492X mutation can cause the loss of the entire carboxyl terminal, altering PINK1 kinase activity [6, 17].

There has been no report on the identification of PINK1 autophosphorylation sites in vitro studies and the effect on physiological functions brought by the changes of these sites. Our study demonstrated that Ser465 was one of the autophosphorylation sites in PINK1. The autophosphorylation of PINK1 protein can affect its kinase activity, protein stability, as well as the interaction with Parkin. *PINK1* causative mutations T313 M and R492X may cause PD by affecting its kinase activity and interaction with Parkin.

Methods

Plasmid construction

293A human embryonic kidney cells, pGEX-5X-1 vector, pKH3-PINK1 and EGFP-Parkin plasmid were provided by the school of Life Science of University of Science and Technology in China. pKH3-PINK1-T313 M, pKH3-PINK1-R492X and pGEX-5X-1-PINK1 plasmids were constructed in our previous work [3, 22]. pGEX-5X-1-PINK1-T313 M, pGEX-5X-1-PINK1-R492X, pGEX-5X-1-PINK1-S465A, pGEX-5X-1-PINK1-S465D, pKH3-PINK1-S465A and pKH3-PINK1- S465D plasmids were all constructed by this study.

Protein expression and purification in *E. coli*

We used the same method to induce prokaryotic plasmid expression and purify protein as described in a previous study [3, 22]. A small amount of GST-PINK1 bacteria (112–581 aa) were inoculated into a 600 mL culture medium (AMP+), incubated at 37 °C, 250 rpm. When OD values reached between 0.4–0.6, 100 μl IPTG was added to the culture and incubated for 3 h under the same condition. Resuspended the culture with 1XPBS, followed by sonication, then a crude supernatant was obtained. The protein extract was purified with G4B purification column. SDS-PAGE was used to identify the purified protein, followed by Coomassie brilliant blue staining.

Kinase assay and mass spectrometry

Autophosphorylation of recombinant PINK1 protein was performed in the reaction system containing 2.4 μL of 10X kinase reaction buffer, 19.6 μL of GST-PINK1 purified protein supernatant, 2 μL of 10 mM ATP. Then the mixture was incubated in 30 °C water bath for 1.5 h. All the phosphorylated proteins were denatured by 5XSDS, heating at 100 °C for 5 min, resolved by SDS-PAGE, followed by brilliant coomassie blue R250 staining for 30 min and decolorizing for 5 min. Excised gel slices containing desired bands, can be stored at 4 °C and sent for mass spectrometry analysis.

Autoradiography

The proteins were purified by the same method described before. 2.4 μL of 10X kinase reaction buffer, 19.6 μL of purified protein supernatant, 10 μCi of [γ^{-32P}] ATP were added, and incubated in 30 °C water bath for 30 min. Then 5XSDS was added, and boiled at 100 °C for 5 min. SDS-PAGE was carried out as described previously, and protein bands were stained with brilliant coomassie blue R250 for 5 min, and decolorized for another 5 min. The plastic wrapped gel and a film in the X-ray film cassette were placed in a dark room. The film was exposed at −80 °C for 8-16 h, followed by developing and fixing.

Cell culture and transfection

The 293A cells were maintained in the medium containing 10% fetal bovine serum, 100 U/ml penicillin and 100 U/ml streptomycin, and incubated at 37 °C in a CO_2 incubator. Plasmid transfection was performed according to the Lipofectamine®2000 protocol.

Immunocytochemistry staining

The immunocytochemical staining of eukaryotic plasmid cells was conducted with the method used in previous articles [3, 22]. The cultured cells were fixed with 4% paraformaldehyde. 0.25% TritonX-100/PBS was used for permeabilization. The samples were blocked in 1% FBS/PBS, and incubated with primary antibody and Rhodamine fluorophores conjugated secondary antibodies. Counterstaining with DAPI, the fluorescence was observed under the inverted fluorescence microscope, then images were captured.

Pulse-chase analysis

After cell transfection for 24-36 h, each well was added with 100 μg/mL CHX (cycloheximide, CHX). Cells were collected at 0 h, 1 h, 2 h and 3.5 h after the addition of CHX. Total protein was extracted for Western analysis to detect the degradation of the interested protein.

Statistical analysis

All statistical data were calculated and analyzed using SPSS Statistics 13.0 software. All error bars were expressed as mean ± s.d.. The statistical significance of differences was evaluated by one-way ANOVA, followed by student's *t*-test.

Results

Identification of PINK1 protein autophosphorylation site(s) with mass spectrometry

We firstly constructed GST-PINK1 plasmid and purified the GST-PINK1 protein in large quantities. The purity of the recombinant protein was verified by SDS-PAGE and followed by coomassie blue staining, as shown in Fig. 1a. To identify the autophosphorylation sites of PINK1, we adopted the well-utilized kinase assay with the purified GST-PINK1 protein as both the kinase and substrate. Afterwards, the phosphorylated mix was separated by SDS-PAGE, and the matched bands were excised for mass spectrometry (provided by Beijing Proteome Research Center) and analyzed with Mascot (UK Matrix Science Co.) (Fig. 1b, c, d). The MS/MS data suggested that the auto-phosphorylation site was located in the 465th amino acid in PINK1, which was demonstrated to be well conserved by the homology detection among nine different species (Fig. 1e).

PINK1 protein autophosphorylation level can be weakened by silencing S465 phosphorylation site

To further confirm whether Ser465 in PINK1 was the autophosphorylation site, we firstly constructed prokaryotic expression vector pGEX-5X-1-PINK1-S465A, in which serine residue (S) was replaced by alanine residue (A) by site-directed mutagenesis, which cannot be phosphorylated. The GST-PINK1-S465A can be expressed in *E. coli* after induction (Fig. 2a). To detect the change of autophosphorylation level of PINK1 protein after Ser465 was silenced, we performed the kinase phosphorylation reaction with the purified fusion proteins as both kinase and substrate meanwhile. With the involvement of [γ^{-32P}] ATP, we can quantify the kinase activity. The experiment was divided into three groups with purified GST, GST-PINK1-WT, GST-PINK1-S465A fusion protein, respectively. The SDS-PAGE was performed after the kinase reaction (Fig. 2b). Autoradiography results were showed in Fig. 2c. No positive bands appeared in the GST only group, which is a negative control; positive bands appeared in both GST-PINK1-WT and GST-PINK1-S465A groups. Compared to the GST-PINK1-WT, the autophosphorylation level of GST-PINK1-S465A was obviously lower (Fig. 2d), implying that the total phosphorylation level was

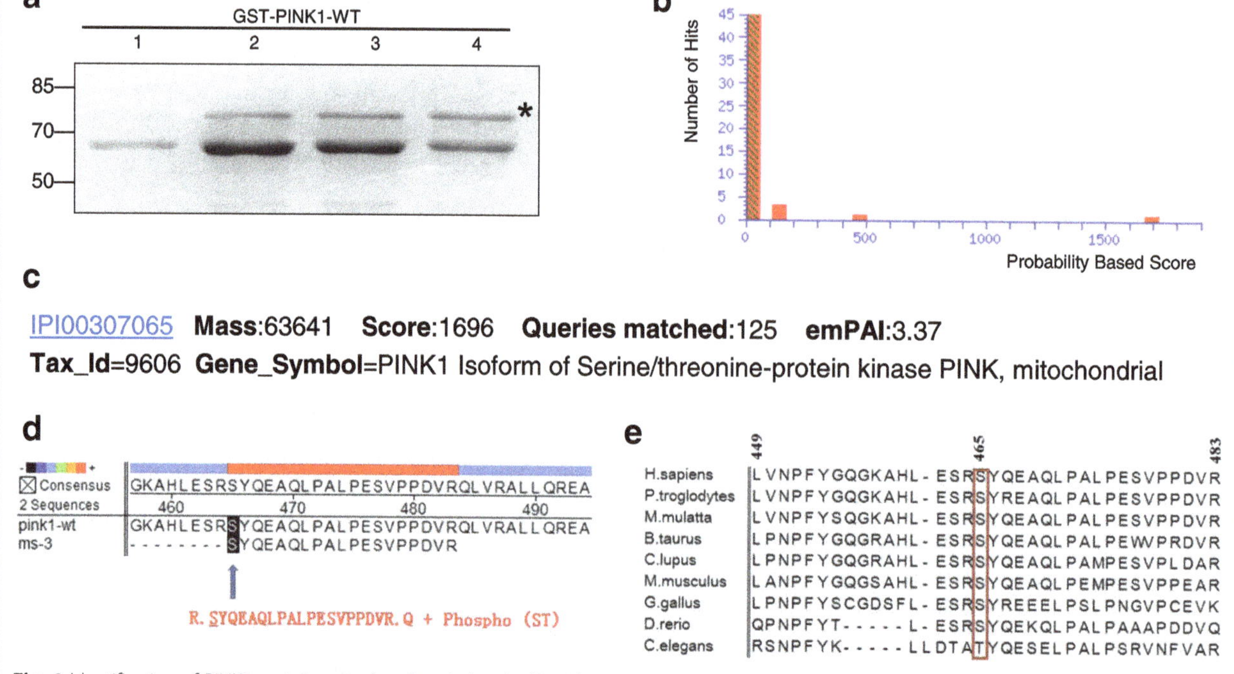

Fig. 1 Identification of PINK1 protein autophosphorylation site(s) with mass spectrometry. **a** Coomassie blue staining of purified GST-PINK1-WT fusion protein. The asterisk indicates the band of PINK1, 77 kDa, equivalent of the molecular weight of GST-PINK1-WT fusion protein. **b** Protein score histogram in Mascot with the mass spectrometry data. The horizontal axis stands for protein match score (a higher score indicating a more reliable result), and the vertical axis represents the number of matched protein. The red bar, located around 1600–1700 at the horizontal axis, suggests the autophosphorylation site. **c** Detailed information of the identified autophosphorylation site. **d** A comparison of the identified sequence with the PINK1 protein sequence (NCBI database). The modified serine site (marked by black square), referring to the autophosphorylation site, is located at the 465th serine site in PINK1. **e** Ser465 (in red) displays highly conserved in nine organisms

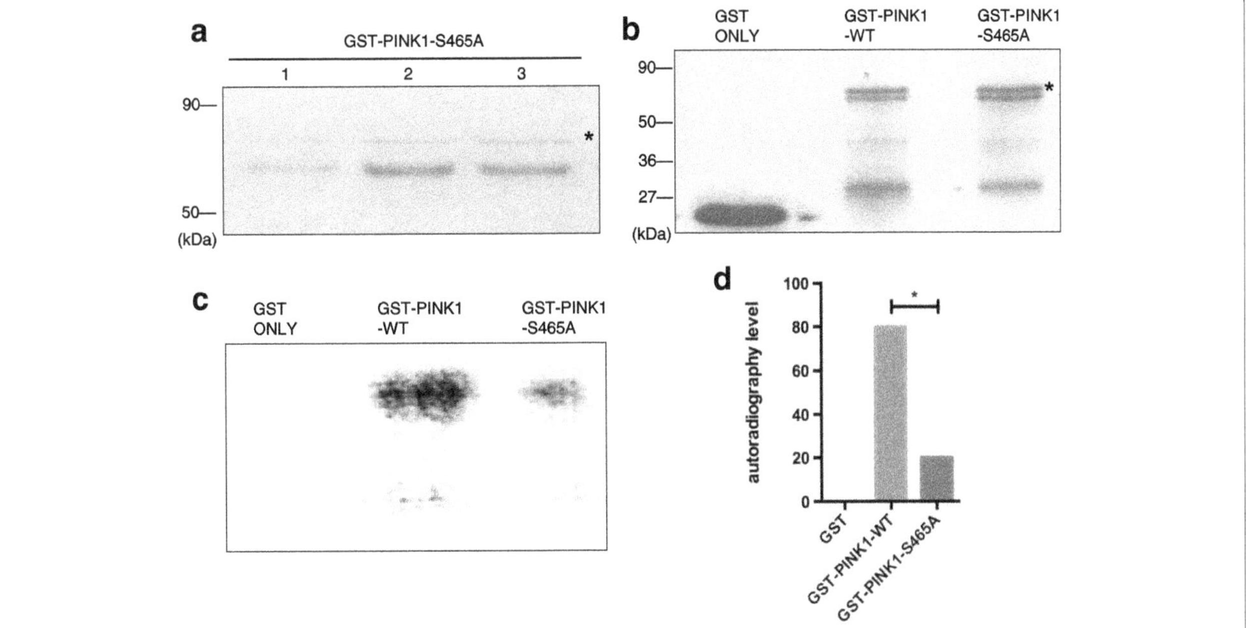

Fig. 2 PINK1 protein autophosphorylation can be weakened by silencing S465 phosphorylation site. **a** Coomassie blue staining of purified GST-PINK1-S465A fusion protein. **b** Coomassie blue staining of three kinase phosphorylation reaction systems (GST, GST-PINK1-WT and GST-PINK1-S465A). GST protein band was shown in lane 1, as a negative control. Visible GST-PINK1-WT and GST-PINK1-S465A fusion protein bands were shown in Lane 2 and lane 3 respectively, as shown by asterisk. **c** Autoradiography results of three groups. Two positive bands were shown in lane 2 and 3, which stands for the autophosphorylation level of the two groups with GST-PINK1-WT and GST-PINK1-S465A as the kinases, respectively. No positive bands in lane 1. **d** Quantification of the autophosphorylation activity of GST-PINK1-WT and GST-PINK1-S465A protein based on the result of autoradiography. Compared to the WT fusion protein, the autophosphorylation level of mutant GST-PINK1-S465A protein was lower. *$P < 0.05$, statistically significant

significantly decreased after Ser465 kinase activity was disabled. The result strongly demonstrated that Ser465 was the autophosphorylation site in PINK1. Even though Ser465 was disabled, there were still some detectable weak signals in the GST-PINK1-S465A group, hinting the existence of other autophosphorylation sites besides Ser465 in PINK1.

Both disease-causing mutant PINK1 protein and Ser465A mutant PINK1 protein decrease its kinase activity

In our previous work, we found two novel *PINK1* homozygous disease-causing mutations, T313 M and R492X, which are mutations on Thr313 and Arg492, respectively. As the two sites are both kinase domain located, they may cause disease by affecting PINK1 kinase activity. In order to investigate whether T313 M and R492X mutations affect its kinase activity, we constructed prokaryotic expression vector of T313 M and R492X PINK1 plasmid, pGEX-5X-1-PINK1-T313 M and pGEX-5X-1-PINK1-R492X (Fig. 3a, b), which were purified as described above (Fig. 3c, d). Ser465A is also the mutant PINK1 protein, which can disable the autophosphorylation activity of Ser465 in PINK1, as described above. Five phosphorylation reaction groups were designed with casein as the common substrate and the fusion proteins as the kinases, respectively, including GST protein, GST-PINK1-WT protein, GST-PINK1-T313 M protein, GST-PINK1-R492X, GST -PINK1-S465A protein. After the phosphorylation reaction, SDS-PAGE was performed (Fig. 3e). The autoradiography results were shown in Fig. 3e. No positive bands appeared in GST only group. The levels of phosphorylated casein were decreased in the three mutant protein groups, GST-PINK1-T313 M, GST-PINK1-R492X and GST-PINK1-S465A, compared with GST-PINK1-WT group. The differences between three mutants and the wild-type PINK1 protein were statistically significant ($P < 0.05$), respectively (Fig. 3f).

S465 has no influence on PINK1 subcellular localization

In order to further clarify the meaning of Ser465 autophosphorylation in eukaryotic cells, we constructed prokaryotic expression vector of S465A and S465D mutant PINK1, pKH3-PINK1-S465A and pKH3-PINK1-S465D. S465A was described as above, which cannot be phosphorylated. In opposite, aspartic acid residues (D) took the place of the serine residue (S), which was phosphorylation-mimic. We then transfected pKH3-PINK1-WT, pKH3-PINK1-S465A, pKH3- PINK1-S465D in HEK293 cells respectively, with the pKH3 vector as a blank control, followed by immunofluorescence staining. The results showed that pKH3-PINK1-WT protein was located in the cytoplasm, punctate distribution, co-

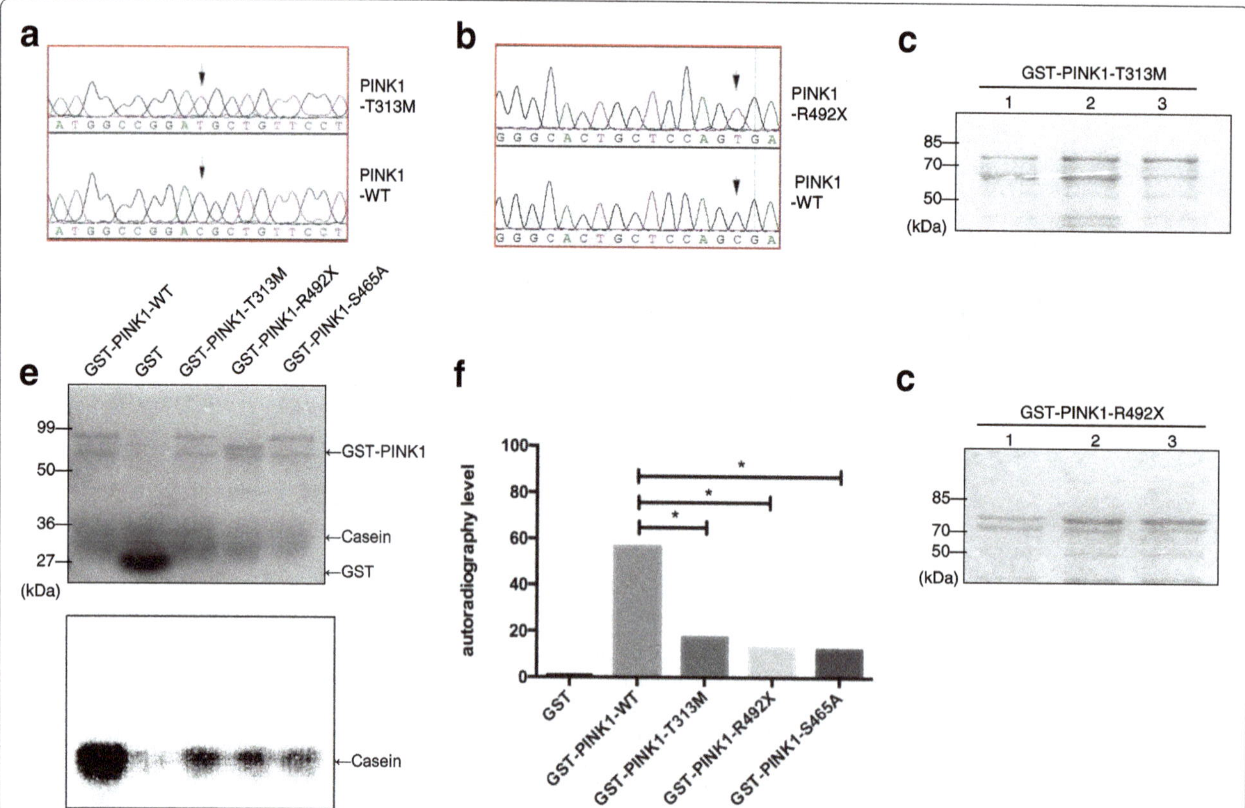

Fig. 3 Both disease-causing mutant PINK1 protein and Ser465A mutant PINK1 protein decreased its kinase activity. **a** Sanger sequencing of T313 M mutant PINK1 and WT PINK1. The arrow indicates that the 938th base mutated from C to T, leading to threonine mutated to methionine. **b** Sanger sequencing of R492X mutant PINK1 and WT PINK1. The arrow indicates that the 1474th base mutated from C to T, leading to arginine mutated to a stop code. (**c, d**) Coomassie blue staining of purified GST-PINK1-T313 M and GST-PINK1-R492X fusion proteins. **e** Wild-type and three mutant GST-PINK1 proteins phosphorylation activity with casein as the common substrate. The upper one is the result of Coomassie Blue staining. Each lane represents GST-PINK1-WT fusion protein, GST protein, GST-PINK1-T313 M fusion protein and GST-PINK1-R492X fusion protein, respectively. The lower one was the result of autoradiography of five groups. Except GST group, four positive signals appeared in the other four groups, standing for the casein phosphorylated by GST-PINK1-WT fusion protein, GST-PINK1-T313 M fusion protein, GST-PINK1-R492X fusion protein and GST-PINK1-S465A fusion protein respectively. **f** Bar graph showing the quantification of phosphorylation activity of the five groups. The difference between three mutant PINK1 proteins and WT protein were statistically significant ($^{*}P < 0.05$)

localized with the Mito staining, showing a typical mitochondrial localization (Fig. 4f); No significant change of subcellular location for the two mutant PINK1 protein, pKH3-PINK1-S465A and pKH3-PINK1-S465D, still displaying the same co-localization with mitochondria in the cytoplasm (Fig. 4i, l).

S465 phosphorylation site affects PINK1 degradation

HA-PINK1-WT, HA-PINK1-S465A and HA-PINK1-S465D plasmids were transfected into HEK293 cells, followed by pulse chase experiment to measure protein degradation. The results showed that degradation half-life time of WT PINK1 protein was about 2 h; For the HA-PINK1-S465A protein and HA-PINK1-S465D protein, the degradation half-life time of both were about 3.5 h, slower than the WT PINK1 protein (Fig. 5). The phosphorylation of S465 may be related to the degradation of PINK1, as both disabled phosphorylation and excessive phosphorylation of Ser465 increase the half-life time and the concentration of PINK1 in cells. The normal phosphorylation of Ser465 may be required to maintain a stable level of PINK1 and cell homeostasis.

Both disease-causing mutant PINK1 protein and Ser465A mutant PINK1 protein affect Parkin subcellular localization

Studies have shown that PINK1 can phosphorylate Parkin protein directly, and translocate Parkin to the mitochondria, which gathers in clusters around the nucleus [10]. It is still unclear whether S465 autophosphorylation site can affect the subcellular localization of Parkin. In our study, we found that EGFP-Parkin protein evenly distributed in the cytoplasm when cells were transfected with pKH3-EGFP-Parkin only (Fig. 6a); when cells were co-transfected EGFP-Parkin with pKH3-PINK1-WT or pKH3-PINK1-S465D, colocalization of Parkin with PINK1 in clustered mitochondrias was observed (Fig. 6a); when

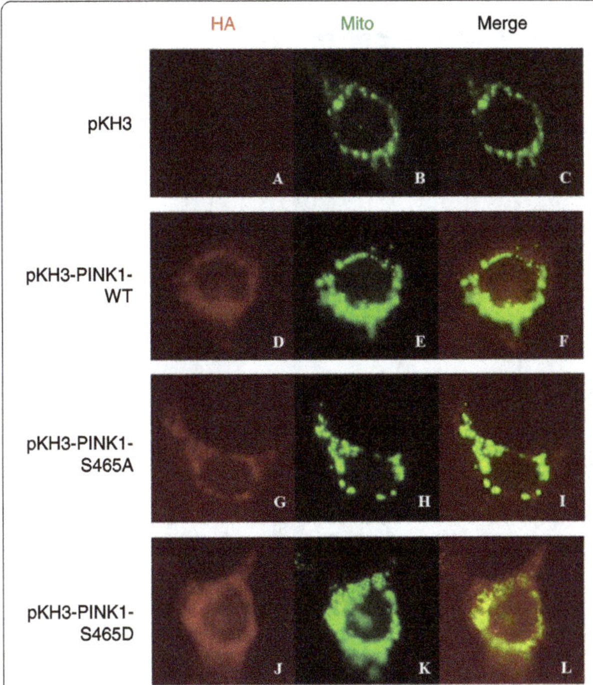

Fig. 4 S465 has no influence on PINK1 subcellular localization. **a**, **b**, **c**, the subcellular localization in HEK 293 cells transfected with pKH3, as negative control; (**d**, **e**, **f**), the subcellular localization in HEK 293 cells transfected with pKH3-PINK1-WT; (**g**, **h**, **i**), the subcellular localization of pKH3-PINK1-S465A transfected cells; (**j**, **k**, **l**), the subcellular localization of pKH3-PINK1-S465D transfected cells. In A, D, G and J, the red fluorescence illustrated the subcellular localization of proteins containing the HA tag; In B, E, H and K, the green fluorescence stood for mitochondria; In C, F, I and L, co-localization (*in yellow*) of both HA-tag containing protein (*in red*) and mitochondria (*in green*)

cells were co-transfected EGFP-Parkin with mutant PINK1, pKH3-PINK1-S465A, pKH3-PINK1-T313 M or pKH3-PINK1-R492X, respectively, EGFP-Parkin evenly distributed in the cytoplasm (Fig. 6a), and each mutant PINK1 protein exhibited scattered distribution in cytoplasm, was located in mitochondria (Fig. 6a). The percentage of cells containing colocalization of PINK1 with Parkin protein was shown in Fig. 6b. We compared the four mutant PINK1 co-transfected with EGFP-Parkin groups and the WT PINK1 group, three of them (pKH3-PINK1-S465A, pKH3-PINK1-T313 M and pKH3- PINK1-R492X) exhibited obvious decreased percentage of positive cells compared with WT PINK1 ($^{*}P < 0.05$), and the difference was not statistically significant ($^{*}P > 0.05$) in pKH3-PINK1-S465D group compared with the WT group (Fig. 6c).

Discussion

The dynamic changes of protein play a key role in life, as they can achieve the physiological function through various post-translational modifications, among which, reversible protein phosphorylation is a common and crucial one. In mammals, there are about 30% of the proteins going on with phosphorylation process. A variety of biological processes are closely related to post-translational protein phosphorylation, which has been playing an on/off regulation in numerous biochemical functions, such as transcriptional regulation, signal transduction, DNA repair, apoptosis regulation. Therefore, the phosphorylation of proteins is an essential part in intracellular signaling transduction.

In our experiment, we used in vitro phosphorylation studies to exclude the possibilities of PINK1 phosphorylated by other proteins, adopted a liquid chromatography mass spectrometry to identify the Ser465 site as the PINK1 protein autophosphorylation site. Since phosphorylation is a reversible process, the loss of phosphate groups was possible under the experimental conditions. In addition, the phosphorylated peptides were relatively little compared with non-phosphorylated peptides, which could be concealed easily when identified in the mass spectrometry, leading to the false negative results. Therefore, besides Ser465 site, there may be other unidentified PINK1 autophosphorylation sites.

In order to identify whether Ser465 was the PINK1 autophosphorylation site or not, we firstly constructed Ser465 autophosphorylation silent type pGEX-5X-1-PINK1-S465A, replacing the serine residue (S) with alanine residue (A) which cannot be phosphorylated, using the site-directed mutagenesis. After Ser465 being silenced, the PINK1 protein autophosphorylation level was decreased, but not completely blocked, indicating that Ser465 is just one of the PINK1 autophosphorylation sites.

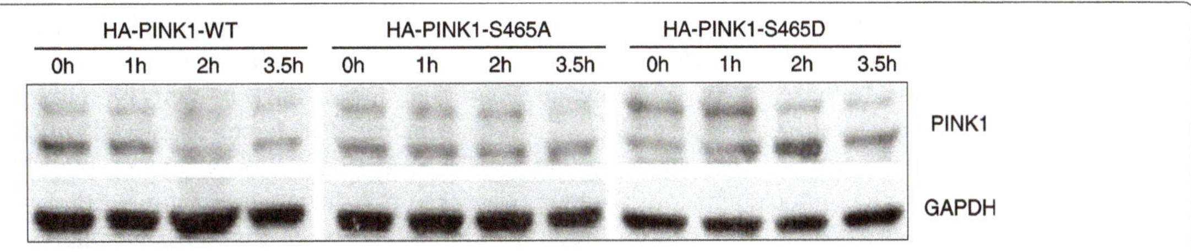

Fig. 5 S465 phosphorylation site affects PINK1 degradation. The first four lanes represented the quantity of HA-PINK1-WT protein in HEK293 cells transfected with pKH3-PINK1-WT plasmid, collected 0 h,1 h, 2, 3.5 h after the addition of actidione. Similarly, the middle and last four lanes represented HA-PINK1-S465A and HA-PINK1-S465D protein, respectively

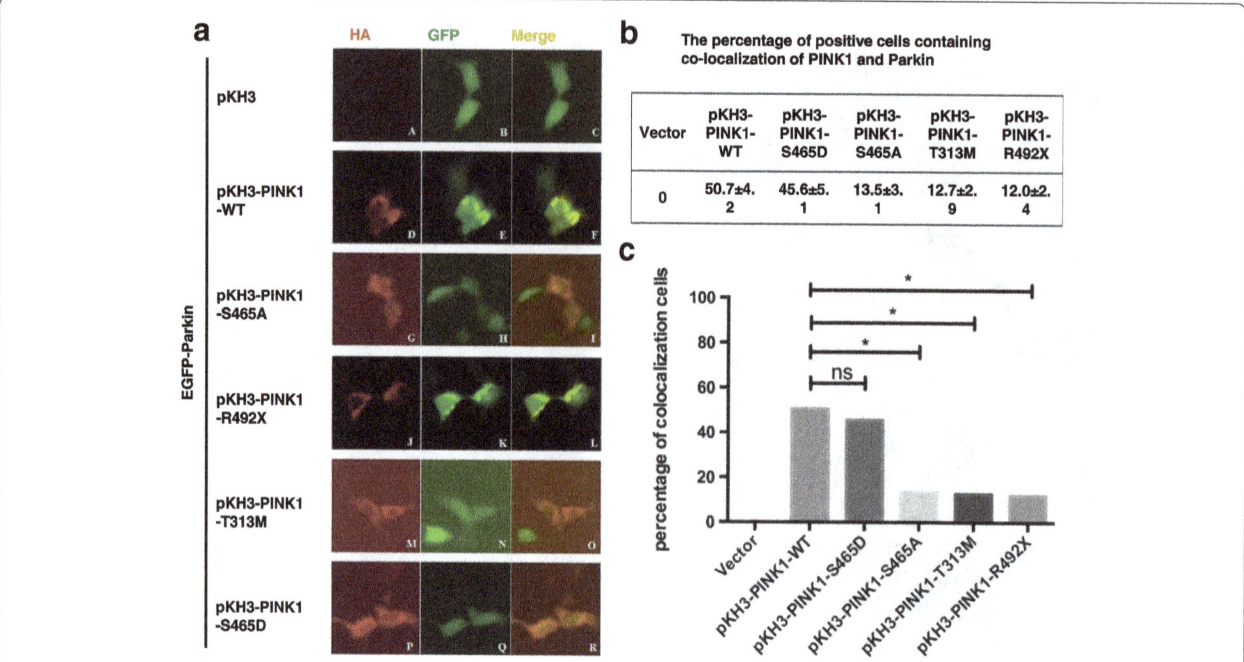

Fig. 6 Both disease-causing mutant PINK1 protein and Ser465A mutant PINK1 protein affects Parkin subcellular localization. **a** The six rows represented the subcellular localization of co-transfection of EGFP-Parkin with pKH3, pKH3-PINK1-WT, pKH3-PINK1-S465A, pKH3-PINK1-S465D, pKH3-PINK1-T313 M and pKH3-PINK1-R492X, respectively. The red fluorescence showed the subcellular localization of PINK1 protein containing HA tag in the first column; The green fluorescence illustrated subcellular localization of Parkin protein containing GFP tag in the second column; The yellow fluorescent showed the co-localization of both PINK1 (*red*) and Parkin (*green*) in the third column. **b** The percentage of positive cells containing colocalization of PINK1 and Parkin in six co-transfection groups of EGFP-Parkin with pKH3 vector, pKH3-PINK1-WT, pKH3-PINK1-S465A, pKH3-PINK1- S465D, pKH3-PINK1-T313 M and pKH3-PINK1-R492X. **c** Quantification of the percentage of PINK1/Parkin colocalization cell. (*$P < 0.05$, statistically significant)

Our study found that the inactivation of Ser465 can down-regulate the kinase activity of PINK1. Together with Ser465A, T313 M and R492X mutant PINK1 also decrease kinase activity in vitro, both of which are disease-causing mutations of PINK1, implying that decreased kinase activity may contribute to PD. However, experiments in vitro cannot fully simulate the phosphorylation process of eukaryotic cells in vivo, and the specific mechanism remains to be further studied.

When we transfected two pKH3-PINK1 mutants in HEK293 cells, HA-PINK1-S465A and HA-PINK1-S465D, there were no significant changes of subcellular localization of PINK1, still displaying the mitochondrial localization. These results suggest that the Ser465 site has no effect on PINK1 subcellular localization. PINK1 protein is an integral membrane protein, mainly located in the mitochondria. It has already shown that PINK1 protein localizes in mitochondria cristae, and both wild-type and mutant (outside the mitochondrial localization domain) PINK1 protein distribute in the same way in cells, indicating that PINK1 mutation outside the mitochondrial localization domain does not affect its subcellular localization [12]. As a mitochondrial-located kinase, PINK1 plays a key role in maintaining the normal function of mitochondria and protecting the mitochondria from oxidative stress.

Our study found that Ser465 phosphorylation was also related to the PINK1 degradation. Both disabled or excessive PINK1 phosphorylation can slow down the PINK1 degradation, increase the intracellular concentration of PINK1. A proper concentration of PINK1 is required to maintain mitochondrial homeostasis. Most studies have found that PINK1 mainly maintains normal mitochondrial morphology and function, reduces mitochondrial dysfunction under stress, inhibits apoptosis, and is a neuron protective protein ([1, 4, 5, 13, 15]). Some studies have demonstrated that PINK1 protein degrades primarily by the ubiquitin-proteasome degradation pathway, but so far the related E3 ligase in the pathway remains unclear [16, 19, 23], which may be associated with the PINK1 autophosphorylation.

Our study also investigated the influence of PINK1 autophosphorylation on Parkin. Both wild-type PINK1 protein and S465D mutant protein can promote the transfer of Parkin to clustered mitochondria, while S465A, T313 M, R492X mutant PINK1 had a relatively weaker role in the interaction with Parkin. S465A mutant can disable the autophosphorylation of PINK1, repressing the transfer process; While mutant S465D possesses the phosphorylation ability, completing the same process as the wild-type protein. We can infer that

PINK1 autophosphorylation contributes to the transit of Parkin to mitochondria. For the S465A, T313 M and R492X mutant protein, the inhibition of transfer process may be related to the reduced kinase activity. Some studies[10] have also confirmed that PINK1 can phosphorylate Parkin and jointly transfer to the mitochondria, which were gathered in clusters around the nucleus. The decreased kinase activity of these mutant PINK1 proteins may lead to the abnormal physiological processes.

Conclusion

In summary, protein phosphorylation is a crucial aspect of intracellular signaling. Our study elucidated that PINK1 protein autophosphorylation can affect its kinase activity and protein stability, and influent PINK1 and Parkin protein interaction. We also included two *PINK1* causative mutations in our study, T313 M and R492X, which can decrease the kinase activity and affect the interaction with Parkin in the same way as Ser465A, hinting that the change of autophosphorylation activity of PINK1 may be one of the mechanisms of the two disease-causing mutations.

Acknowledgements

We would like to thank all individuals participating in the study.

Funding

This work was supported by grant 2016YFC1306000, 2017YFC0909100 from the national key plan for scientific research and development of China, grants 81430023, 81371405, 81571248 from the National Natural Science Foundation of China, grant 2016CX025 from innovation-driven plan of Central South University,grant 2017JJ1037 from Hunan Science Funds for Distinguished Young Scholar.

Authors' contributions

BT, XY and JG conceived of the study, and participated in the coordination and helped to draft the manuscript. LY, QS carried out the identification of the autophosphorylation and following functional study, participated in the data analysis. YC, YY and QX participated in the manuscript draft and interpretation of data. All authors read and approved the final manuscript.

Competing interests

The authors declare that they have no competing interests.

Author details

[1]Department of Neurology, Xiangya Hospital, Central South University, Changsha, Hunan 410008, People's Republic of China. [2]Laboratory of Medical Genetics, Central South University Changsha, Changsha, Hunan 410078, China. [3]National Clinical Research Center for Geriatric Disorders, Changsha, Hunan 410078, China. [4]Key Laboratory of Hunan Province in Neurodegenerative Disorders, Central South University, Changsha, Hunan 410008, China. [5]Parkinson's Disease Center of Beijing Institute for Brain Disorders, Beijing 100069, China. [6]Collaborative Innovation Center for Brain Science, Shanghai 200032, China. [7]Collaborative Innovation Center for Genetics and Development, Shanghai 200433, China.

References

1. Beilina A, Van Der Brug M, Ahmad R, Kesavapany S, Miller DW, Petsko GA, Cookson MR. Mutations in PTEN-induced putative kinase 1 associated with recessive parkinsonism have differential effects on protein stability. Proc Natl Acad Sci U S A. 2005;102:5703–8.
2. Cannon JR, Greenamyre JT. Gene-environment interactions in Parkinson's disease: specific evidence in humans and mammalian models. Neurobiol Dis. 2013;57:38–46.
3. Che X, Tang B, Wang X, Chen D, Yan X, Jiang H, Shen L, Xu Q, Wang G, Guo J. The BAG2 Protein Stabilises PINK1 By Decreasing its Ubiquitinationion. Biochem Biophys Res Commun. 2013;441:488–92.
4. Cookson MR, Dauer W, Dawson T, Fon EA, Guo M, Shen J. The roles of kinases in familial Parkinson's disease. J Neurosci. 2007;27:11865–8.
5. Giasson BI. Mitochondrial injury: a hot spot for parkinsonism and Parkinson's disease? Sci Aging Knowl Environ. 2004;2004:pe42.
6. Guo JF, Xiao B, Liao B, Zhang XW, Nie LL, Zhang YH, Shen L, Jiang H, Xia K, Pan Q, Yan XX, Tang BS. Mutation analysis of Parkin, PINK1, DJ-1 and ATP13A2 genes in Chinese patients with autosomal recessive early-onset Parkinsonism. Mov Disord. 2008;23:2074–9.
7. Kalia LV, Lang AE. Parkinson's disease. Lancet. 2015;386:896–912.
8. Kim Y, Park J, Kim S, Song S, Kwon SK, Lee SH, Kitada T, Kim JM, Chung J. PINK1 controls mitochondriallocalization of Parkin through direct phosphorylation. Biochem Biophys Res Commun. 2008;377:975–80.
9. Matenia D, Hempp C, Timm T, Eikhof A, Mandelkow EM. Microtubule affinity-regulating kinase 2 (MARK2) turns on phosphatase and tensin homolog (PTEN)-induced kinase 1 (PINK1) at Thr-313, a mutation site in Parkinson disease: effects on mitochondrial transport. J Biol Chem. 2012;287:8174–86.
10. Meissner C, Lorenz H, Weihofen A, Selkoe DJ, Lemberg MK. The mitochondrial intramembrane protease PARL cleaves human Pink1 to regulate Pink1 traicking. J Neurochem. 2011;117:856–67.
11. Nakajima A, Kataoka K, Hong M, Sakaguchi M, Huh NH. BRPK, a novel protein kinase showing increased expression in mouse cancer cell lines with higher metastatic potential. Cancer Lett. 2003;201:195–201.
12. Okatsu K, Oka T, Iguchi M, Imamura K, Kosako H, Tani N, Kimura M, Go E, Koyano F, Funayama M, Shiba-Fukushima K, Sato S, Shimizu H, Fukunaga Y, Taniguchi H, Komatsu M, Hattori N, Mihara K, Tanaka K, Matsuda N. PINK1 autophosphorylation upon membrane potential dissipation is essential for Parkin recruitment to damaged mitochondria. Nat Commun. 2012;3:1016.
13. Petit A, Kawarai T, Paitel E, Sanjo N, Maj M, Scheid M, Chen F, Gu Y, Hasegawa H, Salehi-Rad S, Wang L, Rogaeva E, Fraser P, Robinson B, St George-Hyslop P, Tandon A. Wild-typePINK1 prevents basal and induced neuronal apoptosis, a protective effect abrogated by Parkinson disease-related mutation. J Biol Chem. 2005;280:34025–32.
14. Pridgeon JW, Olzmann JA, Chin LS, Li L. PINK1 protects against oxidative stress by Phosphorylating mitochondrial chaperone TRAP1. Plos Bio. 2007;5:1494–503.
15. Schapira AH. Mitochondrial involvement in Parkinson's disease, Huntington's disease, hereditary spastic paraplegia and Friedreich's ataxia. Biochim Biophys Acta. 1999;1410:159–70.
16. Shiba K, Arai T, Sato S, Kubo S, Ohba Y, Mizuno Y, Hattori N. Parkin stabilizes PINK1 through direct interaction. Biochem Biophys Res Commun. 2009;383:331–5.
17. Silvestri L, Caputo V, Bellacchio E, Atorino L, Dallapiccola B, Valente EM, Casari G. Mitochondrial import and enzymatic activity of PINK1 mutants associated to recessive parkinsonism. Hum Mol Genet. 2005;14:3477–92.
18. Sim CH, Lio DS, Mok SS, Masters CL, Hill AF, Culvenor JG, Cheng HC. C-terminal truncation and Parkinson's disease-associated mutations down-regulate the protein serine/threonine kinase activity of PTEN-induced kinase-1. Hum Mol Genet. 2006;15:3251–62.
19. Um JW, Stichel-Gunkel C, Lübbert H, Lee G, Chung KC. Molecular interaction between parkin and PINK1 in mammalian neuronal cells. Mol Cell Neurosci. 2009;40:421–32.
20. Valente EM, Abou-Sleiman PM, Caputo V, Muqit MM, Harvey K, Gispert S, Ali Z, Del Turco D, Bentivoglio AR, Healy DG, Albanese A, Nussbaum R, González-Maldonado R, Deller T, Salvi S, Cortelli P, Gilks WP, Latchman DS, Harvey RJ, Dallapiccola B, Auburger G, Wood NW. Hereditary early-onset Parkinson's disease caused by mutations in PINK1. Science. 2004;304:1158–60.
21. Volta M, Milnerwood AJ, Farrer MJ. Insights from late-onset familial parkinsonism on the pathogenesis of idiopathic Parkinson's disease. Lancet Neurol. 2015;14:1054–64.

22. Wang X, Guo J, Fei E, Mu Y, He S, Che X, Tan J, Xia K, Zhang Z, Wang G, Tang B. BAG5 protects against mitochondrial oxidative damage through regulating PINK1 degradation. PLoS One. 2014;9:e86276.
23. Xiong H, Wang D, Chen L, Choo YS, Ma H, Tang C, Xia K, Jiang W, Ronai Z, Zhuang X, Zhang Z. Parkin, PINK1, and DJ-1 form a ubiquitin E3 ligase complex promoting unfolded protein degradation. Parkin, PINK1, and DJ-1 form a ubiquitinE3 ligase complex promoting unfolded protein degradation. J Clin Invest. 2009;119:650–60.

The role of substantia nigra sonography in the differentiation of Parkinson's disease and multiple system atrophy

Hai-Yan Zhou[1†], Pei Huang[1†], Qian Sun[1], Juan-Juan Du[1], Shi-Shuang Cui[1], Yun-Yun Hu[2], Wei-Wei Zhan[2], Ying Wang[1], Qin Xiao[1], Jun Liu[1], Yu-Yan Tan[1*] and Sheng-Di Chen[1*]

Abstract

Background: The differential diagnosis of Parkinson's disease (PD) and multiple system atrophy (MSA) remains a challenge, especially in the early stage. Here, we assessed the value of transcranial sonography (TCS) to discriminate non-tremor dominant (non-TD) PD from MSA with predominant parkinsonism (MSA-P).

Methods: Eighty-six MSA-P patients and 147 age and gender-matched non-TD PD patients who had appropriate temporal acoustic bone windows were included in this study. All the patients were followed up for at least 2 years to confirm the initial diagnosis. Patients with at least one substantia nigra (SN) echogenic size ≥18 mm^2 were classified as hyperechogenic, those with at least one SN echogenic size ≥25 mm^2 was defined as markedly hyperechogenic.

Results: The frequency of SN hyperechogenicity in non-TD PD patients was significantly higher than that in MSA-P patients (74.1% vs. 38.4%, $p < 0.001$). SN hyperechogenicity discriminated non-TD PD from MSA-P with sensitivity of 74.1%, specificity of 61.6%, and positive predictive value of 76.8%. If marked SN hyperechogenicity was used as the cutoff value (≥ 25 mm^2), the sensitivity decreased to 46.3%, but the specificity and positive predictive value increased to 80.2 and 80.0%. Additionally, in those patients with SN hyperechogenicity, positive correlation between SN hyperechogenicity area and disease duration was found in non-TD PD rather than in MSA-P patients. In this context, among early-stage patients with disease duration ≤3 years, the sensitivity, specificity and positive predictive value of SN hyperechogenicity further declined to 69.8%, 52.2%, and 66.7%, respectively.

Conclusions: TCS could help discriminate non-TD PD from MSA-P in a certain extent, but the limitation was also obvious with relatively low specificity, especially in the early stage.

Keywords: Parkinson's disease, Multiple system atrophy, Atypical parkinsonian disorders, Transcranial sonography, Substantia nigra, Disease duration

Background

The diagnosis of Parkinson's disease (PD) mainly depends on the clinical manifestations [1], which results in the accuracy of diagnosis affected by the physicians' experiences in a great extent. Although as high as 90% accurate diagnosis of PD could be reached in the movement disorders clinics [2, 3], it was already the best scenario. A recent clinical pathology study demonstrated that in the early stage of the disease, only 50% parkinsonian patients received an accurate diagnosis of PD [4]. The most diagnostic confusing diseases are atypical parkinsonian disorders (APD), including progressive supranuclear palsy (PSP), multiple system atrophy (MSA), corticobasal ganglionic degeneration (CBD) and dementia with Lewy bodies (DLB). Those APD share some clinical features with PD, but progress aggressively and have much poorer prognosis. The misdiagnosis not only posed psychosocial and economic burden to patients and their families, but also set up obstacles to the

* Correspondence: yuyantan00@126.com; ruijincsd@126.com
†Hai-Yan Zhou and Pei Huang contributed equally to this work.
[1]Department of Neurology & Institute of Neurology, Ruijin Hospital affiliated to Shanghai Jiao Tong University School of Medicine, No.197 Ruijin 2nd Road, Shanghai 200025, China
Full list of author information is available at the end of the article

neuroprotective or modified therapies for both PD and APD. Therefore, it is currently eager to find a battery of tools to help diagnosis and differential diagnosis. Transcranial sonography (TCS) is a non-invasive, convenient and economic tool. Recent evidence has shown that it not only helps in the diagnosis of PD, but also helps to differentiate it from APD [5, 6]. However, most of evidence came from Caucasians [6]. Moreover, in most previous differentiation studies not only the number of APD recruited was relatively small, but those distinct entities were pooled into one single APD group for comparison [6]. Among those APD, MSA with predominant parkinsonism (MSA-P), a subtype of MSA, presents most similar clinical features with PD and could be most easily confused with non-tremor dominant (non-TD) PD, especially in the early stage [7, 8]. In our study, we collected 86 clinical probable MSA-P and 147 age and gender matched non-TD PD patients who were clinically diagnosed, and explored if TCS could help the differential diagnosis.

Methods

This cross-sectional study was performed at the Movement Disorder Clinic, Department of Neurology, Ruijin Hospital affiliated to Shanghai Jiao Tong University School of Medicine from April 2014 to September 2017.

Subjects

Two hundred and thirty-three Chinese patients with parkinsonism were included, 86 MSA-P and 147 age and gender-matched non-TD PD. All the PD patients met the Movement Disorder Society Clinical Diagnostic Criteria for Parkinson's disease [9]. Among them, 79 (53.7%) patients met clinically established PD and 68 (46.3%) patients met clinically probable PD at the beginning of recruitment. Moreover, they all met the classification criterion of non-TD PD [10]. Briefly, an average global tremor score was calculated as the mean of 9 items. A mean score for the complex of postural instability and gait difficulty (PIGD) was calculated as the mean of 5 items. The non-TD group was defined as patients with a ratio of mean tremor score/mean PIGD score less than 1.5. Also, the established criterion was used for the diagnosis of probable MSA-P [8]. Cases demonstrated identifiable possible causes of other secondary parkinsonism were excluded. All the patients had appropriate temporal acoustic bone windows and were followed for at least 2 years to confirm the initial diagnosis. During the period of follow-up, no clinical diagnosis was changed. At the end of follow-up, 119 (81.0%) patients met clinically established PD and 28 (19.0%) patients met clinically probable PD. We further analyzed a subgroup of early-stage non-TD PD and MSA-P patients, which was defined as the patients with 3 years or less disease duration. For clinical assessment, disease severity was rated using the Hoehn and Yahr (H-Y) stage.

Transcranial sonography

The sonographic examinations were done as previously described [11]. Briefly, it was performed by one experienced sonographer blinded to the clinical data of all patients. TCS was performed by a 2.5 MHz sonographic device (MyLab90, ESAOTE, Italy) with 16 cm depth and 45 dB dynamic range. Initially, the butterfly shaped hypoechogenic midbrain was identified. Then, the one with the hyperechogenic signal at the anatomical region of SN in its maximum extent was stored. Bilateral SN echogenic areas were then manually encircled and measured. Reproducibility of the SN sonographic measurement had been previously validated by two independent investigators [11]. The larger value of bilateral SN echogenicity was defined as SN_L. Those with SN_L less than 18 mm^2 were identified as normal; the others with at least one SN echogenic size ≥18 mm^2 were classified as hyperechogenic as previously described [11]. Besides, to keep consistent with the literatures [5, 12–15], in this study $SN_L \geq 25$ mm^2 was defined as markedly hyperechogenic, and sizes between 18 and 25 mm^2 as moderately hyperechogenic. For intergroup comparisons, the SN_L was used.

Statistical analyses

All analyses were performed using SPSS 18.0. Continuous variables were given as means (± standard deviation, SD). Categorical variables were summarized by counts of patients and percentages. All variables were tested for normality by Kolmogorov-Smirnov. Two-sample T test or Chi-square test was applied for the comparison of clinical data between non-TD PD and MSA-P. For the comparison of the frequency of different echogenic intensity between groups, Chi-square test was used. The sensitivity, specificity, positive predictive value (PPV) and negative predictive value (NPV) of TCS were determined for SN hyperechogenicity as a marker for the differential diagnosis of non-TD PD from MSA-P. Correlation analyses between the variables and SN_L were performed by Spearman correlation coefficients. Adjusted p values were calculated by controlling other confounding factors. The significant level was set at $\alpha = 0.05$.

Results

Demographics

Table 1 presents the demographic data of non-TD PD and MSA-P. Group MSA-P consisted of 57 men and 29 women with clinically probable MSA. Their age was 62.3 ± 7.5 years, onset age 58.7 ± 7.6 years, disease duration 3.6 ± 2.1 years, and H-Y stage 3.5 ± 1.0. Group non-TD PD consisted of 104 men and 43 women. Their age was 62.2 ± 8.4 years,

Table 1 Demographic data and substantia nigra echogenicity of patients

	non-TD PD (n = 147)	MSA-P (n = 86)	P value
Age (y)	62.2 (8.4)	62.3 (7.5)	0.912
Gender (M/F)	104/43	57/29	0.557
Onset age (y)	56.8 (8.9)	58.7 (7.6)	0.096
Disease duration (y)	5.4 (4.4)	3.6 (2.1)	< 0.001*
H-Y stage	2.0 (0.8)	3.5 (1.0)	< 0.001*
SN_L (mm^2)	24.7 (12.8)	12.2 (13.6)	< 0.001*

Non-TD PD non-tremor dominant Parkinson's disease, *MSA-P* multiple system atrophy with predominant parkinsonism, *H-Y* Hoehn and Yahr, SN_L the larger value of bilateral SN hyperechogenicity. Two-sample T test or Chi-square test was applied for the comparisons. *P values below 0.05 were considered significant

onset age 56.8 ± 8.9 years, disease duration 5.4 ± 4.4 years, and H-Y stage 2.0 ± 0.8. The age and gender were matched between those two groups ($p = 0.912$ and $p = 0.557$, respectively). No difference was found in their onset age ($p = 0.096$). However, MSA-P patients had shorter disease duration ($p < 0.001$) and higher H-Y stage ($p < 0.001$).

SN echogenicity of non-TD PD and MSA-P

The mean SN_L of non-TD PD was 24.7 ± 12.8 mm^2, larger than that of MSA-P patients, which was 12.2 ± 13.6 mm^2 ($p < 0.001$). In non-TD PD group, 109 (74.1%) of 147 patients exhibited SN hyperechogenicity. Forty-one (27.9%) were classified as moderate, and 68 (46.3%) as marked. Thirty-eight (25.9%) of 147 non-TD PD patients had normal SN echogenicity. On the contrary, in the MSA-P group, only 33 (38.4%) of 86 patients exhibited SN hyperechogenicity, and the frequency was lower than that in non-TD PD ($P < 0.001$). Among them, 16 (18.6%) patients were classified as moderate, and 17 (19.8%) as marked. Fifty-three (61.6%) patients exhibited normal SN echogenicity (Fig. 1a).

In the subgroup of patients with disease duration ≤3 years ($n = 109$), the mean SN_L of non-TD PD ($n = 63$) was 23.9 ± 12.0 mm^2, also larger than that of MSA-P patients ($n = 46$), which was 15.2 ± 14.9 mm^2 ($p = 0.002$). In non-TD PD group, 44 (69.8%) of 63 patients exhibited SN hyperechogenicity. Eighteen (28.6%) of 63 patients were classified as moderate, and 26 (41.3%) patients as marked. Nineteen (30.2%) of 63 non-TD PD patients had normal SN echogenicity. On the contrary, in the MSA-P group, 24 (52.2%) of 46 patients exhibited normal SN echogenicity and 22 (47.8%) patients exhibited SN hyperechogenicity. Among them, 10 (21.7%) patients were classified as moderate, and 12 (26.1%) patients as marked (Fig. 1b).

SN hyperechogenicity differentiating non-TD PD from MSA-P

Table 2 summarizes SN sonographic findings discriminating non-TD PD from MSA-P. Of all the 233 patients,

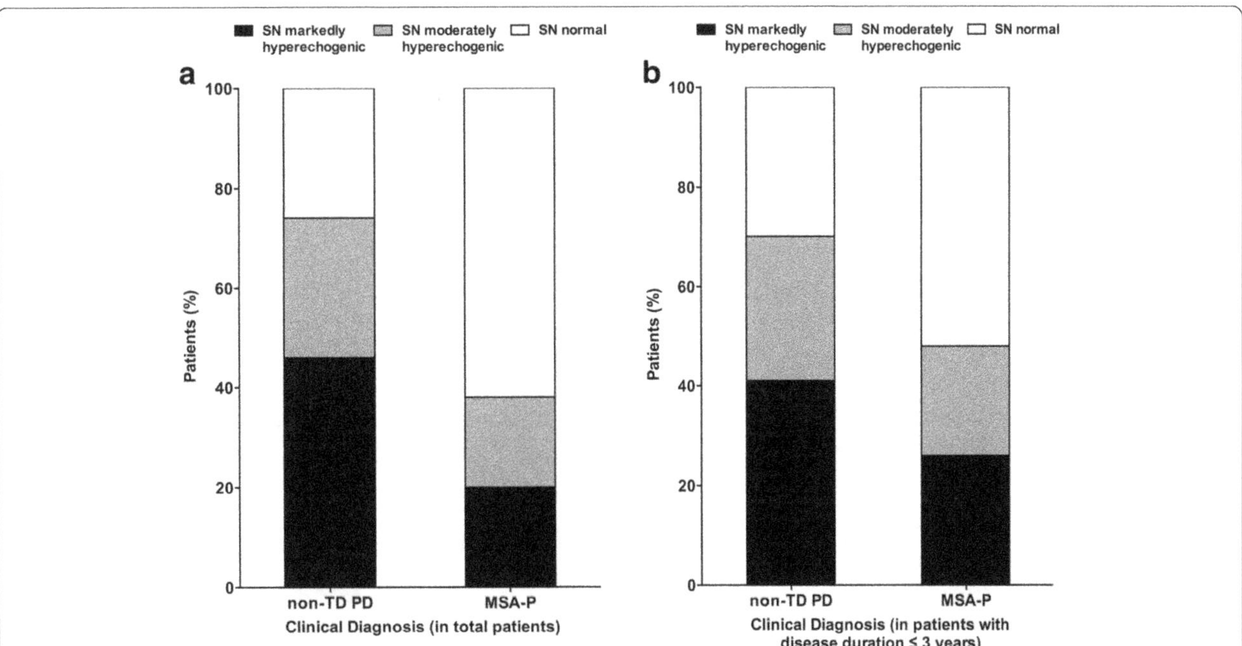

Figure 1 Percentage of patients with different ultrasound findings in the two groups. **a** showed the percentage of cases with different sonographic findings in total patients. **b** showed the percentage of cases with different sonographic findings in the subgroup of patients with disease duration ≤3 years. Black: percentage of patients with a marked substantia nigra (SN) hyperechogenicity; grey: percentage of patients who exhibited a moderate increase in SN echogenicity; and white: percentage of patients with a normal SN echogenicity; non-TD PD, non-tremor dominant Parkinson's disease; MSA-P, parkinsonian variant of multiple system atrophy.

SN echogenicity correctly diagnosed 162 (69.5%) cases as non-TD PD ($n = 109$) or MSA-P ($n = 53$). For the clinical diagnosis of non-TD PD, sensitivity, specificity and PPV of SN hyperechogenicity were 74.1%, 61.6% and 76.8%; while for being diagnosed as MSA-P, normal SN echogenicity had a NPV of 58.2%. For marked SN hyperechogenicity, sensitivity, specificity and PPV for the diagnosis of non-TD PD were 46.3%, 80.2% and 80.0%, respectively. Conversely, normal SN echogenicity indicated MSA-P with 46.6% NPV.

In the subgroup of patients with disease duration ≤3 years ($n = 109$), SN echogenicity correctly diagnosed 68 (62.4%) cases as non-TD PD ($n = 44$) or MSA-P ($n = 24$). SN hyperechogenicity had 66.7% PPV for the clinical diagnosis of non-TD PD and normal SN echogenicity had 55.8% NPV for being diagnosed as MSA-P. Sensitivity and specificity of SN hyperechogenicity for detecting non-TD PD patients decreased to 69.8% and 52.2%. For marked SN hyperechogenicity, sensitivity, specificity, and PPV for non-TD PD were 41.3%, 73.9% and 68.4%. Conversely, normal SN echogenicity indicated MSA-P with 47.9% NPV.

Correlation of SN_L with disease duration in the patients with SN hyperechogenicity

Correlation analysis of SN_L with disease duration was performed in patients with SN hyperechogenicity. The results indicated that SN_L did not correlated with disease duration either in MSA-P ($r = -0.114$, $p = 0.526$) or in non-TD PD patients ($r = 0.137$, $p = 0.156$). However, after controlling onset age and H-Y stage as confounding factors, significant correlation was found only in non-TD PD patients ($r = 0.264$, $p = 0.006$) rather than in MSA-P patients ($r = -0.096$, $p = 0.607$) (Fig. 2).

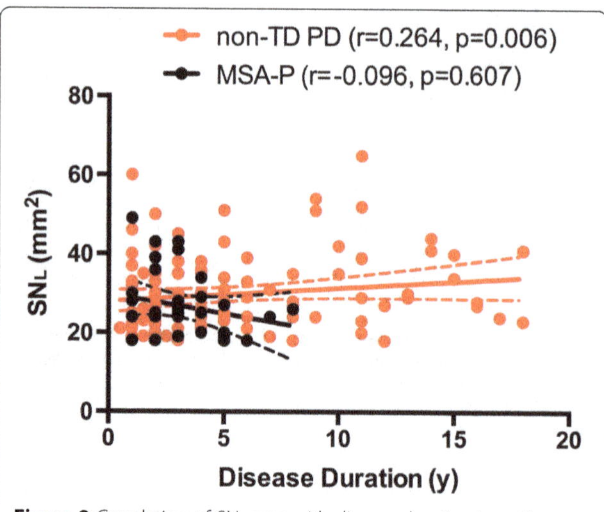

Figure 2 Correlation of SN_L area with disease duration in patients with SN hyperechogenicity

Discussion

Consistent with previous results [12, 15, 16], our present study demonstrated that more percentage of SN hyperechogenicity was detected in non-TD PD patients than in MSA-P patients. However, the sensitivity for the non-TD PD patients in our cohort was only 74.1%, which was lower than most of previous studies performed by other researchers [5, 6, 12–22]. The majority of earlier studies were conducted in Caucasians and the sensitivity was almost more than 90%, even reaching up to 100% [5, 6, 12–19]. Only a few studies were performed in the Asian patients, and the sensitivity varied widely (50%~ 80%) [11, 20–28]. Ethnic differences might not be completely excluded between Caucasians and Asians, but the spectrum bias should be the more reasonable cause. It has been well known that PD is a heterogeneous disorder, and it can be divided into various phenotypes based on the onset age or prominent clinical presentations, such as early or late onset PD, TD PD or non-TD PD [29–31]. Different patterns of SN echogenicity have been shown to be associated with different clinical subtypes [32] and different onset ages [22]. Also, gender and disease duration could affect the SN echogenic pattern [11, 20, 22, 33]. In view of above-mentioned various factors, it was not surprising that varied sensitivity was found in our own studies. Lower sensitivity in our previous studies with a larger number of PD patients could also be due to different patient's enrollment standard [11]. In the current study, PD patients were limited to the non-TD patients, and their ages and genders were strictly matched with that of MSA-P. Finally, the possibility of misdiagnosis could not be absolutely ruled out

Table 2 Substantia nigra sonography findings indicating non-TD PD rather than MSA-P

	Total patients		Patients with disease duration ≤3 years	
	$SN_L \geq 18$ mm^2	$SN_L \geq 25$ mm^2	$SN_L \geq 18$ mm^2	$SN_L \geq 25$ mm^2
Sensitivity, %	74.1	46.3	69.8	41.3
Specificity, %	61.6	80.2	52.2	73.9
PPV, %	76.8	80.0	66.7	68.4
NPV, %	58.2	46.6	55.8	47.9

Non-TD PD non-tremor dominant Parkinson's disease, *MSA-P* multiple system atrophy with predominant parkinsonism, SN_L the larger value of bilateral SN hyperechogenicity, *PPV* positive predictive value, *NPV* negative predictive value since a fairly part of non-TD PD patients were at their early disease stages. However, similar with a recent study conducted in Japanese patients where the sensitivity of SN hyperechogenicity was around 50% [23], all the patients in our cohort were followed up for at least 2 years to confirm the diagnosis. In supporting for the minimum possibility of misdiagnosis, the differing characteristics of non-TD PD and MSA-P in our study were obvious, that is, MSA-P patients had higher H-Y stages with shorter disease duration, which suggesting more aggressive progression.

In contrast, the sensitivity of SN hyperechogenicity for MSA-P was 38.4%. Even only the marked SN hyperechogenicity was considered, the sensitivity was up to 19.8%, which was still higher than most of previous reports [5, 6, 12, 15, 16, 18, 19, 21, 23]. The majority of sensitivity of SN hyperechogenicity for MSA was reported as about 10%, except for two studies, which were 25 and 50%, respectively [12, 27]. Just as occurred in PD, the most probable reason for the discrepancy between earlier studies and ours could be the spectrum bias. In the previous studies, the number of MSA patients enrolled was relatively small and ranged from 8 to 32 [5, 6]. A small sample size could not only affect statistical power, but also influence the statistical results even with a few cases of misdiagnosis. Moreover, there are two variants of MSA, which are MSA with predominant cerebellar ataxia (MSA-C) and MSA-P. No evidence could make sure that their SN hyperechogenicity pattern should be the same. Therefore, to minimum the bias mentioned above, the MSA patients selected in our study were all MSA-P variants and were followed up for at least two years to confirm the diagnosis in the same movement disorder clinic. In addition, the sample size of MSA-P in the present study reached up to 86, which was the largest one so far.

For overall patients, the sensitivity of SN hyperechogenicity for PD was 74.1%, and the specificity was 61.6%. If SN hyperechogenicity was marked, the specificity increased to 80.2%, but the sensitivity decreased to 46.3%. With either cutoff value, the positive predictive value for the diagnosis of non-TD PD was around 80%. However, among the patients with equal to or less than 3 years disease duration, the sensitivity and specificity further declined to 69.8% and 52.2% respectively, so did PPV decrease to 66.7%. The exact reason was not clear, and the possibility of misdiagnosis could not be definitely excluded since a fairly part of patients were at their early stages. However, it might be explained by the fact that there were different patterns between non-TD PD and MSA-P with regard to the correlation of SN hyperechogenicity with disease duration. In non-TD PD, it seems that with disease course prolonged, the area of SN hyperechogenicity became larger, which was discrepant with recent studies indicating that SN hyperechogenicity was stable during disease progression [17, 32, 34, 35]. Although the correlation between SN_L and disease duration was weak, several investigations [20, 22, 33] and our previous study [36] did support this positive correlation. In contrast, a tendency of reversed correlation was found in MSA-P patients, although without statistical significance. Therefore, it could be expected that within shorter disease duration, non-TD PD patients had smaller SN echogenicity, which could lead to lower percentage of SN hyperechogenicity, whereas MSA-P patients might have larger SN echogenicity, which could lead to higher percentage of SN hyperechogenicity. Additionally, this different correlation of SN hyperechogenicity with disease duration might also support the hypothesis about the distinct underlying mechanisms in the pattern of SN echogenicity of PD and MSA. So far, the origin of SN hyperechogenecity was not completely elucidated, nonchelated forms of iron, protein bound iron and microglia activation were all supposed to be involved in the reflection of SN hyperechogenecity signals [33, 37, 38]. Tissue iron has been shown to be elevated in both PD and MSA-P [39], but the detailed iron metabolism and gliosis might be different in PD and MSA [33, 37–39].

Limitations of this study need to be mentioned. Indeed, we could not promise absolutely accurate diagnosis of PD and MSA, since no post-mortem verification was achieved. This also was the problem for the differentiation between MSA and other APD, such as CBD and DLB. SN hyperechogenicity has been reported frequent in CBD and DLB [40, 41], therefore misdiagnosis of those disorders could also contribute to higher sensitivity of SN hyperechogenicity in MSA-P. Additionally, although non-TD PD was considered as the phenotype that was most difficult to discriminate from MSA-P, one should note that non-TD and TD PD subtypes do not necessarily represent different subtypes of PD. TD subtype was much more likely to shift to non-TD subtype during the disease progression [42].

Conclusions

In summary, our present study demonstrated that SN hyperechognicity could help to discriminate non-TD PD from MSA-P; however, both sensitivity and specificity were not satisfactory, particularly in the earlier stage. Combination with other auxiliary tests seemed a necessary way to help differentiation of these two entities.

Abbreviations

APD: Atypical parkinsonian disorders; CBD: Corticobasal ganglionic degeneration; DLB: Dementia with Lewy bodies; H-Y: Hoehn and Yahr; MSA: Multiple system atrophy; MSA-C: MSA with predominant cerebellar ataxia; MSA-P: MSA with predominant parkinsonism; non-TD PD: Non-tremor dominant PD; NPV: Negative predictive value; PD: Parkinson's disease; PIGD: Postural instability and gait difficulty; PPV: Positive predictive value;

PSP: Progressive supranuclear palsy; SN: Substantia nigra; TCS: Transcranial sonography

Funding
This study was supported by Natural Science Fund of China (No. 81430022, 81371407, 81771374), Innovation Program of Shanghai Municipal Education Commission (2017-01-07-00-01-E00046) and Natural Science Foundation of Science and Technology of Shanghai (No. 15ZR1426700).

Authors' contributions
H-YZ was responsible for the conception of the project; design, review and critique of statistical analysis, and writing the first draft. PH was responsible for organization and execution of this project, as well as design and execution of statistical analysis. QS, J-JD and S-SC were responsible for collecting parts of patients' data. Y-YH was responsible for performing ultrasound. W-WZ was responsible for supervising ultrasound. YW, QX and JL provided patient data. Y-YT was responsible for review and critique the manuscript. S-DC was responsible for providing most of the patient data, and was involved in the conception of this project and review and critique the manuscript.

Competing interests
The authors declare that they have no competing interests.

Author details
[1]Department of Neurology & Institute of Neurology, Ruijin Hospital affiliated to Shanghai Jiao Tong University School of Medicine, No.197 Ruijin 2nd Road, Shanghai 200025, China. [2]Department of Ultrasonography, Ruijin Hospital affiliated to Shanghai Jiao Tong University School of Medicine, Shanghai 200025, China.

References

1. Saeed U, Compagnone J, Aviv RI, Strafella AP, Black SE, Lang AE, Masellis M. Imaging biomarkers in Parkinson's disease and parkinsonian syndromes: current and emerging concepts. Transl Neurodegener. 2017;6:8.
2. Hughes AJ, Daniel SE, Kilford L, Lees AJ. Accuracy of clinical diagnosis of idiopathic Parkinson's disease: a clinico-pathological study of 100 cases. J Neurol Neurosurg Psychiatry. 1992;55:181–4.
3. Rizzo G, Copetti M, Arcuti S, Martino D, Fontana A, Logroscino G. Accuracy of clinical diagnosis of Parkinson disease: a systematic review and meta-analysis. Neurology. 2016;86:566–76.
4. Adler CH, Beach TG, Hentz JG, Shill HA, Caviness JN, Driver-Dunckley E, Sabbagh MN, Sue LI, Jacobson SA, Belden CM, et al. Low clinical diagnostic accuracy of early vs advanced Parkinson disease: clinicopathologic study. Neurology. 2014;83:406–12.
5. Bouwmans AE, Vlaar AM, Srulijes K, Mess WH, Weber WE. Transcranial sonography for the discrimination of idiopathic Parkinson's disease from the atypical parkinsonian syndromes. Int Rev Neurobiol. 2010;90:121–46.
6. Shafieesabet A, Fereshtehnejad SM, Shafieesabet A, Delbari A, Baradaran HR, Postuma RB, Lokk J. Hyperechogenicity of substantia nigra for differential diagnosis of Parkinson's disease: a meta-analysis. Parkinsonism Relat Disord. 2017;42:1–11.
7. Geser F, Wenning GK, Seppi K, Stampfer-Kountchev M, Scherfler C, Sawires M, Frick C, Ndayisaba JP, Ulmer H, Pellecchia MT, et al. Progression of multiple system atrophy (MSA): a prospective natural history study by the European MSA study group (EMSA SG). Mov Disord. 2006;21:179–86.
8. Gilman S, Wenning GK, Low PA, Brooks DJ, Mathias CJ, Trojanowski JQ, Wood NW, Colosimo C, Durr A, Fowler CJ, et al. Second consensus statement on the diagnosis of multiple system atrophy. Neurology. 2008;71:670–6.
9. Postuma RB, Berg D, Stern M, Poewe W, Olanow CW, Oertel W, Obeso J, Marek K, Litvan I, Lang AE, et al. MDS clinical diagnostic criteria for Parkinson's disease. Mov Disord. 2015;30:1591–601.
10. Jankovic J, McDermott M, Carter J, Gauthier S, Goetz C, Golbe L, Huber S, Koller W, Olanow C, Shoulson I, et al. Variable expression of Parkinson's disease: a base-line analysis of the DATATOP cohort. The Parkinson study group. Neurology. 1990;40:1529–34.
11. Zhou HY, Sun Q, Tan YY, Hu YY, Zhan WW, Li DH, Wang Y, Xiao Q, Liu J, Chen SD. Substantia nigra echogenicity correlated with clinical features of Parkinson's disease. Parkinsonism Relat Disord. 2016;24:28–33.
12. Behnke S, Berg D, Naumann M, Becker G. Differentiation of Parkinson's disease and atypical parkinsonian syndromes by transcranial ultrasound. J Neurol Neurosurg Psychiatry. 2005;76:423–5.
13. Walter U, Wittstock M, Benecke R, Dressler D. Substantia nigra echogenicity is normal in non-extrapyramidal cerebral disorders but increased in Parkinson's disease. J Neural Transm (Vienna). 2002;109:191–6.
14. Berg D, Siefker C, Ruprecht-Dorfler P, Becker G. Relationship of substantia nigra echogenicity and motor function in elderly subjects. Neurology. 2001;56:13–7.
15. Walter U, Niehaus L, Probst T, Benecke R, Meyer BU, Dressler D. Brain parenchyma sonography discriminates Parkinson's disease and atypical parkinsonian syndromes. Neurology. 2003;60:74–7.
16. Gaenslen A, Unmuth B, Godau J, Liepelt I, Di Santo A, Schweitzer KJ, Gasser T, Machulla HJ, Reimold M, Marek K, et al. The specificity and sensitivity of transcranial ultrasound in the differential diagnosis of Parkinson's disease: a prospective blinded study. Lancet Neurol. 2008;7:417–24.
17. Berg D, Siefker C, Becker G. Echogenicity of the substantia nigra in Parkinson's disease and its relation to clinical findings. J Neurol. 2001;248:684–9.
18. Walter U, Dressler D, Probst T, Wolters A, Abu-Mugheisib M, Wittstock M, Benecke R. Transcranial brain sonography findings in discriminating between parkinsonism and idiopathic Parkinson disease. Arch Neurol. 2007;64:1635–40.
19. Busse K, Heilmann R, Kleinschmidt S, Abu-Mugheisib M, Hoppner J, Wunderlich C, Gemende I, Kaulitz L, Wolters A, Benecke R, et al. Value of combined midbrain sonography, olfactory and motor function assessment in the differential diagnosis of early Parkinson's disease. J Neurol Neurosurg Psychiatry. 2012;83:441–7.
20. Kim JY, Kim ST, Jeon SH, Lee WY. Midbrain transcranial sonography in Korean patients with Parkinson's disease. Mov Disord. 2007;22:1922–6.
21. Okawa M, Miwa H, Kajimoto Y, Hama K, Morita S, Nakanishi I, Kondo T. Transcranial sonography of the substantia nigra in Japanese patients with Parkinson's disease or atypical parkinsonism: clinical potential and limitations. Intern Med. 2007;46:1527–31.
22. Huang YW, Jeng JS, Tsai CF, Chen LL, Wu RM. Transcranial imaging of substantia nigra hyperechogenicity in a Taiwanese cohort of Parkinson's disease. Mov Disord. 2007;22:550–5.
23. Fujita H, Suzuki K, Numao A, Watanabe Y, Uchiyama T, Miyamoto T, Miyamoto M, Hirata K. Usefulness of cardiac MIBG scintigraphy, olfactory testing and substantia Nigra Hyperechogenicity as additional diagnostic markers for distinguishing between Parkinson's disease and atypical parkinsonian syndromes. PLoS One. 2016;11:e0165869.
24. Chen W, Tan YY, Hu YY, Zhan WW, Wu L, Lou Y, Wang X, Zhou Y, Huang P, Gao Y, et al. Combination of olfactory test and substantia nigra transcranial sonopraphy in the differential diagnosis of Parkinson's disease: a pilot study from China. Transl Neurodegener. 2012;1:25.
25. Li DH, Zhang LY, Hu YY, Jiang XF, Zhou HY, Yang Q, Kang WY, Liu J, Chen SD. Transcranial sonography of the substantia nigra and its correlation with DAT-SPECT in the diagnosis of Parkinson's disease. Parkinsonism Rela Disord. 2015;21:923–8.
26. Liu P, Li X, Li FF, Ou-Yang QH, Zhang HX, Feng T. The predictive value of transcranial sonography in clinically diagnosed patients with early stage Parkinson's disease: comparison with DAT PET scans. Neurosci Lett. 2014;582:99–103.
27. Bartova P, Skoloudik T, Fadrna P, Ressner P, Kanovsky P, Herzig R. Substantia nigra evaluation in atypical parkinsonian syndromes and Parkinson's disease. Mov Disord. 2007;22:S140.
28. Luo WF, Zhang YC, Sheng YJ, Fang JC, Liu CF. Transcranial sonography on Parkinson's disease and essential tremor in a Chinese population. Neurol Sci. 2012;33:1005–9.

29. Thenganatt MA, Jankovic J. Parkinson disease subtypes. JAMA Neuro. 2014; 71:499–504.
30. Schrag A, Schott JM. Epidemiological, clinical, and genetic characteristics of early-onset parkinsonism. Lancet Neurol. 2006;5:355–63.
31. van Rooden SM, Heiser WJ, Kok JN, Verbaan D, van Hilten JJ, Marinus J. The identification of Parkinson's disease subtypes using cluster analysis: a systematic review. Mov Disord. 2010;25:969–78.
32. Walter U, Dressler D, Wolters A, Wittstock M, Benecke R. Transcranial brain sonography findings in clinical subgroups of idiopathic Parkinson's disease. Mov Disord. 2007;22:48–54.
33. Becker G, Seufert J, Bogdahn U, Reichmann H, Reiners K. Degeneration of substantia nigra in chronic Parkinson's disease visualized by transcranial color-coded real-time sonography. Neurology. 1995;45:182–4.
34. Behnke S, Runkel A, Kassar HA, Ortmann M, Guidez D, Dillmann U, Fassbender K, Spiegel J. Long-term course of substantia nigra hyperechogenicity in Parkinson's disease. Mov Disord. 2013;28:455–9.
35. Berg D, Merz B, Reiners K, Naumann M, Becker G. Five-year follow-up study of hyperechogenicity of the substantia nigra in Parkinson's disease. Mov Disord. 2005;20:383–5.
36. Zhou HY, Huang P, Sun Q, Du JJ, Cui SS, Tan YY, Hu YY, Zhan WW, Wang Y, Xiao Q et al. Substantia nigra echogenicity associated with clinical subtpes of Parkinson's disease. J Parkinson Dis 2018; doi: https://doi.org/10.3233/JPD-171264.
37. Berg D, Godau J, Riederer P, Gerlach M, Arzberger T. Microglia activation is related to substantia nigra echogenicity. J Neural Transm (Vienna). 2010;117: 1287–92.
38. Berg D, Becker G, Zeiler B, Tucha O, Hofmann E, Preier M, Benz P, Jost W, Reiners K, Lange KW. Vulnerability of the nigrostriatal system as detected by transcranial ultrasound. Neurology. 1999;53:1026–31.
39. Dexter DT, Jenner P, Schapira AH, Marsden CD. Alterations in levels of iron, ferritin, and other trace metals in neurodegenerative diseases affecting the basal ganglia. The Royal Kings and Queens Parkinson's Disease Research Group. Ann Neurol. 1992;32(Suppl):S94–100.
40. Walter U, Dressler D, Wolters A, Probst T, Grossmann A, Benecke R. Sonographic discrimination of corticobasal degeneration vs progressive supranuclear palsy. Neurology. 2004;63:504–9.
41. Walter U, Dressler D, Wolters A, Wittstock M, Greim B, Benecke R. Sonographic discrimination of dementia with Lewy bodies and Parkinson's disease with dementia. J Neurol. 2006;253:448–54.
42. Nutt JG. Motor subtype in Parkinson's disease: different disorders or different stages of disease? Mov Disord. 2016;31:957–61.

CSF $A\beta_{1-42}$ level is associated with cognitive decline in early Parkinson's disease with rapid eye movement sleep behavior disorder

Maowen Ba[1†], Guoping Yu[1†], Min Kong[2*], Hui Liang[2] and Ling Yu[2]

Abstract

Background: Rapid eye movement sleep behavior disorder (RBD) is associated with cognitive decline in early Parkinson's disease (PD). However, the underlying basis for this association remains unclear.

Methods: Parkinson's Progression Marker's Initiative (PPMI) subjects underwent baseline RBD testing with RBD sleep questionnaire (RBDSQ). Serial assessments included measures of motor symptoms, non-motor symptoms (NMS), neuropsychological assessment, blood and cerebrospinal fluid (CSF) biomarkers. Up to three years follow-up data were included. We stratified early PD subjects into PD with RBD (RBDSQ score > 5) and PD without RBD groups. Then, we evaluated baseline biomarkers in each group as a predictor of cognitive decline using Montreal Cognitive Assessment (MoCA) score changes over three years in regression models.

Results: Four hundred twenty-three PD subjects were enrolled at baseline, and a total of 350 PD subjects had completed 3 years of study follow-up with completely serial assessments. We found that at baseline, only CSF β-amyloid 1–42 ($A\beta_{1-42}$) was significantly lower in PD subjects with RBD. On three years follow-up analysis, PD subjects with RBD were more likely to develop incident mild cognitive impairment (MCI) and presented greater cognitive decline in MoCA score. Lower baseline CSF $A\beta_{1-42}$ predicted cognitive decline over 3 years only in PD subjects with RBD ($\beta = -0.03$, $P = 0.003$). A significant interaction between $A\beta_{1-42}$ and the 2 groups confirmed that this effect was indeed higher in PD with RBD than the other individual ($\beta = -2.85$, $P = 0.014$).

Conclusion: These findings indicate that CSF $A\beta_{1-42}$ level is associated with global cognitive decline in early PD with RBD. The addition of CSF $A\beta_{1-42}$ to RBD testing increase the likelihood of identifying those at high risk for cognitive decline in early PD.

Keywords: Parkinson's disease, Rapid eye movement sleep behavior disorder, Cognitive decline, β-Amyloid

Background

Parkinson's disease (PD) is one of age-related neurodegenerative diseases with a wide range of motor and non-motor symptoms (NMS) [1, 2]. Rapid eye movement sleep behavior disorder (RBD) and cognitive impairement are two common NMS manifestations in PD [3–6]. The presence of RBD can predict a greater cognitive decline and a greater risk of developing dementia in advanced PD [7–10]. The relationship between RBD and cognitive decline has also been reported in a preliminary analysis of early PD subjects from the Parkinson's Progression Markers Initiative (PPMI) cohort [11, 12]. However, no prior work has identified the underlying basis of cognitive impairement in early PD with or without RBD.

Recent studies have suggested that several biomarkers including blood apolipoprotein E ε4 (ApoE4) genotype, cerebrospinal fluid (CSF) $A\beta_{1-42}$ (lower) and tau (higher) have been associated with cognitive impairment in PD in cross sectional studies [13–16]. However, the results did

* Correspondence: kk_kmm@sina.com
[†]Maowen Ba and Guoping Yu contributed equally to this work.
[2]Department of Neurology, Yantaishan Hospital, Yantai City, Shandong 264000, People's Republic of China
Full list of author information is available at the end of the article

not clarify the relationship between these biomarkers and RBD for cognitive decline in early PD. It is interesting to explore whether the presence of any of these biomarkers increases the risk of developing cognitive decline in early PD with RBD. So, the aims of this study were to (i) confirm the association between RBD and global cognitive decline in early PD over 3 years follow-up period, and (ii) further assess which biomarker is associated with cognitive decline in early PD with RBD. The PPMI therefore provides an early opportunity to explore relationships between cognitive findings and potentially influencing factors at the early stage of PD in a large, untreated, imaging-confirmed cohort of newly diagnosed PD patients, where medications do not confound motor and NMS measures.

Methods

Study samples

Data used in the preparation of this study were obtained from PPMI database (http://www.ppmi-info.org). The PPMI was a prospective cohort study of PD patients untreated at enrollment and sponsored by The Michael J. Fox Foundation for Parkinson's Research. The primary goal of PPMI is to identify one or more biomarkers of Parkinson's disease progression. This longitudinal study, following over 1000 subjects for up to 8 years, is taking place at 33 clinical sites in the United States, Europe, Israel and Australia. Subjects underwent clinical assessments, imaging and blood and CSF collection at predetermined time points. Further information can be found at http://www.ppmi-info.org.

Standard protocol approvals, registrations, and patient consents

The PPMI study was approved by the Institutional Review Boards of each PPMI site. Informed written consent was obtained from all subjects at each site.

Subject selection

In this study, we selected PD subjects who must meet clinical motor criteria for PD confirmed by dopamine transporter (DAT) imaging deficit with a diagnosis within 2 years and dementia-free based on the site investigator's cognitive evaluation. Further information about the inclusion/exclusion criteria of PD adopted by the PPMI is described in detail at http://www.ppmi-info.org. Data were downloaded from http://www.ppmi-info.org on July 30, 2016 for this analysis. At the time of data acquisition, 423 PD subjects were enrolled, 362 PD subjects had completed 3 years of study follow-up. Eight PD subjects missed CSF data at baseline. Twelve PD subjects missed MoCA data at 3-year follow-up. A total of 350 PD subjects were included with completely clinical and neuropsychological assessments, and lumbar puncture at baseline, and 3 years follow-up visits for the neuropsychological assessments.

RBD sleep assessments

We defined possible RBD individuals in PD with RBD sleep questionnaire (RBDSQ), in which a positive screen was defined as a score > 5 [17]. The RBD data used in this study were obtained from the PPMI files 'REM_Sleep_Disorder_Questionnaire.csv'. According to this definition, the early PD subjects were allocated to PD with RBD and PD without RBD groups.

Cognitive tests

The question 1 on part 1 of the Movement Disorder Society–Unified Parkinson's Disease Rating Scale (MDS-UPDRS1.1) and Montreal Cognitive Assessment (MoCA) data sets used in this study were obtained from the PPMI files 'MDS_UPDRS_Part_I.csv' and 'Montreal_Cognitive_Assessment__MoCA_.csv' respectively. Question 1 on part 1 of the MDS-UPDRS was used to screen for PD reported cognitive impairment. MoCA is a validated global cognition test. The recommended cutoff score of < 26 was used to define mild cognitive impairment (MCI) [18]. Δ%MoCA over 3 years in each group were used to reflect cognitive decline and defined as:

$$\Delta\%\text{MoCA} = \left(\frac{\text{MoCA follow-up} - \text{MoCA baseline}}{\text{MoCA baseline}}\right) \text{x } 100$$

In addition, individual cognitive tests for specific domains have been previously described [19] and included Verbal memory—the Hopkins Verbal Learning Test (HVLT) total recall, HVLT Recognition Discrimination, Visuospatial function—Benton Judgment of Line Orientation, Processing speed /attention—Symbol Digit Modalities Test, Executive function /working memory—Letter-Number Sequencing Test and Semantic Fluency. Mild cognitive impairment was defined as any 2 or more of the above cognitive tests > 1.5 SD below the standardized mean [19]. Δ% individual cognitive tests over 3 years in each group were used to reflect specific cognitive decline and defined as:

$$\Delta\%\text{cognitive test} = \left(\frac{\text{cognitive test follow-up} - \text{cognitive test baseline}}{\text{cognitive test baseline}}\right) \text{x } 100$$

Other clinical characteristics and assessments

The demographic, ApoE4 genotype, education and disease duration data were obtained from PPMI files. Hoehn and Yahr Stage was obtained to measure disease severity. Subscores of MDS-UPDRS part III were also collected at each visit to measure motor function. Assessments of NMS included (i) the University of Pennsylvania Smell Identification Test (UPSIT) with lower scores reflecting worse olfactory function, (ii) the State-Trait

Anxiety Inventory (STAI), (iii) the 15-item Geriatric Depression Scale (GDS-15).

CSF biomarkers

CSF $A\beta_{1-42}$, alpha-synuclein, total tau (t-tau), and phosphorylated-tau at threonine 181 (p-tau) were measured by using Innogenetics (INNO-BIA AlzBio3) immunoassay kit–based reagents in the multiplex xMAPLuminex platform (Luminex). The CSF data used in this study were obtained from the PPMI files 'Biospecimen_Analysis_Results.csv'. Further details of PPMI methods for CSF acquisition, and measurements and quality control procedures can be found at http://www.ppmi-info.org/.

Statistical analysis

Baseline demographic, CSF biomarkers ($A\beta_{1-42}$, t-tau, p-tau, alpha-synuclein), MoCA scores, individual cognitive tests, other motor and non-motor data were compared between two study groups using two-tailed Student *t* test for continuous variables and chi-square ($\chi 2$) tests for categorical variables, respectively. Normality assumptions were checked where appropriate. Kaplan-Meier survival analysis was used to estimate the effects of RBD on the progression to MCI. Seventy five PD subjects met criteria for MCI at baseline by MoCA criteria. Thus, PD subjects with baseline MCI were only excluded from Kaplan-Meier survival analysis.

We analyzed the association between all baseline CSF biomarkers and Δ% MoCA in each group. Linear regression models evaluated the predictive effects of all baseline CSF biomarkers on outcomes of Δ% MoCA over 3 years in each group. We further added an interaction term (CSF biomarkers*group) in the regression models to evaluate the interaction between CSF biomarkers and the 2 groups on the outcomes. Confounding variables based on biological rationality and published data were selected in linear regression model. Because UPDRS part III differed and Geriatric Depression Scale were borderline among the PD RBD and non-RBD subjects, linear regression model was corrected for UPDRS part III scores and Geriatric Depression Scale when analyzing the association between all baseline CSF biomarkers and Δ% MoCA. Age, gender, education, ApoE4 status were also included as covariates for analysis involving cognition. For each model, the coefficient (β) represents the difference in annual rate of change in the MoCA for each 1 point increase in the parameter (dependent variable) for the continuous variables. For the models involving categorical variables, each coefficient represents the difference in annual rate of change of the MoCA between the group. Statistical analysis were performed using SPSS (version 19.0) and a *P*-value < 0.05 was taken as statistically significant.

Results

Baseline demographic and clinical characteristics

Of the 350 early PD subjects analyzed, 136 were PD with RBD and 214 were PD without RBD. There were no differences in gender, age, education, ApoE4 genotype distribution, baseline disease duration, Hoehn and Yahr Stage, UPDRS1.1 positive cognition, MoCA scores and other NMS scores between two groups. There were significant differences detected in the baseline UPDRS part III in PD with RBD group compared to PD without RBD group ($P = 0.044$). The detailed characteristics of all these PD subjects were listed in Table 1.

Baseline performance on the individual cognitive test among PD subjects with vs. without RBD are shown in Table 2. At baseline, those with RBD performed worse on the HVLT total recall ($P = 0.039$) and Symbol Digit Modalities ($P = 0.008$). Baseline Benton Judgment of Line Orientation and Letter-Number Sequencing tests also differed, however, they did not reach significance.

Baseline CSF biomarkers

Baseline CSF biomarker levels by study groups were demonstrated in Table 3. There were no differences at baseline CSF t-tau, p-tau, alpha-synuclein, p-tau/t-tau ratio, and t-tau/$A\beta_{1-42}$ ratio between two groups. CSF $A\beta_{1-42}$ was lower in PD with RBD group compared to PD without RBD group ($P = 0.005$).

Follow-up cognitive decline and conversion to MCI

On 3 year follow-up visits, those in PD with RBD group were more likely to report cognitive impairment (UPDRS1.1) compared to PD without RBD group (52.9% versus 31.8%, $P < 0.001$). The Δ% MoCA of PD subjects with RBD declined more than in those without RBD ($P = 0.004$). In Kaplan-Meier survival analysis with time to conversion to MCI as the dependent variable, there was a suggestion of an effect of RBD on the risk of developing MCI ($P < 0.001$, Fig. 1).

In a separate analysis, we defined MCI by individual cognitive tests criteria. We found that on 3 year follow-up visits, in visuospatial function domain, the Δ%Benton Judgment of Line Orientation of PD subjects with RBD declined more than in those without RBD ($P = 0.016$, Fig. 2). Similarly, PD subjects with RBD presented more MCI prevalence in comparision with PD subjects without RBD, however, they did not reach significance (15.0% versus 8.5%, $P = 0.071$).

Baseline CSF $A\beta_{1-42}$ as a predictor of cognitive decline in PD subjects with RBD

We further found that baseline CSF $A\beta_{1-42}$ predicted global cognitive decline (Δ%MoCA) over 3 years in PD with RBD group ($\beta = -0.03$, $P = 0.003$), but not in the PD without RBD group. For instance, MoCA scores

Table 1 Baseline characteristics of PD stratified by RBD

	PD with RBD (N = 136)	PD without RBD (N = 214)	P value
Age, years	61.22 ± 9.44	60.42 ± 9.88	0.447
Males, n(%)	92(67.6%)	137(64.0%)	0.564
Education, year	15.61 ± 2.91	15.57 ± 2.97	0.890
ApoE4(%)	23.40%	24.50%	0.893
RBD	7.04 ± 1.91	2.53 ± 1.17	< 0.001*
Disease duration (months)	7.51 ± 6.69	7.35 ± 6.29	0.816
Hoehn and Yahr Stage	1.57 ± 0.49	1.51 ± 0.52	0.289
UPDRS part III	21.58 ± 9.41	19.63 ± 8.39	0.044*
UPDRS1.1 Cognition, N (% positive)	39(28.7%)	46(21.5%)	0.159
MoCA	26.98 ± 2.40	27.32 ± 2.21	0.170
UPSIT Total	21.60 ± 8.39	22.33 ± 7.96	0.411
Geriatric Depression Scale	5.39 ± 1.94	5.10 ± 1.37	0.065
Total STAI	93.58 ± 8.49	93.33 ± 7.58	0.771

Results are mean ± (SD). P value was assessed using two-tailed Student t test for each variable except gender, ApoE4 and UPDRS1.1, where chi-square ($\chi 2$) test was performed. *P value statistically significant. The age, education, ApoE4, disease duration, Hoehn and Yahr Stage, UPDRS1.1 Cognition, MoCA, UPSIT Total, depression and total STAI had no difference between two groups. However, the PD with RBD group had relative greater UPDRS part III
Abbreviations: PD Parkinsonr's disease, *RBD* Rapid eye movement sleep behavioral disorder, *ApoE4* Apolipoprotein E ε4, *UPDRS* Unified Parkinson's Disease Rating Scale, *MoCA* Montreal Cognitive Assessment, *UPSIT* University of Pennsylvania Smell Identification Test, *STAI* State Trait Anxiety Inventory

decreased by 0.03 points for every 1 point reduction in CSF $A\beta_{1-42}$ value. For example, a subject with an CSF $A\beta_{1-42}$ value of 354 pg/ml could be expected to experience an additional 2.7 point decline in MoCA score over 3 years compared to a subject with an CSF $A\beta_{1-42}$ value of 384 pg/ml. In addition, a significant interaction between $A\beta_{1-42}$ and the 2 groups ($A\beta_{1-42}$*group) confirmed that this effect was indeed higher in PD subjects with RBD than PD subjects without RBD (β = – 2.85, P = 0.014, Table 4).

Discussion

Based on the present results from PPMI database, we report that RBD is an predictor of cognitive decline in early PD patients and CSF $A\beta_{1-42}$ is associated with cognitive decline in early PD with RBD.

RBD has been reported to be present in 15–72% of PD patients and is associated with poor parkinsonian symptoms, higher daily levodopa dosage, and cognitive impairment in more advanced PD patients [4, 7–10, 20]. However, in the large-scale, untreated, imaging-confirmed early PD cohort, we found that multiple baseline NMS didn't show worse presentation in PD patients with RBD compared with PD patients without RBD, and they also remain relatively stable over 3 years (data not shown). While global cognition deteriorates in 3 years follow-up period in PD patients with RBD. Thus, we confirmed that RBD was still associated with cognitive decline in the early stage of PD.

There are several hypothesis that might explain the association between RBD and cognitive decline in PD [21, 22]. This is the first study to our knowledge exploring the underlying basis for the association between RBD and cognitive decline within the untreated, imaging-confirmed early PD cohort. The ApoE4 is an established risk factor for Alzheimer's disease [23–25] and has also been proposed to be an important risk factor for cognitive impairment in PD [13, 14]. Yet, our results showed that in early

Table 2 Baseline specific cognitive characteristics of PD stratified by RBD

Cognitive domain	Measure	PD with RBD (N = 136)	PD without RBD (N = 214)	P value
Verbal memory	HVLT Total Recall	45.23 ± 10.80	47.69 ± 10.83	0.039*
	HVLT Recognition Discrimination	47.52 ± 13.05	49.70 ± 10.86	0.092
Visuospatial function	Benton Judgment of Line Orientation	12.65 ± 2.82	13.21 ± 2.58	0.058
Processing speed /attention	Symbol Digit Modalities	43.64 ± 9.08	46.36 ± 9.36	0.008*
Executive function /working memory	Letter-Number Sequencing	11.17 ± 2.53	11.72 ± 2.71	0.06
	Semantic Fluency total	50.19 ± 9.24	51.31 ± 10.40	0.305

Results are mean ± (SD). P value was assessed using two-tailed Student t test for each variable. *P value statistically significant. The PD with RBD group performed worse on the HVLT total recall and Symbol Digit Modalities
Abbreviations: PD Parkinsonr's disease, *RBD* Rapid eye movement sleep behavioral disorder, *HVLT* Hopkins Verbal Learning Test

Table 3 Baseline CSF biomarkers of PD stratified by RBD

	PD with RBD ($N = 136$)	PD without RBD ($N = 214$)	P value
$A\beta_{1-42}$ (pg/ml)	354.70 ± 103.45	384.73 ± 90.77	0.005*
t-tau (pg/ml)	43.76 ± 18.75	44.42 ± 16.89	0.736
p-tau (pg/ml)	14.57 ± 7.85	16.31 ± 11.32	0.121
alpha-synuclein (pg/ml)	1811.69 ± 741.35	1860.50 ± 818.55	0.578
p-tau/t-tau	0.35 ± 0.17	0.39 ± 0.25	0.130
t-tau/$A\beta_{1-42}$	0.13 ± 0.07	0.12 ± 0.05	0.056

Results are mean ± (SD). *P* value was assessed using two-tailed Student *t* test for each variable. *P value statistically significant. The PD with RBD patients had significantly lower contents of CSF $A\beta_{1-42}$

Abbreviations: PD Parkinsonr's disease, *RBD* Rapid eye movement sleep behavioral disorder, *CSF* cerebrospinal fluid, *t-tau* total tau, *p-tau* phosphorylated-tau, *Aβ* β-amyloid

PD there was no difference in frequency of ApoE4 occurrence between PD with RBD and PD without RBD. In addition, in ApoE4 positive and ApoE4 negative PD paients with RBD, there was no difference in MoCA score loss (7.48 ± 11.04 versus 3.57 ± 11.05, $P = 0.098$) and Benton Judgment of Line Orientation (18.01 ± 25.03 versus 8.46 ± 29.13, $P = 0.101$). Thus, our data suggest that RBD increases the risk and severity of cognitive impairement in early stage of PD and is independent of ApoE4 status. Recent study even pointed out that ApoE4 did not affect cognitive performance in PD patients [26, 27]. Thus, the presence of ApoE4 does not increase the risk of becoming MCI at least in the first 3 years of early dementia-free PD with RBD.

Alzheimer's disease (AD) pathology has been linked to cognitive decline in PD. Pathologic accumulation of Aβ is associated with PD patients with dementia. Cortical Aβ seem to determine the rate to dementia [28, 29]. Up to one third of patients who develop PD dementia will also meet pathologic criteria for AD, involving β-amyloid plaques and tau-containing neurofibrillary tangles, which may have an additive effect with alpha-synuclein pathology to worsen prognosis. The phosphorylated-tau at threonine 181 is one more specific biomarker for AD and is related to neurofibrillary tangles [30, 31]. CSF biomarkers, such as increased tau and decreased $A\beta_{1-42}$, can reflect the degenerative process and have been associated with cognitive impairment in PD in cross sectional studies [15, 16, 32]. Yet, the relationship between CSF tau or $A\beta_{1-42}$ and RBD in predicting cognitive decline in early PD remains unknown. In the present study, early PD patients were dichotomized into PD with RBD and PD without RBD based on RBD SQ score > 5 [17]. We found that in comparison to PD without RBD, only CSF $A\beta_{1-42}$ was obviously lower in PD with RBD. Regression analysis showed that baseline CSF $A\beta_{1-42}$ could predict cognitive decline over 3 years only in PD subjects with RBD. Similar studies with a relatively small sample of PD subjects have found a relationship between CSF $A\beta_{1-42}$ levels and cognitive status in PD patients [33, 34]. Lower $A\beta_{1-42}$ levels in the spinal fluid may be related to sequestration of the peptide from CSF into amyloid plaques. Lower CSF $A\beta_{1-42}$ levels reflect greater amyloid plaque burden in patients with PD at risk for cognitive decline [35]. Therefore, our data suggest that lower CSF $A\beta_{1-42}$ could be the closely related biomarker in cognitive decline in early PD with RBD. The addition of CSF $A\beta_{1-42}$ to RBD testing may increase the likelihood of identifying those at high risk for cognitive decline in early PD.

Lewy body-type synucleinopathy is the main pathological marker in PD. PD dementia has also two major

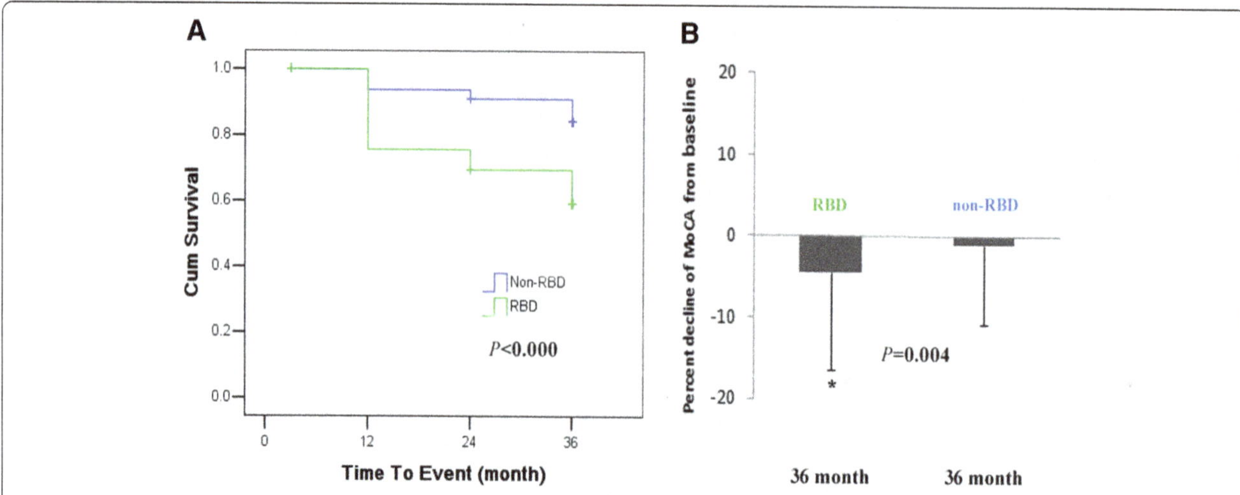

Fig. 1 The effect of RBD on global cognitive decline in early PD subjects. **a** RBD predict conversion to MCI. Kaplan-Meier survival analysis was used to estimate the effects of RBD on the progression to MCI. **b** Cognitive decline by Δ%MoCA from baseline to 36 month in PD with RBD and without RBD. Results are mean ± (SD). *P* value was assessed using two-tailed Student *t* test for each variable. *P value statistically significant. Abbreviations: RBD, Rapid eye movement sleep behavioral disorder

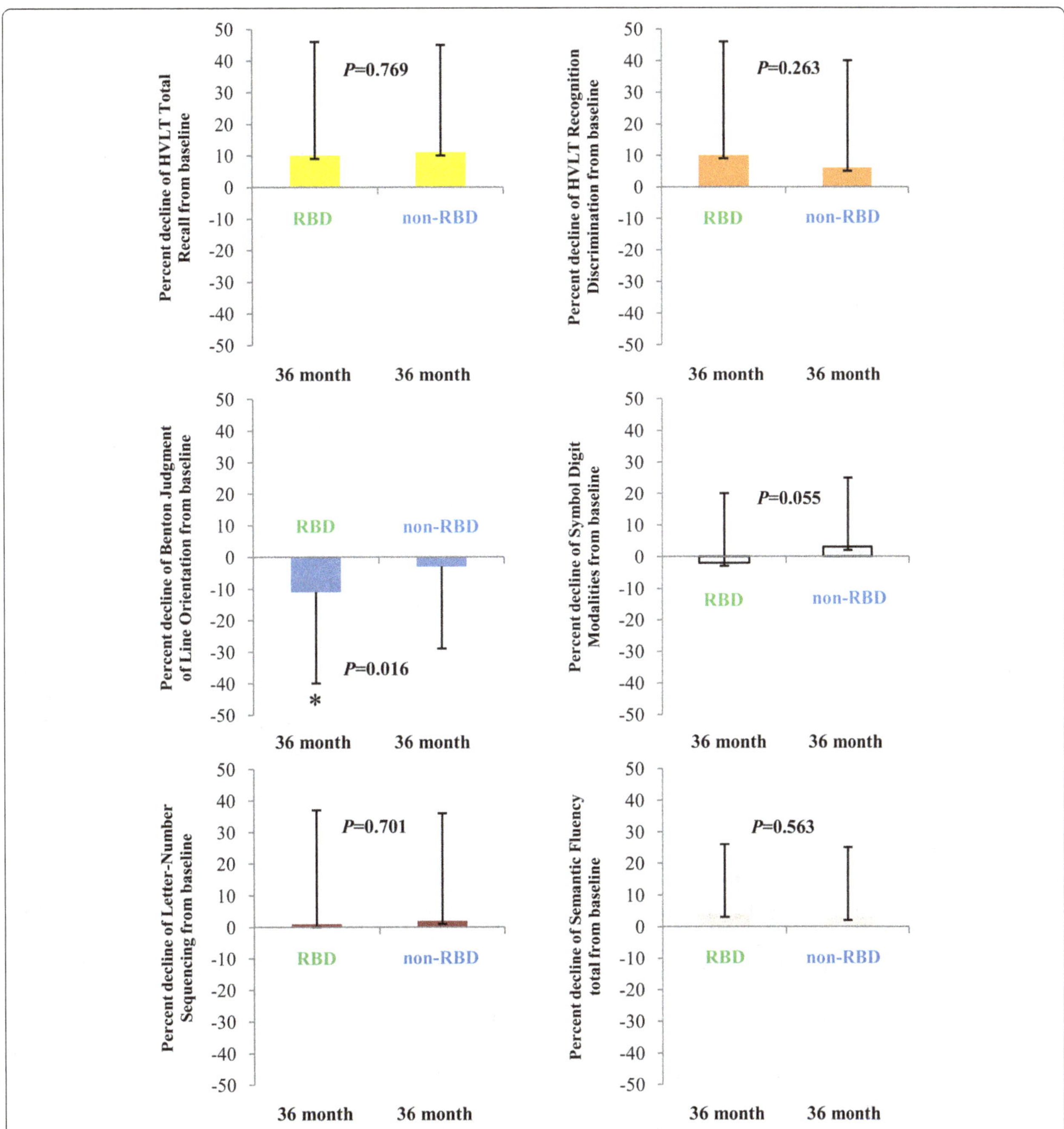

Fig. 2 The effect of RBD on specific cognitive domains in early PD subjects. Cognitive decline by Δ%HVLT total recall, Δ%HVLT Recognition Discrimination, Δ% Benton Judgment of Line Orientation, Δ%Symbol Digit Modalities, Δ% Letter-Number Sequencing and Δ%Semantic Fluency from baseline to 36 month in PD with RBD and without RBD. Results are mean ± (SD). *P* value was assessed using two-tailed Student *t* test for each variable. **P* value statistically significant. Abbreviations: RBD, Rapid eye movement sleep behavioral disorder; HVLT, Hopkins Verbal Learning Test

pathologic subgroups: neocortical synucleinopathy and neocortical synucleinopathy with Aβ deposition [28, 29]. Interestingly, there is inconsistent data about the relationship between CSF alpha-synuclein and cognitive impairment in PD patients. Several research found that high CSF alpha-synuclein correlated with PD dementia [36, 37] and low CSF total-α-synuclein was associated with dysfunction in phonetic-fluency (a frontal-lobe function) and with frontal cortical thinning in RBD [36]. Unlike several previous research, we did not show an association between CSF alpha-synuclein level and cognitive impairment in early PD. For high CSF alpha-synuclein, it is important to note that these previous research have focused on PD patients with dementia [36, 37], and the PPMI sample is relatively young and dementia-free. Our findings were consistent with some previous studies showing no

Table 4 CSF biomarkers and RBD as predictors of global cognitive decline in PD

Variables (Δ%MoCA as dependent variable)	β	*P* value
$A\beta_{1-42}$ (RBD group)	−0.03 ± 0.01	0.003*
$A\beta_{1-42}$ (non-RBD group)	−0.001 ± 0.007	0.944
Group (categorical RBD and non-RBD)	2.95 ± 1.18	0.013*
$A\beta_{1-42}$*Group	−2.85 ± 1.15	0.014*

Data are shown as coefficient (β) ± (SE). In these linear effects models, Δ%MoCA is the dependent variable and $A\beta_{1-42}$, group and $A\beta_{1-42}$*Group are the independent variable, with age, sex, education, ApoE4 status, disease duration and baseline UPDRS part III score as co-variates. *P value statistically significant. Significant interactive effects were observed in $A\beta_{1-42}$ and RBD group

Abbreviations: PD Parkinsonr's disease, *RBD* Rapid eye movement sleep behavioral disorder, *CSF* cerebrospinal fluid, *MoCA* Montreal Cognitive Assessment, *Aβ* β-amyloid

association between CSF alpha-synuclein and cognitive impairment in early PD [32, 38]. Perhaps high CSF alpha-synuclein was more prevalent in PD patients with dementia. Our data supports the conclusion that CSF alpha-synuclein does not increase the risk of becoming MCI at least in the first 3 years of early dementia-free PD with RBD. Longer follow-up duration of PPMI cohort will reveal whether CSF alpha-synuclein is important in more advanced cognitive dysfunction of PD.

There are other baseline factors, including severity of disease, disease duration, education level, male gender, advanced age of onset, and concomitant medication which may be associated with more rapid cognitive decline in PD [39, 40]. However, in the early PD subjects from PPMI cohort, no significant differences were found in Hoehn and Yahr Stage, disease duration, onset age, education level, and male gender. There are few SSRI or SNRI usages in PD subjects in PPMI database. Previous study from PPMI database also demonstrated that the majority of PD patients with clinically significant depression were not treated with antidepressants [11]. So, these confounding factors were actually excluded when we investigated the relationship between CSF $A\beta_{1-42}$ and cognitive decline in early PD with RBD. Meanwhile, there are very few diabetes or metabolic syndrome in these early PD subjects in PPMI cohort, so contribution of diabetes or metabolic syndrome to our findings is likely minimal. Additionally, although GBA mutations were more common in RBD, there are few GBA mutations carriers in PD subjects in PPMI database. Of the 350 early PD subjects analyzed, we identified only 6 PD with p.N370S GBA mutations. The confounding effect of p.N370S GBA mutations to our findings was likely minor.

Of course, we recognize that the present study has several limitations. First, the MoCA is one broadly-used and abbreviated instrument for global cognition assessment. The recommended cutoff scores < 26 was used to determine MCI (PD-MCI level I category). Since comprehensive testing may not always be available, an MCI definition based on an abbreviated assessment is very useful in routine clinical practice. The use of the MoCA alone is one level I category for defining PD-MCI by MDS guidelines and a diagnosis by this criteria is regarded less certain than a diagnosis of PD-MCI by level II category assessment. However, Analysis by MCI level II category assessment based on neuropsychological testing for specific domains (PD-MCI level II) did not reach significance likely due to low progression to MCI event rate as described in the present and previous research [41]. Second, the diagnosis of RBD was only based on clinical interview without sleep laboratory recording [17]. Thus, the diagnosis of RBD might not be formally confirmed. The onset time of RBD with PD was unknown in the PPMI cohort. There is no available data of RBD duration for PD subjects and the present analysis. Future study is still highly desirable in order to is disclose the more possible mechanism of RBD on cognition impairment of PD patients. Third, the neuropathological and neuroimaging correlates of lower CSF $A\beta_{1-42}$ are not clear, which just can reflect the evidences for degeneration [42, 43]. In addition, cholinergic dysfunction is also associated with PD with RBD. However, longitudinal studies on large cohorts are required to gain more insight into the role of cholinergic dysfunction in the emergence of cognition impairment of PD patients with RBD [21]. Further studies based on this preliminary study are still required so as to contribute to a deeper understanding of cognitive impairement in PD with RBD, therapy planning and prognosis prediction for early PD patients with RBD.

Conclusions

Taken together, this study provides evidence that CSF $A\beta_{1-42}$ may play a role in prediction of cognitive impairment among early PD patients with RBD. As single marker, RBD may lack enough specificity. Early testing of CSF $A\beta_{1-42}$ in such PD patients is important for providing more potential diagnostic value and determining next therapies.

Abbreviations

ApoE4: Apolipoprotein E ε4; Aβ: β-amyloid; CSF: cerebrospinal fluid; HVLT: Hopkins verbal learning test; MoCA: Montreal cognitive assessment; PD: Parkinsonr's disease; RBD: Rapid eye movement sleep behavioral disorder; STAI: State Trait Anxiety Inventory; UPDRS: Unified Parkinson's Disease Rating Scale; UPSIT: University of Pennsylvania Smell Identification Test

Acknowledgements

Data used in the preparation of this article were obtained from the Parkinson's Progression Markers Initiative (PPMI) database (www.ppmi-info.org/data). For up-to-date information on the study, visit www.ppmi-info.org. PPMI - a public-private partnership - is sponsored by the Michael J. Fox Foundation (MJFF) for Parkinson's Research and is co-funded by MJFF, Abbvie, Avid Radiopharmaceuticals, Biogen Idec, Bristol-Myers Squibb, Covance, Eli Lilly & Co., F. Hoffman-La Roche, Ltd., GE Healthcare, Genentech, GlaxoSmithKline, Lundbeck, Merck, MesoScale, Piramal, Pfizer, and UCB.

Funding
This Study was funded by Chinese National Natural Science Foundation (No.81571234), Key research and development plan of Shandong Province (2018GSF118235), Shandong Province medical science and technology development projects (2014WS0260) and Yantai Science and Technology Development Project (2014WS035, 2016WS037).

Authors' contributions
MWB pool the data and prepare the manuscript; GPY study concept and design; MK study concept, design and interpretation of data; HL enter the data; LY perform the statistical analysis; All authors read and approved the final manuscript.

Competing interests
The authors declare that they have no competing interests.

Author details
[1]Department of Neurology, the Affiliated Yantai Yuhuangding Hospital of Qingdao University, Yantai City, Shandong 264000, People's Republic of China. [2]Department of Neurology, Yantaishan Hospital, Yantai City, Shandong 264000, People's Republic of China.

References

1. Jankovic J. Parkinson's disease: clinical features and diagnosis. J Neurol Neurosurg Psychiatry. 2008;79:368–76.
2. Chaudhuri KR, Martinez-Martin P, Schapira AH, Stocchi F, Sethi K, Odin P, et al. International multicenter pilot study of the first comprehensive self-completed nonmotor symptoms questionnaire for Parkinson's disease: the NMS quest study. Mov Disord. 2006;21:916–23.
3. Poryazova R, Oberholzer M, Baumann CR, Bassetti CL. REM sleep behavior disorder in Parkinson's disease: aquestionnaire-based survey. J Clin Sleep Med. 2013;9:55–9A.
4. Gagnon JF, Bédard MA, Fantini ML, Petit D, Panisset M, Rompré S, et al. REM sleep behavior disorder and REM sleep without atonia in Parkinson's disease. Neurology. 2002;59:585–9.
5. Aarsland D, Bronnick K, Williams-Gray C, Weintraub D, Marder K, Kulisevsky J, et al. Mild cognitive impairment in Parkinson disease: a multicenter pooled analysis. Neurology. 2010;75:1062–9.
6. Aarsland D, Andersen K, Larsen JP, Lolk A, Kragh-Sørensen P. Prevalence and characteristics of dementia in Parkinson disease: an 8-year prospective study. Arch Neurol. 2003;60:387–92.
7. Postuma RB, Bertrand JA, Montplaisir J, Desjardins C, Vendette M, Rios Romenets S, et al. Rapid eye movement sleep behavior disorder and risk of dementia in Parkinson's disease: a prospective study. Mov Disord. 2012;27:720–6.
8. Sinforiani E, Pacchetti C, Zangaglia R, Pasotti C, Manni R, Nappi G. REM behavior disorder, hallucinations and cognitive impairment in Parkinson's disease: a two-year follow up. Mov Disord. 2008;23:1441–5.
9. Anang JB, Gagnon JF, Bertrand JA, Romenets SR, Latreille V, Panisset M, et al. Predictors of dementia in Parkinson disease: a prospective cohort study. Neurology. 2014;83:1253–60.
10. Kwon KY, Kang SH, Kim M, Lee HM, Jang JW, Kim JY, et al. Nonmotor symptoms and cognitive decline in de novo Parkinson's disease. Can J Neurol Sci. 2014;41:597–602.
11. de la Riva P, Smith K, Xie SX, Weintraub D. Course of psychiatric symptoms and global cognition in early Parkinson disease. Neurology. 2014;83:1096–103.
12. Chahine LM, Xie SX, Simuni T, Tran B, Postuma R, Amara A, et al. Longitudinal changes in cognition in early Parkinson's disease patients with REM sleep behavior disorder. Parkinsonism Relat Disord. 2016;27:102–6.
13. Huang X, Chen P, Kaufer DI, Tröster AI, Poole C. Apolipoprotein E and dementia in Parkinson disease: a meta-analysis. Arch Neurol. 2006;63:189–93.
14. Morley JF, Xie SX, Hurtig HI, Stern MB, Colcher A, Horn S, et al. Genetic influences on cognitive decline in Parkinson's disease. Mov Disord. 2012;27:512–8.
15. Bibl M, Mollenhauer B, Esselmann H, Lewczuk P, Klafki HW, Sparbier K, et al. CSF amyloid-beta-peptides in Alzheimer's disease, dementia with Lewy bodies and Parkinson's disease dementia. Brain. 2006;129:1177–87.
16. Parnetti L, Farotti L, Eusebi P, Chiasserini D, De Carlo C, Giannandrea D, et al. Differential role of CSF alpha-synuclein species, tau, and Aβ42 in Parkinson's disease. Front Aging Neurosci. 2014;6:53.
17. Nomura T, Inoue Y, Kagimura T, Uemura Y, Nakashima K. Utility of the REM sleep behavior disorder screening questionnaire (RBDSQ) in Parkinson's disease patients. Sleep Med. 2011;12:711–3.
18. Litvan I, Goldman JG, Tröster AI, Schmand BA, Weintraub D, Petersen RC, et al. Diagnostic criteria for mild cognitive impairment in Parkinson's disease: Movement Disorder Society task force guidelines. Mov Disord. 2012;27:349–56.
19. Weintraub D, Simuni T, Caspell-Garcia C, Coffey C, Lasch S, Siderowf A, et al. Cognitive performance and neuropsychiatric symptoms in early, untreated Parkinson's disease. Mov Disord. 2015;30:919–27.
20. Lee JE, Kim KS, Shin HW, Sohn YH. Factors related to clinically probable REM sleep behavior disorder in Parkinson disease. Parkinsonism Relat Disord. 2010;16:105–8.
21. Lenka A, Hegde S, Jhunjhunwala KR, Pal PK. Interactions of visual hallucinations, rapid eye movement sleep behavior disorder and cognitive impairment in Parkinson's disease: a review. Parkinsonism Relat Disord. 2016;22:1–8.
22. Postuma RB, Adler CH, Dugger BN, Hentz JG, Shill HA, Driver-Dunckley E, et al. REM sleep behavior disorder and neuropathology in Parkinson's disease. Mov Disord. 2015;30:1413–7.
23. Bu G. Apolipoprotein E and its receptors in Alzheimer's disease: pathways, pathogenesis and therapy. Nat Rev Neurosci. 2009;10:333–44.
24. Yu JT, Tan L, Hardy J. Apolipoprotein E in Alzheimer's disease: an update. Annu Rev Neurosci. 2014;37:79–100.
25. Kim J, Basak JM, Holtzman DM. The role of apolipoprotein E in Alzheimer's disease. Neuron. 2009;63:287–303.
26. Mengel D, Dams J, Ziemek J, Becker J, Balzer-Geldsetzer M, Hilker R, et al. Apolipoprotein E ε4 does not affect cognitive performance in patients with Parkinson's disease. Parkinsonism Relat Disord. 2016;29:112–6.
27. Yarnall AJ, Breen DP, Duncan GW, Khoo TK, Coleman SY, Firbank MJ, et al. Characterizing mild cognitive impairment in incident Parkinson disease: the ICICLE-PD study. Neurology. 2014;82:308–16.
28. Compta Y, Parkkinen L, O'Sullivan SS, Vandrovcova J, Holton JL, Collins C, et al. Lewy- and Alzheimer-type pathologies in Parkinson's disease dementia: which is more important? Brain. 2011;134:1493–505.
29. Kotzbauer PT, Cairns NJ, Campbell MC, Willis AW, Racette BA, Tabbal SD, et al. Pathologic accumulation of α-synuclein and Aβ in Parkinson disease patients with dementia. Arch Neurol. 2012;69:1326–31.
30. Irwin DJ, Lee VM, Trojanowski JQ. Parkinson's disease dementia: convergence of alpha-synuclein, tau and amyloid-beta pathologies. Nat Rev Neurosci. 2013;14:626–36.
31. Buerger K, Ewers M, Pirttilä T, Zinkowski R, Alafuzoff I, Teipel SJ, et al. CSF phosphorylated tau protein correlates with neocortical neurofibrillary pathology in Alzheimer's disease. Brain. 2006;129:3035–41.
32. Terrelonge M Jr, Marder KS, Weintraub D, Alcalay RN. CSF β-amyloid 1-42 predicts progression to cognitive impairment in newly diagnosed Parkinson disease. J Mol Neurosci. 2016;58:88–92.
33. Siderowf A, Xie SX, Hurtig H, Weintraub D, Duda J, Chen-Plotkin A, et al. CSF amyloid {beta} 1-42 predicts cognitive decline in Parkinson disease. Neurology. 2010;75:1055–61.
34. Compta Y, Pereira JB, Ríos J, Ibarretxe-Bilbao N, Junqué C, Bargalló N, et al. Combined dementia-risk biomarkers in Parkinson's disease: a prospective longitudinal study. Parkinsonism Relat Disord. 2013;19:717–24.
35. Clark CM, Xie S, Chittams J, Ewbank D, Peskind E, Galasko D, et al. Cerebrospinal fluid tau and beta-amyloid: how well do these biomarkers reflect autopsy-confirmed dementia diagnoses? Arch Neurol. 2003;60:1696–702.

36. Compta Y, Valente T, Saura J, Segura B, Iranzo Á, Serradell M, et al. Correlates of cerebrospinal fluid levels of oligomeric- and total-α-synuclein in premotor, motor and dementia stages of Parkinson's disease. J Neurol. 2015;262:294–306.
37. Hu Y, Yu SY, Zuo LJ, Cao CJ, Wang F, Chen ZJ, et al. Parkinson disease with REM sleep behavior disorder: features, α-synuclein, and inflammation. Neurology. 2015;84:888–94.
38. Caspell-Garcia C, Simuni T, Tosun-Turgut D, Wu IW, Zhang Y, Nalls M, et al. Multiple modality biomarker prediction of cognitive impairment in prospectively followed de novo Parkinson disease. PLoS One. 2017;12: e0175674.
39. Zhu K, van Hilten JJ, Marinus J. Predictors of dementia in Parkinson's disease; findings from a 5-year prospective study using the SCOPA-COG. Parkinsonism Relat Disord. 2014;20:980–5.
40. Xu Y, Yang J, Shang H. Meta-analysis of risk factors for Parkinson's disease dementia. Transl Neurodegener. 2016;5:11.
41. Fullard ME, Tran B, Xie SX, Toledo JB, Scordia C, Linder C, et al. Olfactory impairment predicts cognitive decline in early Parkinson's disease. Parkinsonism Relat Disord. 2016;25:45–51.
42. Strozyk D, Blennow K, White LR, Launer LJ. CSF Abeta 42 levels correlate with amyloid-neuropathology in a population-based autopsy study. Neurology. 2003;60:652–6.
43. Fagan AM, Mintun MA, Mach RH, Lee SY, Dence CS, Shah AR, et al. Inverse relation between in vivo amyloid imaging load and cerebrospinal fluid Abeta42 in humans. Ann Neurol. 2006;59:512–9.

22

Quercetin prevents spinal motor neuron degeneration induced by chronic excitotoxic stimulus by a sirtuin 1-dependent mechanism

Rafael Lazo-Gomez and Ricardo Tapia*

Abstract

Background: Excitotoxicity is a mechanism of foremost importance in the selective motor neuron degeneration characteristic of motor neuron disorders. Effective therapeutic strategies are an unmet need for these disorders. Polyphenols, such as quercetin and resveratrol, are plant-derived compounds that activate sirtuins (SIRTs) and have shown promising results in some models of neuronal death, although their effects have been scarcely tested in models of motor neuron degeneration.

Methods: In this work we investigated the effects of quercetin and resveratrol in an in vivo model of excitotoxic motor neuron death induced by the chronic infusion of α-amino-3-hydroxy-5-methyl-4-isoxazolepropionic acid (AMPA) into the rat spinal cord tissue. Quercetin and resveratrol were co-infused with AMPA and motor behavior and muscle strength were assessed daily for up to ten days. Then, animals were fixed and lumbar spinal cord tissue was analyzed by histological and immunocytological procedures.

Results: We found that the chronic infusion of AMPA [1 mM] caused a progressive motor neuron degeneration, accompanied by astrogliosis and microgliosis, and motor deficits and paralysis of the rear limbs. Quercetin infusion ameliorated AMPA-induced paralysis, rescued motor neurons, and prevented both astrogliosis and microgliosis, and these protective effects were prevented by EX527, a very selective SIRT1 inhibitor. In contrast, neither resveratrol nor EX527 alone improved motor behavior deficits or reduced motor neuron degeneration, albeit both reduced gliosis.

Conclusions: These results suggest that quercetin exerts its beneficial effects through a SIRT1-mediated mechanism, and thus SIRT1 plays an important role in excitotoxic neurodegeneration and therefore its pharmacological modulation might provide opportunities for therapy in motor neuron disorders.

Keywords: Motor neuron disorder, Quercetin, Resveratrol, Sirtuin, Excitotoxicity

Background

Motor neuron disorders (MNDs) are a heterogeneous group of neurodegenerative diseases pathologically characterized by the loss of MNs, which notably include amyotrophic lateral sclerosis (ALS) and spinal muscular atrophy (SMA). Chronic MN loss leads to gradually increasing weakness and paralysis, and ultimately to respiratory failure and death. These disorders are uniformly fatal, thus it is a priority to characterize the basic mechanisms that cause MN degeneration as a mean to develop appropriate therapeutic interventions [1].

Glutamatergic excitatory neurotransmission is a fundamental process in the mammalian brain, but an excessive activation of glutamate receptors results in excitotoxic neuronal death [2]. Although several hypotheses have been advanced to explain the selective degeneration of MNs, there is ample evidence of a role of excitotoxicity in MND, especially for ALS, although a causal relationship remains to be established (for in-depth reviews see [3, 4]). For example, increased concentrations of glutamate have

* Correspondence: rtapia@ifc.unam.mx
División de Neurociencias, Instituto de Fisiología Celular, Universidad Nacional Autónoma de México, Circuito exterior s/n, Ciudad Universitaria, Coyoacán, 04510 Ciudad de México, Mexico

been found in cerebrospinal fluid of ALS patients [5], and in synaptosomes obtained from human mutated superoxide dismutase G93A gene (hSOD1^{G93A}) transgenic mice, an animal model of familial ALS, an increased basal release of glutamate has been documented [6, 7].

Our group designed an in vivo experimental model of chronic MN death in healthy rats through the infusion of α-amino-3-hydroxy-5-methyl-4-isoxazolepropionic acid (AMPA) directly in the lumbar spinal cord, using osmotic minipumps. With this model we replicated several important characteristics of MND: its chronic course, its onset in adulthood, and the fact that most of the cases are sporadic [8]. This approach has allowed us to study some of the basic mechanisms underlying excitotoxic MN death [9–11], and also to test potential strategies for neuroprotection, such as growth factors [12, 13] and energy substrates [14, 15].

Polyphenols are plant-derived compounds that have emerged as a promising therapeutic approach for several neurodegenerative disorders [16, 17]. This beneficial effect has been attributed to the allosteric activation of sirtuin 1 (SIRT1), the first member of the class III of oxidized nicotine adenine dinucleotide (NAD^+)-dependent histone deacetylases [18].

Among the vast amount of polyphenolic compounds discovered, resveratrol (RSV) and quercetin (QCT) are two of the most promising molecules. RSV is a well-documented sirtuin activating compound (STAC), and has shown neuroprotective effects in in vitro and in vivo models of excitotoxic neuronal degeneration [19]. QCT has been shown to reduce glutamate-induced hippocampal [20] and retinal [21] neuronal death in vitro, as well as neuronal damage in an in vivo model of focal cerebral ischemia [22]. In addition, it was recently reported to be protective in a model of hypoxia-mediated hippocampal neurodegeneration by modulating SIRT1 expression [23]. However, studies on the effects of these compounds in experimental models of MND are scarce. Therefore, we explored the possible neuroprotective effects of RSV and QCT in our established model of chronic AMPA-induced excitotoxic spinal MN degeneration in vivo, and the involvement of SIRT1 as the mechanism of neuroprotection exerted by these polyphenols.

Methods

Animals

Adult Wistar male rats (280–300 g) were used in all of the experiments and were handled in accordance with the Rules for Research and Health Matters (Mexico), with international standards of research animal welfare (including ARRIVE guidelines), and with approval of the Institutional Committee for the Care and Use of Laboratory Animals (protocol approval number RTI21–14). All animals were housed in a controlled laboratory environment with a 12 h light/dark cycle, and fed with regular animal chow and water ad libitum. All surgical procedures were performed under general anesthesia, and every effort was made to minimize the number of animals used, as well as animal suffering during experimental procedures.

Drugs and osmotic minipump preparation

All drugs were dissolved in vehicle solution that consisted in a mixture of isotonic saline solution and 3% *v*/v dimethylsulfoxide. Osmotic minipumps (Alzet model 2004, volume ~250 µL, flow rate 6 µl/day; Durect, Cupertino, CA, USA) were filled with the indicated solutions, which were vehicle only (control group), AMPA [1 mM], and/or RSV, QCT and EX527, at concentrations calculated in such a way that the osmotic minipump delivered 1 nanomole/day (nm/d) or 10 nm/d, or a mixture of drugs, as indicated in Results.

Our group has previously reported that chronic infusion of AMPA into the rat spinal cord in vivo induces paralysis, MN degeneration and astrogliosis [12, 24]. In these studies a 7.5 mM concentration was used and this caused a relatively rapid (~3 days) paralysis and MN death, which makes testing potential neuroprotective drugs difficult. Therefore, we selected a lower concentration (1 mM) that we had previously shown to produce a more gradual and reproducible paralysis, MN degeneration and spinal cord gliosis, features characteristic of MNDs [12]. The concentrations of the remaining drugs were chosen on the basis of preliminary experiments. (R,S)-AMPA was purchased from Tocris Bioscience (Bristol, United Kingdom), and RSV, QCT and EX527 from Sigma Aldrich (St. Louis, MO, USA).

Surgical procedures for osmotic minipump implantation

Osmotic minipumps were prepared 48 h before surgical implantation, and were incubated at 37.0 ° C in saline solution for flow rate stabilization. The procedure for osmotic minipump implantation was performed essentially as previously described [12], with minor modifications. Briefly, animals were anesthetized with 5.0% isofluorane in a 95% O2/5% CO2 mixture and placed in a spinal unit, and isofluorane concentration was gradually diminished to 1.5–2.0% as the surgery was performed. After shaving and disinfection, a median sagittal incision, ~4 cm long, was made in the back and the underlying fascia and muscle tissue were dissected until appropriate visualization of the L3 vertebral lamina was achieved. The spinous process was removed with a drill, and a ~2 mm diameter hole was drilled in the right lamina until the spinal cord tissue was visualized and the meninges were carefully removed with a metallic hook. A stainless-steel screw (3.7 mm long, 1 mm diameter) was fixed in the left lamina. A fused silica capillary (1 mm long, 50 µm internal diameter, 80 µm external diameter; VitroCom Inc.,

Mountain Lakes, NJ, USA) was carefully advanced down into the spinal cord in a vertical fashion 0.8 to 1 mm; this capillary was attached to a plastic tube (cannula) that was connected, and fixed with cyanoacrylate glue, to the osmotic minipump. During all these procedures great care was taken to avoid unnecessary damage to the spinal cord tissue. Dental cement was poured and let dry on the L3 vertebra, to fix both the screw and the cannula on place. Osmotic minipumps were subcutaneously placed in the back of the animal, at the right side of the vertebral column. Finally, the skin incision was closed with surgical stainless-steel clips, anesthesia was withdrawn, and animals received a single intraperitoneal antibiotic shot and were monitored until recovery (see Additional file 1: Figure S1A for details). In addition to control group, where vehicle was infused into the spinal cord tissue, a group of sham surgeries was performed to assess the potential effect of the cannula's glass capillary insertion into the spinal cord on the proliferation of astroglial and microglial cells. These surgical procedures were identical to those previously described until laminectomy completion, except no cannula and no osmotic minipump were implanted. Animals subjected to these sham surgeries were perfused/fixed, as described below, 10 days after the procedure.

Behavioral assessment

Four to five days prior to surgery, rats were trained to walk during 120 s on an accelerating Rotarod (Columbus Instruments, Columbus, OH, USA), starting from 10 rpm (0.2 rpm/s of acceleration). Time to fall from the instrument was recorded, up to a limit of 120 s. Also, grip strength of both hind limbs was measured by placing the animals on their hind limbs on the metallic mesh of a grip strength meter (TSE Systems, Chesterfield, MO, USA) and gently pulling the tail to induce the animals to escape from the examiner; data was disregarded if the animals, when attempting to escape, used their forelimbs. The maximum force displayed by the instrument in every trial was recorded in ponds, and normalized to values obtained the day before surgery (day 0). In both tests the best time, or the greater force, out of three trials was recorded. Great care was taken to avoid excessive distress of the animals, and appropriate time between trials was given to animals for rest. These behavioral motor tasks were assessed daily for 10 days and, on this cutoff time, animals were sacrificed and fixed/perfused for histology.

Perfusion/fixation and Nissl staining

Behavioral assessment was concluded 10 days after minipump implantation, and rats were perfused and fixed for histological analyses as previously described [12]. Briefly, animals were deeply anesthetized with an intraperitoneal injection of pentobarbital, the rib cage was cut to expose the heart, and a wide cut in the right atria was made. A needle, connected to a peristalsis pump, was inserted into the left ventricle and ~250 ml of ice cold normal saline were perfused, followed by ~250 ml of 4% paraformaldehyde in 0.1 M phosphate buffer. The back was dissected, the acrylic implant removed, and the lumbar spinal cord tissue was obtained by pushing it out of the vertebral canal with cold saline solution in a syringe. Tissue was postfixed for 48 h at 4.0 ° C, then dehydrated in increasingly concentrated sucrose solutions (10, 20 and 30%), and the region where the cannula was inserted was visually identified and used for study. Approximately 100 transverse sections (40 μm thick) were obtained in a cryostat, and the slices that showed the cannula's capillary glass track were used for analyses and, of these, 6–8 were processed for immunocytochemistry (see below), and 15 to 20 slices were stained with cresyl violet (Nissl staining) (for further details see Additional file 1: Figure S1B). The number of morphologically healthy MNs (multipolar neurons with clear cytoplasm, soma diameter > 20 μm and distinguishable nucleus) was counted in the ipsilateral and contralateral ventral horns (for a histological comparison of healthy and degenerating MNs see Additional file 1: Figure S1C). Micrographs were obtained with digital Nikon camera attached to a Nikon Eclipse optic microscope (Melville, NY, USA), with a 10X objective, of the ventral gray matter. All images were minimally manipulated *off-line*, with cropping and brightness/contrast adjusted to ensure better visualization of MNs.

Immunocytochemistry and confocal microscopy

To study the expression pattern of SIRT1 in the spinal cord tissue, double immunocytochemistry was performed on floating tissue sections of intact rats for SIRT1 and microtubule associated protein 2 (MAP2), ionized calcium-binding adapter molecule 1 (Iba1), or glial fibrillary acidic protein (GFAP). To perform glial cell counting in treated animals, double immunocytochemistry was performed for GFAP and Iba1 on floating tissue sections. First, sections were permeabilized with PBS 0.1 M/Triton X-100 0.3% *v*/v solution for 10 min; all subsequent procedures were carried on this solution. Then, tissue sections were blocked with bovine albumin 5% *w*/*v* for 120 min, and later incubated in the same blocking solution with primary antibody at 4.0 °C for 48 h with gentle shaking. Primary antibodies were used at the following dilutions: chicken anti-MAP2, 1:1000; chicken anti-GFAP, 1:1000; rabbit anti-Iba1, 1:500; and mouse anti-SIRT1, 1:50. All primary antibodies were purchased from Abcam (Cambridge, MA, USA). Later, primary antibodies were washed thrice, and antibody binding was revealed with the following secondary antibodies in the indicated dilutions: goat anti-chicken IgY

FITC, 1:200; donkey anti-rabbit IgG Alexa Fluor 647, 1:200; goat anti-mouse IgG FITC, 1:200. All secondary antibodies were purchased from Life Technologies (Waltham, MA, USA). Tissue sections were exposed for 120 min to secondary antibodies in the dark and at room temperature, and then they were washed thrice before mounting in xylene-treated glass slides with simple fluorescent mounting medium (Dako Inc., Carpinteria, CA, USA, for glial cell counting) or with DAPI-containing mounting medium (Vector Laboratories; Burlingame, CA, USA, for SIRT1 location assessment). Fluorescence imaging was performed in a Zeiss LSM 710 (Oberkochen, Germany) confocal microscope. Imaging parameters (laser intensity, gain, digital offset, confocal aperture) were manually adjusted initially on tissues obtained from control group, and later on used on all other preparations. For glial cell counting, stacks were composed of images obtained every 2.5 µm that spanned the complete thickness of the tissue, with a 20X objective, of the ventral gray matter, composed of two channels: green for GFAP/FITC imaging and red for Iba1/AlexaFluor 647 imaging. Maximal intensity projections and merged images were obtained off-line with FIJI program [25].

Glial cell counting analysis off-line

An .lsm format composite image was obtained for each side of each slice of spinal cord tissue. At least 3 slices were analyzed per animal of 5 animals per group. Since we observed that cannula insertion, even in control groups, induced astrogliosis (although no microgliosis), we only used the data obtained from the contralateral side to cannulae insertion for analysis. To perform the automated counting of GFAP(+) and Iba1(+) particles, interpreted as astrocytes and microglial cells respectively, an Image J [26] programming language-based macro was designed. This macro instructed FIJI to open and split.lsm image channels (as described above, green for GFAP(+) particles and red for Iba1(+) particles), and to create and save composite 16-bit depth TIFF format images in separate folders, one for GFAP and one for Iba1. Then these TIFF images were subjected to Z-stacking, smoothing, and automated thresholding with the Max Entropy method. Binary versions of each Z-stack TIFF image were obtained, and automated particle analysis was carried on. For astroglial cells, GFAP(+) particles >10 μm^2 were counted, and for microglial cells, Iba1(+) particles >19.5 μm^2 were counted. This threshold was chosen based on the profile of the whole-particle frequency histograms displayed by the Analyze Particles tool of FIJI. In addition, a researcher, blinded to the results of this study, independently and manually counted a sample of the images, with comparable results obtained to those of the automated counting. Also, this macro obtained the area of tissue photographed, using the GFAP/FITC channel TIFF images previously obtained. These images were Z-stacked, smoothened, and the Moments method of automated thresholding was applied. Then, the whole area of the image was quantified with the Measure tool. The number of particles in an area of ($\mu m^2 \times 10^5$) was used to calculate the mean values and standard deviation for each animal.

Statistical analysis

All statistical analyses were carried out in GraphPad Prism 5.0 (La Jolla, CA, USA). After checking data (time to fall, normalized grip strength, MN counting, GFAP+ particle counting and Iba1+ particle counting) followed a normal distribution with the D'Agostino-Pearson omnibus normality test, parametric versions of hypothesis testing were performed. A two-way ANOVA (in the case of behavioral tasks) followed by Tukey's post hoc test, or a one-way ANOVA (for number of healthy MN, and glial cell counting) followed by Tukey's post hoc test were used. A value of $p < 0.05$ was considered statistically significant.

Results

SIRT1 is expressed in neuronal cells in the spinal cord, but is absent in glial cells

We performed double immunohistofluorescence in the spinal cord tissue slices of intact rats to describe the cellular location of SIRT1 expression. We observed that SIRT1 is widely expressed in the ventral gray matter of the spinal cord, especially in the soma and nuclei (DAPI-labeling) of MAP2-positive cells (neurons), but it was not found in GFAP(+) (astrocytes) and Iba1(+) (microglia) cells. (Fig. 1).

Motor behavior tasks changes induced by AMPA, RSV, QCT or EX527

The results of treatment with 1 mM AMPA for 10 days replicated previously reported data [12]. Treated animals showed a gradual, but incomplete, paralysis of the hindlimbs, beginning in the ipsilateral limb and later involving the contralateral one. This change was different from control group performance from day 1 until day 10 of infusion (Fig. 2a, left panel). Also, it is noteworthy that time to fall abruptly diminishes during the first three days (from 65.0 ± 16.0 s at day 1 until 33.5 ± 5.9 s at day 3), and then reaches a plateau value at ~57 s until day 10. As opposed, in the hindlimb grip strength assessment AMPA treatment did not induce significant strength reductions, although a trend towards lower values was observed (~33% reduction from basal conditions at day 5; Fig. 2a, right panel).

RSV-alone infusion (at 10 nm/d) did not change motor behavior performance, as assessed by rotarod or hindlimb strength changes (data not shown). RSV, either at

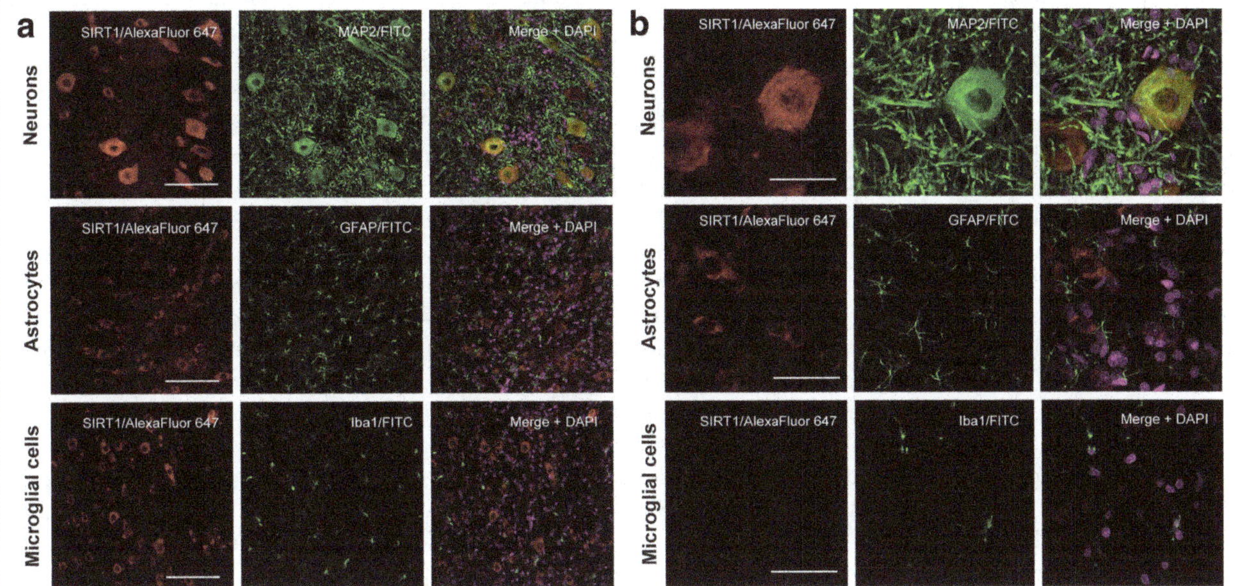

Fig. 1 SIRT1 is expressed in lumbar spinal neuronal somas, including MNs. **a** Representative maximal intensity projections of confocal immunohistofluorescence images of the ventral gray matter of spinal cord sections of intact rats labeled with anti-SIRT1 (red, left and right columns), anti-MAP2 (green, Neurons row), anti-GFAP (green, Astrocytes row) and anti-Iba1 (green, Microglial cells row). Merged images (right column, with DAPI staining in magenta), show that there is co-location of SIRT1 signal only in neuronal somas and nuclei, including MNs (yellow cells). Scale bar, 100 µm. **b** Representative maximal intensity projections of high-magnification confocal immunohistofluorescence images; labeling and color codes are the same as in panel A. In the merged images SIRT1 labeling co-localizes with MAP2 immunostaining (Neurons rows) and is also present in neuronal nuclei. SIRT1 labeling signal was not detected in GFAP (Astrocytes row) or in Iba1 (Microglial cells) immunostained cells. Scale bar, 50 µm. Images were obtained from three spinal cord slices of five animals, all of which yielded similar results

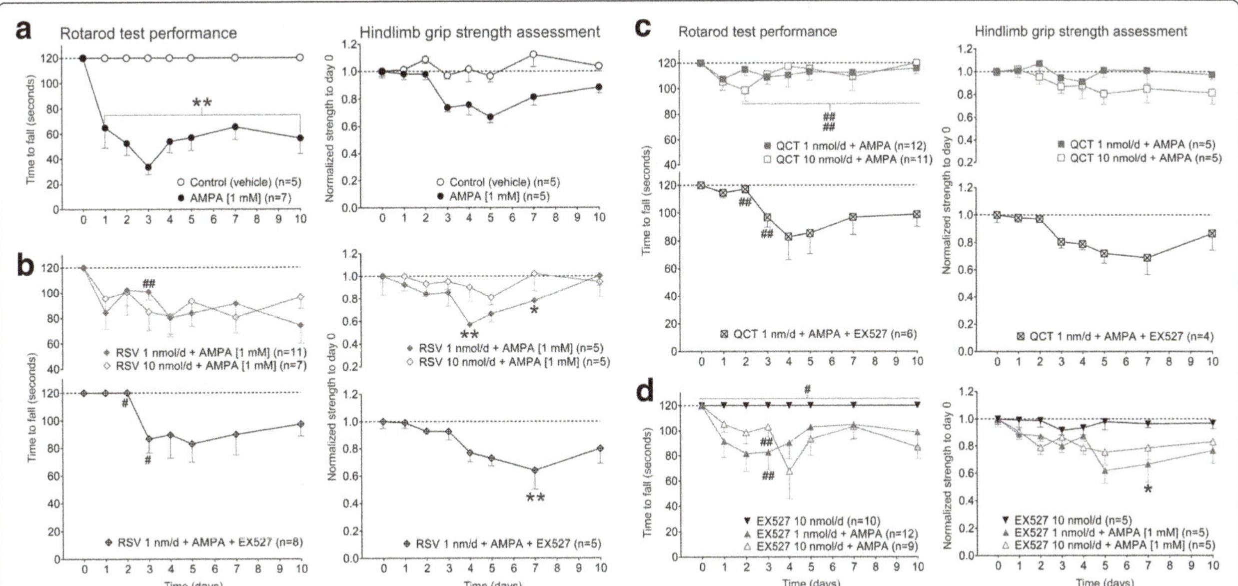

Fig. 2 Effects of RSV, QCT and EX527 on motor behavior tasks during chronic AMPA-induced excitotoxicity. **a** Results of rotarod test and hindlimb grip strength measurement, as indicated, during 10 days of continuous vehicle (control) or AMPA infusions. **b** RSV effects, alone or co-infused with AMPA and EX527, as indicated. **c** QCT effects, alone or co-infused with AMPA or EX527. **d** Effects of EX527 alone or co-infused with AMPA. Number of animals is shown in parentheses. $^{*}p < 0.05$ and $^{**}p < 0.01$ versus control, and $^{\#}p < 0.05$ and $^{\#\#}p < 0.01$ versus AMPA. Two-way ANOVA followed by Tukey's post hoc test

1 nm/d or at 10 nm/d, co-infused with AMPA [1 mM] did not prevent the AMPA-induced decline in rotarod test performance, except for a significant protection ($p < 0.01$) at day 3 with the 1 mM concentration. We further explored the potential contribution of SIRT1 activation by RSV, so we used the very potent and selective inhibitor EX527 [27]. We co-infused RSV at 1 nm/d and AMPA [1 mM] with EX527 at 10 nm/d to ensure SIRT1 remained inhibited while RSV exerted its effects. This co-infusion resulted in a slight and transitory improvement in the time to fall from rotarod as compared to AMPA ($p < 0.05$ only at days 2 and 3), but was not different from the RSV 1 nm/day + AMPA group values (Fig. 2b, left panels). No changes in hindlimb grip strength were observed, although statistical significance was reached as compared to control at days 4 and 7 in the RSV 1 nm/d + AMPA group, and at day 7 in the RSV 1 nm/d + AMPA + EX527 group (Fig. 2b, right panels).

QCT-alone infusion did not induce reductions in time to fall or strength loss throughout the 10 days of infusion (data not shown). We also found that at both doses tested, 1 and 10 nm/d, QCT almost completely prevented the AMPA-induced paralysis, being significantly different from day 2 and throughout the 10 days of infusion ($p < 0.01$ versus AMPA for both concentrations), as assessed by rotarod. SIRT1 role in the QCT-mediated effects was also studied with EX527 at 10 nm/d. EX527 added to the infusion of QCT 1 nm/day + AMPA resulted in a reduced time to fall at days 2 and 3 when compared to AMPA ($p < 0.05$). However, when compared to QCT 1 nm/day + AMPA group values, a clear trend to diminished time to fall is observed from day 4 until day 10, although no signficance was reached (Fig. 2c, left panels). In the hindlimb grip strength assessment (Fig. 2c, right panels), QCT-infusion resulted in no significant differences respect to AMPA or to control values, and a clear trend to reduced strength is noted when EX527 is added to QCT 1 nm/day + AMPA treatment, as well.

EX527-alone treatment did not result in reductions in the time to fall in rotarod test or in the hindlimb strength assessment (Fig. 2d, left panel). EX527 co-infused, at 1 and 10 nm/d, with AMPA did not show an increase in the time to fall from rotarod as compared to AMPA value, although a significant increased value was observed at day 3 ($p < 0.01$). No significant differences were appreciated in the hindlimb grip strength assessment in any group studied, although a clear trend toward reduced strength is observed in both doses when compared to control values ($p < 0.05$ only at day 7) (Fig. 2d, right panels).

Effects of RSV, QCT or EX527 on AMPA-induced MN degeneration

An almost complete absence of MNs in the ipsilateral side to the infusion was observed in Nissl stained sections of the spinal cords of animals treated with AMPA after 10 days of continuous infusion, whereas in the contralateral side only a modest loss was evident (Fig. 3a). When quantified, more than 90% of MNs were lost in the ipsilateral side in the AMPA group (0.4 ± 0.3 versus 14.1 ± 0.6), whereas in the contralateral side remained approximately 60% of MNs as compared to control (8.7 ± 1.0 versus 15.0 ± 0.6, $p < 0.01$; Fig. 3e, left histogram).

RSV-alone infusion did not change ventral spinal cord histology or MN number. RSV did not prevent the neurodegeneration provoked by AMPA after 10 days of infusion (Fig. 3b). MN quantification revealed no changes, both ipsilateral (0.9 ± 0.3 for RSV 1 nm/d and 0.6 ± 0.5 for 10 nm/d) and contralateral (11.8 ± 0.5 for RSV 1 nm/d and 11.5 ± 1.9 for 10 nm/d) to the infusion, when compared to AMPA (Fig. 3e, middle left histogram). Likewise, EX527 treatment in combination with RSV 1 nm/d + AMPA did not change spinal cord histology or MN number when compared to AMPA-alone infusion (0.1 ± 0.0 ipsilateral and 9.3 ± 0.9 contralateral versus 0.4 ± 0.3 ipsilateral and 8.7 ± 1.0 contralateral), although this values were significantly different to control values ($p < 0.05$; Fig. 3e, middle left histogram).

QCT ameliorated histological changes in the spinal cord (Fig. 3c), and prevented excitotoxic MN number diminution, especially in the ipsilateral side to the infusion (0.4 ± 0.3 in AMPA versus 6.4 ± 1.3 for QCT 1 nm/d + AMPA, $p < 0.05$; and 4.8 ± 1.1 for QCT 10 nm/d + AMPA, $p < 0.05$; Fig. 3e, middle right histogram). EX527-added infusion to QCT 1 nm/d + AMPA treatment induced a statistically significant reduction in MN number in the ipsilateral side when compared to QCT 1 nm/d + AMPA (1.3 ± 0.7 versus 6.4 ± 1.3, $p = 0.027$, Fig. 3e, middle right histogram).

EX527-alone at 10 nm/d, even after 10 days of infusion, showed a ventral spinal cord histology (Fig. 3e) and MN number similar to control values (Fig. 3e, right histogram). EX527 co-infused with AMPA resulted in spinal cord histology similar to that of AMPA-treated animals (Fig. 3d), and MN number values not different to the AMPA group values (Fig. 3e, right histogram).

Effects of AMPA, RSV, QCT or EX527 on astrocytes and microglia number

Glial cell counting in the contralateral side revealed that GFAP(+) particle number does not change in control conditions (vehicle infusion for 10 days) as compared to sham (92.3 ± 5.2 versus 101.1 ± 12.9, $p = 0.85$) (Figs. 4 and 5a). However, we observed a more than 2-fold increase in Iba1(+) particle number, which however did not reach significance (48.0 ± 1.4 versus 17.4 ± 2.7, $p = 0.06$) (Figs. 6 and 7a). We expected this change, since glass capillary insertion into the spinal cord tissue might

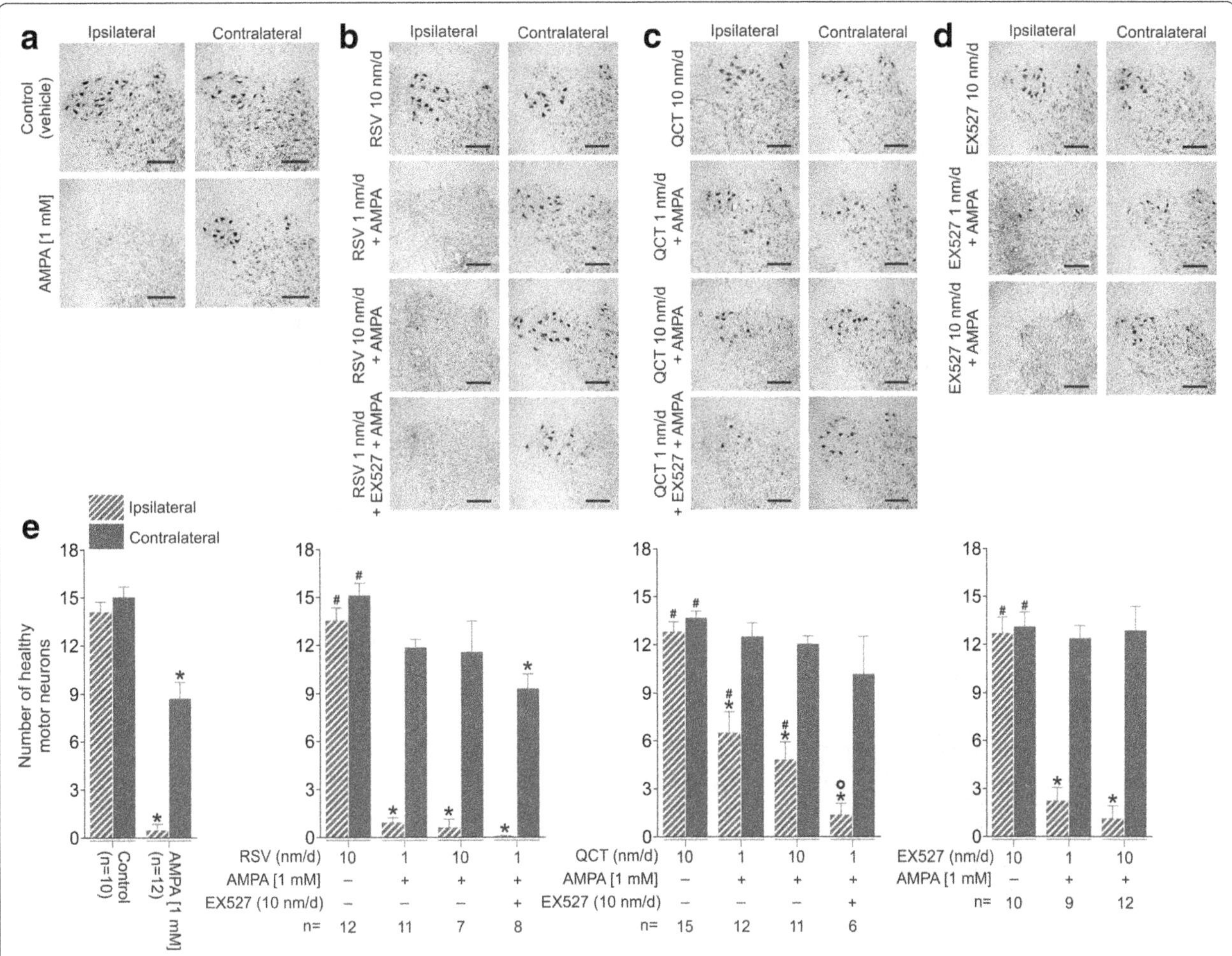

Fig. 3 MN degeneration is prevented by QCT infusion, but not by RSV. Representative photomicrographs of Nissl stained ipsilateral and contralateral lumbar ventral spinal cord of rats after 10 days of continuous infusion of: **a** vehicle or AMPA; **b** RSV alone or co-infused with AMPA and EX527; **c** QCT alone or co-infused with AMPA and EX527; **d** EX527 alone or co-infused with AMPA. Scale bar, 250 μm. **e**. Quantitative analysis of healthy motor neurons. Number of animals is shown in parentheses. *$p < 0.05$ versus control, #$p < 0.05$ versus AMPA, and °$p < 0.05$ versus QCT 1 nm/d + AMPA. One-way ANOVA followed by Tukey's post hoc test

induce cell death and inflammatory signaling, as has previously been described with stiff materials (such as borosilicate glass) implanted in the rodent brain [28]. AMPA treatment, as expected, was associated with a significant ~2-fold increase, as compared to control group values, in GFAP(+) particle (171.7 ± 11.1 versus 101.1 ± 12.9, Figs. 4 and 5a) and Iba1(+) particle (91.9 ± 17.4 versus 48.0 ± 1.4, Figs. 6 and 7a) number.

RSV-alone infusion (at 10 nm/d) did not change GFAP(+) particle (97.5 ± 8.7 versus 101.1 ± 12.9 in control, $p > 0.99$) or Iba1(+) particle numbers. AMPA-induced GFAP(+) particle number increase was prevented by RSV treatment, only at 10 nm/d (171.7 ± 11.1 versus 110.1 ± 8.3, $p = 0.03$; Figs. 4 and 5b), but Iba1(+) particle number was not altered at neither RSV rate of infusion (87.8 ± 14.2 for 1 nm/d and 61.6 ± 18.2 for 10 nm/d versus 91.9 ± 17.4, $p = 0.99$ and 0.593, respectively; Figs. 6 and 7b). In contrast, adding EX527-infusion to RSV 1 nm/d + AMPA treatment prevented GFAP(+) particle number increase ($p < 0.05$ versus AMPA and $p < 0.05$ versus RSV 1 nm/day + AMPA), although no significant changes in Iba1(+) particle number were attained, even when a clear trend towards a reduction was appreciated.

QCT-alone infusion did not cause changes in glial cell number when compared to control values, either in GFAP(+) particles (85.1 ± 4.0 versus 101.1 ± 12.9, $p = 0.97$) or in Iba1(+) particles (57.4 ± 14.4 versus 48.0 ± 1.4, $p = 0.87$). QCT prevented GFAP(+) and Iba1(+) particle number increases induced by AMPA, although only at the 1 nm/d dose (171.7 ± 11.1 versus 109.8 ± 4.5 for GFAP(+) particle number, $p = 0.018$, Figs. 4 and 5c; and 46.3 ± 7.1 versus 91.9 ± 17.4 for Iba1(+) particle number, $p = 0.049$, Figs. 6 and 7c), while the larger dose did not have any effect. Adding EX527-infusion to QCT 1 nm/d + AMPA treatment did not significantly reduce

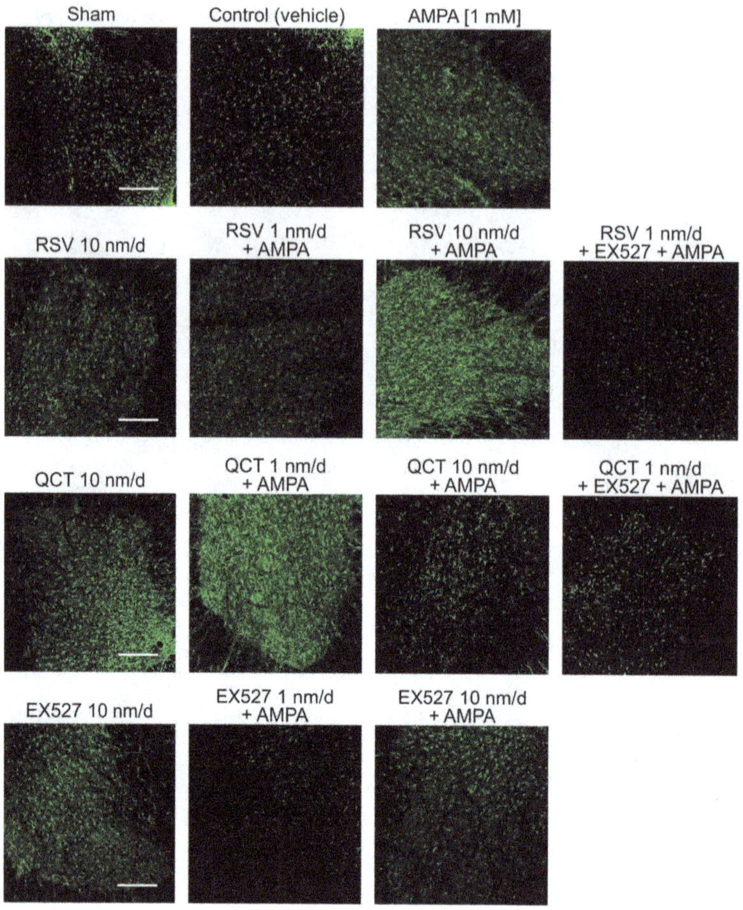

Sham | Control (vehicle) | AMPA [1 mM]

RSV 10 nm/d | RSV 1 nm/d + AMPA | RSV 10 nm/d + AMPA | RSV 1 nm/d + EX527 + AMPA

QCT 10 nm/d | QCT 1 nm/d + AMPA | QCT 10 nm/d + AMPA | QCT 1 nm/d + EX527 + AMPA

EX527 10 nm/d | EX527 1 nm/d + AMPA | EX527 10 nm/d + AMPA

Fig. 4 Effect of RSV, QCT and EX527 on spinal astroglial cell number during chronic AMPA-induced excitotoxicity. Representative maximal intensity projections of fluorescent confocal micrographs of GFAP/FITC-immunostained lumbar ventral spinal cord sections of rats contralateral to the side of infusion after 10 days of the indicated treatments. Quantitative analysis is shown in Fig. 5. Scale bar, 200 μm

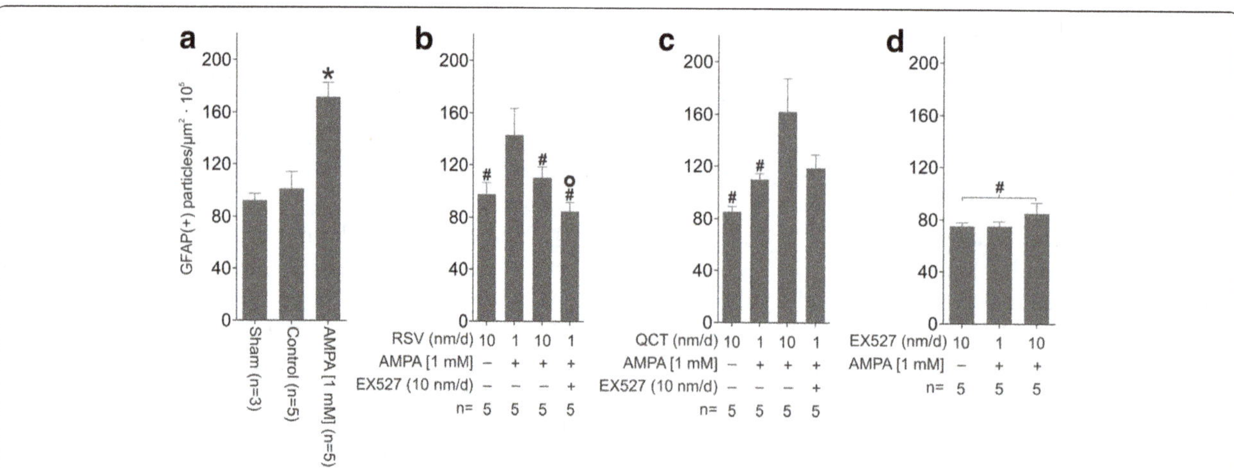

Fig. 5 Quantification of GFAP-labeled particles in the ventral horn contralateral to the infusion site. **a** Sham, and control and AMPA infusions. **b** RSV alone or co-infused with AMPA and EX527. **c** QCT alone or co-infused with AMPA and EX527. **d** EX527 alone or co-infused with AMPA. Number of animals is indicated below each column. $^{*}p < 0.05$ versus control, $^{\#}p < 0.05$ versus AMPA, $^{\circ}p < 0.05$ versus RSV 1 nm/d + AMPA. One-way ANOVA followed by Tukey's post hoc test

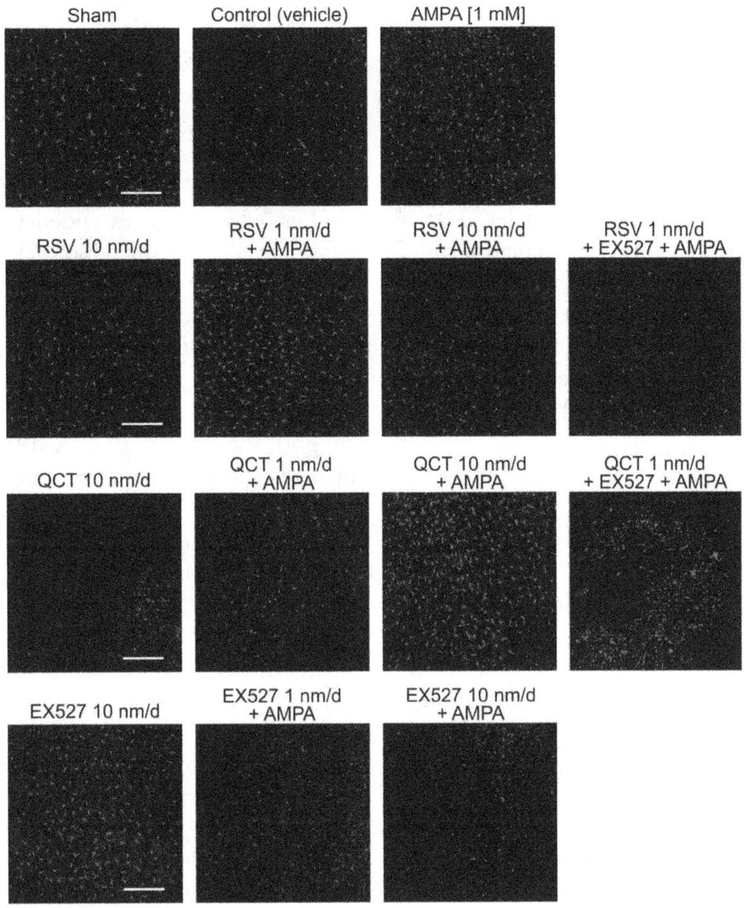

Sham
Control (vehicle)
AMPA [1 mM]
RSV 10 nm/d
RSV 1 nm/d + AMPA
RSV 10 nm/d + AMPA
RSV 1 nm/d + EX527 + AMPA
QCT 10 nm/d
QCT 1 nm/d + AMPA
QCT 10 nm/d + AMPA
QCT 1 nm/d + EX527 + AMPA
EX527 10 nm/d
EX527 1 nm/d + AMPA
EX527 10 nm/d + AMPA

Fig. 6 Effect of RSV, QCT and EX527 on spinal microglial cell number during chronic AMPA-induced excitotoxicity. Representative maximal intensity projections of fluorescent confocal micrographs of Iba1/AlexaFluor 546-immunostained lumbar ventral spinal cord sections of rats contralateral to the side of infusion after 10 days of the indicated treatments. Quantitative analysis is shown in Fig. 7. Scale bar, 200 μm

a
b
c
d
Iba1(+) particles/μm² · 10⁵
ns
p=0.06
ns
p=0.10
Sham (n=3)
Control (n=5)
AMPA [1 mM] (n=5)
RSV (nm/d) 10 1 10 1
AMPA [1 mM] – + + +
EX527 (10 nm/d) – – – +
n= 5 5 5 5
QCT (nm/d) 10 1 10 1
AMPA [1 mM] – + + +
EX527 (10 nm/d) – – – +
n= 5 5 5 5
EX527 (nm/d) 10 1 10
AMPA [1 mM] – + +
n= 5 5 5

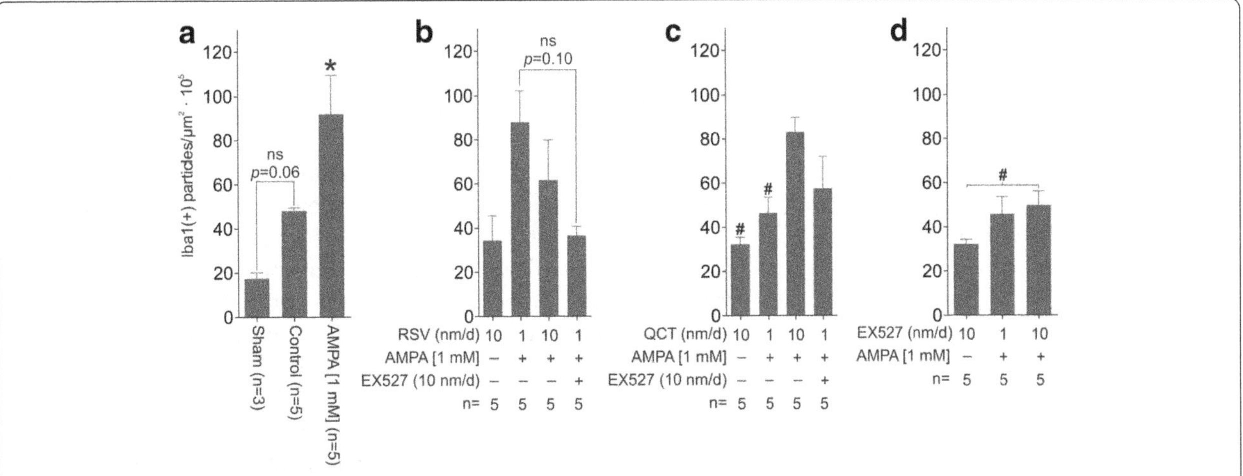

Fig. 7 Quantification of Iba1-labeled particles in the ventral horn contralateral to the infusion site. **a** Sham, and control and AMPA infusions. **b** RSV alone or co-infused with AMPA and EX527. **c** QCT alone or co-infused with AMPA and EX527. **d** EX527 alone or co-infused with AMPA. Number of animals is indicated below each column. $^{*}p < 0.05$ versus control, and $^{\#}p < 0.05$ versus AMPA. One-way ANOVA followed by Tukey's post hoc test

the GFAP(+) particle (118.6 ± 10.1 versus 109.8 ± 4.5 in QCT 1 nm/day + AMPA, $p = 0.99$) or Iba1(+) particle ($p = 0.96$ versus QCT 1 nm/day + AMPA) number, although a clear trend is evident.

EX527-alone treatment resulted in glial number similar to control values (75.0 ± 2.8 versus 101.1 ± 12.9, $p = 0.28$ for GFAP(+) particles, Figs. 4 and 5d; 32.3 ± 2.0 versus 48.0 ± 1.4, $p = 0.66$ for Iba1(+) particles, Figs. 6 and 7d). GFAP(+) and Iba1(+) particle numbers resulted markedly reduced by EX527 treatment in AMPA-induced excitotoxic conditions, without a dose-related effect, reaching values similar to control conditions ($p < 0.01$ versus AMPA for GFAP(+) particle quantification, and $p < 0.05$ versus AMPA for Iba1(+) particle quantification).

Discussion

In this work we investigated the effects of the polyphenols RSV and QCT in our model of excitotoxic MN death and, since polyphenols' efficacy has been attributed to SIRT1 activation [29], we also addressed the involvement of this sirtuin activity to the effects observed.

SIRT1 was located in the nuclei and cytoplasm of neurons, including those of MNs, of the lumbar spinal cord of intact rats. These results are similar to those recently reported in the spinal MNs of transgenic hSOD1^{G93A} mouse [30], whereas data from another group showed that SIRT1 is widely expressed in the brain and spinal cord of healthy humans and rodents, but restricted to the nuclei of neurons [31]. In post-mortem spinal cord tissue of ALS patients SIRT1 mRNA is increased [32], whereas in the hSOD1^{G93A} mouse a study reported increased levels of SIRT in the spinal cord [33], and according to another report this level decreases with disease progression [34]. We did not observe SIRT1 immunolabeling in astrocytes and microglial cells, which differs from the finding that SIRT1 is expressed in cultured mouse astrocytes [35], so this differences might be due to the different species and experimental conditions (in vivo and in vitro). In agreement, an exhaustive study of the expression pattern of sirtuins in the rat nervous tissue found that SIRT1 is present at low concentrations in whole tissue homogenates of the spinal cord, while in vitro is more abundant in neurons than in astrocytes [36].

RSV, classically described as a STAC that preferentially targets SIRT1 [37], did not exert significant protection against AMPA-induced paralysis or MN loss, although it prevented the AMPA-induced increase in the number of astrocytes, while it had no effect on microglial cell number. This was an unexpected result, given the numerous works supporting its potential as a protective agent in models of excitotoxic neuronal death. For example, RSV prevented glutamate-induced neuronal death in brain slices cultures [38], as well as neuronal loss in a model of kainate-induced brain injury in vivo [39]. However, few studies have explored the role of RSV in experimental models of MN loss. RSV was shown to reduce spontaneous degeneration of primary cortical neurons transfected with hSOD1^{G93A} [40], and to upregulate SIRT1 expression in a culture of hSOD1^{G93A}-transfected MN-like cells [41]. This was corroborated in vivo in two studies, where RSV extended the survival of the transgenic hSOD1^{G93A} mice [30, 42], a result attributed to an upregulation of SIRT1 activity and to a prevention in spinal microgliosis and astrogliosis, as well as to an improvement of mitochondrial respiratory function. Although in the present work we did not address mitochondrial function, previous research from our group support the notion that AMPA-induced excitotoxicity involves energy disruption. Indeed, energy substrates administration prevents the alterations of mitochondrial respiratory complexes induced by AMPA in the spinal cord, and this is associated with MN survival and improved motor behavior performance [14, 15]. These findings reinforce the idea that AMPA-mediated chronic excitotoxicity and expression of hSOD1^{G93A} share common mechanisms that prompts MN degeneration.

Regardless of these similarities, RSV was not neuroprotective under our experimental conditions. In this respect, SIRT1 activation by RSV was not confirmed in the studies mentioned previously [30, 40–42], which might imply that RSV effects could be unrelated to SIRT1 expression or activation. In fact, results from recent work suggest that RSV might not be a STAC [43], and that other targets merit consideration, such as AMP-activated protein kinase (AMPK) [44]. Further, it has been suggested that the neuroprotective actions of RSV are not related to SIRT1 activation [45]. We propose that the activation of other molecular pathways by RSV, such as AMPK, might be deleterious for MN survival under AMPA-induced excitotoxic conditions in vivo, as has been shown in the hSOD1^{G93A} transgenic mice [46]. In agreement, it was recently reported that RSV did not protect hippocampal neurons in rat pups treated with kainic acid [47].

QCT exerted a remarkable effect preventing AMPA-induced paralysis, as evidenced by the performance in the rotarod test, as well as a moderate reduction in MN loss. These results were independent of the dose used, and were significant even with the lowest dose of 1 nanomole/day. QCT also diminished the astrogliosis and microgliosis induced by AMPA, but only at the lower dose. Previous studies have demonstrated that QCT is neuroprotective under excitotoxic conditions, albeit these results have been ascribed to the antioxidant capacity of QCT. For example, QCT protected against neuronal death and mitochondrial dysfunction caused by N-methyl-D-aspartate and adenosine diphosphate plus iron in vitro [48]. Also, in a model of cerebral ischemia-reperfusion injury in vivo, QCT diminished infarct volume, improved behavioral deficits and reduced the levels of nitrite and malonyl dialdehyde, both markers of oxidant stress [22]. Whether QCT is a direct scavenger of reactive oxidant species or activates molecular pathways related to oxidant defenses was not addressed in these studies. We consider that the results observed in the present work are independent of QCT antioxidant activity, because we have shown previously that under similar experimental conditions reactive nitrogen species are nearly absent in spinal cord tissue [49] and, more importantly, that classical antioxidant molecules, such as glutathione and ascorbate, do not confer protection against neither acute [15] or chronic [14] excitotoxic damage to spinal cord MNs.

Data on the effects of QCT in the MND setting are very scarce. QCT increased survival of motor neuron 2 gene mRNA in cultured fibroblasts from patients affected by SMA [50], and increased survival of cultured lymphocytes obtained from familial ALS patients caused by the mutated SOD1 [51]. To the best of our knowledge, no studies investigating QCT effects in MND models have been carried out. However, the survival of embryonic spinal MNs from rats was increased by QCT [52].

Interestingly, we found that QCT beneficial effects were partially suppressed by the specific inhibitor of SIRT1, EX527, and that SIRT1 is located in neuronal cells in the spinal cord, specifically in their nucleus and cytoplasm, similarly to previous findings [30]. These results lead us to propose that QCT activates SIRT1, and that this is probably the mechanism of its protective action, rather than its antioxidant activity, as discussed above. In agreement, QCT-mediated survival in cultured neurons in a model of herpes simplex virus 1 infection was ascribed to the increase in SIRT1/AMPK axis activation [53]. In a model of hypobaric-hypoxic brain injury in vivo, QCT prevented cognitive deterioration through SIRT1 upregulation and consequent activation of peroxisome proliferator-activated receptor gamma coactivator 1-alpha (PGC1-α), one of the master regulators of mitochondrial biogenesis [23]. Further, in an in vitro model of dopaminergic neuronal death induced by 6-hydroxydopamine and MitoPark, QCT prevented neuronal death through the activation of the protein kinase D/cAMP response element binding protein/PGC1-α axis, which led to the augmentation of mitochondrial biogenesis and function [54]. These studies suggest that QCT may exert its beneficial effects ultimately improving neuronal energetic state irrespective of its molecular targets.

How does SIRT1 activation protect endangered neurons? Intense research has evidenced that SIRT1 is involved in a vast amount of molecular pathways, most of them intertwined in a complex signaling network that links energetic and metabolic stress to changes in gene expression through epigenetic modifications (histone deacetylation) and modulation of the transcriptional machinery (for a review on the subject see [55]). Which signaling pathway is activated by SIRT1 depends on the experimental model and conditions. Given the relative lack of specificity of the polyphenols, genetic strategies are most suitable to specifically study SIRT1. For example, in a study of double transgenic mice that overexpress SIRT1 in the central nervous system and also harbor the $hSOD1^{G93A}$ mutation, an increased survival was observed, partly due to activation of the heat shock factor 1/inducible heat shock protein 70 chaperone system [56].

Interestingly, the chronic infusion of the SIRT1 inhibitor EX527 alone did not affect motor behavior or induced MN loss. Although SIRT1 expression in the hippocampus seems essential for normal cognitive function and synaptic plasticity in mice [57], no studies have investigated the role of SIRT1 in spinal cord physiology. We hypothesized that EX527 infusion would enhance excitotoxic MN loss and paralysis, since SIRT1 activity would be impaired. Surprisingly, no additional motor behavioral deficits or MN degeneration were observed. Robust experimental evidence in vitro has pointed out that excitotoxicity unequivocally leads to energetic stress, commensurate with reducing amounts of $NAD(P)^+$ [58, 59]. Since NAD^+ is SIRT1's required substrate for its catalytic activity [60], NAD^+ depletion in excitotoxic conditions would result in SIRT1 activity downregulation, which will affect the signaling pathways necessary for survival of the stressed neurons, as has been recently shown [61]. In contrast, SIRT1 activity could also have deleterious effects: consumption of NAD $^+$ in an already energetically compromised neuron may trigger cell death pathways activation, for example through enhanced poly(ADP)ribose polymerase activity [62]. In fact, recent studies have pointed out that SIRT1 inhibition (with nicotinamide) or knock-down may be beneficial for neuronal survival during excitotoxicity [63, 64] or oxidative stress [65]. Therefore, we propose that the lack of enhancement of MN death by EX527 might by due to an increased availability of NAD^+ for other prosurvival pathways, such as energy restoration, as has been suggested in an in vivo model of prion-related neurodegeneration [66].

Besides paralysis and MN loss, we quantitatively confirmed that AMPA infusion induces an increase in astroglial and microglial cells in the spinal cord. This finding was previously reported by our group, but only qualitatively [12]. Numerous studies have already established the crucial role of glial cells in MN degeneration [67]. Our present findings suggest that the abundance of astroglial and microglial cells is not related to neuronal protection, since QCT protection was not accompanied by a reduction in glial cell number. This implies that the molecular pathways modulated by RSV and QCT operate independently on MNs and glial cells, which argues against non-autonomous cell death mechanisms [68].

Conclusions

In summary, chronic AMPA-mediated excitotoxicity in the lumbar spinal cord in vivo induces MN death, manifested as hindlimb paralysis, as well as astrogliosis and microgliosis. The SIRT1 activator QCT prevents excitotoxic MN death, paralysis and gliosis, in part through a SIRT1-dependent mechanism, because the specific inhibitor EX527 partially suppressed QCT-exerted neuroprotective effects. RSV and EX527 had no effect on the AMPA-mediated excitotoxic spinal neurodegeneration. These results contribute to establish polyphenols as promising therapeutic targets in neurodegeneration, and offer insights into their possible mechanisms of action.

Additional file

Additional file 1: Figure S1. Procedure for the chronic infusion of drugs through osmotic minipumps into the L3-L4 segment of the spinal cord and effect of the drugs used. **(A)** Schematic representation of the site of infusion in the rat spinal cord (red dot), viewed from the animal's dorsum; the innervated hindlimb muscles by the respective spinal segments is indicated. **(B)** Representative low-magnification photomicrographs of Nissl stained lumbar spinal cord slices after 10 days of continuous infusion of the indicated treatments. Black arrows indicate the site of the cannula insertion. Note the effects of treatments (nm/d indicates nanomoles/day) on the MNs in the ventral horns, which are shown at higher magnification in Fig. 3. Scale bar, 500 μm. **(C)** Representative high magnification photomicrographs of the healthy MNs of the contralateral side of an AMPA-treated rat (left) and of the degenerating MNs (right, white arrows) of the corresponding infused side (marked by squares in the low magnification micrograph of the AMPA-treated spinal cord). Scale bar, 100 μm. (JPEG 2065 kb)

Abbreviations

ALS: Amyotrophic lateral sclerosis; AMPA: α-Amino-3-hydroxy-5-methyl-4-isoxazolepropionic acid; AMPK: Adenosine mononucleotide phosphate-activated protein kinase; GFAP: Glial fibrillary acidic protein; hSOD1^{G93A}: Human mutated superoxide dismutase, with substituted glycine to alanine in position 93; Iba1: Ionized calcium-binding adapter molecule 1; MAP2: Microtubule associated protein 2; MN: Motor neuron; MNDs: Motor neuron disorders; NAD, NAD(P): Nicotine adenine dinucleotide (phosphate); QCT: Quercetin; RSV: Resveratrol; SIRTs: Sirtuins; SMA: Spinal muscular atrophy; STAC: Sirtuin activating compound

Acknowledgements

Not applicable.

Funding

This work was done under the auspice of Consejo Nacional de Ciencia y Tecnología (CONACyT, protocol approval number 240817) and of Dirección General de Asuntos del Personal Académico (DGAPA), UNAM (protocol approval number IN204516). RLG is recipient of a CONACyT doctoral scholarship.

Authors' contributions

The two authors jointly designed the experiments, analyzed the data and wrote the manuscript. RLG carried out the experiments. RT supervised and approved the general project. All authors read and approved the final manuscript.

Authors' information

RLG is a doctoral student enrolled in Programa de Doctorado en Ciencias Biomédicas at Universidad Nacional Autónoma de México, and this work is part of his doctoral thesis.

Competing interests

The authors declare that they have no competing interests.

References

1. Tiryaki E, Horak HA. ALS and other motor neuron diseases. Contin (Minneap Minn). 2014;20:1185–207.
2. Mehta A, Prabhakar M, Kumar P, Deshmukh R, Sharma PL. Excitotoxicity: bridge to various triggers in neurodegenerative disorders. Eur J Pharmacol. 2013;698:6–18.
3. King AE, Woodhouse A, Kirkcaldie MTK, Vickers JC. Excitotoxicity in ALS: overstimulation, or overreaction? Exp Neurol. 2016;275:162–71.
4. Staats KA, Van den Bosch L. Excitotoxicity and amyotrophic lateral sclerosis. Handb. Neurotox. New York: Springer Science+Business Media; 2014. p. 1209–22.
5. Spreux-Varoquaux O, Bensimon G, Lacomblez L, Salachas F, Pradat PF, Le Forestier N, et al. Glutamate levels in cerebrospinal fluid in amyotrophic lateral sclerosis: a reappraisal using a new HPLC method with coulometric detection in a large cohort of patients. J Neurol Sci. 2002;193:73–8.
6. Milanese M, Zappettini S, Onofri F, Musazzi L, Tardito D, Bonifacino T, et al. Abnormal exocytotic release of glutamate in a mouse model of amyotrophic lateral sclerosis. J Neurochem. 2011;116:1028–42.
7. Bonifacino T, Musazzi L, Milanese M, Seguini M, Marte A, Gallia E, et al. Altered mechanisms underlying the abnormal glutamate release in amyotrophic lateral sclerosis at a pre-symptomatic stage of the disease. Neurobiol Dis. 2016;95:122–33.
8. Tovar-y-Romo LB, Santa-Cruz LD, Tapia R. Experimental models for the study of neurodegeneration in amyotrophic lateral sclerosis. Mol Neurodegener. 2009;4:31.
9. Corona JC, Tapia R. AMPA receptor activation, but not the accumulation of endogenous extracellular glutamate, induces paralysis and motor neuron death in rat spinal cord in vivo. J Neurochem. 2004;89:988–97.
10. Corona JC, Tovar-y-Romo LB, Tapia R. Glutamate excitotoxicity and therapeutic targets for amyotrophic lateral sclerosis. Expert Opin Ther Targets. 2007;11:1415–28.
11. Ramirez-Jarquin UN, Tapia R. Neuropathological characterization of spinal motor neuron degeneration processes induced by acute and chronic excitotoxic stimulus in vivo. Neuroscience. 2016;331:78–90.
12. Tovar-y-Romo LB, Zepeda A, Tapia R. Vascular endothelial growth factor prevents paralysis and motoneuron death in a rat model of excitotoxic spinal cord neurodegeneration. J Neuropathol Exp Neurol. 2007;66:913–22.
13. Tovar-y-Romo LB, Tapia R. Delayed administration of VEGF rescues spinal motor neurons from death with a short effective time frame in excitotoxic experimental models in vivo. ASN Neuro. 2012;4:121–9.
14. Netzahualcoyotzi C, Tapia R. Degeneration of spinal motor neurons by chronic AMPA-induced excitotoxicity in vivo and protection by energy substrates. Acta Neuropathol Commun. 2015;3:27.
15. Santa-Cruz LD, Guerrero-Castillo S, Uribe-Carvajal S, Tapia R. Mitochondrial dysfunction during the early stages of Excitotoxic spinal motor neuron degeneration in vivo. ACS Chem Neurosci. 2016;7:886–96.
16. Ebrahimi A, Schluesener H. Natural polyphenols against neurodegenerative disorders: potentials and pitfalls. Ageing Res Rev. 2012;11:329–45.

17. Del Rio D, Rodriguez-Mateos A, Spencer JP, Tognolini M, Borges G, Crozier A. Dietary (poly)phenolics in human health: structures, bioavailability, and evidence of protective effects against chronic diseases. Antioxid Redox Signal. 2013;18:1818–92.
18. Min SW, Sohn PD, Cho SH, Swanson RA, Gan L. Sirtuins in neurodegenerative diseases: an update on potential mechanisms. Front Aging Neurosci. 2013;5:53.
19. Zhang LN, Hao L, Wang HY, HN S, Sun YJ, Yang XY, et al. Neuroprotective effect of resveratrol against glutamate-induced excitotoxicity. Adv Clin Exp Med. 2015;24:161–5.
20. Yang EJ, Kim GS, Kim JA, Song KS. Protective effects of onion-derived quercetin on glutamate-mediated hippocampal neuronal cell death. Pharmacogn Mag. 2013;9:302–8.
21. Nakayama M, Aihara M, Chen YN, Araie M, Tomita-Yokotani K, Iwashina T. Neuroprotective effects of flavonoids on hypoxia-, glutamate-, and oxidative stress-induced retinal ganglion cell death. Mol Vis. 2011;17:1784–93.
22. Pandey AK, Hazari PP, Patnaik R, Mishra AK. The role of ASIC1a in neuroprotection elicited by quercetin in focal cerebral ischemia. Brain Res. 2011;1383:289–99.
23. Liu P, Zou D, Yi L, Chen M, Gao Y, Zhou R, et al. Quercetin ameliorates hypobaric hypoxia-induced memory impairment through mitochondrial and neuron function adaptation via the PGC-1alpha pathway. Restor Neurol Neurosci. 2015;33:143–57.
24. Lazo-Gomez R, Tapia R. Motor alterations induced by chronic 4-Aminopyridine infusion in the spinal cord in vivo: role of glutamate and GABA receptors. Front Neurosci. 2016;10:200.
25. Schindelin J, Arganda-Carreras I, Frise E, Kaynig V, Longair M, Pietzsch T, et al. Fiji: an open-source platform for biological-image analysis. Nat Methods. 2012;9:676–82.
26. Schneider CA, Rasband WS, Eliceiri KW. NIH image to ImageJ: 25 years of image analysis. Nat Methods. 2012;9:671–5.
27. Gertz M, Fischer F, Nguyen GT, Lakshminarasimhan M, Schutkowski M, Weyand M, et al. Ex-527 inhibits Sirtuins by exploiting their unique NAD+–dependent deacetylation mechanism. Proc Natl Acad Sci U S A. 2013;110:E2772–81.
28. Moshayedi P, Ng G, Kwok JC, Yeo GS, Bryant CE, Fawcett JW, et al. The relationship between glial cell mechanosensitivity and foreign body reactions in the central nervous system. Biomaterials. 2014;35:3919–25.
29. Ayissi VB, Ebrahimi A, Schluesenner H. Epigenetic effects of natural polyphenols: a focus on SIRT1-mediated mechanisms. Mol Nutr Food Res. 2014;58:22–32.
30. Mancuso R, del Valle J, Modol L, Martinez A, Granado-Serrano AB, Ramirez-Nunez O, et al. Resveratrol improves motoneuron function and extends survival in SOD1(G93A) ALS mice. Neurotherapeutics. 2014;11:419–32.
31. Zakhary SM, Ayubcha D, Dileo JN, Jose R, Leheste JR, Horowitz JM, et al. Distribution analysis of deacetylase SIRT1 in rodent and human nervous systems. Anat Rec. 2010;293:1024–32.
32. Korner S, Boselt S, Thau N, Rath KJ, Dengler R, Petri S. Differential sirtuin expression patterns in amyotrophic lateral sclerosis (ALS) postmortem tissue: neuroprotective or neurotoxic properties of sirtuins in ALS? Neurodegener Dis. 2013;11:141–52.
33. Lee JC, Shin JH, Park BW, Kim GS, Kim JC, Kang KS, et al. Region-specific changes in the immunoreactivity of SIRT1 expression in the central nervous system of SOD1(G93A) transgenic mice as an in vivo model of amyotrophic lateral sclerosis. Brain Res. 2012;1433:20–8.
34. Valle C, Salvatori I, Gerbino V, Rossi S, Palamiuc L, Rene F, et al. Tissue-specific deregulation of selected HDACs characterizes ALS progression in mouse models: pharmacological characterization of SIRT1 and SIRT2 pathways. Cell Death Dis. 2014;5:e1296.
35. Cheng Y, Takeuchi H, Sonobe Y, Jin S, Wang Y, Horiuchi H, et al. Sirtuin 1 attenuates oxidative stress via upregulation of superoxide dismutase 2 and catalase in astrocytes. J Neuroimmunol. 2014;269:38–43.
36. Sidorova-Darmos E, Wither RG, Shulyakova N, Fisher C, Ratnam M, Aarts M, et al. Differential expression of sirtuin family members in the developing, adult, and aged rat brain. Front Aging Neurosci. 2014;6:333.
37. Kaeberlein M, McDonagh T, Heltweg B, Hixon J, Westman EA, Caldwell SD, et al. Substrate-specific activation of sirtuins by resveratrol. J Biol Chem. 2005;280:17038–45.
38. Moldzio R, Radad K, Krewenka C, Kranner B, Duvigneau JC, Rausch WD. Protective effects of resveratrol on glutamate-induced damages in murine brain cultures. J Neural Transm. 2013;120:1271–80.
39. Wang Q, Yu S, Simonyi A, Rottinghaus G, Sun GY, Sun AY. Resveratrol protects against neurotoxicity induced by kainic acid. Neurochem Res. 2004;29:2105–12.
40. Kim D, Nguyen MD, Dobbin MM, Fischer A, Sananbenesi F, Rodgers JT, et al. SIRT1 deacetylase protects against neurodegeneration in models for Alzheimer's disease and amyotrophic lateral sclerosis. EMBO J. 2007;26:3169–79.
41. Wang J, Zhang Y, Tang L, Zhang N, Fan D. Protective effects of resveratrol through the up-regulation of SIRT1 expression in the mutant hSOD1-G93A-bearing motor neuron-like cell culture model of amyotrophic lateral sclerosis. Neurosci Lett. 2011;503:250–5.
42. Song L, Chen L, Zhang X, Li J, Le W. Resveratrol ameliorates motor neuron degeneration and improves survival in SOD1(G93A) mouse model of amyotrophic lateral sclerosis. Biomed Res Int. 2014;2014:483501.
43. Beher D, Wu J, Cumine S, Kim KW, SC L, Atangan L, et al. Resveratrol is not a direct activator of SIRT1 enzyme activity. Chem Biol Drug Des. 2009;74:619–24.
44. Dasgupta B, Milbrandt J. Resveratrol stimulates AMP kinase activity in neurons. Proc Natl Acad Sci U S A. 2007;104:7217–22.
45. Tang BL. Resveratrol is neuroprotective because it is not a direct activator of Sirt1-a hypothesis. Brain Res Bull. 2010;81:359–61.
46. Lim MA, Selak MA, Xiang Z, Krainc D, Neve RL, Kraemer BC, et al. Reduced activity of AMP-activated protein kinase protects against genetic models of motor neuron disease. J Neurosci. 2012;32:1123–41.
47. Friedman LK, Goldstein B, Rafiuddin A, Roblejo P, Friedman S. Lack of resveratrol neuroprotection in developing rats treated with kainic acid. Neuroscience. 2013;230:39–49.
48. Silva B, Oliveira PJ, Dias A, Malva JO. Quercetin, kaempferol and biapigenin from Hypericum Perforatum are neuroprotective against excitotoxic insults. Neurotox Res. 2008;13:265–79.
49. Santa-Cruz LD, Tapia R. Role of energy metabolic deficits and oxidative stress in excitotoxic spinal motor neuron degeneration in vivo. ASN Neuro. 2014;6:83–93.
50. Uzunalli G, Bora-Tatar G, Dayangac-Erden D, Erdem-Yurter H. Effects of flavonoid quercetin on survival of motor neuron gene expression. Cell Biol Int. 2015;39:350–4.
51. Said Ahmed M, Hung WY, JS Z, Hockberger P, Siddique T. Increased reactive oxygen species in familial amyotrophic lateral sclerosis with mutations in SOD1. J Neurol Sci. 2000;176:88–94.
52. Ternaux JP, Portalier P. Effect of quercetine on survival and morphological properties of cultured embryonic rat spinal motoneurones. Neurosci Lett. 2002;332:33–6.
53. Leyton L, Hott M, Acuna F, Caroca J, Nunez M, Martin C, et al. Nutraceutical activators of AMPK/Sirt1 axis inhibit viral production and protect neurons from neurodegenerative events triggered during HSV-1 infection. Virus Res. 2015;205:63–72.
54. Ay M, Luo J, Langley M, Jin H, Anantharam V, Kanthasamy A, et al. Molecular mechanisms underlying protective effects of Quercetin against mitochondrial dysfunction and progressive Dopaminergic Neurodegeneration in cell culture and MitoPark transgenic mouse models of Parkinson's disease. J Neurochem. 2017;141:766–82.
55. Ng F, Wijaya L, Tang BL. SIRT1 in the brain-connections with aging-associated disorders and lifespan. Front Cell Neurosci. 2015;9:64.
56. Watanabe S, Ageta-Ishihara N, Nagatsu S, Takao K, Komine O, Endo F, et al. SIRT1 overexpression ameliorates a mouse model of SOD1-linked amyotrophic lateral sclerosis via HSF1/HSP70i chaperone system. Mol Brain. 2014;7:62.
57. Michan S, Li Y, Chou MM, Parrella E, Ge H, Long JM, et al. SIRT1 is essential for normal cognitive function and synaptic plasticity. J Neurosci. 2010;30:9695–707.
58. Schuchmann S, Buchheim K, Meierkord H, Heinemann U. A relative energy failure is associated with low-Mg2+ but not with 4-aminopyridine induced seizure-like events in entorhinal cortex. J Neurophysiol. 1999;81:399–403.
59. Heinemann U, Buchheim K, Gabriel S, Kann O, Kovacs R, Schuchmann S. Cell death and metabolic activity during epileptiform discharges and status epilepticus in the hippocampus. Prog Brain Res. 2002;135:197–210.
60. Feldman JL, Dittenhafer-Reed KE, Denu JM. Sirtuin catalysis and regulation. J Biol Chem. 2012;287:42419–27.
61. Wang S, Yang X, Lin Y, Qiu X, Li H, Zhao X, et al. Cellular NAD depletion and decline of SIRT1 activity play critical roles in PARP-1-mediated acute epileptic neuronal death in vitro. Brain Res. 2013;1535:14–23.
62. Martire S, Mosca L, D'Erme M. PARP-1 involvement in neurodegeneration: a focus on Alzheimer's and Parkinson's diseases. Mech Ageing Dev. 2015;146–148:53–64.
63. Liu D, Gharavi R, Pitta M, Gleichmann M, Mattson MP. Nicotinamide prevents NAD+ depletion and protects neurons against excitotoxicity and cerebral ischemia: NAD+ consumption by SIRT1 may endanger energetically compromised neurons. NeuroMolecular Med. 2009;11:28–42.
64. Liu D, Pitta M, Mattson MP. Preventing NAD(+) depletion protects neurons against excitotoxicity: bioenergetic effects of mild mitochondrial uncoupling and caloric restriction. Ann N Y Acad Sci. 2008;1147:275–82.

65. Li Y, Xu W, McBurney MW, Longo VD. SirT1 inhibition reduces IGF-I/IRS-2/Ras/ERK1/2 signaling and protects neurons. Cell Metab. 2008;8:38–48.
66. Zhou M, Ottenberg G, Sferrazza GF, Hubbs C, Fallahi M, Rumbaugh G, et al. Neuronal death induced by misfolded prion protein is due to NAD+ depletion and can be relieved in vitro and in vivo by NAD+ replenishment. Brain. 2015;138:992–1008.
67. Lasiene J, Yamanaka K. Glial cells in amyotrophic lateral sclerosis. Neurol Res Int. 2011;2011:718987.
68. Ilieva H, Polymenidou M, Cleveland DW. Non-cell autonomous toxicity in neurodegenerative disorders: ALS and beyond. J Cell Biol. 2009;187:761–72.

23

Intranasal rapamycin ameliorates Alzheimer-like cognitive decline in a mouse model of Down syndrome

Antonella Tramutola[1†], Chiara Lanzillotta[1†], Eugenio Barone[1,2], Andrea Arena[1], Ilaria Zuliani[1], Luciana Mosca[1], Carla Blarzino[1], D. Allan Butterfield[3], Marzia Perluigi[1*] and Fabio Di Domenico[1*]

Abstract

Background: Down syndrome (DS) individuals, by the age of 40s, are at increased risk to develop Alzheimer-like dementia, with deposition in brain of senile plaques and neurofibrillary tangles. Our laboratory recently demonstrated the disturbance of PI3K/AKT/mTOR axis in DS brain, prior and after the development of Alzheimer Disease (AD). The aberrant modulation of the mTOR signalling in DS and AD age-related cognitive decline affects crucial neuronal pathways, including insulin signaling and autophagy, involved in pathology onset and progression. Within this context, the therapeutic use of mTOR-inhibitors may prevent/attenuate the neurodegenerative phenomena. By our work we aimed to rescue mTOR signalling in DS mice by a novel rapamycin intranasal administration protocol (InRapa) that maximizes brain delivery and reduce systemic side effects.

Methods: Ts65Dn mice were administered with InRapa for 12 weeks, starting at 6 months of age demonstrating, at the end of the treatment by radial arms maze and novel object recognition testing, rescued cognition.

Results: The analysis of mTOR signalling, after InRapa, demonstrated in Ts65Dn mice hippocampus the inhibition of mTOR (reduced to physiological levels), which led, through the rescue of autophagy and insulin signalling, to reduced APP levels, APP processing and APP metabolites production, as well as, to reduced tau hyperphosphorylation. In addition, a reduction of oxidative stress markers was also observed.

Discussion: These findings demonstrate that chronic InRapa administration is able to exert a neuroprotective effect on Ts65Dn hippocampus by reducing AD pathological hallmarks and by restoring protein homeostasis, thus ultimately resulting in improved cognition. Results are discussed in term of a potential novel targeted therapeutic approach to reduce cognitive decline and AD-like neuropathology in DS individuals.

Keywords: mTOR, Autophagy, Rapamycin, Down syndrome, Alzheimer disease, APP, Tau, Oxidative stress

Background

Down syndrome (DS) is the most common genetic cause of intellectual disability due to total or partial triplication of chromosome 21 (trisomy 21) [1]. The increased risk to develop Alzheimer-like dementia in DS individuals is becoming a key issue to manage the extension of the lifespan of DS population. Indeed, if from one side the improved quality of life and the longer life expectancy are significant achievements of both social and medical care, the overall increase of mean age of DS individuals is associated with an elevated risk to develop age-associated disorders, among which Alzheimer disease (AD) [2]. The neuropathological conditions of DS subjects are complex and involve: deposition of senile plaques and neurofibrillary tangles, dysfunctional mitochondria, defective neurogenesis, increased oxidative stress and altered proteostasis [3]. Approximately two-thirds of individuals with DS develop dementia and brain pathological hallmarks in their 50s, but severity varies significantly among DS population [1]. The triplication of amyloid precursor protein (APP) is considered the major pathological event in both AD and

* Correspondence: marzia.perluigi@uniroma1.it; fabio.didomenico@uniroma1.it
†Antonella Tramutola and Chiara Lanzillotta contributed equally to this work.
[1]Department of Biochemical Sciences, Sapienza University of Rome, P.le Aldo Moro 5, 00185 Rome, Italy
Full list of author information is available at the end of the article

DS with AD, but it is likely that several other triplicated genes contribute to the neurodegenerative process [2, 4–6]. Our previous studies investigated the molecular mechanisms responsible for early onset of AD in DS, focusing attention on the mechanisms that lead to the impairment of protein quality control (PQC) pathways, including the ubiquitin proteasome system (UPS) and autophagy [7, 8]. We showed, in the frontal cortex from DS individuals before and after development of AD neuropathology, that key components of the PQC are irreversibly oxidatively modified resulting in aberrant protein functionality [7, 9]. In agreement, we observed, in young DS subjects, the early accumulation of polyubiquitinylated proteins before the appearance of AD symptoms [10, 11]. These data suggest that impairment of protein degradative system may play a crucial role in the early accumulation of amyloid beta (Aβ) and tau toxic protein aggregates, thus accelerating the neurodegenerative process. Collecting studies suggest that, in AD brain and animal models thereof, the reduced autophagy is strongly associated with the hyperactivation of the PI3K/AKT/mTOR axis, leading to the accumulation of protein aggregates [12, 13]. In the central nervous system (CNS), mTOR and its downstream signalling pathways are involved in synaptic plasticity, memory retention, neuroendocrine regulation, puberty, and neuronal recovery [14–16]. Dysregulation of the mTOR pathway is emerging as a leitmotif in a large number of human diseases, including cancer, metabolic syndromes, and neurological disorders. In the last decade, great attention has been dedicated to the role of mTOR in the development of AD. mTOR hyperactivity is observed in AD brains from human and mouse models, and strong evidence demonstrated that alterations of mTOR may be one of the leading events contributing to the formation of toxic aggregates during AD pathology [17–20]. Recent studies from our laboratory and others employing specimens from DS individuals and DS mouse models confirmed that aberrant mTOR signalling is an early degenerating event in the brain that contributes to acceleration of Aβ and tau deposition and to the development of AD-like cognitive decline [7, 9, 13, 21, 22]. In particular, we investigated the status of the PI3K/AKT/mTOR pathway in the frontal cortex from DS autopsy cases without AD neuropathology (typically under the age of 40 years) and DS with AD neuropathology [13]. Our results showed the hyperactivation of the PI3K/AKT/mTOR axis in the brains of subjects with DS with or without AD pathology in comparison to healthy individuals. These data were associated with decreased autophagosome formation and increased levels of Aβ and p-tau.

These findings represent a strong rationale to test therapeutic strategies aimed to restore the functionality of PQC or prevent its gradual loss. Among drug candidates, mTOR inhibitors led to enormous interest as potential AD-modifying agents [20, 23–28], thus representing an appealing potential approach against neurodegeneration. Evidence showing the positive effects on memory of orally administered rapamycin demonstrated the concomitant reduction, of AD pathological markers, including Aβ and tau levels, in Tg mouse models of AD [16, 19, 27, 29–32]. In the present work, we employed a novel therapeutic strategy using rapamycin, a selective inhibitor of mTOR, delivered by intranasal route in order to avoid peripheral accumulation. Our treatment supports the pathological role of aberrant mTOR/autophagy axis in DS mice and propose/confirm mTOR as a valuable target to prevent/slow the development of AD-related cognitive decline in DS as well as in the general population.

Methods

Mouse colony

Ts65Dn (B6EiC3Sn a/A-Ts(1716)65Dn/J), a well-established mouse model of DS, carries a reciprocal translocation that is trisomic for approximately 104 genes (56%) on Mmu16, from Mrpl39 to the distal telomere, with homologues on HSA21. Mice were generated by repeatedly backcrossing Ts65Dn trisomic females with (B6EiC3SnF1/J) F1 hybrid males. The parental generations were purchased from Jackson Laboratories (Bar Harbour, ME, USA). These breeding pairs produce litters containing both trisomic (Ts65Dn) and euploid (Eu) offsprings. The pups were genotyped to determine trisomy using standard PCR, as described by Reinoldth [33]. In addition, the recessive retinal degeneration 1 mutation (Pdebrd1), which segregates in the colony and results in blindness in homozygotes, was analyzed for all trisomic animals used in the present study by standard PCR. Animals expressing the mutant gene were excluded from the behavioral studies. Mice were housed in clear Plexiglas cages (20 × 22 × 20 cm) under standard laboratory conditions with a temperature of 22 ± 2 °C and 70% humidity, a 12-h light/dark cycle and free access to food and water. Littermates were spliced among age groups to avoid littermates/dam-specific effects. Mice characteristics are reported in Table 1. Mice were sacrificed by cervical dislocation. Trunk blood was collected from the site where the animal was decapitated. Animals were perfused with saline and one brain hemisphere was dissected for immunochemical analysis while the other brain hemisphere was fixed and collected for immunofluorescence staining. All the experiments were performed in strict compliance with the Italian National Laws (DL 116/92), the European Communities Council Directives (86/609/EEC). Experimental protocol was approved by Italian Ministry of Health authorization n° 1183/2016-PR. All efforts were made to minimize the number of animals used in the study and their suffering. All samples were flash-frozen and stored at – 80 °C until utilization.

Table 1 Mouse samples characteristics and experimental use

Treatment	Genotyping	n	Gender (m/f)	Weight (AVG ± SD)	Pde6b	Experimental Use (n)			
						Behavioral Tests	WB	IF	Q-PCR
Vehicle	Eu	10	6/4	31.5 ± 7.2	0	10	8	4	6
	Ts65Dn	10	5/5	25.7 ± 3.2	0	10	8	4	6
InRapa	Eu	10	6/4	31.8 ± 6.8	0	10	8	4	6
	Ts65Dn	10	6/4	28.9 ± 5.6	0	10	8	4	6

InRapa treatment

6-month old Ts65Dn mice and euploid were administered intranasal rapamycin (InRapa; Rapamune, Pfizer, New York, NY, USA) and Vehicle (Veh; saline with 1% DMSO) for 12 weeks. Mice were divided in 4 experimental groups euploid and Ts65Dn treated with vehicle or rapamycin ($n = 10$ per group). The treatment was conducted 3 times per week, with a dose of 0.1 μg/μl of rapamycin solution or vehicle (Fig. 1) in 10 μl (1 μg/mouse). The treatment was well tolerated and no change in body weight or in the consumption of drinking water was observed. The rapamycin dose was chosen from a dose-response pilot study performed before the treatment. In the dose–response treatment the animals were divided in three groups ($n = 6$ per group) and treated with 0.01, 0.05, 0.1 and 0.2 μg/μl of rapamycin. Our data demonstrated that the dose of rapamycin administered during the treatment, 0.1 μg/μl, was able to partially inhibit mTOR (Ser2448) phosphorylation in mice hippocampus and frontal cortex (see Additional file 1). Rapamycin distribution in brain and plasma was investigated before treatment by UPLC-MS analysis. Briefly 6 euploids mice were treated by single intranasal delivery of rapamycin, with the dose of 1 μg/mouse (0.05 mg/Kg/mouse), or by single intraperitoneal injection (i.p.) with the dose of 50 μg/mouse (2.5 mg/kg/mouse). 4 h after the treatment brain and blood were collect for analysis. In particular, for plasma isolation blood was collected in presence of EDTA and then centrifuged at 3000×g for 15 min at 4 °C.

Ultra-performance/pressure liquid chromatography- mass spectrometry (UPLC-MS) analysis

For the quantification of rapamycin in brain and plasma, a UPLC-MS analysis method was utilized. Collected biological specimens were prepared as follows. Brain samples (≈100 mg) were homogenized by 20 strokes of a Wheaton tissue homogenizer using 200 μl of a lysis buffer (30 mM Tris-HCl, 0.1 M NaCl, pH 7.4). Further homogenization was obtained through sonication of the samples for 10 s 3-times in ice. Homogenized brain and isolated plasma (100 μl) samples were then purified using an Ostro™ Pass-through Sample Preparation Plate (Waters) to remove proteins and phospholipids, by following the instructions provided by the manufacturer. The samples were finally dried under vacuum at low temperature. The residue was resuspended in 50 μl of water/acetonitrile (20:80) and 40 μl were injected onto the instrument. Chromatographic separation was performed on a Waters Acquity H-Class UPLC system (Waters, Milford, MA, USA), including a quaternary solvent manager (QSM), a sample manager with flow through needle system (FTN), a photodiode array detector and a single-quadruple mass detector with electrospray ionization source (ACQUITY QDa). The column was a Zorbax Eclipse-Plus C8 (4.6 × 50 mm, 1.8 μm particle size). The mobile phase was composed of a 5 mM ammonium formate aqueous solution (Solvent A) and 0.1% formic acid in methanol (Solvent B). A gradient elution program was performed starting with 30% solvent A and 70% solvent B for 3 min, up to 100% B

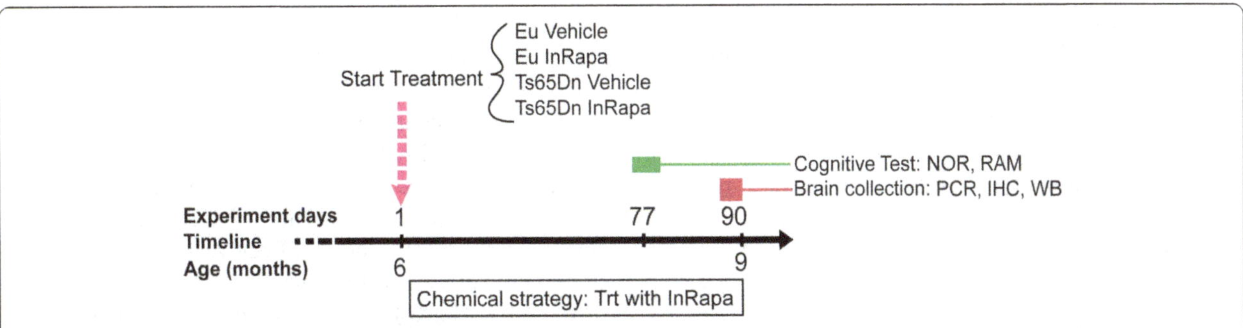

Fig. 1 Schematic of InRapa treatment. 6-month old Ts65Dn mice and euploid (Eu) were administered with intranasal rapamycin (InRapa; Rapamune, Pfizer) 1 μg/mouse and Vehicle (Veh; saline with 1% DMSO) for 90 days total. At day 77 cognitive tests (NOR and RAM) has been initiated while at day 90 mice has been sacrificed to perform PCR, IHC and WB on collected brain samples

in 3 min, followed by 2 min at 100% B. The column was re-equilibrated to 30% A/70% B for 4 min. In these conditions rapamycin has a retention time of 5.4 min. Mass spectrometric detection was set in the positive electrospray ionization mode using nitrogen as nebulizer gas. Analyzes were performed in Total Ion Current (TIC) mode in the mass range 400–1000 m/z. Capillary voltage was 0.8 kV, cone voltage 30 V, ion source temperature 120 °C and probe temperature 600 °C. QDa analysis detected the presence of rapamycin adducts with potassium, sodium and ammonium ions ($[M + K]^+ m/z = 952.45$, $[M + Na]^+ m/z = 936.45$, $[M + NH_4]^+ m/z = 931.45$). The quantification of rapamycin adducts was performed by automatic peak area integration using a dedicated software (Empower3). A calibration curve was plotted using different amounts of rapamycin (0.5 pmoles to 200 pmoles), treated with the same procedure used for the samples. The curves (11 data points in duplicate) were linear with an R^2 value of ≈ 1.00.

Novel object recognition (NOR)

The Novel Object Recognition (NOR) task is used to evaluate cognition, particularly recognition memory, in rodent models of CNS disorders. All experimental groups (Eu Veh, Ts65Dn Veh, Eu InRapa and Ts65Dn InRapa) were involved in the test procedures. This test is based on the spontaneous tendency of rodents to spend more time exploring a novel object than a familiar one. The task procedure consists of three phases: habituation, familiarization, and test phase. In the habituation phase at 1st day, each animal is allowed 10 min to freely exploring the open-field arena (50 cm deep × 30 cm widths × 30 cm height) in the absence of objects. During the familiarization phase on the 2nd day, a single animal is placed in the open-field arena containing two identical objects (two balls), for 10 min. To prevent coercion to explore the objects, rodents are released against the center of the opposite wall with its back to the objects. The experimental context is not drastically different during the familiarization and the test phase. In the test phase after 24 h, the animal is returned to the open-field arena with two objects, one is the familiar object and the other is novel (ball + plastic brick) [34, 35]. The discrimination index and preference index percentage are recorded. Discrimination index (DI), allows discrimination between the novel (TN) and familiar (TF) objects [DI = (TN − TF)/(TN + TF)]. The preference index (PI) is a ratio of the amount of time spent exploring any one of the two objects in training phase (A, B) or the novel one in test phase (C) over the total time spent exploring both objects, i.e., A, B or C/(A, B + C) × 100 (%) in the test phase. Therefore, a preference index above 50% indicates novel object preference, below 50% familiar object preference, and 50% no preference [35].

Radial arms maze (RAM)

The Radial Arms Maze is composed of a central octagonal platform with eight arms extending from it like the spokes of a wheel [36]. All animals were familiarized with the maze for 3 days before training (Eu Veh, Ts65Dn Veh, Eu InRapa and Ts65Dn InRapa; $n = 10$). On these 3 days, they were placed in the maze for 10 min and could eat food rewards that were scattered throughout the maze. In our protocol, the version of the task was an alternated- baited maze procedure, where mice had to learn to visit only all the baited arms. Mice were given daily training sessions (one trial per session) over a 9-day period and day 10th was considered a Test Day. A daily training session started with the animal placed in the central area, once the mouse explored the baited arm and came back into the central area, the trial was ended. For all groups, a trial ended when one of the following conditions was reached: (i) the animal visited all baited arms, or (ii) the trial lasted for more than 10 min. The maze was cleaned with absorbing paper between each animal to minimize the olfactory intra-maze cues. We evaluated the total number of working memory errors (WME), reference memory errors (RME) and latency to finish a trial made by the animals with respect to the training sessions. Distance travelled between groups have been recorded and analyzed showing no significant differences (Additional file 2).

RNA extraction and quantitative real-time RT-PCR

RNA was extracted from the frozen hippocampus in the all groups ($n = 6$/group) using Tissue Total RNA Kit according to manufacturer's instructions (Fisher Molecular biology, Rome, Italy). RNA was quantified using the Biospec Nano spectrophotometer (Shimadzu, Columbia, MD, USA), and RNA was reverse transcribed using the cDNA High Capacity kit (Applied Biosystems, Foster City, CA, USA), including reverse transcriptase, random primers and buffer according to manufacturer's instructions. The cDNA was produced through a series of heating and annealing cycles in the MultiGene OPTIMAX 96-well Thermocycler (LabNet International, Edison, NJ, USA). Real time PCR (Q-PCR) using the following cycling conditions: 35 cycles of denaturation at 95 °C for 20 s; annealing and extension at 60 °C for 20 s, using the SensiFAST™ SYBR® No-ROX Kit (Bioline, London, UK). PCR reactions were carried out in a 20 μl reaction volume in a CFX Connect Real Time PCR machine (Bio-Rad Laboratories, Hercules, CA, USA). Primers used for the evaluation of gene expression are reported in Table 2. Relative mRNA concentrations were calculated from the take-off point of reactions (threshold cycle, Ct) using the comparative quantification method performed by Bio-Rad software and based upon the ΔΔCt method. Ct values for GAPDH expression served as a normalizing signal [37].

Sample preparation for Western blot and immunofluorescence

Brain tissues of Ts65Dn and euploid mice ($n = 8$ per group) after treatment were sagittally divided in right and left hemispheres. The right portion was used for Immunofluorescence studies and the left portion was used for molecular biology studies. For western blot and slot blot, the left-hippocampus were thawed in RIPA buffer (pH 7.4) containing 50 mM Tris-HCl (pH 7.4), 150 mM NaCl, 1% NP-40, 0.25% sodium deoxycholate,1 mM EDTA, 0,1% SDS, 1 mM PMSF, 1 mM NaF and 1 mM Na_3VO_4. Brains were homogenized by 20 strokes of a Wheaton tissue homogenizer. All the samples homogenate was centrifuged at 14,000×g for 10 min to remove cellular debris. The supernatant was extracted to determine the total protein concentration by the BCA method (Pierce, Rockford, IL, USA).

Western blot

For Western blot, 30 μg of proteins were prepared by adding in 2X Laemmli Buffer (Bio-Rad Laboratories, Hercules, CA, USA). The sample was heated at 100 °C for 10 min. Electrophoresis was performed on the samples using a Criterion TGX Stain-Free 4–15% 18-well gel in a Criterion large format electrophoresis cell (Bio-Rad Laboratories, Hercules, CA, USA) in TGS Running Buffer (Bio-Rad Laboratories, Hercules, CA, USA), for 60 min at 100 V. Immediately after electrophoresis, the gel was placed on a Chemi/UV/Stain-Free tray and then placed into a ChemiDoc MP imaging System (Bio-Rad Laboratories, Hercules, CA, USA) and UV-activated based on the appropriate settings with Image Lab Software (Bio-Rad Laboratories, Hercules, CA, USA). For gels that would be later used in blotting, the software-selected activation time was 45 s. Following electrophoresis and gel imaging, the proteins were transferred via the TransBlot Turbo semi-dry blotting apparatus (Bio-Rad Laboratories, Hercules, CA, USA) onto a nitrocellulose membrane. After transfer, the blot was imaged using the ChemiDoc MP imaging system using the Stain-Free Blot settings. This total protein signal was used as the basis for total protein normalization. Membranes were blocked with 3% of bovine serum albumin (SERVA Electrophoresis GmbH, Heidelberg, Germany) and incubated over night at 4 °C with primary antibody. An additional table shows the antibody details (see Additional file 3). All the membranes were incubated for 1 h at room temperature with secondary antibody horseradish peroxidase-conjugated anti-rabbit, anti-mouse or anti-goat IgG (1:5000, Sigma–Aldrich, St Louis, MO, USA). The blot was then imaged via the ChemiDoc MP imaging system using the Chemiluminescence settings. Subsequent determination of relative abundance via total protein normalization was calculated using Image Lab 6.0 software (Bio-Rad Laboratories, Hercules, CA, USA).

Slot blot

For the analysis of total 3-nitrotyrosine (3-NT) and 4-hydroxy-2-nonenal (HNE)-bound protein levels, 10 μl of hippocampus homogenate were incubated with 10 μl of Laemmli buffer containing 0.125 M Tris base pH 6.8, 4% (*v/v*) SDS, and 20% (v/v) glycerol. The resulting samples (250 ng per well) were loaded onto a nitrocellulose membrane with a slot-blot apparatus under vacuum pressure. The membrane was blocked for 2 h with a solution of 3% (*w/v*) bovine serum albumin in PBS containing 0.01% (w/v) sodium azide and 0.2% (v/v) Tween 20 and incubated respectively with primary antibodies anti-HNE (Alpha diagnostic, San Antonio, TX, USA) and anti-3NT (Santa Cruz Biotechnology, Dallas, TX, USA) for 2 h at RT. Membranes were washed and incubated with anti-rabbit or mouse IgG alkaline phosphatase secondary antibodies (Sigma-Aldrich, St Louis, MO, USA) for 1 h at room temperature. The membrane was developed with Sigma fast tablets (5-bromo-4-chloro-3-indolyl phosphate/nitroblue tetrazolium substrate [BCIP/NBT substrate], Sigma-Aldrich, St Louis, MO, USA). Membranes were dried and the image was acquired using ChemiDoc XP image system and analyzed using Image Lab software (Bio-Rad Laboratories, Hercules, CA, USA).

Immunofluorescence

Brains were removed and immersed in 4% paraformaldehyde for 24 h at 4 °C. Fixed brains were cryoprotected in successive 48 h with a solution of 20% sucrose and 0.02% NaN_3 at 4 °C. Brains were frozen on a temperature-controlled freezing stage, coronal sectioned (20 μm) on a sliding cryostat (Leica Biosystems, Wetzlar, Germany), and stored in a solution of PBS containing 0.02% NaN_3 at 4 °C. Brain sections were mounted on glass slide. Once dried, sections were blocked with a solution containing 10% normal goat serum, 0.02% NaN_3, and 0.2% Triton X-100 in TBS. Slides were then incubated overnight at 4 °C with following antibodies: p(Ser 2448)-mTOR (mouse 1:500), p(Ser416)-tau (rabbit 1:500), amyloid-β (B-4) (rabbit 1:500) (Bio-Rad Laboratories, Hercules, CA, USA; Santa Cruz Biotechnology, Dallas, TX, USA). Slides were then washed with TBS and then incubated with Alexa Fluor -488 nm and -594 nm secondary antibodies (Invitrogen Corporation, Carlsbad, CA, USA) at 1:1500 for 2 h at room temperature. Slides were then washed again and incubated with DAPI (1:10.000). One slide per group was stained omitting primary antibodies to establish nonspecific background signal. Cover slips were placed using a drop of Fluorimount (Sigma-Aldrich, St Louis, MO, USA).

All slides were imaged using Zeiss AXio (Carl Zeiss, Oberkochen, Germany). All immunolabeling acquisition intensities, field sizes, and microscopy settings were kept consistent across all images. Images were analyzed using

ImageJ. Image montages for Figures were collated in Illustrator and Photoshop Cs6 (Adobe System, San Josè, CA, USA) software programs and were based upon cells that most closely approximated the group means.

Experimental size and statistical analysis

Behavioural tests (NOR and RAM) were performed using 10 mice per group (Ts65Dn Veh and Rapa; Eu Veh and Rapa). Q-PCR was achieved one time with cDNA from 6 mice per group (Ts65Dn Veh and Rapa; Eu Veh and Rapa). Each immunoblot experiment was performed at least three times using 8 samples per group. Immunohistochemistry analyzes were performed using at least 10 sections per brain of 4 mice per group. Details on sample size are summarized in Table 1). All statistical analyses were performed using a non-parametric one-way ANOVA with post hoc Bonferroni t-test. Further to determine how our data are affected by genotype (DS), treatment (InRapa) and their interaction we accomplished a two-way ANOVA analysis (data are reported in a table as Additional file 4). Data are expressed as mean ± SD per group. All statistical analyzes were performed using Graph Pad Prism 7.0 software (GraphPad, La Jolla, CA, USA).

Results

Intranasal delivery reduces peripheral rapamycin concentration

To test the advantage of intranasal delivery in comparison to intraperitoneal (i.p.) injection, we treated mice once by the intranasal route, with the dose of 1 μg/mouse (0.05 mg/Kg/mouse), and by i.p. 50 μg/mouse (2.5 mg/kg/mouse) as previously reported [20]. To note, InRapa dose is about 50-times lower than i.p injection dose. After 4 h of treatment we sacrificed mice and analyzed brain and plasma, from InRapa and i.p. treated animals, by UPLC-MS, to evaluate rapamycin distribution. Our analysis demonstrates that InRapa treated mice showed a brain concentration of rapamycin of 5.0 ± 1.0 ng/g after 4 h, while the plasma concentration was 6.7 ± 1.3 ng/ml (see Additional file 5). In contrast, animals treated by i.p. injection showed a rapamycin brain concentration of 11.1 ± 1.7 ng/g and a plasma concentration of 890.5 ± 98.1 ng/ml (see Additional file 5). Collectively, our data demonstrate that rapamycin delivered by intranasal route reached a therapeutic brain concentration comparable to that obtained by i.p. injection but with an extremely lower distribution at plasma level. Therefore, these results, coupled with the analysis by WB of mTOR inhibition in liver and heart tissue, which showed no changes between Ts65Dn rapamycin and vehicle treated groups (see Additional file 6), suggest that InRapa delivery might not yield consistent side effects in peripheral organs.

InRapa improves cognitive performances in Ts65Dn mice

To evaluate the effects of InRapa treatment on cognitive performances mice were subjected before the end of the treatment to hippocampal-based tasks, novel object recognition test (NOR) and eight-arms radial arms maze test (RAM), to test spatial learning and working memory, at first, to assess memory status differences between treated (InRapa) and untreated (Veh) animals, we performed the NOR tests. Our data show that Eu animals, both vehicle and rapamycin treated groups, demonstrate a PI above 50%, while Ts65Dn mice treated with vehicle exhibit a PI slightly below 50% as result of hippocampal alterations. Interestingly, InRapa treatment is able to recover PI in Ts65Dn mice (increased about 70%; $p = 0.04$) and present a significant difference with Ts65Dn Veh mice, suggesting a recovery of hippocampal functions after InRapa administration (Fig. 2a). In addition, the impairment of cognition in Ts65Dn Veh is demonstrated by the significant reduction of DI (20%; $p = 0.08$) (Fig. 2b) when compared to Eu Veh, while Ts65Dn InRapa group, demonstrate increased DI in comparison with Ts65Dn Veh group (about 20%, $p = 0.019$). The analysis of data by two-way ANOVA demonstrate that PI values are not affected by genotype or treatment variables, while their interaction account for the 17.90% ($p < 0.024$) of the total variance. As far as DI results, genotype significantly account for the 25.92% (0.0016) of the total variance, while InRapa treatment do not affect data. The interaction between genotype and treatment significantly account for the 21.02% (0.0039) of the total variance.

The effects of InRapa on the working and reference memory was further evaluated by the radial arm maze (RAM) test. In 9 days of trial and in the test-day (day 10) we measured three different parameters (i) the time that all mice spend to reach all the 4 beads (Latency, min) (Fig. 2c, d); (ii) the reference memory errors, entry to an empty arm (Fig. 2e, f); (iii) the working memory errors, repeat entries to arms of the maze already visited (Fig. 2g, h). At day 1 all the mice spent an equal time to reach the beads and they showed no significant differences in latency and reference memory errors. At the day 10 Ts65Dn Veh showed poor acquisition ability, measured as increased in latency (50%, $p = 0.0015$) and as well as in working (80%, $p = 0.042$) and reference (40%, $p = 0.021$) memory compared to Eu Veh group. On the other hand, the number of errors (working and reference memory) and the latency was lowest for Eu Veh, Eu InRapa and Ts65Dn InRapa groups and this effect was persistent during testing and was evident especially at day 10. Indeed, if the attention is focused on day 10 (considered as Test Day), Ts65Dn treated with InRapa showed a decreased latency (45%; $p = 0.07$) as show in Fig. 2d and reference memory errors (40%, $p = 0.013$) (Fig. 2h) compared to Ts65Dn Veh. A

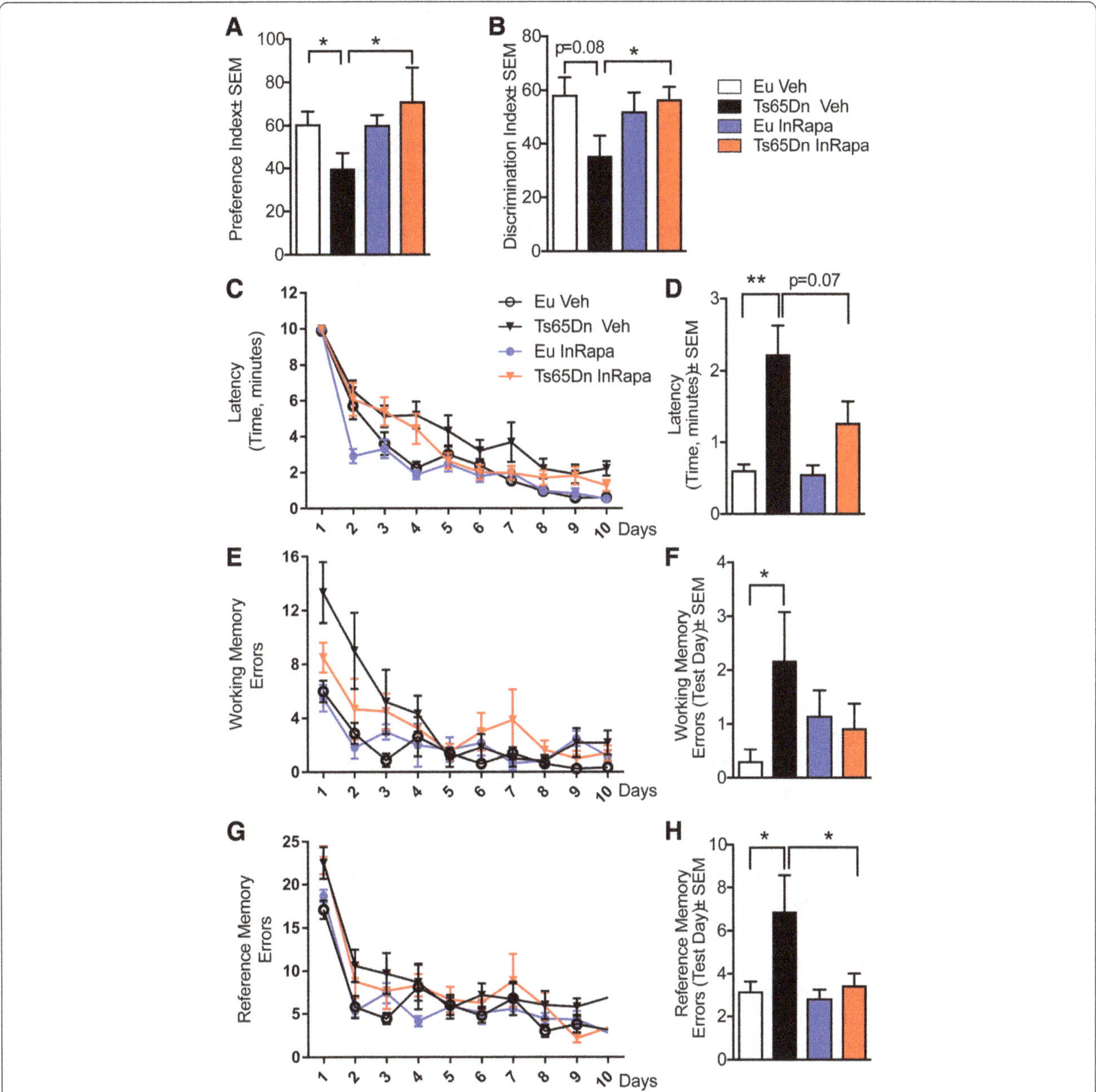

Fig. 2 InRapa improves cognitive performances in TS65Dn mice. Panel **a** and **b** represent data of the novel object recognition test. Values shown in the bar graph are in (**a**) Preference index and in (**b**) Discrimination index (data presented are mean ± SEM $n = 10$/ group). Statistical significance was determined using one–way ANOVA and post hoc Bonferroni t-test (*$p < 0.05$, **$p < 0.01$). Panels from **c** to **h** represent Radial Arm Maze (RAM) results for our treatment groups of treatment. The red and black triangles are data from Ts65Dn mice treated with InRapa and Veh solution. The blue filled circles are data from Eu mice treated with InRapa and the empty circle are data from Eu mice treated with Veh solution. Panel **c** represents the latency of the mice on each trial (one trial per day). Panel **d** represents bar diagram showing latency during the test day (day 10). Panel **e** represents the working memory errors committed by mice on each trial (one trial per day). Panel **f** represents bar diagram showing working memory error during the test day (day 10). Panel **g** represents the reference memory errors committed by mice on each trial (one trial per day). Panel **h** represents bar diagram showing reference memory error during the test day (day 10) values shown in the bar graph are the mean of 10 samples per each group

decreasing trend (not significant) for working memory errors (50%; $p = 0.12$) was evident in Ts65Dn treated with InRapa (Fig. 2f) compared to Ts65Dn Veh. These results showed a partial recovery in cognition for Ts65Dn treated with InRapa. The analysis of RAM results by Two-way ANOVA show that genotype significantly account for the 35.71% ($p = 0.0004$) and the 21.71% (0.0034) of the total variance of latency and reference memory results, respectively, while InRapa treatment significantly account for the 20.91% ($p = 0.0039$) of the total variance of reference memory results. The interaction between genotype and treatment significantly account for the 13.45% (0.0171) of the total variance of reference memory data only.

The results obtained by NOR and RAM tests demonstrate a significant effect of InRapa in Ts65Dn group compared to Veh group, supporting that a targeted rapamycin treatment is able to partially restore memory in Ts65Dn mice.

InRapa decreases mTOR hyperactivation and induces autophagy

We recently showed a pathological mTOR hyper-activation in Ts65Dn mice at 6 months of age compared with euploid controls [22]. Since long-term mTOR activation leads to neuronal dysfunction and cell death, we hypothesized that inhibition of p-mTOR in Ts65Dn mice would ameliorate the detrimental effects of chronic over-activation. Overall, our data show that intranasal delivery of the mTOR inhibitor rapamycin was able to target and modulate mTOR kinase activity in the hippocampus (Fig. 3 A-D) without affecting body weight as reported in Table 1. In particular, the biochemical analysis performed in the four groups of comparison demonstrate at first that Ts65Dn Veh mice compared with Eu Veh mice show an increase of mTOR phosphorylation at Ser2448 (69%; $p = 0.036$) (Fig. 3d). Similarly, p-mTOR (Ser2448) staining in the neuronal layer of CA3 in Ts65Dn mice Veh is significantly increased compared with Eu mice treated with Veh (101%; $p = 0.021$) (Fig. 3a.1–5, B). The administration of InRapa in Ts65Dn mice is able to partially decrease mTOR phosphorylation at Ser2448 in comparison with Ts65Dn Veh mice (82%; $p = 0.014$) rescuing the activity of mTORC1 to physiological levels as demonstrated by the comparison with Eu mice (Fig. 3d). Such results are confirmed by IF analysis that show a decrease of p-mTOR in Ts65Dn mice after InRapa of about 98% ($p = 0.002$) (Fig. 3a.5–7, B). Accordingly, the analysis of dentate gyrus, by IF, demonstrate a trend of increase of mTOR phosphorylation in Ts65Dn mice Veh compared to euploids, which decrease after the treatment. The two-way ANOVA analysis of mTOR phosphorylation data show that genotype accounts for the 12.46% of the total variance ($p = 0.022$), while InRapa treatment significantly accounts for the 20.38% of the total variance, no significant interaction between the two factor is present. Results on the reduced mTOR activation in Ts65Dn treated with rapamycin are confirmed also by real-time PCR. Indeed, Ts65Dn Veh mice compared with Eu Veh mice show a significant increase of mTOR gene expression (30%; $p = 0.024$); in contrast, rapamycin administration is able to decrease the mTOR gene expression in Ts65Dn by 30% ($p = 0.019$) and this reduction is comparable to Eu groups (Fig. 3h). However, alteration in mTOR gene expression do not yield changes in protein levels between groups. Rapamycin is considered a strong and specific inhibitor of mTORC1 activity, mTORC2 was originally considered insensitive to rapamycin administration. However, prolonged treatment with rapamycin also was shown to be able to inhibit mTORC2 [38]. Our analysis of mTORC2 activity, indexed by phosphorylation of mTOR at Ser2481, show no alteration between Eu and Ts65Dn mice either with or without InRapa administration (10.3% $p = 0.8$ and 21.9% $p = 0.23$ respectively), supporting the low sensitivity of mTORC2 to rapamycin treatment (Fig. 3d).

mTORC1 is directly involved in regulating the activity of two components of the protein synthesis machinery, including the ribosomal S6 kinase 1 (S6 K1) and the eukaryotic translation initiation factor 4E-BP1. Active mTORC1 leads to the phosphorylation of p70S6K at Thr389, which in turn can exert its kinase activity on the S6 ribosomal protein, involved in protein translation [8]. Our data show, that hyperphosphorylated mTORC1 lead to the hyperphosphorylation of p70S6K in Ts65Dn mice compared to Eu animals (57%; $p = 0.0002$), while InRapa, despite an increase of protein levels, is able to reduce p70S6K activation to Eu values, suggesting the full restoration of the mTOR pathway (90%; $p = 0.0007$) (Fig. 3e). The two-way ANOVA analysis shows that genotype do not significantly account for the total variance of p-P70S6K, while InRapa treatment significantly accounts for the 53.30% ($p < 0.0001$). The interaction between genotype and treatment accounts for the 21.14% of the total variance ($p < 0.001$).

In parallel, mTORC1 is a negative regulator of autophagy by directly phosphorylating and suppressing the kinase complex Ulk1/Atg13/FIP200 required to promote autophagosome formation [39]. Autophagy plays a crucial role in the removal of toxic/aggregated proteins, such as Aβ and p-tau aggregates, and damaged organelles. The alteration of autophagy is reported in various neurodegenerative and lysosomal storage disorders and has been extensively demonstrated in DS [39–42]. A common molecular marker to evaluate the rate of autophagosome formation is represented by the ratio of the isoform II to isoform I of LC3, a microtubule associated protein, involved in phagophore elongation and closure [43]. Our results support the idea that, mTORC1 hyper-phosphorylation lead to decreased autophagosome formation as observed by reduced LC3 II (33%; $p = 0.04$) and also, its gene expression (about 50%; $p = 0.07$) in Ts65Dn mice (Veh) compared with Eu animals. InRapa treatment in Ts65Dn was able to rescue the LC3 II protein levels, as demonstrated by its increase about 27% ($p = 0.012$) when compared to Ts65Dn Veh mice, therefore retrieving autophagy function to physiological condition (Eu Veh) (Fig. 3F). The two-way ANOVA analysis shows that genotype significantly accounts for the 17.38% ($p < 0.034$) of the total variance of p-P70S6K, while treatment has not significant effect ($p = 0.067$). The interaction between genotype and

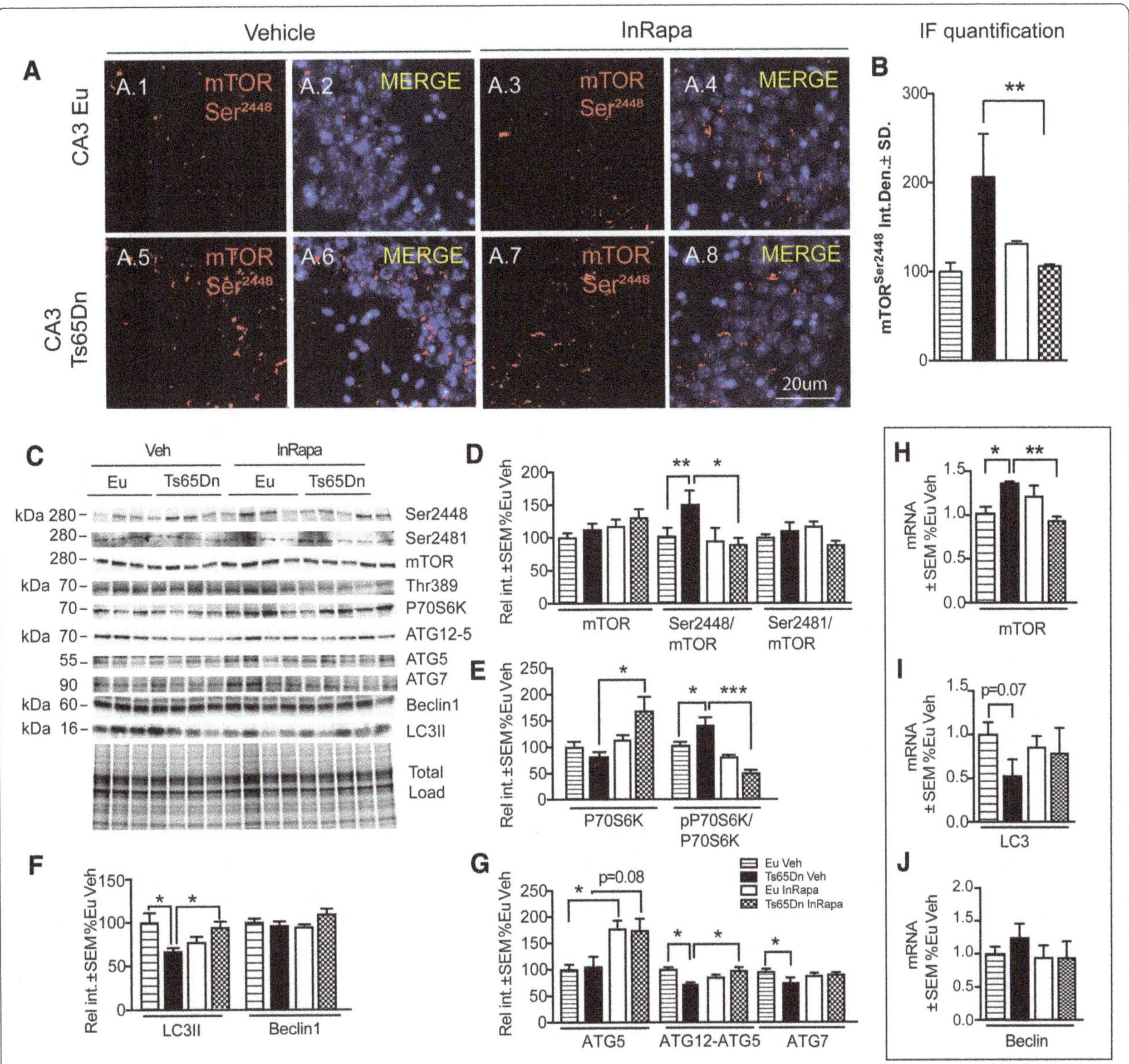

Fig. 3 InRapa recovers mTOR hyperactivation and induce autophagy. (**a** 1–8) Representative immunofluorescent images showing p-mTOR(Ser2448) signal in the CA3 region of the hippocampus from euploid mice treated with Veh and InRapa (A1–4), and Ts65Dn mice treated with Veh and InRapa (A5–8). DAPI (blue) was used to identify cell nuclei. Scale bar represent 20 μm. (**b**) Quantification of fluorescence signal. (**c**) Representative WB showing hippocampal p-mTOR (Ser 2448,2481) and mTOR total protein levels, p-P70S6K and P70S6K total protein levels, Atg5, Atg7, Beclin, LC3II protein levels. (**d**) Quantification of panel C showing mTOR protein levels, p-mTOR (Ser2448)/mTOR ratio and p mTOR (Ser2481)/mTOR ratio. (**e**) Quantification of panel C showing P70S6K and p-P70S6K/ P70S6K ratio. (**f**) Quantification of panel C showing LC3II and Beclin protein levels. (**g**) Quantification of panel C showing Atg5, Atg7 protein levels and quantification of the complex Atg5-Atg12. (**h-j**) Quantification of mRNA levels of mTOR (**h**), LC3 (**i**) and Beclin (**j**) analyzed by RT-PCR analysis. Densitometry values shown in the bar graph are the mean of 8 (WB) and 6 (RT-PCR) samples per each group normalized per total load and are given as percentage of Eu Veh, set as 100%. (*$p < 0.05$, **$p < 0.01$, ***$p < 0.001$)

treatment accounts for the 35.12% ($p < 0.001$) of the total variance.

In addition, this result is supported by an increasing trend (not significant, $p = 0.09$) for LC3 gene expression in Ts65Dn treated with rapamycin (Fig. 3I). So far, the molecular levels of Beclin1, involved in autophagosome induction, and of Atg7, Atg5 and Atg12/Atg 5 complex, involved in autophagosome elongation, are currently employed as further indices of autophagy induction [43]. We show a significant reduction in Ts65Dn Veh mice compared to Eu Veh for both Atg7 levels (26%; $p = 0.043$) and Atg5/Atg12 complex levels (25%; $p = 0.0038$) (Fig. 3G). InRapa treatment in Ts65Dn was able to recover the alteration of these autophagy-related markers to levels observed in euploid animals, despite Atg7 levels. Indeed, we found a 22% ($p = 0.0097$) increase in Ts65Dn mice InRapa compared with Ts65Dn Veh for Atg12/Atg5 complex levels and a 68% ($p = 0.08$) trend of increase in Ts65Dn mice InRapa compared with Ts65Dn Veh for Atg5 protein levels (Fig. 3g). The analysis of Atg12/Atg5 complex data by two-way ANOVA show, as well as for LC3 II, that genotype significantly accounts for the 10.27% ($p < 0.0065$) of the total variance, while treatment has not significant effects ($p = 0.086$). The interaction between genotype and treatment accounts for the 52.76% of the total variance ($p < 0.001$). No alterations of Beclin1 were observed both in gene expression and protein (Fig. 3J). Therefore, intranasal treatment by inhibiting mTOR phosphorylation allowed the recovery of autophagy-related markers alterations to the levels observed in Eu animals.

InRapa reduces aberrant APP levels and APP processing

The DS population demonstrate that the early accumulation of Aβ peptide plays a key toxic role in the brain resulting in AD-like cognitive decline [1, 2, 5, 44, 45]. Aβ is the product of the proteolytic cleavage of APP, which, among the triplicated genes in DS, is considered the most toxic candidate that contributes to the pathogenesis of AD in DS individuals. The overexpression of APP in DS was shown by previous studies in both humans and mouse samples [4–6, 46]. We analyzed the hippocampus of Ts65Dn and Eu mice after InRapa treatment to investigate changes in APP gene expression, APP protein levels and its metabolites, and Aβ peptide levels. At first, we employed the IF technique with the anti-Aβ (B4) antibody, which recognize both Aβ peptides and APP gene product. This analysis shows an increase of fluorescence in Ts65Dn mice compared to Eu mice (Veh groups) in the CA3 region (90%, $p = 0.014$; Fig. 4a.1–5, B) and in the dentate gyrus (53%, $p = 0.08$). While InRapa treatment decreases the levels of about 103% ($p = 0.0017$; Fig. 4a.5–8, B) in the CA3 region and of about 55% ($p = 0.027$, Additional file 7) in the dentate gyrus. In order to evaluate the contribution of APP or Aβ to IF signal changes, we performed a WB analysis using a different array of antibodies (Fig. 4b). The specific analysis of APP shows, as expected, an increase (26%; $p = 0.025$) in Ts65Dn mice compared to euploids but a restoration of the signal (32% reduction; $p = 0.0065$) in the same animals after InRapa treatment (Fig. 4d). The analysis of Aβ oligomers (at 25 and 50 kD) demonstrated an increase in Ts65Dn mice (about 50% and 30% respectively; $p = 0.06$ and $p = 0.048$), which was significantly reduced by InRapa treatment (70% $p = 0.035$ and 40% $p = 0.029$) (Fig. 4f). These data are particularly intriguing since previous studies showed conflicting results about increased Aβ levels in Ts65dn mice at any age [47–49]. In order to investigate whether the decrease of APP protein levels after InRapa treatment were associated with reduced gene expression, we performed RT-PCR analysis demonstrating the same trend observed by IF and WB analysis: a 90% increase ($p = 0.08$) in Ts65Dn mice Veh compared to Eu Veh, while a 102% reduction ($p = 0.031$) in Ts65Dn after InRapa administration (Fig. 4g). The two-way ANOVA analysis of Aβ data show that InRapa treatment account for the 14.67% ($p < 0.0192$) of the total variance of Aβ 25 kD oligomers and for the 15.59% (0.0097) of the total variance of Aβ 50 kD oligomers.

Interactions account for the 15.50% (0.0164) and the 26.53% (0.0011) of the total variance of Aβ oligomers at 25 and 50 kD respectively.

The APP processing can follow two different pathways that produce either non-amyloidogenic or amyloidogenic peptides. The non-amyloidogenic pathway is controlled by α-secretases and lead to the formation of s-APPα and α-CTF, while the amyloidogenic pathways lead to the formation of s-APPβ and β-CTF, which can be furtherly cleaved by γ secretase to form Aβ [50]. The analysis of APP processing products demonstrates, in accordance with APP overexpression, the increased formation of α-CTF (29%; $p = 0.030$) and β–CTF peptides (23%; $p = 0.048$) in Ts65Dn compared to Eu mice treated both with Veh solution. The increased expression of α-CTF and β–CTF, as observed for total APP levels, was recovered significantly by InRapa administration in Ts65Dn mice of about 31% ($p = 0.029$) and 29% ($p = 0.018$), respectively, when compared to Ts65Dn Veh (Fig. 4D). The two-way ANOVA analysis demonstrate that genotype account significantly for the 17.20% ($p < 0.0064$), the 13.74% ($p = 0.0103$) and the 26.95% ($p < 0.0001$) of the total variance of App, App α-CTF and App β-CTF respectively, while InRapa treatment account for the 29.58% ($p = 0.0006$), the 20.98% ($p = 0.0021$) and the 40.05% ($p < 0.0001$) of the total variance of App, App α-CTF and App β-CTF. The interaction between genotype and treatment is significant only for App α-CTF that account for the 14.42% ($p = 0.0088$) of the total variance.

In addition, the levels of β-secretase (BACE1), the rate-limiting enzyme in β–CTF and Aβ generation, were reduced after rapamycin treatment, in both Ts65Dn and Eu animals, suggesting that its expression is susceptible to rapamycin administration in a strain-independent manner (Fig. 4E). The two-way ANOVA analysis demonstrated indeed that InRapa treatment account for the 49.83% ($p < 0.0001$) of the total variance.

InRapa modulates tau hyper-phosphorylation and the expression of tau kinases

To further investigate the efficacy of InRapa treatment to reduce AD-related pathological features in DS animals, we examined tau hyper-phosphorylation and the activation of the main kinases involved in its aberrant

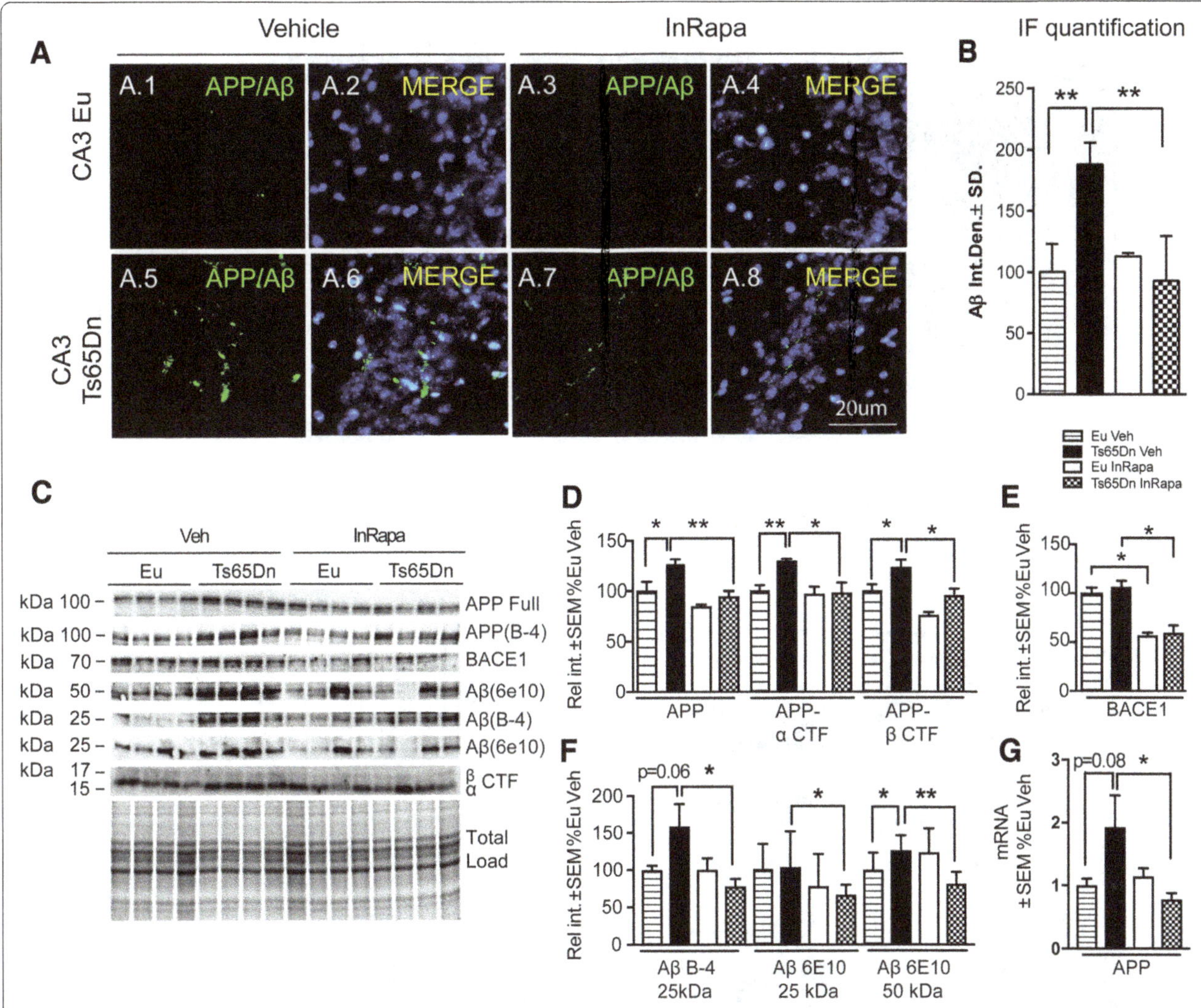

Fig. 4 InRapa reduces APP expression levels, APP metabolites and APP processing. (**a** 1–8) Representative immunofluorescent images showing APP/Aβ (B-4) signal in the CA3 region of the hippocampus from euploid mice treated with Veh and InRapa (**a**.1–4), and Ts65Dn mice treated with Veh and InRapa (A.5–8). DAPI (blue) was used to identify cell nuclei. Scale bar represent 20 μm. (**b**) Quantification of fluorescence signal. (**c**) Representative WB showing total hippocampal levels of APP (full and B-4), BACE1, Aβ oligomers (25 and 50 kDa) and β and α CTF. (**d**) Quantification of panel C showing APP, β and α CTF and BACE1 levels. (**e**) Quantification of panel C showing BACE1 levels. (**f**) Quantification of panel C showing Aβ oligomers (25 and 50 kDa) levels. (**g**) Quantification of mRNA levels of APP analyzed by RT-PCR analysis. Densitometry values shown in the bar graph are the mean of 8 (WB) and 6 (RT-PCR) samples per each group, normalized per total load and given as percentage of Eu Veh, set as 100%

phosphorylation. The Ts65Dn mice show increased phosphorylation of tau on Ser416 (70%; $p = 0.027$) compared with Eu (Fig. 5d). InRapa treatment on Ts65Dn mice, despite showing a slight increase of levels of tau proteins, demonstrate a robust decrease of tau phosphorylation, in Ser416, when compared to the same mouse strain treated with Veh (80%; $p = 0.011$) (Fig. 5d). Similarly, p-tau (Ser416) staining in the neuronal layer of CA3 (Fig. 5a.1–5, B) and dentate gyrus (Additional file 7) are increased in Ts65Dn Veh mice compared with Eu Veh (45%, $p = 0.033$ and 106%, $p = 0.002$). InRapa administration in Ts65Dn mice demonstrates the reduction of tau hyper-phosphorylation in Ts65Dn mice both CA3 (90%, $p = 0.015$; Fig. 5a.5–8, B) and dentate gyrus (95%, $p = 0.004$; Additional file 7) regions. The two-way ANOVA analysis of p-tau demonstrated that InRapa treatment, only account for the 16.64% ($p = 0.0184$) of the total variance. Several proteins are involved in tau phosphorylation, such as GSK3β and DYRK1A, that function as direct kinases of tau, or RCAN1 that operate through the inhibition of calcineurin [51–55]. Akt is known to directly regulate GSK3β by phosphorylation of its inhibitory serine residue (Ser9). GSK3β kinase activity on tau phosphorylation, relies on protein levels and on the balance between the phosphorylation of its activatory (Tyr216) and inhibitory (Ser9) residues. GSK3β expression levels were higher in Ts65Dn cases compared to the appropriate Eu treated with Veh (20%; $p = 0.017$). With

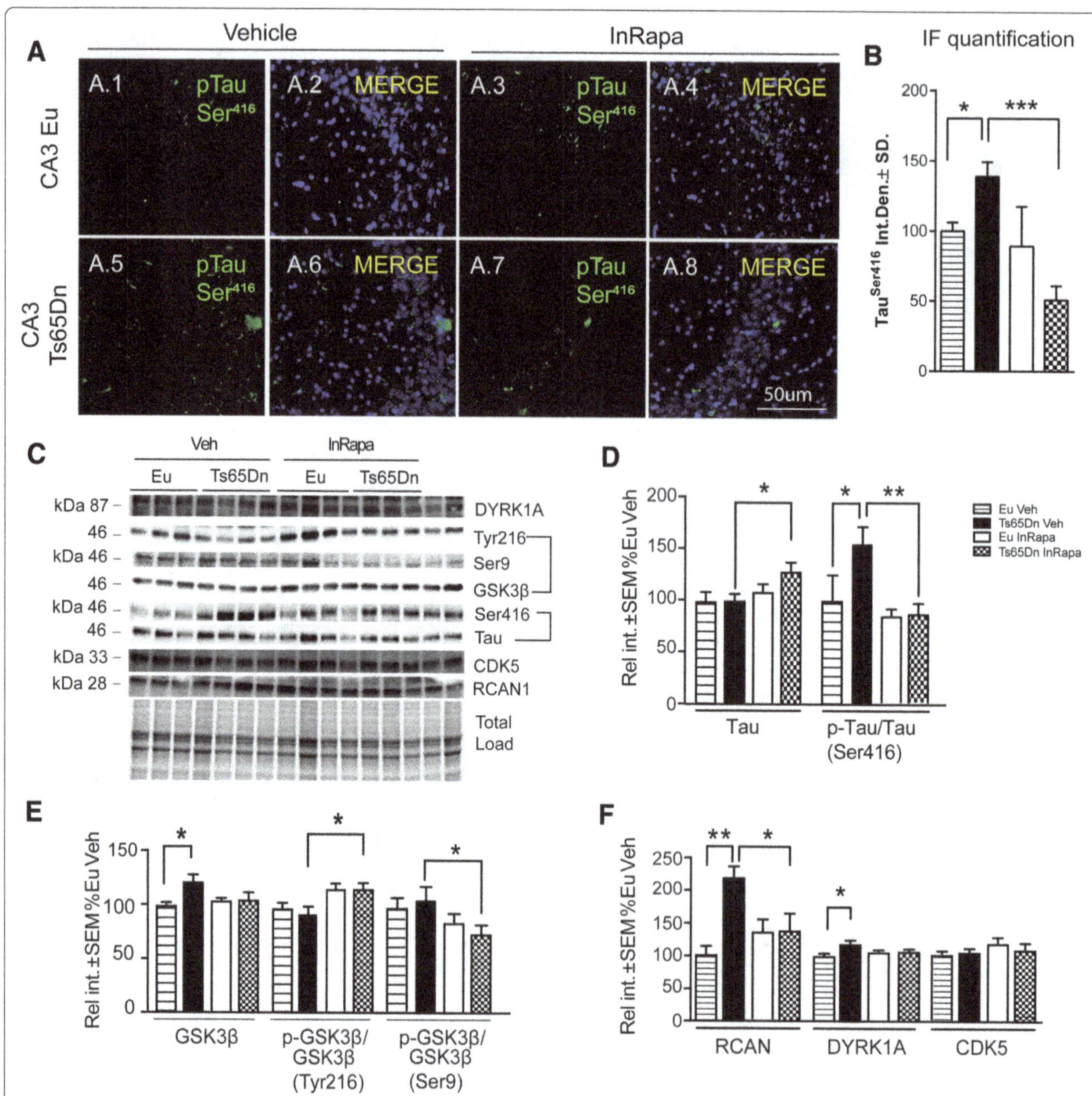

Fig. 5 InRapa decreases tau hyper-phosphorylation and expressions of tau kinases. (**a** 1–8) Representative immunofluorescent images showing tau phosphorylation at Ser416 signal in the CA3 region of the hippocampus from euploid mice treated with Veh and InRapa (**a**.1–4), and Ts65Dn mice treated with Veh and InRapa (**a**.5–8). DAPI (blue) was used to identify cell nuclei. Scale bar represent 50 μm. (**b**) Quantification of fluorescence signal (**c**) Representative WB showing hippocampal p-tau (Ser416), total tau levels, GSK3β levels and phosphorylation (Tyr216 and Ser9), DYRK1A, CDK5 and RCAN1 protein levels. (**d**) Quantification of panel C showing levels of tau and p-tau (Ser416)/tau ratio in Eu and Ts65Dn mice treated with InRapa and Veh. (**e**) Quantification of panel C showing GSK3β, p-GSK3β (Ser9)/GSK3β ratio and p-GSK3β (Tyr216)/GSK3β ratio (**f**) Quantification of panel C showing levels of RCAN1, DYRK1A and CDK5 total protein levels. Densitometry values shown in the bar graph are the mean of 8 (WB) samples per each group normalized per total load, and given as percentage of Eu Veh, set as 100%

regard to GSK3β phosphorylation, we show slight but not significant increase of Ser9 and decrease of, while InRapa administration was able to improve GSK3β kinase activity by increasing Tyr216 and decreasing Ser9 phosphorylation (20% $p = 0.038$ and 25% $p = 0.031$) (Fig. 5e). The two-way ANOVA analysis of GSK3β phosphorylation levels show that InRapa treatment account for the 16.33% (p = 0.03) and the 27.60% (0.041) of the total variance of Ser9 and Tyr216 respectively.

As previously noted, tau phosphorylation could be induced directly or indirectly by DYRK1A and RCAN1, which are both encoded on chromosome 21. DYRK1A is expressed in fetal and adult brain and target tau at different serine residues, leading to its aberrant phosphorylation. Tau hyper-phosphorylation occurring in the brain from both Ts65Dn mice and DS subjects correlates with DYRK1A hyperactivation [56]. Our data confirm the over expression of DYRK1A in Ts65Dn mice (19%; $p = 0.035$) due to Chr16 triplication, however this condition was not restored by InRapa administration, (Fig. 5f). DYRK1A data are affected by genotype, which account for the 13.62% of the total variance. Moreover, RCAN1 (regulator of calcineurin 1) is able to control tau dephosphorylation through the regulation of calcineurin. Increased RCAN1 levels result in decreased calcineurin activity and tau hyperphosphorylation. Our data report, as expected, the overexpression of RCAN1 in Ts65Dn Veh compared with Eu Veh (118%; p = 0.004), while InRapa treatment was able to reduce RCAN1 expression levels of Ts65Dn about 79% (% p = 0.03) when compared to Ts65Dn Veh (Fig. 5F). The two-way ANOVA analysis of RCAN1 levels show that genotype treatment account for the 21.52% ($p = 0.0033$) of the total variance. In addition, CDK5 promotes p-tau accumulation in DS [57]. Increased levels of CDK5 was previously reported in the brains of young Ts65Dn [58], however our data show no significant alterations of CDK5 in Ts65Dn mice compared with Eu in both InRapa and Veh groups (Fig. 5f).

InRapa leads to the recovery of mTOR upstream signalling

mTORC1 is regulated upstream by positive inputs such as growth factors, hormones, chemokines, nutrients (e.g., glucose or amino acids), and cell energy status (ATP/AMP ratio). The regulation of mTORC1 by growth factors mainly involves insulin, which binds to insulin receptor (IR) and triggers the activation of the insulin receptor substrate 1 (IRS1). The phosphorylation of IRS1 on its activatory (Tyr632) or inhibitory (Ser307) residue modulates PI3K activation, which is negatively regulated by PTEN, a phosphatase protein and tensin homolog [8]. PI3K activation lead to increased PIP_3 levels that recruit Akt, to the membrane, where the latter is activated by phosphorylation of Thr308 and Ser473 residues. In turn, Akt positively regulates mTORC1 activity. Moreover, through a negative-feedback mechanism, mTORC1/p70S6K mediates the inhibitory phosphorylation of IRS1 on a serine residue uncoupling the PI3K/Akt axis from insulin receptor signals [8].

The analysis of mTOR upstream signalling regulation shows no differences in levels and phosphorylation of PI3K (subunit p85; Tyr508) and increased levels of Akt in Ts65Dn Veh compared to Eu Veh (40%; $p = 0.022$), but no differences in phosphorylation (Ser473) between all groups (Fig. 6b, c). Intriguingly, increased p-PTEN (Ser380/Thr382/383)/PTEN was found to be statistically significant in Ts65Dn InRapa compared with Ts65Dn Veh (37%; $p = 0.049$) suggesting that despite decreased expression, PTEN activation is induced by InRapa, perhaps to better promote a correct regulation of the signal (Fig. 6d). The two-way ANOVA analysis show that genotype and interaction account for the 42.93% ($p < 0.0001$) and for the 14.22% ($p = 0.005$) of the total variance of Akt.

The analysis of the foregoing member of IRS1 pathway demonstrates that, despite increased protein levels of IRS1 in Ts65Dn mice compared to Eu (45%; p = 0.049), a trend of inactivation in Ts65Dn mice, as indexed by decreased phosphorylation of its activation residue (Tyr632) and increased phosphorylation of its inhibitory residue (Ser307), is shown. Rapamycin delivered intranasally is able to reduce the inhibition (exerted by mTORC1 and p70S6K) on IRS1 by increasing its activation residue of phosphorylation (80%; $p = 0.03$) and decreasing its inhibitory phosphorylation (52%; $p = 0.012$) in Ts65Dn InRapa compared to Ts65Dn Veh animals (Fig. 6e). The two-way ANOVA analysis of IRS1 phosphorylation levels show that InRapa treatment account for the 62.94% ($p < 0.001$) and the 13.89% (0.0476) of the total variance of Ser307and Tyr632, respectively.

The AMP-activated protein kinase (AMPK) is a key energy sensor and regulates cellular metabolism to maintain energy homeostasis. AMPK is an upstream signal of mTOR and its activation results in the inhibition of mTOR signalling, thereby suppressing protein synthesis, which is an important pathway by which AMPK conserves cellular energy during low energy states. In turn, prolonged mTOR hyper-phosphorylation on Ser2448 reduces AMPK activation [59]. Ts65Dn mice, in the presence of mTOR hyperphosphorylation, do not show increased pAMPK/AMPK signal, while InRapa treatment was able to reactivate AMPK as indexed by increased activatory phosphorylation on Thr172, of about 30% (p = 0.02) (Fig. 6f).

InRapa increases the expression levels of STX 1A and PSD95 synaptic proteins

Prenatal and early post-natal synaptic defects have been largely documented several brain regions including the neocortex, hippocampus and cerebellum of fetuses with Down's syndrome and of mouse models of the disease [60–64]. Decreased numbers of presynaptic and postsynaptic terminals were previously observed during development in Ts65Dn hippocampus and Ts65Dn dentate gyrus has been shown to have a reduced number of neurons and deficient LTP [60, 65, 66]. To determine whether InRapa treatment result in the rescue of synapse failure, we examined the expression levels of syntaxin1A (STX1A) and PSD 95 in euploid and Ts65Dn mice. STX1A is neuronal plasma membrane protein that belongs to the soluble N-ethylmaleimide-sensitive factor attachment protein receptor (SNARE) family and is

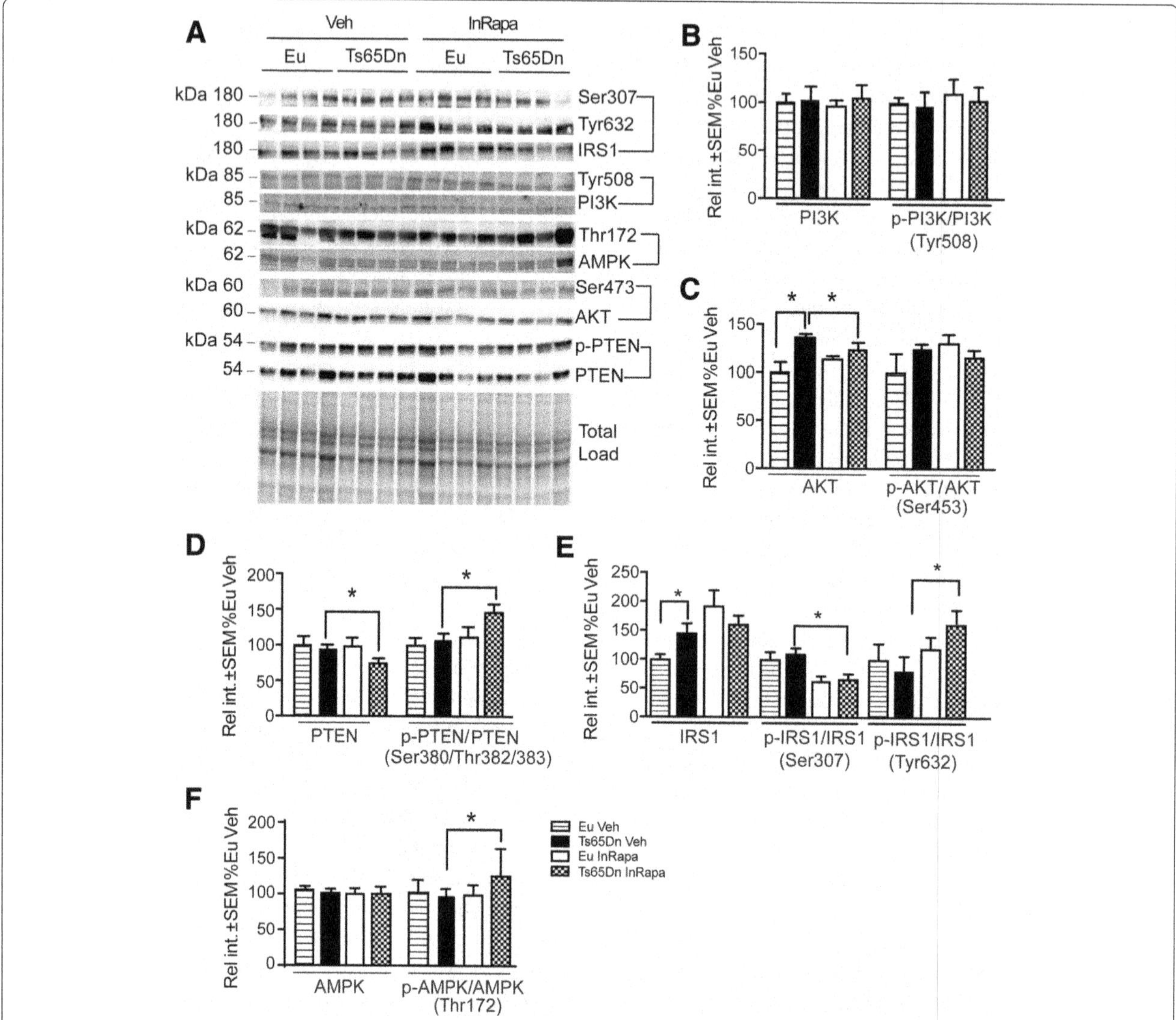

Fig. 6 InRapa recovers mTOR upstream signalling. **a** Representative WB showing hippocampal p-IRS (Ser307), p-IRS1 (Tyr632) and total IRS1 levels, p-PI3K(Tyr508) and total PI3K levels, p-AKT (Ser473) and total AKT levels, and p-PTEN (Ser380/Thr382/383) and total PTEN, p-AMPK (Ser172) and total AMPK. **b** Quantification of panel **a** showing hippocampal levels of PI3K and p-PI3K(Tyr508)/PI3K ratio. **c** Quantification of panel **a** showing AKT and p-AKT(Ser473)/AKT ratio. **d** Quantification of panel **a** showing levels of PTEN and p-PTEN (Ser380/Thr382/383)/PTEN ratio. **e** Quantification of panel **a** showing p-IRS1 (Ser307), p-IRS1 (Tyr632) and total IRS1 levels in Eu and Ts65Dn mice treated with InRapa and Veh. **f** Quantification of panel **a** showing AMPK and p-AMPK(Thr172)/AMPK ratio. Densitometry values shown in the bar graph are the mean of 8 samples per each group, normalized per total load and given as percentage of Eu Veh, set as 100%

involved in vesicle trafficking, docking and/or fusion, playing a key role in neurotransmitter release. PSD 95, a membrane-associated guanylate kinase, is the major scaffolding protein in the excitatory postsynaptic density (PSD) and a potent regulator of synaptic strength. Thought the phosphorylation of 4EBP1 and p70S6K mTOR is able to regulates protein synthesis, influencing the expression of synaptic proteins. Our results show for STX1A expression a significant decrease in Ts65Dn Veh compared to euploid animals (35%, $p = 0.0137$), which is partially rescued (20%, ns) after rapamycin administration (Fig 7a-b). As far as PSD 95 we demonstrate a trend of decrease for its expression levels in Ts65Dn Veh mice compared to euploid Veh (18%, ns), while rapamycin treatment induces the overexpression of PSD 95 in both Ts65Dn (50%, $p = 0.045$) and Euploids (22%, ns) (Fig. 7c-d). Our results are in line with previous studies showing reduced levels of synaptic protein in Ts65Dn mice and their induction after disease-modifying treatment leading to improved cognition [67–69]. Intriguingly, the two-way anova analyses of PSD95 show indeed that the treatment account for the 37.7% ($p = 0.0077$) of the total variance.

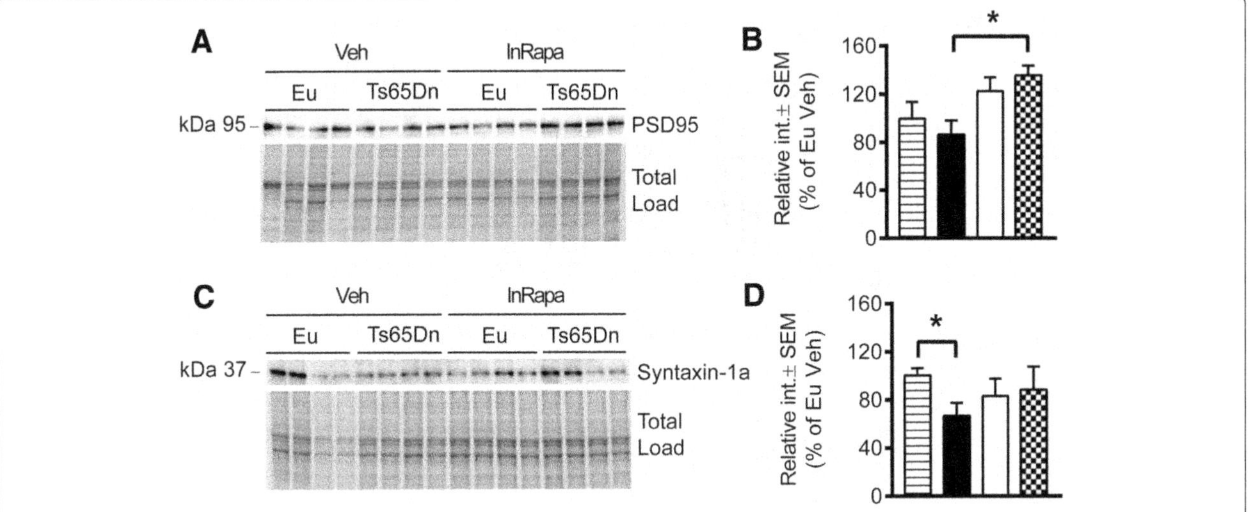

Fig. 7 InRapa increases the levels of PSD95 and STX1A synaptic proteins. **a** Representative WB showing hippocampal PSD95 levels. **b** Quantification of panel **a** showing hippocampal the expression levels of PSD95. **c** Representative WB showing hippocampal STX1A levels. **d** Quantification of panel **c** showing levels of STX1A. Densitometry values shown in the bar graph are the mean of 8 samples per each group, normalized per total load and given as percentage of Eu Veh, set as 100%

InRapa modulates protein oxidative damage and Lys63 poly-ubiquitinylation

Previous studies by our group and others demonstrated that in DS brain alteration of autophagy is associated with increased oxidative stress (OS), which plays an important role in DS neuropathology [7, 9, 13, 22, 70]. However, the link between OS and autophagy is intricate, and increasing evidence suggests that the mTOR/autophagy axis plays a dual role in the cellular response to OS [71, 72] . We evaluated the levels of two protein oxidation markers, 4-hydroxy-2-nonenal protein adducts (HNE) and protein-bound 3-nitrotyrosine (3-NT) in the hippocampus of Ts65Dn and Eu. We found a significant elevation of total 3-NT levels in Ts65Dn mice compared with Eu treated with Veh (28%; $p = 0.021$), and such increase was reduced with InRapa treatment (23%; $p = 0.06$) (Fig. 8a). Further, a trend of increased HNE adducts to proteins was observe between Eu Veh and Ts65Dn Veh, and treatment with InRapa was able to significantly reduce such increase (43%; $p = 0.015$) (Fig. 8a). The two-way ANOVA analysis of 3NT levels show that genotype significantly account for the 31.05% ($p = 0.0007$) of the total variance, while if we consider protein-bound HNE levels InRapa treatment and interaction account for the 47.01 ($p < 0.0001$) and for the 7.19% ($p = 0.043$) of the total variance, respectively.

We also investigated the status of the ubiquitin-dependent proteolysis pathway through analysis of total protein poly-ubiquitinylation and the levels of chain linkage Lys48, considered to be a key signal for proteasome degradation, and chain linkage Lys63, known to have a role in protein degradation through the autophagy-lysosomal system [73]. However, we showed that Lys63 protein poly-ubiquitinylation might have a primary role in protein signalling in addition to protein degradation [10]. With regards to total protein poly-ubiquitinylation, no significant alteration was observed between DS and Eu animals with and without rapamycin treatment (Fig. 8c). However, if we discriminate the lysine residue of poly-ubiquitinylation we observed increased levels of Lys63 poly-ubiquitinylated proteins in Ts65Dn Veh mice compared to Eu Veh (13%; $p = 0.024$), which are reduced in Ts65Dn InRapa compared to Veh (24%; $p = 0.0012$) (Fig. 8c). No significant changes were detected, among groups, for Lys48 poly-ubiquitinylated proteins. The two-way ANOVA analysis of Lys63 poly-Ub levels demonstrate that InRapa treatment and interaction account for the 32.71 ($p = 0.0001$) and for the 20.84% ($p = 0.0013$) of the total variance, respectively.

Discussion

In the last decades, a significant increase of life expectancy has been observed in DS individuals due to improvement in health care. However, improved lifespan in DS is associated with an increased incidence of developing AD-like dementia [2, 74]. The triplication of APP represents a strong evidence on the influence of HSA21 trisomy in the progression to AD-like cognitive decline in DS population. In addition, the triplication of tau kinases, such as DYRK1A and RCAN1, which act in parallel with aberrant mTOR pathway activation, contributes to increased tau phosphorylation and NFT formation [72, 75, 76]. The exact mechanisms by which triplication of genes on HSA21 lead to the early onset of AD in DS population remain still to be fully elucidated.

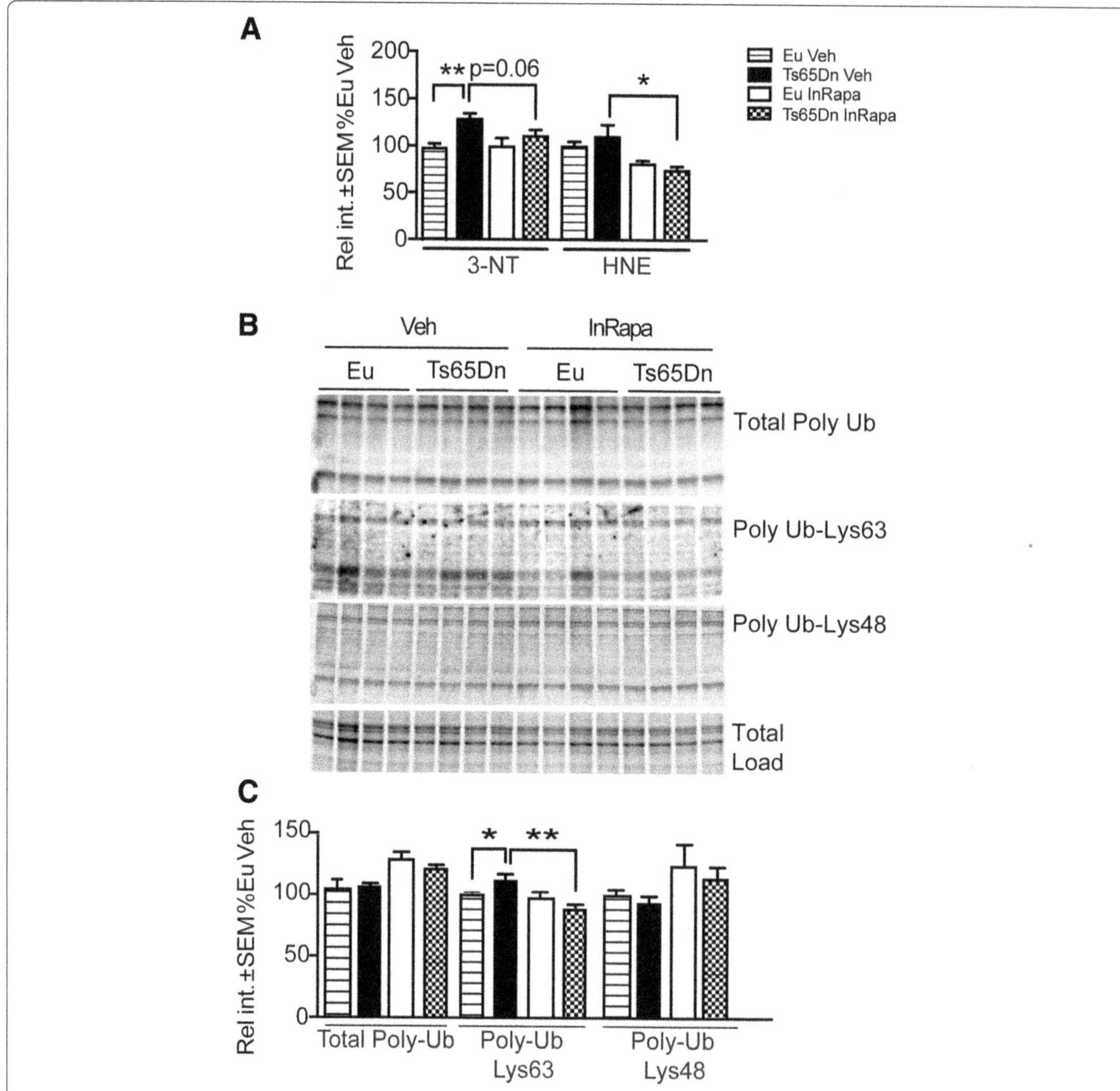

Fig. 8 InRapa reduces protein oxidative damage and K63 poly-ubiquitinylation. In panel **a** are shown the total hippocampal protein-bound 3-NT and HNE of Ts65Dn mice and Eu treated with Veh and InRapa analyzed by slot blot assay. In panel **b** are shown the hippocampal total poly-ubiquitin, poly-ubiquitin Lys63 and poly-ubiquitin Lys48 levels analyzed by Western blot. In panel **c** the quantification of panel **b** is reported. Densitometry values of each lane is the result of the sum of all the bands, analyzed by Image lab software as previously reported [10]. Graph values are the mean of 8 samples per each group, normalized per total load and given as percentage of Eu Veh, set as 100%

Previous studies by our group and others demonstrated the hyper-activation of mTOR pathway in human brain from DS population and in Ts65Dn mouse model of the disease [13, 21, 22, 56, 77]. mTOR hyper-activation was found to be strongly associated with reduced autophagosome formation (most likely leading to impaired autophagy induction), increased Aβ deposition and increased tau hyper-phosphorylation. Data collected by our studies support the key role of aberrant mTOR signalling in mediating the early progression of AD in DS population. Within this frame, the rescue of mTOR signalling by the administration of rapamycin, which has been previously tested in AD mouse models demonstrating favorable outcomes [19, 27, 29–31, 78–81], represents a potentially valuable therapeutic strategy. Indeed, evidence obtained by the Oddo and Galvan laboratories [19, 31] corroborated the positive effects of mTOR inhibition on hippocampal memory rescue in AD mice. In particular, the authors reported that chronic oral rapamycin treatment was able to prevent cognitive loss in two different transgenic mouse models of

AD, 3xTg-AD and J20, if given before robust plaque and tangle deposition. Memory improvement was associated with reduced Aβ levels and tau-aggregation, as well as microglial activation [19, 31]. Based on these evidences, the initiation of an early treatment schedule is necessary to achieve brain protection in DS individuals, known to be at high risk of developing AD-like dementia. Moreover, the use of the intranasal route for the delivery of rapamycin to the brain holds a great potential as a non-invasive practical approach that circumvents systemic alterations and permits to maximal drug concentrations in the CNS, thereby avoiding the rapamycin-related immunosuppressant effects in the periphery [82–85]. This issue is particularly critical in DS pathological phenotypes, since trisomic individuals show depletion of immune system and lymphopenia [86–89]. In this scenario, by UPLC-MS analysis we were able to demonstrate that intranasal administration of rapamycin concentrated the drug in the CNS, where it exerted its inhibitory effects by reducing hippocampal mTORC1 hyper-phosphorylation of about 50%, while, as expected, no effects were observed in peripheral organs analyzed. Of note, the rapamycin dosage delivered to the hippocampus of Ts65Dn was selected to not abolish mTOR activation but to rescue the signal at physiological levels, thus abrogating the pathological increase of mTOR and p70S6K phosphorylation along with the reduction of autophagy.

The restoration of mTORC1 activity after treatment demonstrated a significant effect on cognitive performance in Ts65Dn mice as indexed by RAM and NOR tests. Indeed, the RAM test revealed that mice were able to improve reference and working memory after rapamycin treatment. As well, the NOR test showed the improvement of mice preference index supporting the recovery of novelty-discriminating ability after rapamycin administration. Further, we suggest that the improved cognition, exerted by InRapa, is associated with the rescue of synaptic abnormalities previously observed in DS [60, 69]. Therefore, as previously proven in AD, our data support the capability of rapamycin, if delivered chronically and intranasally before consistent brain damage, to improve memory and reduce cognitive decline in DS mice [31]. In order to understand the mechanisms leading to improved cognition after InRapa treatment we investigated the status of downstream targets of mTOR and the pathological features of AD-like neurodegenerative process.

Human and mouse studies suggest that APP is dosage sensitive as a function of aging and of brain regionalism [4, 6, 46, 50]. In contrast, Aβ accumulation becomes significant in humans only in the second/third decade of life, with some exceptions in a few childhood post- mortem observations [2, 75, 76]. Moreover, published data on Aβ peptides levels in the brain of Ts65Dn mice are conflicting. This discrepancy might depend on the diversity of techniques, brain area analyzed and age of the samples. We observed an increase of Aβ oligomers at 25 and 50 kD only, while previous studies focused on the identification of plaques, which are formed only at a very late stage of the disease. Within this scenario, our data suggest a primary role for APP and its processing in the neurodegenerative process occurring in DS [33, 47, 49, 50, 90]. Indeed, in Ts65Dn mouse, which develops AD-like neuronal endosomal pathology, the increase of APP-αCTF and APP-βCTF between 6 and 12 months of age is likely to underlie the failure of NGF-mediated trophic support [6], and contribute to cognitive failure. Our analysis shows increased levels of APP in Ts65Dn mice at 9 months of age both in total hippocampus as well as in the CA3 region, together with the increased APP metabolites APP-αCTF and APP-βCTF. InRapa administration is able to significantly reduce APP levels in the hippocampus of Ts65Dn mice and to decrease APP metabolites, suggesting the re-establishment of proper APP processing. Surprisingly, we also observed increased Aβ oligomers in Ts65Dn mice and the reduction of such increase due to InRapa treatment. Two main mechanisms can be directly involved in the reduction of APP, APP metabolites and Aβ in Ts65Dn mice after rapamycin treatment: i) the reduction of APP gene expression; ii) the rescue of protein synthesis/degradation pathways; ii) the restoration of key signalling pathways, including BACE1, PI3K/Akt, GSK-3β, AMPK and IRS1, that regulate APP processing products formation/clearance [8, 12, 14, 39, 72, 91] . Our data show, as expected, the increase of APP mRNA in Ts65Dn mice as a result of trisomy that demonstrate a significant decrease after InRapa treatment. In general, mTORC1 inhibition by rapamycin results in a reduction in global mRNA, indeed mTOR is able to bind a number of transcription factors (e.g. STAT3; PGC1α) that can regulate the expression of a broad range of target genes, comprising mTOR itself, whose aberrant modulation is known to be involved in neurodegeneration [92]. In agreement, our data supports a role for rapamycin in the down-regulation of APP transcription process. The transcription factor ETS2, encoded on Chr21, was demonstrated to transactivate the APP promoter, leading to its overexpression [93]. Previous studies revealed that the expression levels of ETS2 can be modulated by the mTOR pathway; therefore, rapamycin-induced mTOR inhibition, through the reduction of ETS2 levels, might reduce APP overexpression levels [94]. Besides, it is indeed equally important to highlight the significant increase of autophagosome formation observed in Ts65Dn mice after InRapa treatment. Our data demonstrate that mTOR inhibition lead to increased LC3II and Atg 12/5 levels supporting a crucial role for rapamycin in restoring the aberrant control of mTOR on autophagy. The observed induction of autophagosome formation in rapamycin treated DS mice is associated with the reduction of toxic aggregates burden and misfolded/oxidized proteins accumulation. Therefore, our results are in agreement with previous studies demonstrating that rapamycin-dependent stimulation of autophagy is likely one of the principal mechanisms by which the reduction of toxic protein aggregates, comprised of Aβ, aberrantly expressed APP and APP metabolites, is achieved in the brains of Tg-AD mice [18, 19, 23, 26, 31, 40, 79, 95]. Furthermore, the analysis of molecular pathways involved in APP processing demonstrated that rapamycin lead to the reduction of BACE1 levels and to the recovery of IRS1 signaling. Conversely, we obtained conflicting results concerning PI3K/Akt and GSK3β that suggest their modest involvement in APP metabolite reduction. The increased BACE1 activation is required for the cleavage of APP and the production of the neurotoxic Aβ peptide during neurodegeneration, as demonstrated in AD mice and in our DS model [4, 5]. On one side we could suppose that the reduction of BACE1 levels, observed after InRapa treatment, could be most likely related with the reduction of the APP substrate, accomplished by re-balanced synthesis/degradation. However, because such reduction is observed in both Ts65Dn and Eu mice, it is tempting to presume a close interaction between rapamycin/ mTOR and BACE1. The direct interaction of mTOR with IRS1 have been previously demonstrated and was shown to be deeply involved in the development of AD [13, 20, 21, 96–98]. Indeed, the failure of energy metabolism associated with the increase of brain insulin resistance are well-recognized contributors to AD neurodegeneration [96, 97, 99]. Our previous studies demonstrated that mTOR hyperphosphorylation and the subsequent overactivation of p70S6K kinase activity target IRS1 by increasing the phosphorylation on its inhibitory serine residues, which lead to the inactivation of the protein. Such effects contribute to the uncoupling of IRS1 from PI3K/Akt signalling and to the development of brain insulin resistance [13]. The rescue of mTOR signalling in Ts65Dn mice after InRapa leads to reduced IRS1 inhibitory phosphorylation sites; therefore, a proper insulin signalling is reinstated that contributes to decreased metabolic failure and conceivably reduced APP processing products in DS [84, 97, 100, 101].

As noted above, AMPK signalling is a major inducer of autophagy associated with the reduction of energy metabolism [59]. The loss of sensitivity of AMPK activation to cellular stress impairs metabolic regulation, increases oxidative stress and reduces autophagic clearance. Recent studies confirmed that the responsiveness of AMPK to different insults is clearly suppressed in aged tissues during mTOR overactivation. In line with this proposed scenario, AMPK signal is dampened in Ts65Dn mice. Intriguingly, the inhibition of mTOR, by InRapa treatment, lead to increased phosphorylation of AMPK on its activatory residue rescuing signalling induction. Noteworthy, previous reports demonstrated that AMPK activation is able to induce autophagy by also phosphorylating Ulk1, beyond inhibiting mTOR signalling [102].

The sequence of pathological mechanisms of DS neurodegeneration in Ts65Dn mice include aberrant tau phosphorylation, associated with the increased activation state of different tau kinases. Among these, DYRK1A and RCAN1 encoded on HSA21, and GSK3β and CDK5 seem to have a prominent role in tau hyper-phosphorylation occurring in the brain of AD and DS subjects [72].

Substantial evidence supports the critical role of mTOR in tau-related pathological progress in DS. A number of studies sustain that the activation of mTOR signalling promotes tau hyper-phosphorylation, while its inhibition prevents this phenomenon [27–29, 32, 95]. In particular, the mechanisms by which altered mTOR signalling lead to tau hyper-phosphorylation include the aberrant regulation of tau kinases and the reduction of autophagy. Ts65Dn mice after InRapa treatment demonstrate a robust and significant reduction of tau phosphorylation in the hippocampus, both total and CA3 region-specific. The reduction is associated with significantly decreased expression of RCAN1 and with a trend of decreased DYRK1A levels. No alteration is shown for CDK5 in Ts65Dn prior or after the treatment, while an opposite trend is reported for GSK3β, as previously reported also in human studies [13]. Despite the reduction of tau kinases, lowered levels of hyperphosphorylated tau cannot be observed after InRapa administration without the increase of autophagosome formation, which play a key role in the clearence of intracellular toxic tau aggregates. These results suggest that rapamycin is able to reduce the degree of tau phosphorylation by modulating the expression of certain tau kinases, and to improve hyperphosphorylated tau degradation through the induction of autophagy [103–105].

A further intriguing outcome observed after InRapa treatment is represented by the reduction of protein oxidative damage in Ts65Dn mice. Increased oxidative stress is a characteristic feature of DS neuropathology in humans and mice [3, 74, 106]. Data collected in DS human brain indicated that oxidative damage targeted specific components of the proteostasis network, resulting in dysfunctional activation of autophagy and the ubiquitin proteasome system [7, 9, 70]. Previous studies by our laboratory demonstrated that the chronic increase of OS in Ts65Dn mice with aging, in parallel with reduced autophagy, leads to the accumulation of total protein-bound HNE and protein nitration levels [22]. Therefore, a vicious cycle that involves the prolonged failure of protein degradation systems and the chronic build-up of oxidized protein may exist in DS. The rescue of mTOR activity, by InRapa treatment, likely induces the autophagy-driven degradation of oxidized proteins as demonstrated through the decrease of total protein-bound HNE levels and total protein nitration. In addition, studies on DS human brain reported that the accumulation of oxidative damage is coupled with increased levels of poly-ubiquitinylated proteins, prior to and after the development of AD [10]. Despite, Ts65Dn did not recapitulate the same profile of protein poly-ubiquitinylation observed in humans an increase in poly-Lys63 ubiquitinylation levels were observed. These data suggest that impairment of the proteasome system in Ts65Dn mice is less pronounced compared with humans, supporting the concept that the failure of protein degradation is related to the impairment of the autophagy pathway rather than to the impairment of the UPS. Noteworthy, InRapa treatment was able to reduce the poly-ubiquitinylation of Lys63 residues supporting the restoration of autophagy and implying a certain degree the crosstalk between mTOR and UPS.

Conclusions

Overall, we demonstrated that rapamycin, administered for 3 months by intranasal route, led to improved cognition in DS mice with no effects at peripheral organs. The favorable outcomes of rapamycin treatment seem to rely on its ability to rescue molecular pathways associated with aberrant mTOR phosphorylation, whose alteration accelerate the age-related neurodegenerative process and increase the risk of AD development in DS. Therefore, InRapa treatment represents an attractive therapeutic strategy to reduce the early development of neuropathology in DS population and delay the onset of AD. At final, this therapeutic strategy may be also translated to different neuronal disorders that share, as a common pathological mechanism, the alteration of mTOR/autophagy axis.

Additional files

Additional file 1: List of antibodies used for WB and IF analysis. For each antibody employed in the study is reported the brand, the catalogue number and the dilution employed in the study. (PPTX 146 kb)

Additional file 2: Bar graph reporting mice distance traveled during RAM test. The distance travelled was measured for 10 min at the end of the test days in all experimental groups, no differences were found between the groups. (PPTX 2553 kb)

Additional file 3: Pilot studies to assess InRapa therapeutic dose. Mice were treated by InRapa daily for 1 week after which brain regions were collected and analyzed. Phosphorylation levels of mTOR in both hippocampus and cortex are reported for each of the dose tested, 0.01 μg/μl (0.1 μg/mouse), 0.05 μg/μl (0.5 μg/mouse), 0.1 μg/μl (1 μg/mouse) and 0.2 μg/μl (2 μg/mouse). Each value is the mean of 6 replicate ± SEM. Our data demonstrate that the InRapa dosage of 0.1 μg/μl (1 μg/mouse) is able to inhibit mTOR phosphorylation when compared to vehicle. (PPTX 1203 kb)

Additional file 4: Table reporting 2-way ANOVA data analysis. For 2-way ANOVA analysis only proteins showing changes before and after the InRapa treatment have been taken under consideration. (PPTX 844 kb)

Additional file 5: Rapamycin distribution by UPLC-MS. Chromatograms of rapamycin in plasma (A) and brain (B) from animals treated by single I.P. injection of 50 μg/mouse (2,5 mg/kg/mouse) 4 h before sacrifice. Chromatograms of rapamycin in plasma (C) and brain (D) from animals treated by single InRapa administration of 1 μg/mouse (0.05 mg/Kg/mouse) 4 h before sacrifice. (PPTX 50 kb)

Additional file 6: Western blot analysis of mTOR and p70S6K phosphorylation in liver and heart tissue after InRapa treatment. Graph bars are reported as percentage in respect to euploid vehicle group, which is set as 100%. Data Show no significant alteration in Ts65Dn undergoing rapamycin (black bar) or vehicle (checquered bars) after intranasal delivery supporting no effects of InRapa treatment at peripheral level. (PPTX 72 kb)

Additional file 7: Immunofluorescence staining of Dentate gyrus in Eu and Ts65Dn mice. Representative immunofluorescent images showing (A) p-mTOR at serine 2448, (B) at Ser416 and (C) APP/Ab levels in the dentate gyrus region of the hippocampus from euploid mice treated with Veh and InRapa (A.1–4), and Ts65Dn mice treated with Veh and InRapa (A.5–8). DAPI (blue) was used to identify cell nuclei. Scale bar represent 20 μm. On the right of each panel a graph of the quantification of fluorescence signal is reported. (PPTX 16410 kb)

Abbreviations

3-NT: 3-Nitrotyrosine; AD: Alzheimer's Disease; AMPK: AMP-activated protein kinase; APP: Amyloid Precursor Protein; Atg: Autophagy related proteins; Aβ: Amyloid-β; BACE1: Beta-secretase 1; CDK5: cyclin dependent kinase 5; CNS: Central Nervous System; Ct: threshold cycle; DI: Discrimination Index; DS: Down Syndrome; DYRK1A: Dual specificity tyrosine-phosphorylation-regulated kinase 1A; Eu: Euploid; GAPDH: Glyceraldehyde-3-Phosphate Dehydrogenase; GSK3β: glycogen synthase kinase 3 isoforms β; HNE: 4-Hydroxynonenal; Hsa21: human chromosome 21; InRapa: Intranasal Rapamycin; IRS-1: Insulin Receptor Substrate-1; LC3: Microtubule-associated protein 1A/1B-light chain 3; mTOR: mammalian Target Of Rapamycin; NFT: Neurofibrillary Tangles; NOR: Novel Object Recognition; OS: Oxidative Stress; P70S6K: ribosomal p70S6 kinase; Pdebrd1: Recessive Retinal Degeneration 1 Mutation; PI: preference Index; PI3K: Phosphoinositide-3-Kinase; PQC: Protein Quality Control; PTEN: phosphatase and tensin homolog; RAM: Radial Arm Maze; Rapa: Rapamycin; RCAN1: Regulator of Calcineurin 1; RME: reference memory errors; RNS: Reactive Nitrogen Species; ROS: Reactive Oxygen Species; RT-PCR: Real time Polymerase Chain Reaction; Tg: Transgenic; UPLC: Ultra-performance/pressure Liquid Chromatography analysis; UPS: Ubiquitin Proteasome System; Veh: Vehicle; WME: working memory errors

Acknowledgements

Not applicable.

Funding

This work was supported by the Ministry of Instruction, Universities and Research (MIUR) under the SIR program n° RBSI144MT to FDD, Jerome Lejeune Foundation with the grant # PERLUIGI/1484-PM2016A to MP and Fondi di Ateneo Progetti Grandi # RG116154C9214D1A from Sapienza University of Rome to FDD.

Authors' contributions

FDD and MP were involved in designing the study and the experimental procedure, and in the preparation of the manuscript; AT, CL, EB, AA and IZ were involved in animal treatment and in performing the experimental procedures; LM was involved in UPLC/MS analysis; CB was involved in manuscript preparation and correction; DAB was involved in study design and manuscript revising. All authors read and approved the final manuscript.

Authors' information
Not applicable

Competing interests
The authors declare that they have no competing interests.

Author details
[1]Department of Biochemical Sciences, Sapienza University of Rome, P.le Aldo Moro 5, 00185 Rome, Italy. [2]Universidad Autònoma de Chile, Instituto de Ciencias Biomédicas, Facultad de alud, Avenida Pedro de Valdivia 425, Providencia, Santiago, Chile. [3]Department of Chemistry and Sanders-Brown Center on Aging, University of Kentucky, Lexington, KY 40506-0055, USA.

References
1. Wiseman FK, Al-Janabi T, Hardy J, Karmiloff-Smith A, Nizetic D, Tybulewicz VL, Fisher EM, Strydom A. A genetic cause of Alzheimer disease: mechanistic insights from Down syndrome. Nat Rev Neurosci. 2015;16:564–74.
2. Head E, Powell D, Gold BT, Schmitt FA. Alzheimer's disease in Down syndrome. Eur J Neurodegener Dis. 2012;1:353–64.
3. Perluigi M, Di Domenico F, Buttterfield DA. Unraveling the complexity of neurodegeneration in brains of subjects with Down syndrome: insights from proteomics. Proteomics Clin Appl. 2014;8:73–85.
4. Cheon MS, Dierssen M, Kim SH, Lubec G. Protein expression of BACE1, BACE2 and APP in Down syndrome brains. Amino Acids. 2008;35:339–43.
5. Jiang Y, Mullaney KA, Peterhoff CM, Che S, Schmidt SD, Boyer-Boiteau A, Ginsberg SD, Cataldo AM, Mathews PM, Nixon RA. Alzheimer's-related endosome dysfunction in Down syndrome is Abeta-independent but requires APP and is reversed by BACE-1 inhibition. Proc Natl Acad Sci U S A. 2010;107:1630–5.
6. Salehi A, Delcroix JD, Belichenko PV, Zhan K, Wu C, Valletta JS, Takimoto-Kimura R, Kleschevnikov AM, Sambamurti K, Chung PP, et al. Increased app expression in a mouse model of Down's syndrome disrupts NGF transport and causes cholinergic neuron degeneration. Neuron. 2006;51:29–42.
7. Di Domenico F, Coccia R, Cocciolo A, Murphy MP, Cenini G, Head E, Butterfield DA, Giorgi A, Schinina ME, Mancuso C, et al. Impairment of proteostasis network in Down syndrome prior to the development of Alzheimer's disease neuropathology: redox proteomics analysis of human brain. Biochim Biophys Acta. 1832;2013:1249–59.
8. Perluigi M, Di Domenico F, Butterfield DA. mTOR signaling in aging and neurodegeneration: at the crossroad between metabolism dysfunction and impairment of autophagy. Neurobiol Dis. 2015;84:39–49.
9. Di Domenico F, Pupo G, Tramutola A, Giorgi A, Schinina ME, Coccia R, Head E, Butterfield DA, Perluigi M. Redox proteomics analysis of HNE-modified proteins in Down syndrome brain: clues for understanding the development of Alzheimer disease. Free Radic Biol Med. 2014;71:270–80.
10. Tramutola A, Di Domenico F, Barone E, Arena A, Giorgi A, di Francesco L, Schinina ME, Coccia R, Head E, Butterfield DA, Perluigi M. Polyubiquitinylation profile in Down syndrome brain before and after the development of Alzheimer neuropathology. Antioxid Redox Signal. 2017;26:280–98.
11. Tramutola A, Triani F, Di Domenico F, Barone E, Cai J, Klein JB, Perluigi M, Butterfield DA. Poly-ubiquitin profile in Alzheimer disease brain. Neurobiol Dis. 2018;118:129–41.
12. O' Neill C. PI3-kinase/Akt/mTOR signaling: impaired on/off switches in aging, cognitive decline and Alzheimer's disease. Exp Gerontol. 2013;48:647–53.
13. Perluigi M, Pupo G, Tramutola A, Cini C, Coccia R, Barone E, Head E, Butterfield DA, Di Domenico F: Neuropathological role of PI3K/Akt/mTOR axis in Down syndrome brain. Biochim Biophys Acta 2014, 1842:1144–1153.
14. Hoeffer CA, Klann E. mTOR signaling: at the crossroads of plasticity, memory and disease. Trends Neurosci. 2010;33:67–75.
15. Laplante M, Sabatini DM. mTOR Signaling. Cold Spring Harb Perspect Biol. 2012;4:1-3.
16. Ma T, Hoeffer CA, Capetillo-Zarate E, Yu F, Wong H, Lin MT, Tampellini D, Klann E, Blitzer RD, Gouras GK. Dysregulation of the mTOR pathway mediates impairment of synaptic plasticity in a mouse model of Alzheimer's disease. PLoS One. 2010;5:1-10.
17. Cai Z, Chen G, He W, Xiao M, Yan LJ. Activation of mTOR: a culprit of Alzheimer's disease? Neuropsychiatr Dis Treat. 2015;11:1015–30.
18. Oddo S. The role of mTOR signaling in Alzheimer disease. Front Biosci. 2012; 4:941–52.
19. Spilman P, Podlutskaya N, Hart MJ, Debnath J, Gorostiza O, Bredesen D, Richardson A, Strong R, Galvan V. Inhibition of mTOR by rapamycin abolishes cognitive deficits and reduces amyloid-beta levels in a mouse model of Alzheimer's disease. PLoS One. 2010;5:e9979.
20. Tramutola A, Lanzillotta C, Di Domenico F. Targeting mTOR to reduce Alzheimer-related cognitive decline: from current hits to future therapies. Expert Rev Neurother. 2017;17:33–45.
21. Iyer AM, van Scheppingen J, Milenkovic I, Anink JJ, Adle-Biassette H, Kovacs GG, Aronica E. mTOR Hyperactivation in Down syndrome hippocampus appears early during development. J Neuropathol Exp Neurol. 2014;73:671–83.
22. Tramutola A, Lanzillotta C, Arena A, Barone E, Perluigi M, Di Domenico F. Increased mammalian target of rapamycin signaling contributes to the accumulation of protein oxidative damage in a mouse model of Down's syndrome. Neurodegener Dis. 2016;16:62–8.
23. Cai Z, Zhao B, Li K, Zhang L, Li C, Quazi SH, Tan Y. Mammalian target of rapamycin: a valid therapeutic target through the autophagy pathway for Alzheimer's disease? J Neurosci Res. 2012;90:1105–18.
24. Franco R, Martinez-Pinilla E, Navarro G, Zamarbide M. Potential of GPCRs to modulate MAPK and mTOR pathways in Alzheimer's disease. Prog Neurobiol. 2017;149-150:21–38.
25. Chong ZZ, Shang YC, Zhang L, Wang S, Maiese K. Mammalian target of rapamycin: hitting the bull's-eye for neurological disorders. Oxidative Med Cell Longev. 2010;3:374–91.
26. Richardson A, Galvan V, Lin AL, Oddo S. How longevity research can lead to therapies for Alzheimer's disease: the rapamycin story. Exp Gerontol. 2015; 68:51–8.
27. Siman R, Cocca R, Dong Y. The mTOR inhibitor rapamycin mitigates Perforant pathway neurodegeneration and synapse loss in a mouse model of early-stage Alzheimer-type Tauopathy. PLoS One. 2015;10:e0142340.
28. Tang Z, Bereczki E, Zhang H, Wang S, Li C, Ji X, Branca RM, Lehtio J, Guan Z, Filipcik P, et al. Mammalian target of rapamycin (mTor) mediates tau protein dyshomeostasis: implication for Alzheimer disease. J Biol Chem. 2013;288:15556–70.
29. Caccamo A, Majumder S, Richardson A, Strong R, Oddo S. Molecular interplay between mammalian target of rapamycin (mTOR), amyloid-beta, and tau: effects on cognitive impairments. J Biol Chem. 2010;285:13107–20.
30. Caccamo A, Maldonado MA, Majumder S, Medina DX, Holbein W, Magri A, Oddo S. Naturally secreted amyloid-beta increases mammalian target of rapamycin (mTOR) activity via a PRAS40-mediated mechanism. J Biol Chem. 2011;286:8924–32.
31. Majumder S, Richardson A, Strong R, Oddo S. Inducing autophagy by rapamycin before, but not after, the formation of plaques and tangles ameliorates cognitive deficits. PLoS One. 2011;6:e25416.
32. Oddo S, Vasilevko V, Caccamo A, Kitazawa M, Cribbs DH, LaFerla FM. Reduction of soluble Abeta and tau, but not soluble Abeta alone, ameliorates cognitive decline in transgenic mice with plaques and tangles. J Biol Chem. 2006;281:39413–23.
33. Reinholdt LG, Ding Y, Gilbert GJ, Czechanski A, Solzak JP, Roper RJ, Johnson MT, Donahue LR, Lutz C, Davisson MT. Molecular characterization of the translocation breakpoints in the Down syndrome mouse model Ts65Dn. Mamm Genome. 2011;22:685–91.
34. Ennaceur A. One-trial object recognition in rats and mice: methodological and theoretical issues. Behav Brain Res. 2010;215:244–54.
35. Antunes M, Biala G. The novel object recognition memory: neurobiology, test procedure, and its modifications. Cogn Process. 2012;13:93–110.
36. Vorhees CV, Williams MT. Assessing spatial learning and memory in rodents. ILAR J. 2014;55:310–32.
37. Livak KJ, Schmittgen TD. Analysis of relative gene expression data using real-time quantitative PCR and the 2(T)(−Delta Delta C) method. Methods. 2001;25:402–8.
38. Sarbassov DD, Ali SM, Kim DH, Guertin DA, Latek RR, Erdjument-Bromage H, Tempst P, Sabatini DM. Rictor, a novel binding partner of mTOR, defines a rapamycin-insensitive and raptor-independent pathway that regulates the cytoskeleton. Curr Biol. 2004;14:1296–302.
39. Jung CH, Ro SH, Cao J, Otto NM, Kim DH. mTOR regulation of autophagy. FEBS Lett. 2010;584:1287–95.
40. Orr ME, Oddo S. Autophagic/lysosomal dysfunction in Alzheimer's disease. Alzheimers Res Ther. 2013;5:53.

41. Nixon RA. Autophagy, amyloidogenesis and Alzheimer disease. J Cell Sci. 2007;120:4081–91.
42. Nixon RA, Yang DS. Autophagy failure in Alzheimer's disease--locating the primary defect. Neurobiol Dis. 2011;43:38–45.
43. Klionsky DJ, Abdelmohsen K, Abe A, Abedin MJ, Abeliovich H, Acevedo Arozena A, Adachi H, Adams CM, Adams PD, Adeli K, et al. Guidelines for the use and interpretation of assays for monitoring autophagy (3rd edition). Autophagy. 2016;12:1–222.
44. Webb RL, Murphy MP. beta-Secretases, Alzheimer's Disease, and Down Syndrome. Curr Gerontol Geriatr Res. 2012;2012:362839.
45. Mori C, Spooner ET, Wisniewsk KE, Wisniewski TM, Yamaguch H, Saido TC, Tolan DR, Selkoe DJ, Lemere CA. Intraneuronal Abeta42 accumulation in Down syndrome brain. Amyloid. 2002;9:88–102.
46. Seo H, Isacson O, Abnormal APP. Cholinergic and cognitive function in Ts65Dn Down's model mice. Exp Neurol. 2005;193:469–80.
47. Lomoio S, Scherini E, Necchi D. Beta-amyloid overload does not directly correlate with SAPK/JNK activation and tau protein phosphorylation in the cerebellar cortex of Ts65Dn mice. Brain Res. 2009;1297:198–206.
48. Hunter CL, Bimonte-Nelson HA, Nelson M, Eckman CB, Granholm AC. Behavioral and neurobiological markers of Alzheimer's disease in Ts65Dn mice: effects of estrogen. Neurobiol Aging. 2004;25:873–84.
49. Yu T, Li ZY, Jia ZP, Clapcote SJ, Liu CH, Li SM, Asrar S, Pao A, Chen RQ, Fan N, et al. A mouse model of Down syndrome trisomic for all human chromosome 21 syntenic regions. Hum Mol Genet. 2010;19:2780–91.
50. Choi JH, Berger JD, Mazzella MJ, Morales-Corraliza J, Cataldo AM, Nixon RA, Ginsberg SD, Levy E, Mathews PM. Age-dependent dysregulation of brain amyloid precursor protein in the Ts65Dn Down syndrome mouse model. J Neurochem. 2009;110:1818–27.
51. Liu F, Liang Z, Wegiel J, Hwang YW, Iqbal K, Grundke-Iqbal I, Ramakrishna N, Gong CX. Overexpression of Dyrk1A contributes to neurofibrillary degeneration in Down syndrome. FASEB J. 2008;22:3224–33.
52. Ryoo SR, Jeong HK, Radnaabazar C, Yoo JJ, Cho HJ, Lee HW, Kim IS, Cheon YH, Ahn YS, Chung SH, Song WJ. DYRK1A-mediated hyperphosphorylation of tau. A functional link between Down syndrome and Alzheimer disease. J Biol Chem. 2007;282:34850–7.
53. Jung MS, Park JH, Ryu YS, Choi SH, Yoon SH, Kwen MY, Oh JY, Song WJ, Chung SH. Regulation of RCAN1 protein activity by Dyrk1A protein-mediated phosphorylation. J Biol Chem. 2011;286:40401–12.
54. Ermak G, Harris CD, Battocchio D, Davies KJ. RCAN1 (DSCR1 or Adapt78) stimulates expression of GSK-3beta. FEBS J. 2006;273:2100–9.
55. Ermak G, Sojitra S, Yin F, Cadenas E, Cuervo AM, Davies KJ. Chronic expression of RCAN1-1L protein induces mitochondrial autophagy and metabolic shift from oxidative phosphorylation to glycolysis in neuronal cells. J Biol Chem. 2012;287:14088–98.
56. Sheppard O, Plattner F, Rubin A, Slender A, Linehan JM, Brandner S, Tybulewicz VL, Fisher EM, Wiseman FK. Altered regulation of tau phosphorylation in a mouse model of Down syndrome aging. Neurobiol Aging. 2012;33:828 e831–44.
57. Swatton JE, Sellers LA, Faull RLM, Holland A, Iritani S, Bahn S. Increased MAP kinase activity in Alzheimer's and Down syndrome but not in schizophrenia human brain. Eur J Neurosci. 2004;19:2711–9.
58. Pollonini G, Gao V, Rabe A, Palminiello S, Albertini G, Alberini CM. Abnormal expression of synaptic proteins and neurotrophin-3 in the Down syndrome mouse model Ts65Dn. Neuroscience. 2008;156:99–106.
59. Xu J, Ji J, Yan XH. Cross-talk between AMPK and mTOR in regulating energy balance. Crit Rev Food Sci. 2012;52:373–81.
60. Chakrabarti L, Galdzicki Z, Haydar TF. Defects in embryonic neurogenesis and initial synapse formation in the forebrain of the Ts65Dn mouse model of Down syndrome. J Neurosci. 2007;27:11483–95.
61. Lorenzi HA, Reeves RH. Hippocampal hypocellularity in the Ts65Dn mouse originates early in development. Brain Res. 2006;1104:153–9.
62. Contestabile A, Fila T, Ceccarelli C, Bonasoni P, Bonapace L, Santini D, Bartesaghi R, Ciani E. Cell cycle alteration and decreased cell proliferation in the hippocampal dentate gyrus and in the neocortical germinal matrix of fetuses with Down syndrome and in Ts65Dn mice. Hippocampus. 2007;17:665–78.
63. Contestabile A, Fila T, Bartesaghi R, Ciani E. Cell cycle elongation impairs proliferation of cerebellar granule cell precursors in the Ts65Dn mouse, an animal model for Down syndrome. Brain Pathol. 2009;19:224–37.
64. Guidi S, Bonasoni P, Ceccarelli C, Santini D, Gualtieri F, Ciani E, Bartesaghi R. Neurogenesis impairment and increased cell death reduce total neuron number in the hippocampal region of fetuses with Down syndrome. Brain Pathol. 2008;18:180–97.
65. Insausti AM, Megias M, Crespo D, Cruz-Orive LM, Dierssen M, Vallina IF, Insausti R, Florez J. Hippocampal volume and neuronal number in Ts65Dn mice: a murine model of Down syndrome. Neurosci Lett. 1998;253:175–8.
66. Kleschevnikov AM, Belichenko PV, Villar AJ, Epstein CJ, Malenka RC, Mobley WC. Hippocampal long-term potentiation suppressed by increased inhibition in the Ts65Dn mouse, a genetic model of Down syndrome. J Neurosci. 2004;24:8153–60.
67. Guidi S, Stagni F, Bianchi P, Ciani E, Giacomini A, De Franceschi M, Moldrich R, Kurniawan N, Mardon K, Giuliani A, et al. Prenatal pharmacotherapy rescues brain development in a Down's syndrome mouse model. Brain. 2014;137:380–401.
68. Giacomini A, Stagni F, Trazzi S, Guidi S, Emili M, Brigham E, Ciani E, Bartesaghi R. Inhibition of APP gamma-secretase restores sonic hedgehog signaling and neurogenesis in the Ts65Dn mouse model of Down syndrome. Neurobiol Dis. 2015;82:385–96.
69. Stagni F, Raspanti A, Giacomini A, Guidi S, Emili M, Ciani E, Giuliani A, Bighinati A, Calza L, Magistretti J, Bartesaghi R. Long-term effect of neonatal inhibition of APP gamma-secretase on hippocampal development in the Ts65Dn mouse model of Down syndrome. Neurobiol Dis. 2017;103:11–23.
70. Di Domenico F, Pupo G, Mancuso C, Barone E, Paolini F, Arena A, Blarzino C, Schmitt FA, Head E, Butterfield DA, Perluigi M. Bach1 overexpression in Down syndrome correlates with the alteration of the HO-1/BVR-a system: insights for transition to Alzheimer's disease. J Alzheimers Dis. 2015;44:1107–20.
71. Lanzillotta C, Tramutola A, Meier S, Schmitt F, Barone E, Perluigi M, Di Domenico F, Abisambra JF. Early and selective activation and subsequent alterations to the unfolded protein response in Down syndrome mouse models. J Alzheimers Dis. 2018;62:347–59.
72. Di Domenico F, Tramutola A, Foppoli C, Head E, Perluigi M, Butterfield DA. mTOR in Down syndrome: role in ass and tau neuropathology and transition to Alzheimer disease-like dementia. Free Radic Biol Med. 2018;114:94–101.
73. Korolchuk VI, Menzies FM, Rubinsztein DC. Mechanisms of cross-talk between the ubiquitin-proteasome and autophagy-lysosome systems. FEBS Lett. 2010;584:1393–8.
74. Butterfield DA, Di Domenico F, Swomley AM, Head E, Perluigi M. Redox proteomics analysis to decipher the neurobiology of Alzheimer-like neurodegeneration: overlaps in Down's syndrome and Alzheimer's disease brain. Biochem J. 2014;463:177–89.
75. Head E, Lott IT, Wilcock DM, Lemere CA. Aging in Down syndrome and the development of Alzheimer's disease neuropathology. Curr Alzheimer Res. 2016;13:18–29.
76. Lemere CA, Blusztajn JK, Yamaguchi H, Wisniewski T, Saido TC, Selkoe DJ. Sequence of deposition of heterogeneous amyloid beta-peptides and APO E in Down syndrome: implications for initial events in amyloid plaque formation. Neurobiol Dis. 1996;3:16–32.
77. Troca-Marin JA, Alves-Sampaio A, Montesinos ML. Deregulated mTOR-mediated translation in intellectual disability. Prog Neurobiol. 2012;96:268–82.
78. Andrade-Talavera Y, Benito I, Casanas JJ, Rodriguez-Moreno A, Montesinos ML. Rapamycin restores BDNF-LTP and the persistence of long-term memory in a model of Down's syndrome. Neurobiol Dis. 2015;82:516–25.
79. Caccamo A, Majumder S, Deng JJ, Bai Y, Thornton FB, Oddo S. Rapamycin rescues TDP-43 mislocalization and the associated low molecular mass neurofilament instability. J Biol Chem. 2009;284:27416–24.
80. Lin AL, Zheng W, Halloran JJ, Burbank RR, Hussong SA, Hart MJ, Javors M, Shih YY, Muir E, Solano Fonseca R, et al. Chronic rapamycin restores brain vascular integrity and function through NO synthase activation and improves memory in symptomatic mice modeling Alzheimer's disease. J Cereb Blood Flow Metab. 2013;33:1412–21.
81. Ramirez AE, Pacheco CR, Aguayo LG, Opazo CM. Rapamycin protects against Abeta-induced synaptotoxicity by increasing presynaptic activity in hippocampal neurons. Biochim Biophys Acta. 1842;2014:1495–501.
82. Lochhead JJ, Thorne RG. Intranasal delivery of biologics to the central nervous system. Adv Drug Deliv Rev. 2012;64:614–28.
83. Barone E, Tramutola A, Triani F, Calcagnini S, Di Domenico F, Ripoli C, Gaetani S, Grassi C, Butterfield DA, Cassano T, Perluigi M. Biliverdin Reductase-A Mediates the beneficial effects of intranasal insulin in Alzheimer disease. Mol Neurobiol. 2018; https://doi.org/10.1007/s12035-018-1231-5.
84. Chen Y, Zhao Y, Dai CL, Liang Z, Run X, Iqbal K, Liu F, Gong CX. Intranasal insulin restores insulin signaling, increases synaptic proteins, and reduces Abeta level and microglia activation in the brains of 3xTg-AD mice. Exp Neurol. 2014;261:610–9.
85. Freiherr J, Hallschmid M, Frey WH, Brunner YF, Chapman CD, Holscher C, Craft S, De Felice FG, Benedict C. Intranasal insulin as a treatment for

Alzheimer's disease: a review of basic research and clinical evidence. Cns Drugs. 2013;27:505–14.
86. Ram G, Chinen J. Infections and immunodeficiency in Down syndrome. Clin Exp Immunol. 2011;164:9–16.
87. Carsetti R, Valentini D, Marcellini V, Scarsella M, Marasco E, Giustini F, Bartuli A, Villani A, Ugazio AG. Reduced numbers of switched memory B cells with high terminal differentiation potential in Down syndrome. Eur J Immunol. 2015;45:903–14.
88. Kusters MA, Verstegen RH, Gemen EF, de Vries E. Intrinsic defect of the immune system in children with Down syndrome: a review. Clin Exp Immunol. 2009;156:189–93.
89. Cuadrado E, Barrena MJ. Immune dysfunction in Down's syndrome: primary immune deficiency or early senescence of the immune system? Clin Immunol Immunopathol. 1996;78:209–14.
90. Butterfield DA, Galvan V, Lange MB, Tang H, Sowell RA, Spilman P, Fombonne J, Gorostiza O, Zhang J, Sultana R, Bredesen DE. In vivo oxidative stress in brain of Alzheimer disease transgenic mice: requirement for methionine 35 in amyloid beta-peptide of APP. Free Radic Biol Med. 2010;48:136–44.
91. Zhao J, Garcia GA, Goldberg AL. Control of proteasomal proteolysis by mTOR. Nature. 2016;529:E1–2.
92. Laplante M, Sabatini DM. Regulation of mTORC1 and its impact on gene expression at a glance. J Cell Sci. 2013;126:1713–9.
93. Wolvetang EW, Bradfield OM, Tymms M, Zavarsek S, Hatzistavrou T, Kola I, Hertzog PJ. The chromosome 21 transcription factor ETS2 transactivates the beta-APP promoter: implications for Down syndrome. Biochim Biophys Acta. 2003;1628:105–10.
94. Li M, Zhang Z, Hill DL, Wang H, Zhang RW. Curcumin, a dietary component, has anticancer, chemosensitization, and radiosensitization effects by down-regulating the MDM2 oncogene through the PI3K/mTOR/ETS2 pathway. Cancer Res. 2007;67:1988–96.
95. Caccamo A, Magri A, Medina DX, Wisely EV, Lopez-Aranda MF, Silva AJ, Oddo S. mTOR regulates tau phosphorylation and degradation: implications for Alzheimer's disease and other tauopathies. Aging Cell. 2013;12:370–80.
96. Barone E, Di Domenico F, Cassano T, Arena A, Tramutola A, Lavecchia MA, Coccia R, Butterfield DA, Perluigi M. Impairment of biliverdin reductase-a promotes brain insulin resistance in Alzheimer disease: a new paradigm. Free Radic Biol Med. 2016;91:127–42.
97. Bedse G, Di Domenico F, Serviddio G, Cassano T. Aberrant insulin signaling in Alzheimer's disease: current knowledge. Front Neurosci. 2015;9:204.
98. Haruta T, Uno T, Kawahara J, Takano A, Egawa K, Sharma PM, Olefsky JM, Kobayashi M. A rapamycin-sensitive pathway down-regulates insulin signaling via phosphorylation and proteasomal degradation of insulin receptor substrate-1. Mol Endocrinol. 2000;14:783–94.
99. Butterfield DA, Di Domenico F, Barone E. Elevated risk of type 2 diabetes for development of Alzheimer disease: a key role for oxidative stress in brain. Biochim Biophys Acta. 1842;2014:1693–706.
100. Mao YF, Guo Z, Zheng T, Jiang Y, Yan Y, Yin X, Chen Y, Zhang B. Intranasal insulin alleviates cognitive deficits and amyloid pathology in young adult APPswe/PS1dE9 mice. Aging Cell. 2016;15:893–902.
101. Solano DC, Sironi M, Bonfini C, Solerte SB, Govoni S, Racchi M. Insulin regulates soluble amyloid precursor protein release via phosphatidyl inositol 3 kinase-dependent pathway. FASEB J. 2000;14:1015–22.
102. Kim J, Kundu M, Viollet B, Guan KL. AMPK and mTOR regulate autophagy through direct phosphorylation of Ulk1. Nat Cell Biol. 2011;13:132–41.
103. Cardenas AM, Ardiles AO, Barraza N, Baez-Matus X, Caviedes P. Role of tau protein in neuronal damage in Alzheimer's disease and Down syndrome. Arch Med Res. 2012;43:645–54.
104. Lee MJ, Lee JH, Rubinsztein DC. Tau degradation: the ubiquitin-proteasome system versus the autophagy-lysosome system. Prog Neurobiol. 2013;105: 49–59.
105. Wang Y, Martinez-Vicente M, Kruger U, Kaushik S, Wong E, Mandelkow EM, Cuervo AM, Mandelkow E. Tau fragmentation, aggregation and clearance: the dual role of lysosomal processing. Hum Mol Genet. 2009;18:4153–70.
106. Barone E, Head E, Butterfield DA, Perluigi M. HNE-modified proteins in Down syndrome: involvement in development of Alzheimer disease neuropathology. Free Radic Biol Med. 2017;111:262–9.

24

Dopaminergic neurons show increased low-molecular-mass protein 7 activity induced by 6-hydroxydopamine in vitro and in vivo

Ming-Shu Mo[1†], Gui-Hua Li[1†], Cong-Cong Sun[2†], Shu-Xuan Huang[1], Lei Wei[1], Li-Min Zhang[3], Miao-Miao Zhou[1], Zhuo-Hua Wu[1], Wen-Yuan Guo[1], Xin-Ling Yang[4], Chao-Jun Chen[5], Shao-Gang Qu[6], Jian-Xing He [7*] and Ping-Yi Xu[1,4*]

Abstract

Background: Abnormal expression of major histocompatibility complex class I (MHC-I) is increased in dopaminergic (DA) neurons in the substantia nigra (SN) in Parkinson's disease (PD). Low-molecular-mass protein 7 (β5i) is a proteolytic subunit of the immunoproteasome that regulates protein degradation and the MHC pathway in immune cells.

Methods: In this study, we investigated the role of β5i in DA neurons using a 6-hydroxydopamine (6-OHDA) model in vitro and *vivo*.

Results: We showed that 6-OHDA upregulated β5i expression in DA neurons in a concentration- and time-dependent manner. Inhibition and downregulation of β5i induced the expression of glucose-regulated protein (Bip) and exacerbated 6-OHDA neurotoxicity in DA neurons. The inhibition of β5i further promoted the activation of Caspase 3-related pathways induced by 6-OHDA. β5i also activated transporter associated with antigen processing 1 (TAP1) and promoted MHC-I expression on DA neurons.

Conclusion: Taken together, our data suggest that β5i is activated in DA neurons under 6-OHDA treatment and may play a neuroprotective role in PD.

Keywords: Parkinson's disease, 6-hydroxydopamine, Immunoproteasome, TAP1

Background

Oxidative stress, accumulation of aggregated and misfolded protein aggregates, and neuroinflammation have been suggested to play roles in the pathogenesis of Parkinson's disease (PD) [1, 2] These factors impair the ubiquitin-proteasome system (UPS) which is critical for protein metabolic homeostasis [3–5], and they promote the replacement of constitutive proteasome subunits β1, β2 and β5 by the respective immunoproteasome catalytic subunits β1i/ low-molecular-mass protein 2 (LMP2, PSMB9), β2i/multicatalytic endo- peptidase complex-like 1 (MECL1, PSMB10) and β5i (LMP7, PSMB8) [6–8]. The immunoproteasome helps to degrade abnormal proteins, present cleaved peptides as antigens to major histocompatibility complex (MHC) molecules and regulate neuroinflammation [9, 10].

Immunoproteasome expression is low in normal young human brains but higher in brain specimens from older normal subjects and Alzheimer's disease (AD) patients [11, 12]. LMP2 knockout mice show classic AD-like symptoms and severe oxidative stress involved in Aβ aggregation [12, 13]. In Huntington's disease (HD), immunoproteasomes may contribute to the metabolism of huntingtin protein, which is not easily degraded by classical proteasomes [14].

* Correspondence: drjianxing.he@gmail.com; pingyixu@sina.com
†Ming-Shu Mo, Gui-Hua Li, and Cong-Cong Sun contributed equally to this work.
[7]Department of Thoracic Surgery, First Affiliated Hospital of Guangzhou Medical University, Guangzhou 510120, Guangdong China
[1]Department of Neurology, First Affiliated Hospital of Guangzhou Medical University, Guangzhou 510120, Guangdong, China
Full list of author information is available at the end of the article

β5i also plays an important role in the regulation of oxidative stress in chronic epilepsy and stroke [15, 16]. β5i expression and changes in proteasomal structure have been found in tyrosine hydroxylase (TH^+) cells in postmortem brains of people with PD-like synucleinopathies such as multiple system atrophy (MSA) and progressive supranuclear palsy (PSP) [17]. β5i is known to shape the antigenic repertoire presented on MHC-I. A recent study demonstrated that catecholamine neurons were more responsive to MHC-I expression under γ-interferon (IFN) treatment and that these neurons were more susceptible to neurotoxicity in neuroinflammatory conditions than in control conditions [18, 19]. However, whether β5i contributes to DA neuronal neurotoxicity remains unclear. In this study, we further explored the role of β5i in the loss of dopaminergic (DA) neurons under 6-hydroxydopamine (6-OHDA) insult in vitro and *vivo*.

Methods

Cell culture

SN4741 cells derived from embryonic substantia nigra and maintained in Dulbecco's-modified Eagle's high-glucose medium (DMEM, Life Technologies, Rockville, MD, USA) supplemented with 10% fetal calf serum (FCS, Irvine Scientific, Santa Ana, CA, USA), 1% glucose (Sigma, St. Louis, MO, USA), 1% penicillin–streptomycin (Gibco™, Invitrogen, China) and 2 mmol/L l-glutamine (Gibco™, Invitrogen, China). SN4741 cells were kindly provided by Prof. Qian-Yang of the Fourth Military Medical University [20]. Cells were grown at 37 °C in 5% CO_2 and subcultured every 3 days as described previously [21].

Cell viability, reactive oxygen species (ROS) and chymotrypsin-like function

CCK-8 (Dojindo, Kumamoto, Japan) was used to analyze cell viability under different treatment conditions according to the manufacturer's recommendations. Cells were trypsinized, suspended and cultured in 96-well plates at a concentration of 5×10^3 cells/well. Each sample was made in triplicate. The plate contained blank, positive and negative control wells. PR-957 (Selleck, Houston, CA, USA) was used as a selective inhibitor of β5i in SN4741 cells [22]. Cells were treated with 6-OHDA or PR-957 overnight or for 48 h, respectively, or with control solution. At different time points, 10 μl cell counting kit-8 (CCK-8) (Dojindo, Kumamoto, Japan) solution dissolved in 100 μl DMEM (Life Technologies, Rockville, MD, USA) replaced the drug in each well. The incubation continued for another 0.5, 1, or 2 h at 37 °C following the manufacturer's instructions. The optical density (OD) value at 450 nm was measured to calculate cell viability using the formula: cell viability (%) = [OD (Sample)-OD (blank control)]/ [OD (negative control)-OD (blank control)] by an ELISA microplate reader (ELX800, BioTeK, USA).

Rhodamine 123 (Sigma-Aldrich, St Louis, MO, USA) was used to measure the mitochondrial membrane potential disruption. Cells were suspended and cultured in 6-well plates. After overnight incubation, groups were exposed to 6-OHDA, PR-957 or control solution. Cells were washed 3 times with PBS and reincubated with 100 μl DMEM (Life Technologies, Rockville, MD, USA) containing 10 μg/mL rhodamine 123 at 37 °C for 30 mins. The fluorescence of rhodamine 123 was detected by a fluorescence spectrophotometer (Shimadzu, Matsuyama, Japan, RF5000U) at 490 nm excitation (Ex) and 520 nm emission (Em).

2′, 7′-Dichlorofluorescin diacetate (DCFH-DA; Sigma-Aldrich, St Louis, MO, USA) was used to measure ROS level following manufacturer's recommendations. Cells were treated with 6-OHDA or PR-957 at different concentrations and exposure durations. After the cells were washed 3 times with PBS, DCFH-DA diluted in DMEM to 10 μM was added and incubated at 37 °C for 20 min. Cells were washed 3 times with DMEM, and the resultant optical density was measured at 488 nm excitation and 525 nm emission by a microplate reader (Spectramax Gemini XS, Molecular Devices, Pennsylvania, USA). The amount of generated ROS was calculated using the formula: [OD (Sample)-OD (Negative control)]/ OD (Negative control).

The chymotrypsin-like activity (CTL) of the immunoproteasome was assayed with Suc-LLVY-AMC [2]. Cells were seeded at a concentration of 1×10^4 cells/well in 96-well plates. Each test was performed in 4 replicates. After treatment with different concentrations of 6-OHDA, cells were harvested and lysed in proteolysis buffer (50 mM Tris-HCl pH 7.4, 5 mM MgCl2, 1 mM DTT ± 0.25 mM ATP). Then, 100 μl containing 2 μg cell lysate was mixed with 50 μM Suc-LLVY-AMC (Sigma-Aldrich, St Louis, MO, USA). After 1 h of equilibration, fluorescence was monitored for 3 h using a SpectraMax M5 plate reader (Molecular Devices, Pennsylvania, USA, Ex/Em: 370 nm/460 nm).

Overexpression plasmid and shRNA transfection

The β5i overexpression plasmid was synthesized by GeneCopoeia (Product ID: EX-Mm34282-M29, GeneCopoeia, Guangzhou, China). This sequence was inserted into a p-EZ-M29 vector containing neomycin as a stable selection marker. The insertion was confirmed by sequencing. The mU6 vector contained the mCherryFP gene as a marker to identify transfection efficiency (Product ID: CSHCTR001, GeneCopoeia, Guangzhou, China). PSMB8 was suppressed by specific shRNA in the mU6 vector (Product ID: RSH052242-mU6, GeneCopoeia, Guangzhou, China) with target sequences GGAATGCAGCCCACTGAATTC, GGAAGGTTCAGATTGAAATGG, GCAGGAAGTTACATTGCTACC and GCCA

AGGAATGCAGGCTATAC and the hairpin loop sequence TCAAGAG. The mU6-pri vector (Product ID: CSHCTR001-mU6, GeneCopoeia, Guangzhou, China) without the target gene and an empty plasmid were used in the negative control (NC) and mock (M) groups, respectively. First, we detected β5i mRNA by qQT-PCR and then confirmed β5i protein expression by Western blot.

Transfection was performed based on manufacturer's instructions (Invitrogen, Grand Island, NY, USA). Cells were suspended and seeded in 24-well plates at a 50% cell density after counting. After 24 h of culture, transfection was performed as follows. Solution A contained 20 pmol shRNA dissolved in 50 μl Opti-MEM without serum, and B solution contained 1 μl lipofectamine 3000 (Invitrogen, Grand Island, NY, USA) dissolved in 50 μl Opti-MEM without serum. Solution A and B were mixed and kept at room temperature for 20 min. The culture medium for each well was replaced with 400 μl serum-free medium. Cells were incubated in this mixture (serum-free medium containing solutions A and B) for 6 h for transfection, which was then replaced with serum medium. Transfection efficiency was assessed by fluorescence on the following day.

Partial 6-OHDA lesion and behavioral test

Forty male Sprague Dawley (SD) rats, ranging from 280 to 300 g in weight, were bred and maintained in the Specific Pathogen-Free Laboratory Animal Center at Guangzhou Medical University (Guangzhou, China). Weight-matched rats were randomly assigned to four groups: the sham group, 6-OHDA (Sigma-Aldrich, St Louis, MO, USA) group, PR-957 (Adooq Bioscience, CA, USA) group and 6-OHDA plus PR-957 group. Rats were anesthetized with ketamine (10%) /xylazine (2%) (Sigma Aldrich, St Louis, MO, USA) and injected with 8 μg 6-OHDA in 4 μl solvent [0.9% *w*/*v* NaCl with 0.1% ascorbic acid (Sigma-Aldrich, St Louis, MO, USA)] into the left anterior medial bundle (Coordinates: AP: - 4.0 mm, ML: - 1.5 mm, DV: - 7.8 mm). Animals in the 6-OHDA plus PR-957 group were given the same dose of 6-OHDA followed by 4 μl PR-957 (50 nM) injected into the lateral ventricle. The sham group was given the same volume of solvent [0.9% *w*/*v* NaCl with 0.1% ascorbic acid]. At 4 weeks after the 6-OHDA injection, rats were tested in the rotation test. Rotation asymmetry was calculated for 30 min after intraperitoneal injection of 0.6 mg/kg apomorphine (Sigma-Aldrich, St Louis, MO, USA) as described previously [23]. All animal studies followed the institutional guidelines for animal experiments of Guangzhou Medical University. All procedures were approved by the Institutional Animal Care and Use Committee of Guangzhou Medical University.

Western blot

After electrophoresis of proteins from SN4141 cells or the midbrain of rats and blocking with 0.5% BSA in PBS, the PVDF membranes (Pall Corporation, Pensacola, FL, USA) were incubated with primary antibodies such as anti-β5i (1:800, Abcam, Cambridge, MA, USA), anti-β5 (1:1000, Abcam, Cambridge, MA, USA) or anti-β-actin (1:2000, CST, Danvers, MA, USA) at 4 °C overnight. The primary antibodies were diluted in blocking solution (LI-COR Biosciences, Lincoln, NE, USA). After the membranes were washed, they were incubated with fluorescent-conjugated secondary antibodies (1: 15000; LI-COR Biosciences, Lincoln, NE, USA) for 1 h in the dark. The Odyssey infrared fluorescence detection system (LI-COR Biosciences, Lincoln, NE, USA) was used for scanning and analysis. For traditional Western blot, secondary antibodies conjugated with horseradish peroxidase (HRP, Santa Cruz Biotechnology, Santa Cruz, CA, USA) and the chemical luminescence detection method (ECL, Pierce Biotechnology, Rockford, IL, USA) were used. Data were scanned and analyzed using the GE 600 system (GE Healthcare, Piscataway, NJ, USA).

Following the protocol used by Goyal et al. [24], 1.0×10^4 cells were inoculated in 96-well plates (Corning, Sigma-Aldrich, Dorset, UK) for the in-cell western assay. Cells were cultured in DMEM with 10% FCS (Irvine Scientific, Santa Ana, CA, USA) for 48 h, which was then replaced with 6-OHDA dissolved in FCS-free DMEM, but the control group was cultured in FCS-free DMEM. Then, each well was washed with PBS and fixed in 4% formaldehyde for 1 h. Formaldehyde was washed away with PBS, and cells were incubated with 0.1% Triton X-100 in PBS (3 times, 5 min each). Then, cells were treated with blocking solution (LI-COR Biosciences, Lincoln, NE, USA) and incubated with mouse anti-β5i (1:800, Abcam, Cambridge, MA, USA) and rabbit anti-β5i (1:800, Abcam, Cambridge, MA, USA) overnight at 4 °C. After the cells were washed, fluorescent-conjugated secondary antibodies (LI-COR Biosciences, Lincoln, NE, USA), diluted at 1: 1000 in PBS, were added, and the cells were incubated for 1 h in the dark at room temperature. Cells were with PBS three times in the dark. Then, plates were imaged on an Odyssey infrared scanner (LI-COR Biosciences, Lincoln, NE, USA).

Immunofluorescence staining and immunohistochemistry

Brain tissue was cut at a thickness of 15 μm and stored at – 20 °C. Primary antibodies used for immunohistochemistry included mouse monoclonal anti-tyrosine hydroxylase (TH) (1:500, MAB318, Merck Millipore, Billerica, MA, USA), anti-β5i (1:500, Abcam, Cambridge, MA, USA) and anti-TAP-1 (1:500, ab10356; Abcam, Cambridge, MA, USA). TAP-1 is a downstream protein that receives peptides provided by the immunoproteasome [25]. After overnight incubation with primary antibodies, the tissue or cells were incubated with secondary antibodies such as Cy3-conjugated anti-mouse IgG (1:400, Jackson Immunoresearch laboratory, PA, USA) and/or Alexa 488-conjugated anti-rabbit IgG (1:400, Molecular Probes, Eugene, OR, USA). Images were acquired using a fluorescence microscope (BX51, Olympus, Fujinon, Japan). For immunohistochemistry, the secondary antibody used was a horseradish peroxidase (HRP)-conjugated goat anti-mouse IgG (1:1000, Kangcheng, Shanghai, China). Sections were stained with 3, 3′-diaminobenzidine (DAB) kits (Wuhan Boster Bioengineering Co., Ltd., Wuhan, China). Images were acquired under a microscope (Olympus AX70; Olympus, Tokyo, Japan). Four images at 200× magnification were taken, with each image covering an area of the SN or striatum, and combined into one figure. Images were analyzed by ImageJ software (version 1.45; National Institutes of Health, Bethesda, Maryland, USA).

Fast TH staining and laser capture microdissection (LCM)

To reduce RNA degradation, we used fast TH staining to detect DA neurons. Slices were fixed in acetone-methanol solution at − 20 °C for 10 min, washed with PBS containing 1% Triton X-100, incubated with the TH antibody (MAB318, Merck Millipore, Billerica, MA, USA) at a 1:100 dilution for 10 min, rinsed in PBS with Triton twice, and incubated with the goat antirabbit antibody with HRP (1:100, Kangcheng, Shanghai, China) for 5 min. Immunohistochemistry staining was done by DAB kits (Wuhan Boster Bioengineering Co., Ltd., Wuhan, China). The stained slices were dehydrated in RNase-free solutions as follows: 100% acetone for 5 min, 75% ethanol, 95 and 100% ethanol for 1 min each, and then xylene twice for 1 min and 5 min.

As described previously [26, 27], nonfixed fresh brain tissue was rapidly frozen and cut into 8-μm-thick slices. Slices were collected on to polyethylene naphthalate membrane-coated glass slides (Life Technologies, Grand Island, NY, USA). After fast tyrosine hydroxylase staining, TH^+ neurons in the substantia nigra were captured by the Arcturus XT system (Life Technologies, CA, USA). Laser power was set at 70 mW and 150 mV. Approximately 300–450 TH^+ neurons were collected, and total RNA was extracted using the mirVana PARIS Kit (PN AM1556, Austin, TX, Ambion, USA) and converted into cDNA by a Reverse Transcription Kit (Takara, Shiga, Japan). RT1A (rat monomorphic MHC class I antigen) binds the peptide or antigens translocated by TAP into the ER, and its mRNA level in DA neurons was detected by qRT-PCR. The PCR primers (TIANGEN Biotech, China) used were as follows: GAPDH-F: 5'-TACTAGCGGTTTTACGGGCG-3′ and GAPDH-R: 5'-TCG-AACAGGAGGAGCAGAGAGCGA-3′; TAP-1-F: 5'-GGCAGACTCAGTTC-CTCTCAC-3′ and TAP-1-R: 5'-CAGAACGGGTTGGGGATCAA-3'; RT1A (Rat monomorphic MHC class I antigen) -F: 5'-GCTC ACACTCGCTGCGGTAT-3′ and RT1A-R: 5'-GCCA TACATCTCCTGGATGG-3′. GAPDH was used as an internal control, and mRNA expression was analyzed using the $2^{-\Delta\Delta CT}$ method [28].

Statistical analysis

All experiments were repeated at least 3 times. Data are shown as the mean ± SD. ANOVA was followed by Tukey's or Student-Newman-Keuls (SNK) post hoc testing. $P < 0.05$ was considered statistically significant. All analyses were performed using SPSS.13 and STATA software (Version 14; StataCorp, College Station, TX, USA).

Results

6-Hydroxydopamine upregulates immunoproteasome expression in DA neurons

SN4741 cells were treated with different concentrations of 6-OHDA for 24 h. The in-cell western assay showed that β5 was upregulated upon treatment with 6-OHDA for 3–18 h and then downregulated after 24 h, whereas β5i was upregulated by 100–300 nM 6-OHDA for 24 h (Fig. 1a, b). The Western blot data further confirmed that β5 and β5i expression were dose-dependently upregulated when the concentration of 6-OHDA was higher than 50 nM (Fig. 1c, d). In the antigen presentation pathway, the expression of glucose-regulated protein (Bip), a regulator involved in protein translocation into the ER [29], and TAP1, a transporter associated with antigen presentation [30], was increased as a dose-dependent manner under 6-OHDA treatment for 24 h (Fig. 1e, f). In the apoptosis pathway, the expression of proapoptotic proteins, such as Bax, Caspase-3 and cleaved-Caspase-3, was upregulated, and the expression of antiapoptotic proteins, such as Bcl-2, was downregulated significantly by 6-OHDA treatment for 24 h (Fig. 1g, h).

When SN4741 cells were treated with 200 nM 6-OHDA for different exposure times, β5 was upregulated, reaching a peak expression at 12 h (Additional file 1: Figure S1. A, B), whereas β5i, TAP1 and Bip expression were significantly increased upon 6-OHDA treatment at 24 h (Additional file 1: Figure S1. A-D). In vivo, increased expression of β5, β5i, TAP1 and Bip was further confirmed in the SN of the rat after 6-OHDA treatment for 24 h (Fig. 2a-d) and was accompanied by an increased percent of neurons with β5i and TH^+ expression (Fig. 2e).

β5i dysfunction inhibits antigen presentation in DA neurons

SN4741 cells were then treated with 50 nM PR-957 [22]. We noted that CTL associated with β5i function decreased more than 50% but had no significant neurotoxicity in vitro

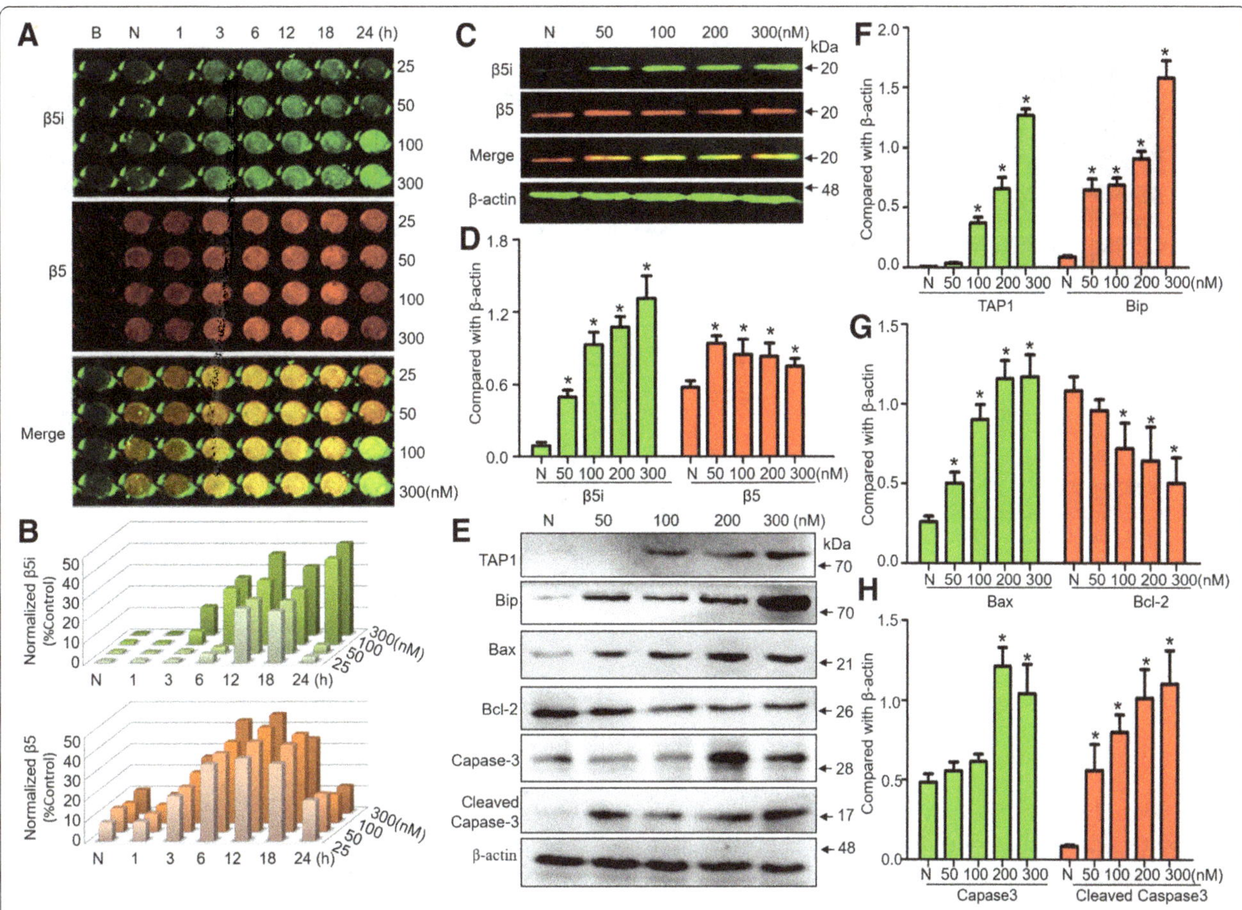

Fig. 1 6-Hydroxydopamine activates immunoproteasomes in DA neurons in a dose-dependent manner. **a** The expression of β5 and β5i in SN4741 cells under 6-OHDA treatment by in-cell western assay and (**b**) the fluorescence intensity in each group after normalization to that in the normal group are shown. **c-h** The expression of β5, β5i, TAP1, Bip, Bax, Bcl-2, Caspase-3 and Cleaved Caspase-3 in SN4741 cells after different concentrations of 6-OHDA treatment for 24 h. Data are presented as the mean ± SD; $n = 4$ experiments; two-way ANOVA and post hoc SNK t-test

(Fig. 3a). TAP1 expression was decreased after 50 nM PR-957 treatment for 3 h (Fig. 3b, c). PR-957 at 100 nM induced neurotoxicity, with significant upregulation of Bax and Bip and downregulation of TH after 24 h treatment (Fig. 3d-f). In vivo, 50 nM PR-957 was stereotaxically injected into the left anterior medial bundle in SD rats. After 24 h, TAP1 and Bip expression in the lesioned side of the SN significantly decreased and increased, respectively (Fig. 3g-h), but TH expression was not changed (Fig. 3i). Our data suggested that 50 nM PR-957 for 24 h may be optimal for β5i inhibition without significant neurotoxicity in vitro and in vivo.

β5i inhibition exacerbates 6-hydroxydopamine-induced DA neuronal damage

Cell morphology, viability and apoptosis were not significantly affected by treatment with PR-957 alone in vitro. However, cotreatment with PR-957 and 6-OHDA dramatically induced cell shrinkage and pyknosis, accompanied by a significant increase in ROS and decrease in cell viability compared to treatment with 6-OHDA alone (Fig. 4a, b). Treatment with PR-957 alone did not affect Caspase-3 or cleaved Caspase-3 expression, but cotreatment significantly exacerbated the 6-OHDA-induced activation of Caspase-3 and cleaved Caspase-3 (Fig. 4c, d). In vivo, we examined the additional loss of DA neurons in the 6-OHDA hemilesioned rats after inhibition of β5i by PR-957 4 weeks after treatment. The number of TH$^+$ cells in the lesioned side did not change after treatment with PR-957 alone. The 6-OHDA-induced hemilesion in the SN was partial in this 6-OHDA model. Compared to 58.3% loss of TH$^+$ cells under 6-OHDA treatment alone, a 74.2% loss of TH$^+$ cells was observed in the lesioned side of rats with DA neuronal damage exacerbated by PR-957, and these rats also exhibited a significant increase in apomorphine-induced rotation (Fig. 4e-g). In the striatum, the TH level on the lesioned side was only at 13.8% of that

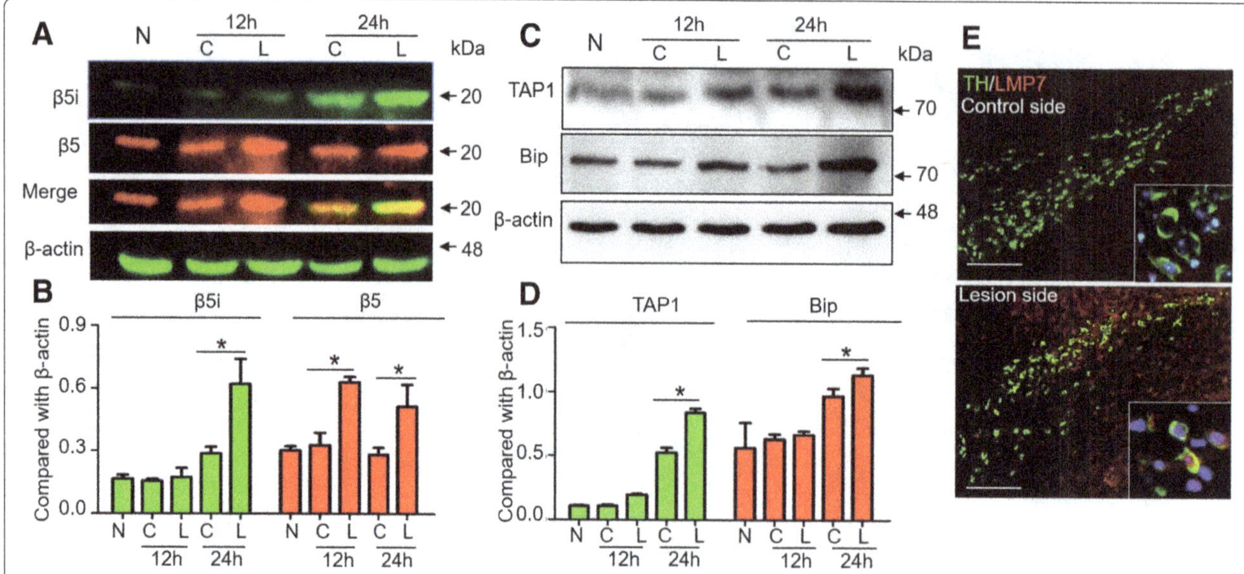

Fig. 2 6-Hydroxydopamine activates immunoproteasomes in DA neurons in vivo. The expression of β5, β5i (**a, b**), TAP1 and Bip (**c, d**) in the SN of the 6-OHDA hemilesioned rat model. **e** The colocalization of β5i on TH neurons in the SN at 1 day after 6-OHDA treatment. Scale bar = 100 μm. * $P < 0.05$, compared with control. N, normal group without treatment. C, control side of the brain. L, lesioned side of the brain. Data are presented as the mean ± SD; $n = 4$ experiments; one-way ANOVA and post hoc SNK t-test

on the control side in the cotreatment group, which was significantly lower than the 21.5% in the group given 6-OHDA treatment alone (Additional file 2: Figure S2).

Downregulated β5i expression impairs antigen presentation in DA neurons under 6-OHDA treatment

CTL function was significantly impaired and enhanced in SN4741 cells after β5i mRNA down- and upregulation, respectively (Fig. 5a). β5i expression was manipulated by RNAi in the normal condition (Fig. 5b, c) and with 6-OHDA treatment (Fig. 5d, e). In vitro, the upregulation of β5i mRNA significantly promoted TAP1 expression and inhibited Bip expression under 6-OHDA treatment, and downregulation of β5i mRNA had an inverse effect (Fig. 5f, g). After β5i function was inhibited by PR-957, the 6-OHDA-induced upregulation of TAP1 was significantly inhibited, and Bip expression was slightly increased in SN4741 cells (Fig. 5h, i) and rats (Fig. 6b, c). Immunofluorescence result showed that the 6-OHDA-induced increase in TAP1 expression was colocalized with TH^+ cells and was attenuated by PR-957 (Fig. 6a). Laser capture microscopy was used to capture TH^+ neurons from the SN of rats administered 6-OHDA (Fig. 6d). A significant increase in TAP1 and RT1A (MHC-I) mRNA expression in laser-captured TH^+ neurons was found at 24 h after 6-OHDA treatment, which was inhibited by PR-957 (Fig. 6e).

Discussion

Immunoproteasome and MHC molecules are minimally expressed in the healthy brain, and their activation and upregulation are indicative of a pathological status in the central nervous system (CNS) [12, 19, 31, 32]. The examination of brain specimens from people with neurodegenerative disorders such as AD, HD, and amyotrophic lateral sclerosis (ALS) have revealed dysfunctions in immunoproteasome activity [12, 33, 34], and these phenomena have also been found in those with autoimmune encephalomyelitis (EAE) and epilepsy [8, 15]. A similar failure in proteolytic mechanisms, as well as increases in oxidative stress and neuroinflammation, have also been reported in PD [35]. We propose the following scenario to describe the role of β5i in PD pathogenesis. Initially, ROS and the unfolded protein response (UPR) induce ER stress and neuronal damage in DA neurons. Then, Bip is activated and ships abnormal proteins from the ER to the UPS. The overloaded proteins induce the activation of β5i and transformation of the immunoproteasome to have an updated and expanded proteasome capacity. Consequently, the ubiquitinated proteins are degraded to peptides by β5i and recognized by MHC-I. Here, our study revealed that β5i is activated in DA neurons exposed to 6-OHDA, and upregulation of β5i or other immunoproteasome components might play a neuroprotective role against ROS-mediated damage in PD.

The UPS is a key factor in the proteostasis network [36]. Different subunit configurations of the UPS, such as the

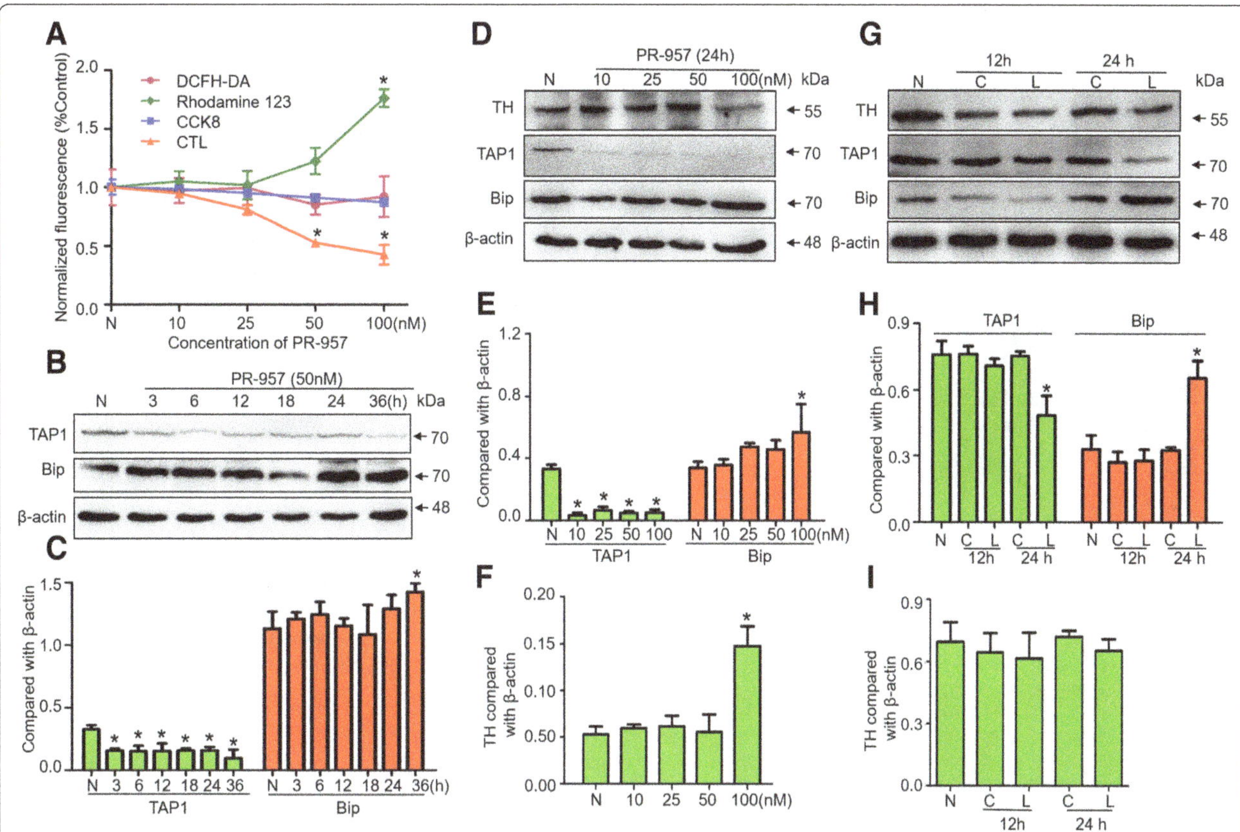

Fig. 3 β5i inhibition impairs antigen presentation in DA neuron. **a** The cytotoxic effect and chymotrypsin-like proteasome activity in the SN4741 cell line treated with PR-957 for 24 h were estimated by various methods such as DCFH-DA, rhodamine 123, CCK8 and CTL tests ($n = 5$ experiments). DCFH-DA, rhodamine 123 and CCK-8 were respectively used to measure ROS, the mitochondrial membrane potential and cell viability. A CTL assay was used to detect the chymotrypsin-like activity of cells. (**b, c**) Western blot analysis of TAP1 and Bip in SN4741 cells after treatment with 50 nM PR-957. Western blot analysis of TH, TAP1 and Bip in SN4741 cells 24 h after PR-957 treatment (**d-f**) and in PD model rats (**g-i**). CTL, chymotrypsin-like proteasome activity. N, normal group without treatment. C, control side of the rat brain. L, lesioned side of the rat brain. Data presented as the mean ± SD; $n = 4$ experiments; * $P < 0.05$, compared with the control; one-way ANOVA and post hoc SNK t-test

standard proteasome, immuneoproteasome, mixed-type proteasome, thymoproteasome and spermatoproteasome, acquire different proteolytic capacities [37]. The immunoproteasomes activated by ROS, lipopolysaccharide (LPS) and IFN-γ have strong capabilities to clear protein deposits and alleviate ROS impairment [8, 38]. The overloading of damaged proteins and insufficient proteolytic capacity may trigger immunoproteasomes to replace impaired proteasome subunits [39]. X-ray crystallography studies have shown that the enzyme active center of the immunoproteasome (iUPS) provides a larger space than the enzyme active center of other proteasomes to accommodate and degrade misfolded or oxidized proteins [40]. For example, the immunoproteasome eliminates the extended huntingtin proteins of HD, Aβ aggregates of AD and mutant SOD1 deposition of ALS more efficiently [14, 41, 42]. Under normal conditions, oxidized cytoplasmic and nuclear proteins are generally degraded by the proteasome [43]. The 20S proteasome, immunoproteasome and PA28αβ regulator are all upregulated under H_2O_2-induced oxidative stress, and the immunoproteasome may degrade oxidized proteins more selectively than the other proteasomes [43]. Some studies have suggested that the enhanced proteolytic activity of the immunoproteasome more efficiently clears aggregated proteins and is important for cell viability under IFN-γ treatment [8]. Others have suggested that the function of the immunoproteasome to bind and degrade ubiquitin conjugates is similar to that of constitutive proteasomes [44]. Recently, we reported that Chinese females carrying the rs17587-G/G mutation of PSMB9 are at a higher risk of PD [35]. The rs17587 variation at exon 4 of PSMB9 affects the glutamyl peptide hydrolyzing activity associated with proteolytic function [45]. As an immunoproteasome subunit, β5i has been found to be involved in proteinopathies and the innate immune response [37]. In this study, we further explored the role of β5i in the 6-OHDA model of PD. Our results showed that β5i was activated and upregulated in a

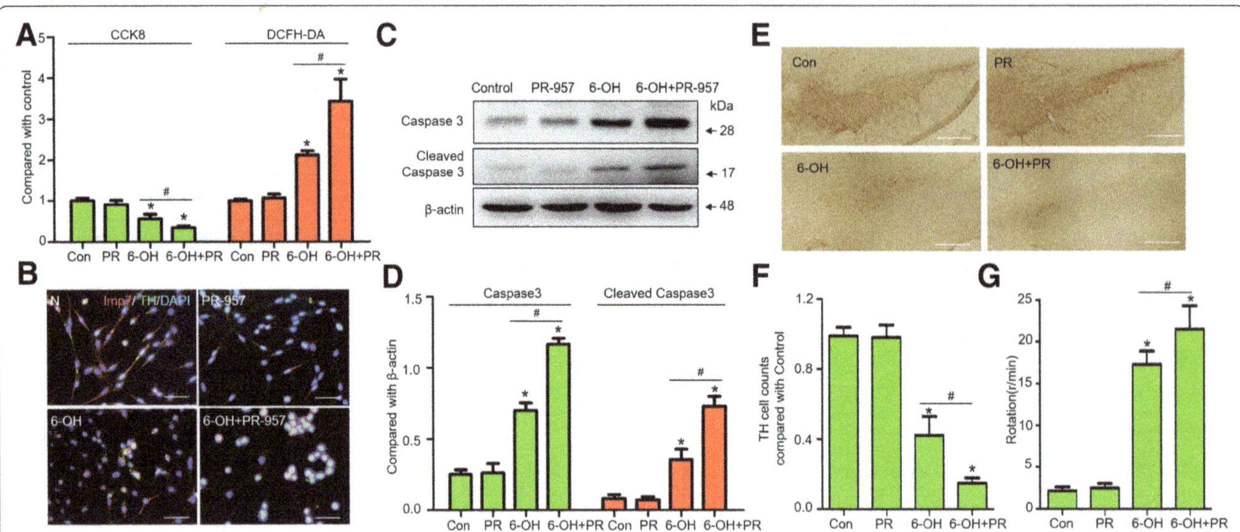

Fig. 4 β5i inhibition exacerbates 6-hydroxydopamine-induced DA neuronal damage. **a** Cytotoxic effect on the SN4741 cell line of different treatments for 24 h analyzed by CCK8 and DCFH-DA tests (n = 5 experiments). **b** Immunofluorescence staining of β5i in SN4741 cells. Scale bar = 100 μm. **c, d** The expression of Caspase-3 and cleaved Caspase-3 in SN4741 cells after treatment with 6-OHDA or PR-957 for 24 h. **e, f** Immunohistochemistry of TH^+ cells in rats after 6-OHDA treatment for 4 weeks. Scale bar = 200 μm. **g** Apomorphine-induced rotation scores after 6-OHDA treatment for 4 weeks (*n* = 6 experiments). Data are presented as the mean ± SD; n = 4 experiments; * $P < 0.05$, compared with control; # $P < 0.05$, compared with the 6-OHDA group; one-way ANOVA

dose- and time-dependent manner after 6-OHDA treatment in a DA neuron cell line, and this was further confirmed in the 6-OHDA hemilesioned rat model of PD. ER stress and oxidative stress have been suggested to contribute to the loss of DA neurons in PD [46]. Compared to the standard proteasome, the immunoproteasome is thought to be more resistant to oxidative stress and ER stress [8]. When protein homeostasis is impaired in neurons, misfolded proteins aggregate in the ER and induce ER stress [47]. Bip is upregulated and binds aggregated proteins for transportation from the ER to the UPS [29]. If the UPS and immunoproteasome system are deficient, neurons are more susceptible to apoptosis due to the stress from the accumulation of oxidized proteins [8, 48]. In aging-related sporadic inclusion body myositis, intracellular protein aggregation was accompanied by ER stress and proteasome dysfunction [49]. A study from X-linked adrenoleukodystrophy revealed that β5i was significantly elevated and recruited to mitochondria in response to oxidative stress where it participated in mitochondrial protein quality control [3]. Recently, IFN-γ-induced oxidative stress was found to upregulate β5i expression with increased poly-Ub substrate degradation efficiency [8]. In this study, we used a 6-OHDA model to induce massive oxidative stress and the unfolded protein response in DA neurons [50]. ROS and ER stress occurred in a dose- and time-dependent manner following 6-OHDA treatment [51]. We found that inhibition and downregulation of β5i resulted in DA neurons with increased sensitivity to 6-OHDA toxicity, suggesting that the neuroprotective effect of β5i may be related to ROS regulation and ER stress at the early stage of PD.

Immunoproteasomes still play an important role in the regulation of neuroinflammation [13, 52]. In the peripheral immune system, immunoproteasome subunits degrade proteins to peptides, which present to TAP1 as antigens [25]. As a peptide transporter protein, TAP1 loads antigenic peptides into the ER where MHC molecules recognize antigens and present them to the cell membrane [30, 53]. IFN-γ-signaling has been proven to promote MHC class I antigen presentation, and IFN-γ-regulated inflammation in proteasome-associated autoinflammatory syndromes (PRAAS) was partly reduced after inhibition of proteolytic function [54, 55]. As a highly selective inhibitor of β5i, PR-957 was shown to reduce the release of IL-23 and TNF-α from inflammatory cells by 90 and 50%, respectively [22]. PR-957 also inhibits inflammation in MOG35–55-induced experimental autoimmune encephalomyelitis [56]. Notably, neurodegenerative diseases predominantly display disorders of neuroinflammation. In transgenic mouse models of AD and human postmortem tissue, immunoproteasome activities and HLA-DR expression are strongly increased and accompanied by overactivated microglia in the cortex. [57, 58] Previously, neurons were considered to be 'immunoprivileged' without antigen presentation capabilities [59, 60]; now MHC-1 expression has been demonstrated on DA neurons in

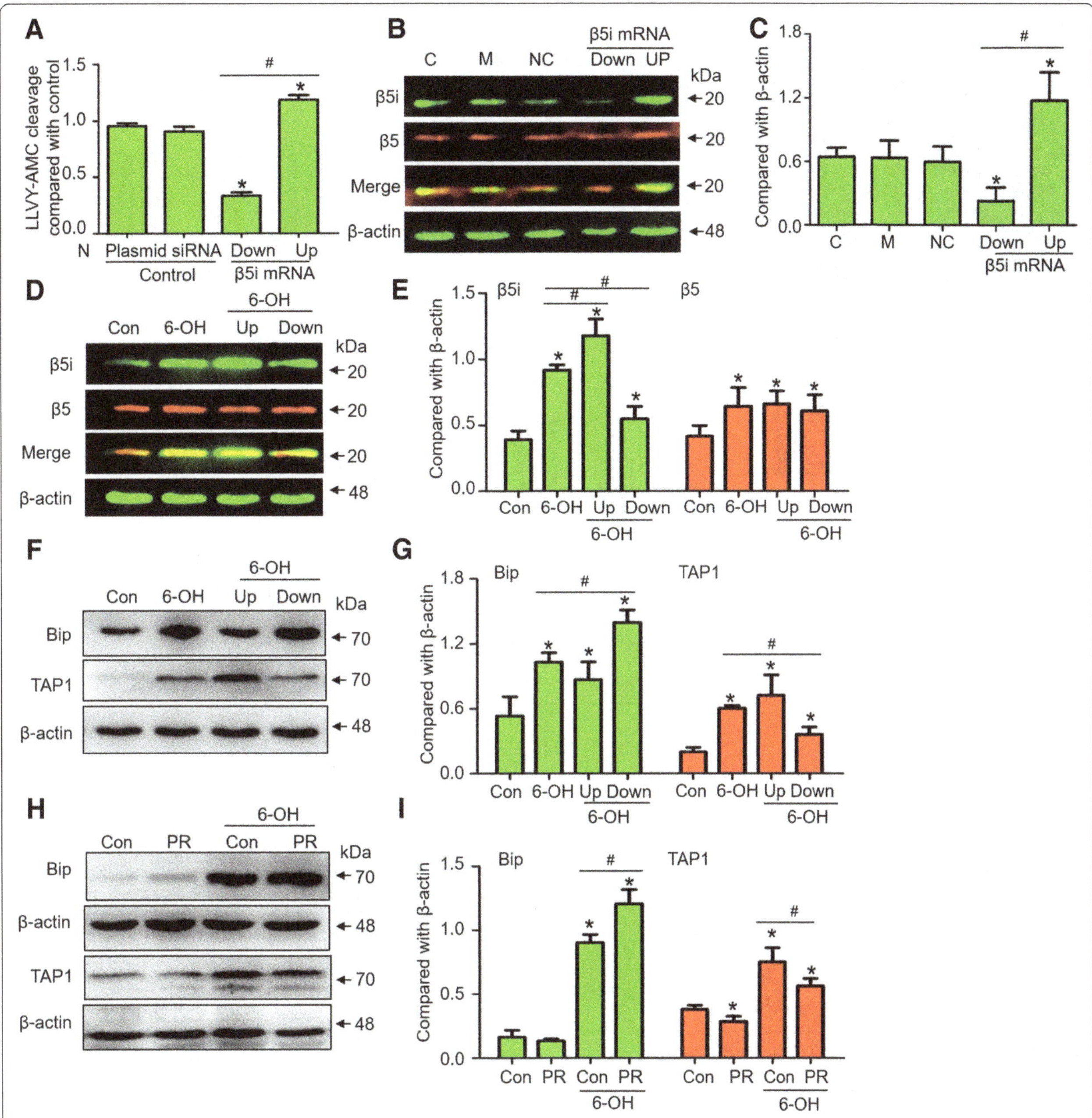

Fig. 5 β5i regulates antigen presentation on DA neurons under 6-hydroxydopamine in vitro. **a** Chymotrypsin-like proteasome activity on SN4741 cell line was assessed by proteasome activity assays ($n = 5$ experiments). The expression of β5 and β5i in SN4741 cells at 24 h after the regulation of β5i by RNAi under normal conditions (**b, c**) and 6-OHDA treatment (**d, e**). The expression of Bip and TAP1 in SN4741 cells at 24 h after β5i downregulation by RNAi (**f, g**), and inhibition with PR-957 (**h, i**). N, normal group without treatment. C, normal condition. M, treated with an empty plasmid. NC, treated with the siRNA negative control. Up, upregulated β5i by overexpression plasmid. Down, downregulated β5i by shRNA. Data are presented as the mean ± SD; n = 4 experiments; * $P < 0.05$, compared with control; # $P < 0.05$, compared with the 6-OHDA group; one-way ANOVA

the rodent and human brain [18, 19]. The catecholaminergic neurons expressing MHC-1 have been shown to be more susceptible to apoptosis induction, suggesting that these neurons may be targeted by ROS during the development of PD [19]. In this study, our results revealed significant upregulation of MHC-I and TAP1 accompanied by increased expression of β5i on DA neurons under 6-OHDA treatment and that MHC-I and TAP1 mRNA levels were decreased after β5i inhibition. These findings suggest that β5i may regulate the TAP1/MHC-I pathway in DA neurons under oxidative stress.

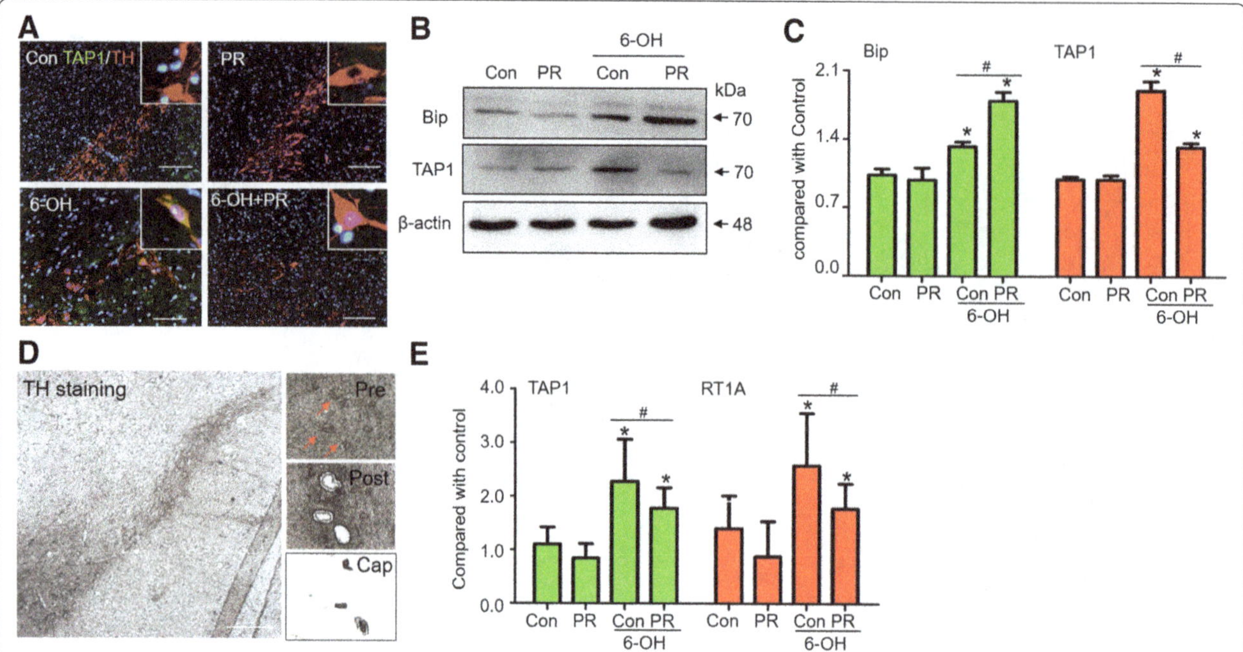

Fig. 6 β5i regulates antigen presentation on DA neurons under 6-OHDA in vivo. **a** The expression and collocation of TAP1 after 6-OHDA for 1 day in the rat. **b, c** The expression of Bip and TAP1 at 24 h after inhibition with PR-957 in the 6-OHDA hemilesioned rats. **d** TH^+ neurons in the SN were collected by LCM. The precaptured (Pre), postcaptured (Post) and captured (Cap) images are shown in the right column, and TH^+ cells are indicated with red arrows. Scale bar = 100 μm. **e** qRT-PCR result of captured TH^+ cells ($n = 6$ experiments). Error bars represent SD. * $P < 0.05$, compared with control; # $P < 0.05$, compared with 6-OHDA treatment but without PR-957

Conclusions

In conclusion, our data showed that β5i was activated by 6-OHDA-induced oxidative stress in DA neurons both in vitro and in vivo and may play a neuroprotective role in the survival of DA neurons. Our data might provide new evidence for the consideration of the immunoproteasome as a potential therapeutic target for PD.

Additional files

Additional file 1: Figure S1. 6-Hydroxydopamine activates immunoproteasomes in DA neurons in a time-dependent manner. The expression of β5, β5i (A-B), TAP1 and Bip (C-D) in SN4741 cells after different durations of exposure to 200 nM 6-OHDA. * $P < 0.05$, compared with the normal condition. Data are presented as the mean ± SD; $n = 4$; one-way ANOVA and post hoc SNK t-test. (TIF 518 kb)

Additional file 2: Figure S2. β5i inhibition exacerbates 6-hydroxydopamine-induced damage in the striatum. (A) Immunostaining of TH in the rat striatum after 6-OHDA treatment for 4 weeks. Scale bar = 200 μm. (B) Quantification of TH immunoreactivity in the striatum. Data are presented as the mean ± SD; n = 4 experiments; * $P < 0.05$, compared with the control; # $P < 0.05$, compared with the 6-OHDA group; one-way ANOVA. (TIF 1137 kb)

Acknowledgements

This work was supported by research grants from National Key R&D Program of China (2016YFC1306600, SQ2017YFSF110116), National Natural Science Foundation of China (81701254, 81471292, U1603281, U1503222, 81430021, 81501100, NO.8187050204), Science Foundation of Guangdong of China (2015A030311021, 2018A030313649), a technology project of Guangzhou (201504281820463), Shandong Provincial Natural Science Foundation (BS2015YY041), International Project of Science and Technology for Guangdong (2016A050502025), Science and Technology of Guangdong of China (2013B022000026) and Collaborative Innovation Foundation of Guangzhou Science and Technology Bureau (2018-1202-SF-0019).
We thank Dr. Madhuvika Murugan, You-Sheng Xiao, Luan Chen, Li Zhang, Ming Lei, Chao-Hao Yang, Xiang Chen, Qin-Hui Huang, Wei-Guo Liu, Long-Jun Wu and Prof. Kai-Ping Li for their help to improve this manuscript. We thank Prof. Qian Yang provide SN4741 cells.

Funding

National Key R&D Program of China, National Natural Science Foundation of China, Science Foundation of Guangdong of China, Technology project of Guangzhou, Shandong Provincial Natural Science Foundation, International Project of Science and Technology for Guangdong, Science and Technology of Guangdong of China and the Collaborative Innovation Foundation of Guangzhou Science and Technology Bureau.

Authors' contributions

M-MS, H-JX and X-PY mainly conceived, designed study and drafted manuscript. The major experiments included the 6-OH DA model in vivo was performed by L-GH and S-CC, and in vitro was performed by H-SX. Z-MM provided technical supports on in-cell western assay and color western blot, W-ZH and G-WY helped to the part on animal behavior and TH staining, Y-XL provided technical supports on LCM and qRT-PCR, Z-LM and W-L contributed to data analysis. Q-SG and C-CJ were involved in revising manuscript and experiment guide. Q-SG drew figures and tables, modified the manuscript. All authors read and approved final manuscript to be published.

Competing interests

Authors have no conflict of interest to declare.

Author details
[1]Department of Neurology, First Affiliated Hospital of Guangzhou Medical University, Guangzhou 510120, Guangdong, China. [2]Department of Neurology, Qilu Hospital of Shandong University, Jinan 250012, Shandong, China. [3]Department of Neurology, First Affiliated Hospital of Sun Yat-sen University, Guangzhou 510080, Guangdong, China. [4]Department of Neurology, Second Affiliated Hospital of Xinjiang Medical University, Urumchi 830011, Xinjiang, China. [5]Clinic Brain Center, Guangzhou Hospital of Integrated Traditional and Western Medicine, Guangzhou 510800, Guangdong, China. [6]Department of Blood Transfusion, Fifth Affiliated Hospital Southern Medical University, Guangzhou 510900, Guangdong, China. [7]Department of Thoracic Surgery, First Affiliated Hospital of Guangzhou Medical University, Guangzhou 510120, Guangdong China.

References

1. Chu Y, Kordower JH. Age-associated increases of α-synuclein in monkeys and humans are associated with nigrostriatal dopamine depletion: is this the target for Parkinson's disease? Neurobiol Dis. 2007;25(1):134–49.
2. Taylor JM, Main BS, Crack PJ. Neuroinflammation and oxidative stress: co-conspirators in the pathology of Parkinson's disease. Neurochem Int. 2013; 62(5):803–19.
3. Launay N, Ruiz M, Fourcade S, Schlüter A, Guilera C, Ferrer I, et al. Oxidative stress regulates the ubiquitin–proteasome system and immunoproteasome functioning in a mouse model of X-adrenoleukodystrophy. Brain. 2013; 136(3):891–904.
4. Bence NF, Sampat RM, Kopito RR. Impairment of the ubiquitin-proteasome system by protein aggregation. Science. 2001;292(5521):1552–5.
5. Wang J, Maldonado MA. The ubiquitin-proteasome system and its role in inflammatory and autoimmune diseases. Cell Mol Immunol. 2006;3(4):255–61.
6. Ciechanover A, Brundin P. The ubiquitin proteasome system in neurodegenerative diseases: sometimes the chicken, sometimes the egg. Neuron. 2003;40(2):427–46.
7. Dasuri K, Zhang L, Keller JN. Oxidative stress, neurodegeneration, and the balance of protein degradation and protein synthesis. Free Radic Biol Med. 2013;62:170–85.
8. Seifert U, Bialy LP, Ebstein F, Bech-Otschir D, Voigt A, Schröter F, et al. Immunoproteasomes preserve protein homeostasis upon interferon-induced oxidative stress. Cell. 2010;142(4):613–24.
9. Kincaid EZ, Che JW, York I, Escobar H, Reyes-Vargas E, Delgado JC, et al. Mice completely lacking immunoproteasomes show major changes in antigen presentation. Nat Immunol. 2012;13(2):129–35.
10. Chen S, Kammerl IE, Vosyka O, Baumann T, Yu Y, Wu Y, et al. Immunoproteasome dysfunction augments alternative polarization of alveolar macrophages. Cell Death Differ. 2016;23(6):1026.
11. Vilchez D, Saez I, Dillin A. The role of protein clearance mechanisms in organismal ageing and age-related diseases. Nat Commun. 2014;5(5):5659.
12. Mishto M, Bellavista E, Santoro A, Stolzing A, Ligorio C, Nacmias B, et al. Immunoproteasome and LMP2 polymorphism in aged and Alzheimer's disease brains. Neurobiol Aging. 2006;27(1):54–66.
13. Orre M, Kamphuis W, Dooves S, Kooijman L, Chan ET, Kirk CJ, et al. Reactive glia show increased immunoproteasome activity in Alzheimer's disease. Brain. 2013;136(5):1415–31.
14. Díaz-Hernández M, Martín-Aparicio E, Avila J, Hernández F, Lucas JJ. Enhaced induction of the immunoproteasome by interferon gamma in neurons expressing mutant huntingtin. Neurotox Res. 2004;6(6):463–8.
15. Mishto M, Raza ML, de Biase D, Ravizza T, Vasuri F, Martucci M, et al. The immunoproteasome β5i subunit is a key contributor to ictogenesis in a rat model of chronic epilepsy. Brain Behav Immun. 2015;49:188–96.
16. Chen X, Zhang X, Wang Y, Lei H, Su H, Zeng J, et al. Inhibition of immunoproteasome reduces infarction volume and attenuates inflammatory reaction in a rat model of ischemic stroke. Cell Death Dis. 2015;6(1):e1626.
17. Bukhatwa S, Zeng B-Y, Rose S, Jenner P. A comparison of changes in proteasomal subunit expression in the substantia nigra in Parkinson's disease, multiple system atrophy and progressive supranuclear palsy. Brain Res. 2010;1326:174–83.
18. Nardo G, Trolese MC, Bendotti C. Major histocompatibility complex I expression by motor neurons and its implication in amyotrophic lateral sclerosis. Front Neurol. 2016;7:89.
19. Cebrián C, Zucca FA, Mauri P, Steinbeck JA, Studer L, Scherzer CR, et al. MHC-I expression renders catecholaminergic neurons susceptible to T-cell-mediated degeneration. Nat Commun. 2014;5:3633.
20. Huang L, Xue Y, Feng DY, Yang RX, Nie T, Zhu G, et al. Blockade of RyRs in the ER attenuates 6-OHDA-induced calcium overload, Cellular Hypo-Excitability and Apoptosis in Dopaminergic Neurons. Frontiers in Cellular Neuroscience. 2017;11:52.
21. Zhang S, Gui X-H, Huang L-P, Deng M-Z, Fang R-M, Ke X-H, et al. Neuroprotective effects of β-asarone against 6-hydroxy dopamine-induced parkinsonism via JNK/Bcl-2/Beclin-1 pathway. Mol Neurobiol. 2016;53(1):83–94.
22. Nijholt DA, De Kimpe L, Elfrink HL, Hoozemans JJ, Scheper W, et al. A selective inhibitor of the immunoproteasome subunit LMP7 blocks cytokine production and attenuates progression of experimental arthritis. Nat Med. 2009;15(7):781–7.
23. Ungerstedt U. Postsynaptic supersensitivity after 6-hydroxy-dopamine induced degeneration of the nigro-striatal dopamine system. Acta Physiol Scand. 1971;82(S367):69–93.
24. Goyal A, Pal N, Concannon M, Paul M, Doran M, Poluzzi C, et al. Endorepellin, the Angiostatic module of Perlecan, interacts with both the α2β1 integrin and vascular endothelial growth factor Receptor 2 (VEGFR2) a DUAL RECEPTOR ANTAGONISM. J Biol Chem. 2011;286(29):25947–62.
25. Hwang L-Y, Lieu PT, Peterson PA, Yang Y. Functional regulation of immunoproteasomes and transporter associated with antigen processing. Immunol Res. 2001;24(3):245–72.
26. Kummari E, Guo-Ross SX, Eells JB. Laser capture microdissection-a demonstration of the isolation of individual dopamine neurons and the entire ventral tegmental area. J Vi. Exp. 2015;96(96):e52336–e52336.
27. Fend F, Emmert-Buck MR, Chuaqui R, Cole K, Lee J, Liotta LA, et al. Immuno-LCM: laser capture microdissection of immunostained frozen sections for mRNA analysis. Am J Pathol. 1999;154(1):61–6.
28. Livak KJ, Schmittgen TD. Analysis of relative gene expression data using real-time quantitative PCR and the 2− **ΔΔ**CT method. *methods*. 2001;**25**(4):402–8.
29. Wang T, Yuan Y, Zou H, Yang J, Zhao S, Ma Y, et al. The ER stress regulator Bip mediates cadmium-induced autophagy and neuronal senescence. Sci Rep. 2016;6:38091.
30. Lawand M, Abramova A, Manceau V, Springer S, van Endert P. TAP-dependent and-independent peptide import into dendritic cell Phagosomes. J Immunol. 2016;197(9):3454–63.
31. Lindå H, Hammarberg H, Piehl F, Khademi M, Olsson T. Expression of MHC class I heavy chain and β2-microglobulin in rat brainstem motoneurons and nigral dopaminergic neurons. J Neuroimmunol. 1999;101(1):76–86.
32. Ferrington DA, Hussong SA, Roehrich H, Kapphahn RJ, Kavanaugh SM, Heuss ND, et al. Immunoproteasome responds to injury in the retina and brain. J Neurochem. 2008;106(1):158–69.
33. Song S, Miranda CJ, Braun L, Meyer K, Frakes AE, Ferraiuolo L, et al. MHC class I protects motor neurons from astrocyte-induced toxicity in amyotrophic lateral sclerosis (ALS). Nat Med. 2016;22(4):397.
34. Díaz-Hernández M, Hernández F, Martín-Aparicio E, Gómez-Ramos P, Morán MA, Castaño JG, et al. Neuronal induction of the immunoproteasome in Huntington's disease. J Neurosci. 2003;23(37):11653–61.
35. Mo M-S, Huang W, Sun C-C, Zhang L-M, Cen L, Xiao Y-S, et al. Association analysis of proteasome subunits and transporter associated with antigen processing on Chinese patients with Parkinson's disease. Chin Med J. 2016; 129(9):1053.
36. Nijholt D, De Kimpe L, Elfrink H L, Hoozemans J JM, Scheper W. Removing protein aggregates: the role of proteolysis in neurodegeneration. Curr Med Chem. 2011;18(16):2459–76.
37. Brehm A, Krüger E. Dysfunction in protein clearance by the proteasome: impact on autoinflammatory diseases. Semin Immunopathol. 2015: Springer; 2015:323–33.
38. Reis J, Hassan F, Guan XQ, Shen J, Monaco JJ, Papasian CJ, et al. The immunoproteasomes regulate LPS-induced TRIF/TRAM signaling pathway in murine macrophages. Cell Biochem Biophys. 2011;60(1–2):119–26.
39. Aiken CT, Kaake RM, Wang X, Huang L. Oxidative stress-mediated regulation of proteasome complexes. Molecular & Cellular Proteomics. 2011;**10**(5):R110. 006924.
40. Unno M, Mizushima T, Morimoto Y, Tomisugi Y, Tanaka K, Yasuoka N, et al. The structure of the mammalian 20S proteasome at 2.75 Å resolution. Structure. 2002;10(5):609–18.

41. Aso E, Lomoio S, López-González I, Joda L, Carmona M, Fernández-Yagüe N, et al. Amyloid generation and dysfunctional immunoproteasome activation with disease progression in animal model of familial Alzheimer's disease. Brain Pathol. 2012;22(5):636–53.
42. Cheroni C, Marino M, Tortarolo M, Veglianese P, De Biasi S, Fontana E, et al. Functional alterations of the ubiquitin-proteasome system in motor neurons of a mouse model of familial amyotrophic lateral sclerosis†. Hum Mol Genet. 2009;18(1):82–96.
43. Pickering AM, Koop AL, Teoh CY, et al. The immunoproteasome, the 20S proteasome and the PA28αβ proteasome regulator are oxidative-stress-adaptive proteolytic complexes. Biochem J. 2010;432(3):585–95.
44. Nathan JA, Spinnenhirn V, Schmidtke G, et al. Immuno-and constitutive proteasomes do not differ in their abilities to degrade ubiquitinated proteins. Cell. 2013;152(5):1184–94.
45. Haroon N, Maksymowych WP, Rahman P, Tsui FW, O'Shea FD, Inman RD. Radiographic severity of ankylosing spondylitis is associated with polymorphism of the large multifunctional peptidase 2 gene in the Spondyloarthritis research consortium of Canada cohort. Arthritis Rheum. 2012;64(4):1119–26.
46. Mercado G, Castillo V, Vidal R, Hetz C. ER proteostasis disturbances in Parkinson's disease: novel insights. Front Aging Neurosci. 2015;7:39.
47. Ugunklusek A, Tatham MH, Elkharaz J, Constantinteodosiu D, Lawler K, Mohamed H, et al. Continued 26S proteasome dysfunction in mouse brain cortical neurons impairs autophagy and the Keap1-Nrf2 oxidative defence pathway. Cell Death Dis. 2017;8(1):e2531.
48. Ebstein F, Kloetzel P-M, Krüger E, Seifert U. Emerging roles of immunoproteasomes beyond MHC class I antigen processing. Cell Mol Life Sci. 2012;69(15):2543–58.
49. Askanas V, Engel WK. Inclusion-body myositis a myodegenerative conformational disorder associated with Aβ, protein misfolding, and proteasome inhibition. Neurology. 2006;66(1 suppl 1):S39–48.
50. Ryu EJ, Harding HP, Angelastro JM, Vitolo OV, Ron D, Greene LA. Endoplasmic reticulum stress and the unfolded protein response in cellular models of Parkinson's disease. J Neurosci. 2002;22(24):10690–8.
51. Tao K, Wang B, Feng D, Zhang W, Lu F, Lai J, et al. Salidroside protects against 6-Hydroxydopamine-induced cytotoxicity by attenuating ER stress. Neurosci Bull. 2016;32(1):61–9.
52. Basler M, Mundt S, Muchamuel T, Moll C, Jiang J, Groettrup M, et al. Inhibition of the immunoproteasome ameliorates experimental autoimmune encephalomyelitis. EMBO Mol Med. 2014;6(2):226–38. e201303543
53. Shastri N, Nagarajan N, Lind KC, Kanaseki T. Monitoring peptide processing for MHC class I molecules in the endoplasmic reticulum. Curr Opin Immunol. 2014;26:123–7.
54. McDermott A, Jacks J, Kessler M, Emanuel PD, Gao L. Proteasome-associated autoinflammatory syndromes: advances in pathogeneses, clinical presentations, diagnosis, and management. Int J Dermatol. 2015;54(2):121–9.
55. McDermott A, de Jesus AA, Liu Y, Kim P, Jacks J, Sanchez GAM, et al. A case of proteasome-associated auto-inflammatory syndrome with compound heterozygous mutations in PSMB8. J Am Acad Dermatol. 2013;69(1):e29.
56. Basler M, Mundt S, Bitzer A, Schmidt C, Groettrup M. The immunoproteasome: a novel drug target for autoimmune diseases. Clin Exp Rheumatol. 2015;33:74–9.
57. Mangold CA, Masser DR, Stanford DR, Bixler GV, Pisupati A, Giles CB, et al. CNS-wide sexually dimorphic induction of the major histocompatibility complex 1 pathway with aging. J Gerontol A Biol Sci Med Sci. 2016;72(1): 16–29. glv232
58. McGeer P, Itagaki S, Boyes B, McGeer E. Reactive microglia are positive for HLA-DR in the substantia nigra of Parkinson's and Alzheimer's disease brains. Neurology. 1988;38(8):1285.
59. Meuth SG, Herrmann AM, Simon OJ, Siffrin V, Melzer N, Bittner S, et al. Cytotoxic CD8+ T cell–neuron interactions: perforin-dependent electrical silencing precedes but is not causally linked to neuronal cell death. J Neurosci. 2009;29(49):15397–409.
60. Neumann H, Cavalie A, Jenne DE, Wekerle H. Induction of MHC class I genes in neurons. Science. 1995;269(5223):549.

Permissions

All chapters in this book were first published in TN, by BioMed Central; hereby published with permission under the Creative Commons Attribution License or equivalent. Every chapter published in this book has been scrutinized by our experts. Their significance has been extensively debated. The topics covered herein carry significant findings which will fuel the growth of the discipline. They may even be implemented as practical applications or may be referred to as a beginning point for another development.

The contributors of this book come from diverse backgrounds, making this book a truly international effort. This book will bring forth new frontiers with its revolutionizing research information and detailed analysis of the nascent developments around the world.

We would like to thank all the contributing authors for lending their expertise to make the book truly unique. They have played a crucial role in the development of this book. Without their invaluable contributions this book wouldn't have been possible. They have made vital efforts to compile up to date information on the varied aspects of this subject to make this book a valuable addition to the collection of many professionals and students.

This book was conceptualized with the vision of imparting up-to-date information and advanced data in this field. To ensure the same, a matchless editorial board was set up. Every individual on the board went through rigorous rounds of assessment to prove their worth. After which they invested a large part of their time researching and compiling the most relevant data for our readers.

The editorial board has been involved in producing this book since its inception. They have spent rigorous hours researching and exploring the diverse topics which have resulted in the successful publishing of this book. They have passed on their knowledge of decades through this book. To expedite this challenging task, the publisher supported the team at every step. A small team of assistant editors was also appointed to further simplify the editing procedure and attain best results for the readers.

Apart from the editorial board, the designing team has also invested a significant amount of their time in understanding the subject and creating the most relevant covers. They scrutinized every image to scout for the most suitable representation of the subject and create an appropriate cover for the book.

The publishing team has been an ardent support to the editorial, designing and production team. Their endless efforts to recruit the best for this project, has resulted in the accomplishment of this book. They are a veteran in the field of academics and their pool of knowledge is as vast as their experience in printing. Their expertise and guidance has proved useful at every step. Their uncompromising quality standards have made this book an exceptional effort. Their encouragement from time to time has been an inspiration for everyone.

The publisher and the editorial board hope that this book will prove to be a valuable piece of knowledge for researchers, students, practitioners and scholars across the globe.

List of Contributors

Wang Zheng, Guoxiang Liu, Xi Chen, Carmelo Sgobio, Lixin Sun, Chengsong Xie and Huaibin Cai
Transgenics Section, Laboratory of Neurogenetics, National Institute on Aging, National Institutes of Health, Building 35, Room 1A112, MSC 3707, 35 Convent Drive, Bethesda, MD 20892-3707, USA

Namratha Sastry
Transgenics Section, Laboratory of Neurogenetics, National Institute on Aging, National Institutes of Health, Building 35, Room 1A112, MSC 3707, 35 Convent Drive, Bethesda, MD 20892-3707, USA
Present addresses: Feinberg School of Medicine, Northwestern University, Chicago, IL 60611, USA

Helen Wang
Transgenics Section, Laboratory of Neurogenetics, National Institute on Aging, National Institutes of Health, Building 35, Room 1A112, MSC 3707, 35 Convent Drive, Bethesda, MD 20892-3707, USA
Present addresses: Swarthmore College, Swarthmore, PA 19081, USA

Parth Contractor
Transgenics Section, Laboratory of Neurogenetics, National Institute on Aging, National Institutes of Health, Building 35, Room 1A112, MSC 3707, 35 Convent Drive, Bethesda, MD 20892-3707, USA
Present addresses: George Washington University, Washington, DC 20052, USA

Michael Cai
Unit on Synapse Development Plasticity, Clinical Brain Disorder Branch, National Institute of Mental Health, National Institutes of Health, Bethesda, MD 20892, USA
Present addresses: Centennial High School, Elicott City, MD 21042, USA

Wei Chen and Günther Deuschl
Department of Neurology, Shanghai Ninth People's Hospital affiliated to Shanghai Jiao Tong University School of Medicine, 200011 Shanghai, China

Franziska Hopfner and Jos Steffen Becktepe
Department of Neurology, Universitätsklinikum Schleswig-Holstein, Kiel Campus, Christian-Albrechts-University, Rosalind Franklinstr.10, 24105 Kiel, Germany

Shi-Fu Xiao, Xiang Lin, Tao Wang, Qi Qiu, Min-Jie Zhu and Xia Li
Alzheimer's Disease and Related Disorders Center, Department of Geriatric Psychiatry, Shanghai Mental Health Center, Shanghai Jiao Tong University School of Medicine, Shanghai, China

Chun-Xia Ban
Alzheimer's Disease and Related Disorders Center, Department of Geriatric Psychiatry, Shanghai Mental Health Center, Shanghai Jiao Tong University School of Medicine, Shanghai, China
Mental Health Center of Jiading District in Shanghai, Shanghai, China

Tingting Xiao, Weiwei Zhang, Bin Jiao, Chu-Zheng Pan and Xixi Liu
Department of Neurology, Xiangya Hospital, Central South University, Changsha, China

Lu Shen
Department of Neurology, Xiangya Hospital, Central South University, Changsha, China
State Key Laboratory of Medical Genetics, Changsha, China
Key Laboratory of Hunan Province in Neurodegenerative Disorders, Central South University, Changsha, China

Anjli Venkateswaran, Antti Nurmi and Robert Hodgson
Discovery Services, Charles Rivers Laboratories, Wilmington, MA, USA

Patrick Sweeney
Discovery Services, Charles Rivers Laboratories, Wilmington, MA, USA
Royal Veterinary College, University of London, London, UK

Hyunsun Park
Health and Life Science Consulting, Los Angeles, CA, USA

Marc Baumann
Biochemistry and Developmental Biology, University of Helsinki, Helsinki, Finland

John Dunlop
Neuroscience Innovation Medicines, Astra Zeneca, Cambridge, MA, USA

Judith Frydman and Ron Kopito
Stanford University, Stanford, CA, USA

Alexander McCampbell
Neurology, Biogen Idec, Cambridge, MA, USA

Gabrielle Leblanc
Leblanc Bioscience Consulting, Berkeley, CA, USA

Hong-Fu Li and Zhi-Ying Wu
Department of Neurology and Research Center of Neurology in Second Affiliated Hospital, and the Collaborative Innovation Center for Brain Science, Zhejiang University School of Medicine, 88 Jiefang Rd, Hangzhou 310009, China

Marcela Cruz-Haces, Jonathan Tang and Joseph Fernandez
Weldon School of Biomedical Engineering, Purdue University, West Lafayette, IN 47907, USA

Riyi Shi
Weldon School of Biomedical Engineering, Purdue University, West Lafayette, IN 47907, USA
Department of Basic Medical Sciences, Purdue University, West Lafayette, USA

Glen Acosta
Department of Basic Medical Sciences, Purdue University, West Lafayette, USA

Gary Leung
Department of Basic Medical Sciences, College of Veterinary Medicine, Purdue University, West Lafayette, IN 47907, USA

Jonathan Tang and Riyi Shi
Department of Basic Medical Sciences, College of Veterinary Medicine, Purdue University, West Lafayette, IN 47907, USA
Weldon School of Biomedical Engineering, Purdue University, West Lafayette, IN 47907, USA

Melissa Tully
Weldon School of Biomedical Engineering, Purdue University, West Lafayette, IN 47907, USA
MSTP program, Indiana University School of Medicine, Indianapolis, IN, USA

Shengxi Wu
Department of Neurobiology, Fourth Military Medical University, Xi'an, China

Shuang-shuang Yang, Rui Zhang and Yong-fang Zhang
Department of Pharmacology, Institute of Medical Sciences, School of Medicine, Shanghai Jiao Tong University, 280 South Chongqing Road, Shanghai 200025, China

Gang Wang
Department of Neurology Ruijin Hospital, School of Medicine, Shanghai Jiao Tong University, Ruijin 2nd Road 197, Shanghai 200025, China

Fangyi Dong, Dunhui Li, Shengdi Chen and Jun Liu
Department of Neurology and Institute of Neurology, Ruijin Hospital affiliated to Shanghai Jiaotong University School of Medicine, Shanghai, China

Wenyan Kang
Department of Neurology and Institute of Neurology, Ruijin Hospital affiliated to Shanghai Jiaotong University School of Medicine, Shanghai, China
Department of Neurology, Ruijin Hospital North affiliated to Shanghai Jiaotong University School of Medicine, Shanghai, China

Thomas J. Quinn
Department of Radiation Oncology, Beaumont Health System, Royal Oak, MI 48073, USA

Lih-Shen Chin and Lian Li
Department of Pharmacology and Center for Neurodegenerative Disease, Emory University School of Medicine, Atlanta, GA 30322, USA

Xue-mei Qi and Jian-fang Ma
Department of Neurology and Institute of Neurology, Ruijin Hospital Affiliated to Shanghai Jiaotong University School of Medicine, Shanghai 200025, China

Lin-lin Gao and Tao Wu
Department of Neurobiology, Key Laboratory on Neurodegenerative Disorders of Ministry of Education, Beijing Institute of Geriatrics, Xuanwu Hospital, Capital Medical University, Beijing 100053, China
Beijing Key Laboratory on Parkinson's Disease, Parkinson Disease Center of Beijing Institute for Brain Disorders, Beijing, China

Xue-Ping Wang, Ming Wei and Qin Xiao
Department of Neurology and Institute of Neurology, Ruijin Hospital affiliated to Shanghai Jiao Tong University School of Medicine, Shanghai, China

Ann J. Jones
New Zealand Brain Research Institute, 66 Stewart Street, Christchurch 8011, New Zealand
Department of Psychology, University of Canterbury, Christchurch, New Zealand

Kyla Horne
New Zealand Brain Research Institute, 66 Stewart Street, Christchurch 8011, New Zealand
Department of Psychology, University of Canterbury, Christchurch, New Zealand

Department of Medicine, University of Otago, Christchurch, New Zealand

Leslie Livingston, Daniel Myall, Michael MacAskill and Toni Pitcher
New Zealand Brain Research Institute, 66 Stewart Street, Christchurch 8011, New Zealand
Department of Medicine, University of Otago, Christchurch, New Zealand

John C. Dalrymple-Alford
New Zealand Brain Research Institute, 66 Stewart Street, Christchurch 8011, New Zealand
Department of Psychology, University of Canterbury, Christchurch, New Zealand
Department of Medicine, University of Otago, Christchurch, New Zealand
Brain Research New Zealand Centre of Research Excellence, Christchurch, New Zealand

Tim J. Anderson
New Zealand Brain Research Institute, 66 Stewart Street, Christchurch 8011, New Zealand
Department of Medicine, University of Otago, Christchurch, New Zealand
Department of Neurology, Christchurch Hospital, Christchurch, New Zealand
Brain Research New Zealand Centre of Research Excellence, Christchurch, New Zealand

Roeline G. Kuijer
Department of Psychology, University of Canterbury, Christchurch, New Zealand

Paul T. Barrett
Department of Psychology, University of Canterbury, Christchurch, New Zealand
Cognadev, UK Ltd., Sandton, South Africa

Yuyan Tan, Dunhui Li, Xiaoli Liu and Jianqing Ding
Department of Neurology, and Institute of Neurology, Ruijin Hospital Affiliated to Shanghai Jiao Tong University School of Medicine, Shanghai 200025, China

Shengdi Chen
Department of Neurology, and Institute of Neurology, Ruijin Hospital Affiliated to Shanghai Jiao Tong University School of Medicine, Shanghai 200025, China
Parkinson's Disease Center, Beijing Institute for Brain Disorders, Beijing 100069, China

Li Wu
Department of Neurology, Shanghai Ninth People's Hospital Affiliated to Shanghai Jiao Tong University School of Medicine, Shanghai 200011, China

Yi Liu and Xiongwei Zhu
Department of Pathology, Case Western Reserve University, Cleveland, OH, USA

Kaicheng Li, Xiao Luo, Qingze Zeng, Yeerfan Jiaerken, Xiaojun Xu, Peiyu Huang, Zhujing Shen, Jingjing Xu, Chao Wang and Min-Ming Zhang
Department of Radiology, 2nd Affiliated Hospital of Zhejiang University School of Medicine, No.88 Jie-fang Road, Shang-cheng District, Hangzhou 310009, China

Jiong Zhou
Department of Neurology, 2nd Affiliated Hospital of Zhejiang University School of Medicine, Zhejiang, China

Ling-yan Yao, Qi-ying Sun, Yi-ting Cui, Yang Yang and Qian Xu
Department of Neurology, Xiangya Hospital, Central South University, Changsha, Hunan 410008, People's Republic of China

Bei-sha Tang
Department of Neurology, Xiangya Hospital, Central South University, Changsha, Hunan 410008, People's Republic of China
Laboratory of Medical Genetics, Central South University Changsha, Changsha, Hunan 410078, China
National Clinical Research Center for Geriatric Disorders, Changsha, Hunan 410078, China
Key Laboratory of Hunan Province in Neurodegenerative Disorders, Central South University, Changsha, Hunan 410008, China
Parkinson's Disease Center of Beijing Institute for Brain Disorders, Beijing 100069, China
Collaborative Innovation Center for Brain Science, Shanghai 200032, China
Collaborative Innovation Center for Genetics and Development, Shanghai 200433, China

Ji-feng Guo
Department of Neurology, Xiangya Hospital, Central South University, Changsha, Hunan 410008, People's Republic of China
Laboratory of Medical Genetics, Central South University Changsha, Changsha, Hunan 410078, China
National Clinical Research Center for Geriatric Disorders, Changsha, Hunan 410078, China
Key Laboratory of Hunan Province in Neurodegenerative Disorders, Central South University, Changsha, Hunan 410008, China

Xin-xiang Yan
Department of Neurology, Xiangya Hospital, Central South University, Changsha, Hunan 410008, People's Republic of China

National Clinical Research Center for Geriatric Disorders, Changsha, Hunan 410078, China
Key Laboratory of Hunan Province in Neurodegenerative Disorders, Central South University, Changsha, Hunan 410008, China

Hai-Yan Zhou, Pei Huang, Qian Sun, Juan-Juan Du, Shi-Shuang Cui, Ying Wang, Qin Xiao, Jun Liu, Yu-Yan Tan and Sheng-Di Chen
Department of Neurology and Institute of Neurology, Ruijin Hospital affiliated to Shanghai Jiao Tong University School of Medicine, No.197 Ruijin 2nd Road, Shanghai 200025, China

Yun-Yun Hu and Wei-Wei Zhan
Department of Ultrasonography, Ruijin Hospital affiliated to Shanghai Jiao Tong University School of Medicine, Shanghai 200025, China

Maowen Ba and Guoping Yu
Department of Neurology, the Affiliated Yantai Yuhuangding Hospital of Qingdao University, Yantai City, Shandong 264000, People's Republic of China

Min Kong, Hui Liang and Ling Yu
Department of Neurology, Yantaishan Hospital, Yantai City, Shandong 264000, People's Republic of China

Rafael Lazo-Gomez and Ricardo Tapia
Divisiön de Neurociencias, Instituto de Fisiología Celular, Universidad Nacional Autónoma de México, Circuito exterior s/n, Ciudad Universitaria, Coyoacán, 04510 Ciudad de México, Mexico

Antonella Tramutola, Chiara Lanzillotta, Andrea Arena, Ilaria Zuliani1, Luciana Mosca, Carla Blarzino, Marzia Perluigi and Fabio Di Domenico
Department of Biochemical Sciences, Sapienza University of Rome, P.le Aldo Moro 5, 00185 Rome, Italy

Eugenio Barone
Department of Biochemical Sciences, Sapienza University of Rome, P.le Aldo Moro 5, 00185 Rome, Italy
Universidad Autònoma de Chile, Instituto de Ciencias Biomédicas, Facultad de alud, Avenida Pedro de Valdivia 425, Providencia, Santiago, Chile

D. Allan Butterfield
Department of Chemistry and Sanders-Brown Center on Aging, University of Kentucky, Lexington, KY 40506-0055, USA

Ming-Shu Mo, Gui-Hua Li, Shu-Xuan Huang, Lei Wei, Miao-Miao Zhou, Zhuo-Hua Wu and Wen-Yuan Guo
Department of Neurology, First Affiliated Hospital of Guangzhou Medical University, Guangzhou 510120, Guangdong, China

Ping-Yi Xu
Department of Neurology, First Affiliated Hospital of Guangzhou Medical University, Guangzhou 510120, Guangdong, China
Department of Neurology, Second Affiliated Hospital of Xinjiang Medical University, Urumchi 830011, Xinjiang, China

Cong-Cong Sun
Department of Neurology, Qilu Hospital of Shandong University, Jinan 250012, Shandong, China

Li-Min Zhang
Department of Neurology, First Affiliated Hospital of Sun Yat-sen University, Guangzhou 510080, Guangdong, China

Xin-Ling Yang
Department of Neurology, Second Affiliated Hospital of Xinjiang Medical University, Urumchi 830011, Xinjiang, China

Chao-Jun Chen
Clinic Brain Center, Guangzhou Hospital of Integrated Traditional and Western Medicine, Guangzhou 510800, Guangdong, China

Shao-Gang Qu
Department of Blood Transfusion, Fifth Affiliated Hospital Southern Medical University, Guangzhou 510900, Guangdong, China

Jian-Xing He
Department of Thoracic Surgery, First Affiliated Hospital of Guangzhou Medical University, Guangzhou 510120, Guangdong China

Index

www.ingramcontent.com/pod-product-compliance
Lightning Source LLC
Chambersburg PA
CBHW080526200326
41458CB00012B/4345
9781632427236